Implant Therapy

Clinical Approaches and Evidence of Success

Implant Therapy
Clinical Approaches and Evidence of Success
Volume 2

Edited by

Myron Nevins, DDS
Diplomate, American Board of Periodontology
Director, Institute for Advanced Dental Studies
Swampscott, Massachusetts

Associate Clinical Professor of Periodontology
Harvard School of Dental Medicine
Boston, Massachusetts

Adjunct Professor
Department of Periodontics, School of Dentistry
University of North Carolina at Chapel Hill
Chapel Hill, North Carolina

James T. Mellonig, DDS, MS
Diplomate, American Board of Periodontology
Professor, Head Specialist Division and
Director Advanced Education Program
Department of Periodontics
The University of Texas Health Science Center at San Antonio
San Antonio, Texas

Associate Editor
Joseph P. Fiorellini, DMD, DMSc
Assistant Professor of Periodontology
Harvard School of Dental Medicine
Boston, Massachusetts

Quintessence Publishing Co, Inc
Chicago, Berlin, London, Tokyo, Paris, Barcelona,
São Paulo, Moscow, Prague, and Warsaw

Library of Congress Cataloging-in-Publication Data

Implant therapy : clinical approaches and evidence of success / edited
    by Myron Nevins, James T. Mellonig ; associate editor, Joseph P.
    Fiorellini.
            p. cm.
        Called vol. 2 of companion vol. : Periodontal therapy.
        Includes bibliographical references and index.
        ISBN 0-86715-341-5
        1. Dental implants.   I. Nevins, Myron.   II. Mellonig, James T.
    III. Fiorellini, Joseph P.   IV. Periodontal therapy.
        [DNLM: 1. Dental Implants.   2. Dental Implantation—methods.   WU
    640 I34 1998]
    RK667.I45I466   1998
    617.6'9—dc21
    DNLM/DLC
    for Library of Congress   98-4259
                                                                        CIP

©1998 by Quintessence Publishing Co, Inc

Quintessence Publishing Co, Inc
551 Kimberly Drive
Carol Stream, Illinois 60188

Editor: Betsy Solaro
Production: Michael Shanahan and Timothy M. Robbins
Cover design: Michael Shanahan

Printed in Japan

Periodontal Therapy: Clinical Approaches and Evidence of Success, Volume I
    ISBN 0-86715-309-1

Implant Therapy: Clinical Approaches and Evidence of Success, Volume II
    ISBN 0-86715-341-5

Volume I and Volume II Set
    ISBN 0-86715-342-3

CONTENTS

Preface   viii

Contributors   ix

1   A Changed Paradigm of Treatment: The Natural Tooth or a Dental Implant   1
Myron Nevins, DDS

2   The Efficacy of Osseointegration for the Partially Edentulous Patient   23
Ulf Lekholm, DDS, PhD

3   Using Computerized Tomography to Develop Realistic Treatment Objectives for the Implant Team   29
Alan L. Rosenfeld, DDS, and Richard A. Mecall, DDS, MScD

4   Biomechanical Interaction Between Implants and Teeth   47
Burton Langer, DMD, MSD, and Bo Rangert, Mech Eng, PhD

5   Guided Bone Regeneration and Dental Implants   53
James T. Mellonig, DDS, MS, and Myron Nevins, DDS

6   Use of Guided Bone Regeneration to Facilitate Ideal Prosthetic Placement of Implants   83
Richard H. Shanaman, DDS

7   Protected Space Development for Bone Formation Using Reinforced Barrier Membranes   91
Sascha A. Jovanovic, DDS, MS

8   Guided Bone Regeneration for Vertical Ridge Augmentation Associated With Osseointegrated Implants   99
Massimo Simion, MD, DDS, Paolo Trisi, DDS, and Adriano Piattelli, MD, DDS

9 The Placement of Maxillary Anterior Implants 111
Myron Nevins, DDS, and James M. Stein, DMD

10 The Placement of Mandibular Anterior Implants 129
Myron Nevins, DDS

11 The Placement of Mandibular Posterior Implants 141
Myron Nevins, DDS

12 The Placement of Maxillary Posterior Implants 153
Myron Nevins, DDS, and Joseph P. Fiorellini, DMD, DMSc

13 The Maxillary Sinus Floor Augmentation Procedure to Support Implant
Prostheses 171
Myron Nevins, DDS, and Joseph P. Fiorellini, DMD, DMSc

14 Implant Use in the Tuberosity, Pterygoid, and Palatine Region: Anatomic and
Surgical Considerations 197
Gary M. Reiser, DDS

15 Osseous Regeneration With Bone Harvested from the Anterior Mandible 209
R. Gilbert Triplett, DDS, PhD, and Sterling R. Schow, DMD

16 The Esthetic Management of Dental Implants 219
Burton Langer, DMD, MSD

17 The Need for Keratinized Tissue for Implants 227
Yoshihiro Ono, DDS, Myron Nevins, DDS, and Emil G. Cappetta, DMD

18 Implant Therapy for Patients With Refractory Periodontal Disease 239
James T. Mellonig, DDS, MS, and Myron Nevins, DDS

Index 251

DEDICATION

This effort has been made possible by the patience and encouragement of my wife, soul mate, and best friend, Marcy, the wind beneath my wings. She and my sons, Michael and Marc, have understood and encouraged my fascination with periodontics, an occupation and an avocation.

—Ron Nevins

To my wife Karen, the love of my life and sage counsel, who allowed me, without any reservation, to pursue every goal in periodontics I dreamed possible and to my children, Tim, Amy, and Kim, who light up my life.

—Jim Mellonig

Dentistry has undergone many changes during the past quarter century; however, no changes have been more profound than those in the field of implant dentistry. Successful endoseous alloplastic implants can be found dating back to AD 600, but the surge in implants for tooth replacement did not flourish until the middle of the 1900s. These early efforts were met with exuberance, bravado, and an emphasis of the mechanical over the biological. It is important to note the contributions of pioneers, such as Aaron Gershkoff, and their continuing struggle to resolve the indignities of the edentulous patient. The success stories were more or less limited to the resorbed mandibular edentulous patient who presented for treatment with the proverbial box of failed implants.

It was not until the biological aspect was emphasized over the mechanical factors that implants were routinely considered more than just a passing fad. The research results emerging from P.I. Brånemark and Associates captured the attention of dentistry. It is worth noting that the research took place over a considerable period of time without marketing a product until the many unknowns were resolved. A root form design, a precise surgical procedure, and an undisturbed healing time suddenly elevated endosseous dental implants to the realm of a highly successful and acceptable predictable procedure. Dentistry was presented with scientific studies that were difficult to refute. Once again, the early emphasis was centered on the edentulous patient but attention turned toward the partially dentate patient after the Toronto conference in the early 1980s. Still, the placement of implants was limited by the demands of an adequate ridge form to house the implants. The periodontist or surgeon was a prisoner of the size and form of the bone. In 1989, the first reports of simultaneous delivery of an implant into an extraction wound were published. The same time frame shared information about growing bone over implant fenestrations or dehiscenses and eventually led to the development of guided bone regeneration, which suddenly expanded the population of candidates for treatment by correction of anatomic obstacles.

Reports surfaced about the efficacy of implant treatment in the maxillary and mandibular posterior regions where previous attempts were thought to be questionable. Three-dimensional radiography provided information to help avoid or alter anatomic obstacles. Grafting of the floor of the maxillary sinus, nerve transposition of the inferior alveolar nerve, and eventually, vertical growth of bone all provided corrections that were previously thought impossible. To quote Sir Anthony Eden, "every succeeding scientific discovery makes greater nonsense of old-time conceptions of sovereignty."

Contemporary dentistry continues to demonstrate the strength of the research results of the pioneers of root form implantology. This form of dentistry offers a remarkable base of evidence to support tradition and evidence the continued need for intellectual innovation.

The major issue today is the clinical question: Can we or should we preserve the remaining natural dentition or do implants offer a more predictable prognosis? This text meets the challenge of confronting this moment of decision on a geographic basis for each area of the dentition. It uses the evidence that is now available for both paths of treatment and directs the well-informed reader toward resolution. We expect to affect the thinking process of the discriminating dentist who is willing to invest time in the decision-making process.

CONTRIBUTORS

Emil G. Cappetta, DMD
Diplomate, American Board of Periodontology
Private Practice
Summit, New Jersey

Clinical Professor
University of Medicine and Dentistry of New Jersey
Newark, New Jersey

Sascha A. Jovanovic, DDS, MS
School of Dentistry
University of California, Los Angeles
Los Angeles, California

Burton Langer, DMD, MSD
Diplomate, American Board of Periodontology
Private Practice
New York, New York

Ulf Lekholm, DDS, PhD
Professor and Chairman
The Brånemark Clinic
Gothenburg, Sweden

Richard A. Mecall, DDS, MScD
Diplomate, American Board of Periodontology
Private Practice
Park Ridge, Illinois

Yoshihiro Ono, DDS
Private Practice
Osaka, Japan

Adriano Piattelli, MD, DDS
Professor
Department of Oral Pathology
University of Chieti
Chieti, Italy

Bo Rangert, Mech Eng, PhD
Director, Clinical Research
Biomedical Engineering
Nobel Biocare AB
Gothenburg, Sweden

Gary M. Reiser, DDS
Diplomate, American Board of Periodontology
Assistant Clinical Professor
Department of Periodontology
Tufts University School of Dental Medicine
Boston, Massachusetts

Institute for Advanced Dental Studies
Swampscott, Massachusetts

Alan L. Rosenfeld, DDS
Diplomate, American Board of Periodontology
Private Practice
Park Ridge, Illinois

Sterling R. Schow, DMD
Professor and Director of Graduate Education
Baylor College of Dentistry
Dallas, Texas

Richard H. Shanaman, DDS
Private Practice
Wyomissing Hills, Pennsylvania

Massimo Simion, MD, DDS
Consultant Professor
University of Milan School of Dentistry
San Raffaele Hospital
Milan, Italy

James M. Stein, DMD
Private Practice
Lecturer
Harvard School of Dental Medicine
Boston, Massachusetts

R. Gilbert Triplett, DDS, PhD
Professor and Chairman
Department of Oral and Maxillofacial Surgery
   and Pharmacology
Baylor College of Dentistry
Dallas, Texas

Paolo Trisi, DDS
Biomaterial Clinical Research Association
Pescara, Italy

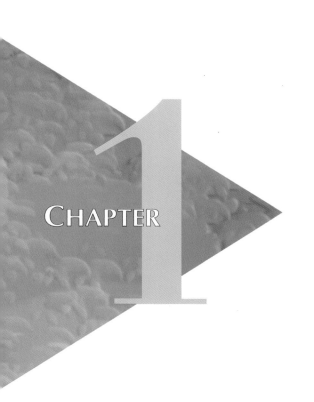

CHAPTER 1

A Changed Paradigm
of Treatment:
The Natural Tooth
or a Dental Implant

Myron Nevins, DDS

The contemporary hallmark of a superior clinician is the ability to make decisions that have predictable and long-lasting results. The question of whether to save a tooth or replace it with a dental implant is multifaceted, and the assessment requires a multidisciplinary approach to dental care.[1]

The decision as to whether to reconstruct the natural dentition with conventional fixed restorative dentistry to replace teeth for the partially dentate patient is greatly influenced by the geographic region of the mouth in question. Anatomic obstacles, single-rooted vs multirooted teeth, the esthetic zone, the difficulty of gaining treatment access, the size of the alveolar process, and the perceived need to replace missing teeth must be considered. Issues at the core of the decision-making process are tooth restorability, esthetics, embrasures, loss of periodontium, mobility, drifting, the maxillomandibular occlusal relationship, and the strategic value of the tooth.

Maintenance of the Natural Dentition

The recent past has not only witnessed the introduction of predictable implant dentistry, but also evidenced major improvements in periodontal regenerative techniques.[2-6] The tooth or teeth that present as candidates for the latter treatment preclude the necessity of implants and indeed will provide patient satisfaction. This is especially true in areas proximal to the inferior alveolar nerve and the maxillary sinus. Periodontal regeneration also may avoid the need to replace an isolated molar with an implant restoration.

It is of paramount importance to recognize at the outset that it is possible, and in some instances preferable, to use the time-honored therapeutic approaches of conventional restorative dentistry. Although it is tempting to note the lack of controlled studies in the discipline of periodontal prostheses, there is a paucity of significant randomized controlled human studies to support the clinical application of many periodontal and prosthetic approaches. There is, however, overwhelming clinical evidence gathered through observation of treated patients, which has to be considered.[7-9] Patients who have periodontal prostheses are characterized by a compromised periodontium that results in mobile and drifting teeth and eventually missing teeth (Fig 1-1a). Such patients require a treatment plan that provides predictability over an extended time frame (Figs 1-1b and 1-1c). The dictating factor for decision making is the clinical root, that portion of the tooth that resides in the alveolar process.

Initial decisions establish which teeth are reasonable candidates for treatment and dictate strategic extractions.[10] The first phase of therapy provides a resolution of the superficial inflammatory disease, focuses on the occlusal traumatic issues (Figs 1-1d and 1-1e), and establishes meaningful plaque control because it is only possible to evaluate the response to this first phase of treatment after these issues are resolved. The hopeless teeth are eliminated and a biologic trial restoration that will provide invaluable information for the construction of the final prosthesis is delivered[11] (Fig 1-1). The provisional prosthesis will not only replace missing teeth, but also stabilize the mobile teeth and help to determine the form of the teeth, the embrasure contours, esthetics, the desired occlusal scheme,

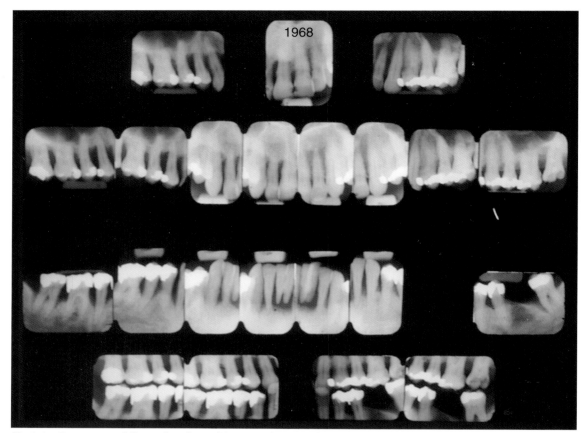

Fig 1-1a Pretreatment full-mouth radiographic survey (1968). Advanced loss of bone is evidenced throughout. It is necessary to select appropriate abutment teeth for the prosthesis with an impossible prognosis.

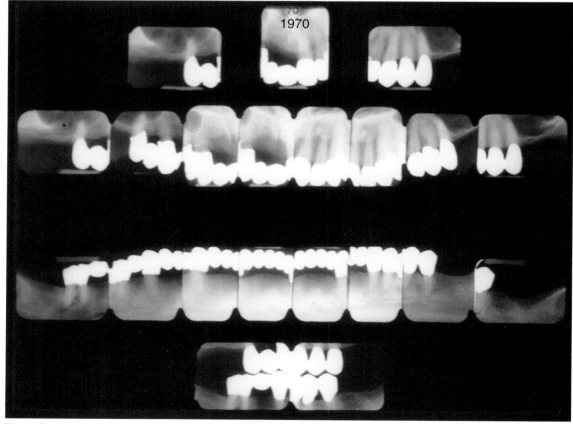

Fig 1-1b Posttreatment full-mouth radiographic survey (1970). The maxilla and mandible are restored with one-piece prostheses that supply missing teeth and stabilize mobile teeth.

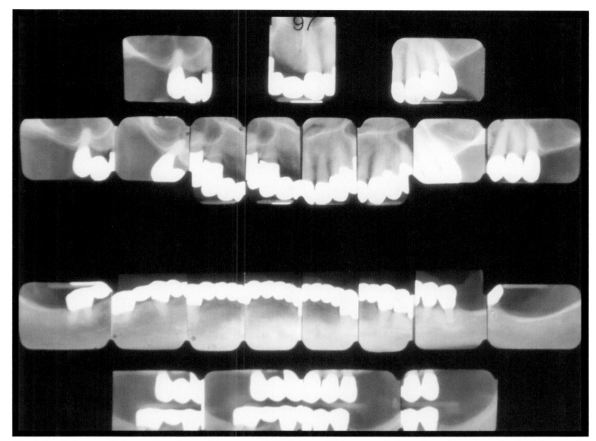

Fig 1-1c Follow-up full-mouth radiographic survey (1997). No additional teeth have been lost since the initial strategic extractions. The restorative margins serve as markers of the osseous levels and allow comparison for a period of 29 years.

and the distal extension of the arch (Figs 1-1f and 1-1g).

The cervical margins of the final restorations serve as a marker of the level of the interproximal bone and as radiographic markers against which bone levels can be measured.[12] A comparison of full-mouth radiographic surveys over meaningful time periods reveals the periodontal fate of abutment teeth, as well as the fate of the restorative procedures (Figs 1-1a to 1-1c). Severely compromised dentitions that require splinting of long clinical crowns and have long edentulous spans are infrequently treated successfully through traditional means. Such treatment plans require an

effort to retain the largest possible area of periodontal ligament to support fixed prostheses and compensate for the multiple missing teeth, but frequently err by retaining teeth with an unrealistic prognosis.[10]

Although the categories of failure for periodontal prostheses include caries, endodontics, occlusion, and recurrent periodontal inflammatory disease, this treatment regimen has been successful for many decades and should not be discarded simply because dental implants are available. It is possible to examine patients with prostheses that continue to function 25 years after placement (Fig 1-1c).

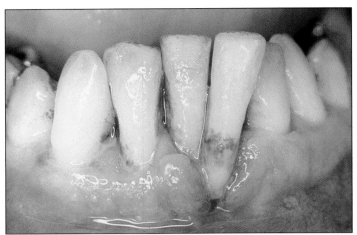

Fig 1-1d Mandibular incisors on the day of presentation. The patient has not been able to incise food for 20 years.

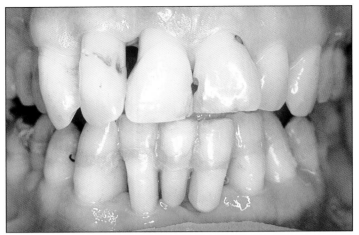

Fig 1-1e Clinical view after debridement and stabilization procedures. There is evidence of desire and dexterity on the part of the patient, and the treatment plan can proceed.

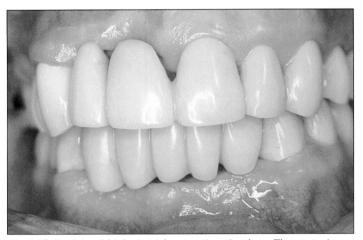

Fig 1-1f Provisional biologic trial restorations in place. The strategic extractions have been accomplished.

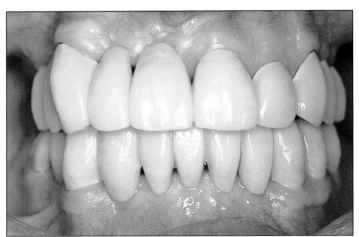

Fig 1-1g Final prostheses in place. Treatment decisions were made based on evidence gathered by the use of the provisional prostheses. (Prosthetic dentistry by Dr Howard M. Skurow.)

Placement of Dental Implants

The recent history of implant placement has remarkably influenced the treatment plan for the partially dentate patient. Contemporary approaches to devastated dentitions reduce the need for long edentulous spans that make it difficult to execute restorative dentistry (Figs 1-2a to 1-2d). Retrospective reports have established osseointegration as a predictable form of therapy for the edentulous patient, and recent and emerging publications seem to show similar results for the partially dentate patient.[13–17] (Fig 1-2b).

Although conventional dental procedures can adequately rehabilitate many dentitions, implants may offer the solution of choice. It appears that contemporary root-form implants outperform their predecessors (Figs 1-3a to 1-3e);

however, predictability can become tainted when the criterion for success becomes confused with implant survival.[18] No one argues the need for the implant to be immobile and without periapical radiolucencies, but some continue to debate the degree of bone loss that is acceptable. Many implants suffer the loss of minimal marginal bone during early loading, but a continued loss over a period of observation must be stopped before it is excessive and precludes additional implant replacement and/or results in exaggerated crown-root ratios.

Many intraosseous blade-vent implants appear to be successful when examined with conventional periapical radiographs, but reexamination with computerized tomography (CT) reveals obvious spacing between the metal surface and the encasing jaw (Figs 1-4a and 1-4b).

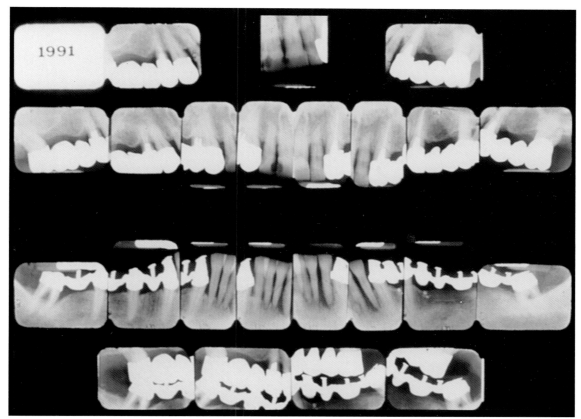

Fig 1-2a Pretreatment full-mouth radiographic survey (1991). The essential treatment will follow the pattern of Figs 1-1a to 1-1g, but the final prosthesis can be segmented by using implants.

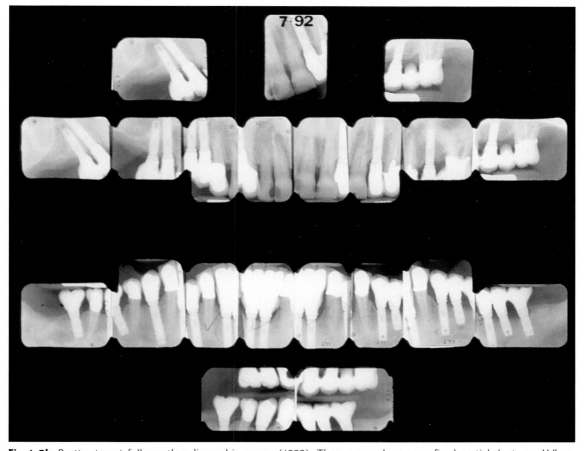

Fig 1-2b Posttreatment full-mouth radiographic survey (1992). There are no long-span fixed partial dentures. Where possible, the implant prosthesis are freestanding.

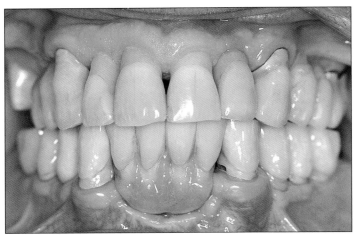

Fig 1-2c All four mandibular incisors are replaced with an implant prosthesis. The posterior teeth are supplemented by a freestanding implant prosthesis on the left side and by four single-tooth restorations on the right. The maxillary left lateral incisor is replaced by an implant, but the other three incisors are unrestored. (Prosthetic dentistry by Dr James Stein.)

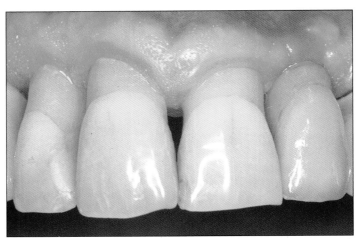

Fig 1-2d The maxillary left lateral incisor is a single-tooth implant that is inconspicuous in the presence of the three remaining natural incisors.

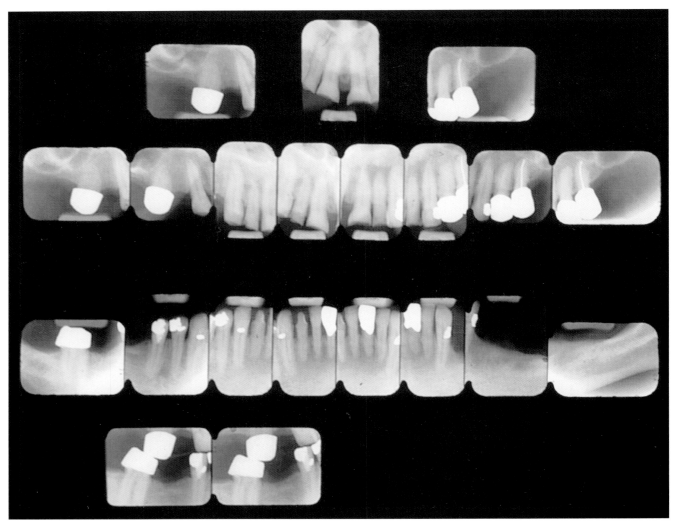

Fig 1-3a Pretreatment full-mouth radiographic survey (1969). Note the edentulous mandibular left posterior quadrant.

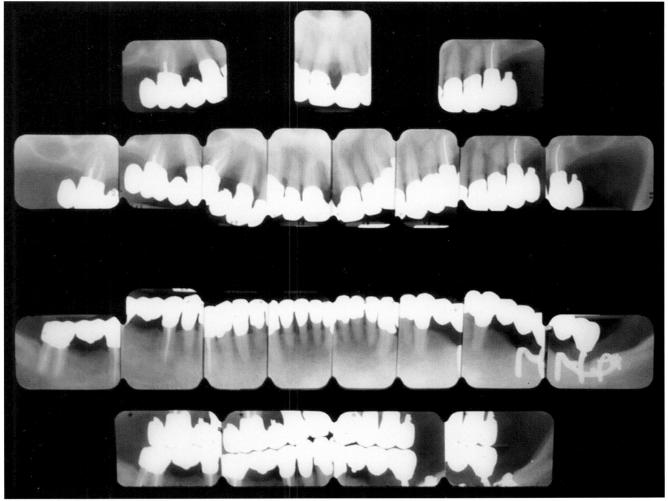

Fig 1-3b Posttreatment full-mouth radiographic survey (1992). The unilateral subperiosteal implant serviced the patient until death.

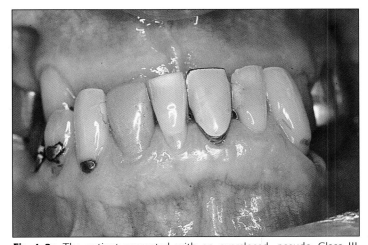

Fig 1-3c The patient presented with an overclosed, pseudo–Class III Angle malocclusion.

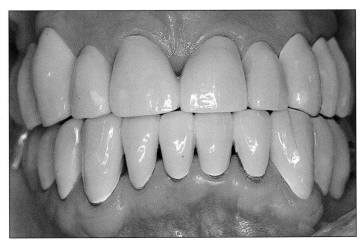

Fig 1-3d Final restorations in place. The overclosed vertical dimension has been restored without infringing on the interocclusal freeway space. (Prosthetic dentistry by Dr Howard M. Skurow.)

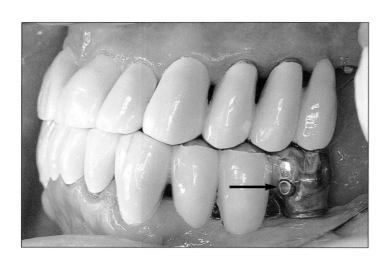

Fig 1-3e Left posterior occlusion with the implant in place. Note the screw-retained crown on the implant *(arrow)*.

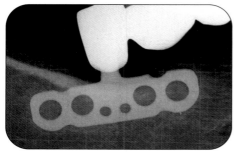

Fig 1-4a In the periapical radiograph, this blade-vent implant appears to be securely positioned.

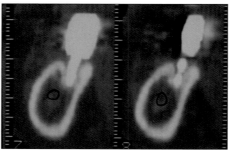

Fig 1-4b The sagittal sections of the CT scan reveal measurable space between the implant surface and the surrounding bone.

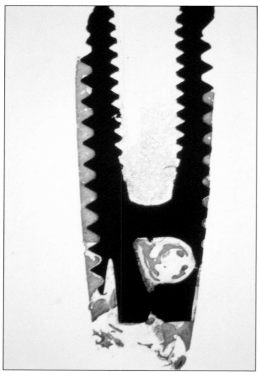

Fig 1-5a Human biopsy specimen of a screw-type, titanium-finish implant that was removed with a trephine. Note the number of consecutive threads in contact with bone.

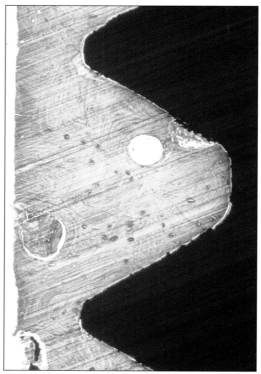

Fig 1-5b An enlargement of the bone-implant contact area demonstrates mature bone in contact with the implant (light microscope). There is no connective tissue between the bone and the implant.

Osseointegration is the mechanical retention of the root-form implant by intimate contact of bone and titanium (as viewed with a light microscope). Little connective tissue is interposed, and with time there appears to be a maturation of the bone (Figs 1-5a and 1-5b). Human biopsy information obtained from a patient who died 10 weeks after implants were placed suggests that loading these implants at the first surgery is precarious[19] (Figs 1-6a and 1-6b). The risk involved with proposed immediate loading must be explained to even the most demanding patient.[20] The original protocol for osseointegration has enjoyed long-term success and remarkable predictability that has bolstered both professional and patient confidence (Figs 1-7 and 1-8).

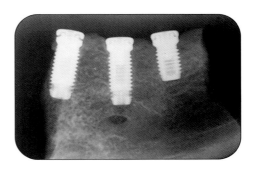

Fig 1-6a Radiograph of human biopsy specimen taken after the patient died, 10 weeks after first-stage surgery.

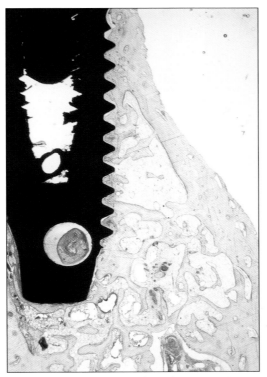

Fig 1-6b Histologic section from the same patient as in Fig 1-6a. Note the large marrow spaces and the bone developing in the screw-threaded areas.

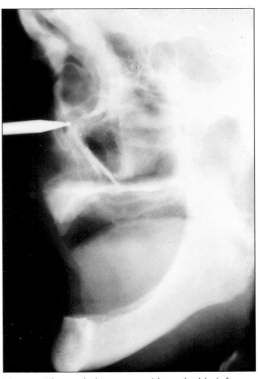

Fig 1-7 The cephalogram provides valuable information about the volume of bone in the maxillary anterior region.

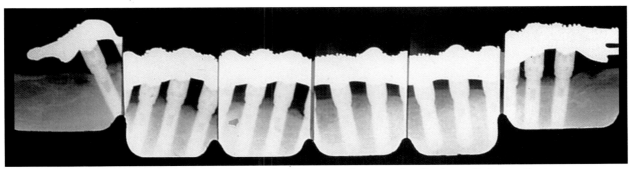

Fig 1-8 Six osseointegrated dental implants provide predictable support for a complete fixed mandibular prosthesis.

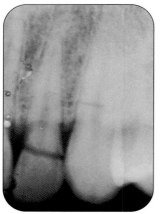 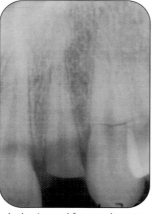

Fig 1-9 The lateral incisor has suffered a horizontal fracture because of trauma. Crown-lengthening surgery will remove periodontium from adjacent teeth and open embrasures. Either orthodontic eruption or a single implant is a better treatment choice.

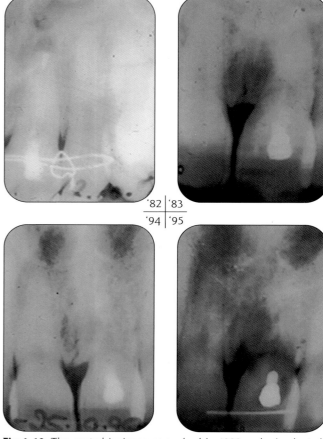

Fig 1-10 The central incisor was avulsed in 1982 and reimplanted. Ankylosis and root resorption resulted in the need to extract the tooth and the loss of crestal alveolar process in 1995. This is detrimental to the long-term future of the area.

Selection of the Optimal Form of Treatment

A tooth that has been compromised by extensive caries, root resorption, or fracture needs to be considered in the context of the adjacent teeth. The possibilities for restoration will be different for single-rooted and multirooted teeth, if there is agreement to end the new restoration on sound tooth structure. Surgical crown-lengthening procedures that are necessary to expose interproximal margins, when treating a tooth in the maximum esthetic zone, result in open spaces (black triangles) interproximally.[20] This tooth may benefit from orthodontic supraeruption if it has a long root or may be better replaced with a dental implant as a single restoration to provide optimum esthetics (Fig 1-9). A multirooted tooth may be a poor candidate for crown-lengthening surgery that would remove bone from the interradicular area. When adjacent teeth require restorations, a traditional fixed partial denture with the replacement of the damaged or missing tooth becomes a strong consideration. Crowded teeth with limited interproximal embrasures must be assessed for esthetics, cleanliness, and prosthetic management of marginal fit before they are irreversibly altered.

Avulsed teeth that are reimplanted too frequently evidence root resorption and ankylosis (Fig 1-10). The immediate and pleasing resolution of the problem belies difficulties later in life, when the tooth must be extracted, and results in a damaged alveolar process at the site of ankylosis. Implants may not be possible, or extensive efforts with guided bone regeneration will be necessary to construct an edentulous ridge that can support a properly placed implant. Similar decisions are necessary when apicoectomy procedures become extensive or repetitive. There is a moment when the least destructive and most conservative treatment is extraction, because it will preserve bone and allow more options to be pursued successfully.

Two-dimensional radiographs do not offer a complete analysis to determine when it would be appropriate for extraction and a change to an implant prosthesis. The easy decision occurs when the tooth structure and/or the periodontium is severely compromised and the pendulum of predictability swings completely to implants (Figs 1-11a and 1-11b). Despite this fact, the clinician must not ignore the successful track record for retention of periodontally compromised dentitions (Figs 1-12a to 1-12e); compliant patients have retained such teeth in a state of health for decades.[9,10,11,21] It should also be stated that the number of patients with refractory periodontal disease in any practice is minimal[22] (Fig 1-13).

Traditional radiographs may confirm which teeth are periodontally compromised, but computerized tomography (three-dimensional radiographs) will allow insight into the future use of implants (Figs 1-14a to 1-14f). The key question: If the tooth or teeth were to be extracted at this time, would implant effectiveness be enhanced? The maxillary incisor that has lost considerable bone will be problematic esthetically now or in the future, but what volume of bone exists apically to the tooth apex? If sufficient, the teeth can be retained for now with little risk for the future use of implants (Figs 1-14c and 1-14d).

The maxillary molar region that demonstrates the loss of interradicular periodontium probably will present inadequate bone volume for an implant (Figs 1-14e and 1-14f). Maintenance of such teeth and continued loss of bone will result in an increased crown-root ratio if implants are implemented in the future. Such teeth must be closely monitored and extracted if bone loss continues. Root resection is a very viable alternative when only one furcation is invaded by inflammatory disease, but is less dependable for a trifurcated tooth if the end point goal is to preserve the tooth and the remaining alveolus (see Chapter 14). If very little bone remains, the decision to remove the maxillary molar may have little influence on the future success or failure of implants in the region. This patient will require a sinus elevation procedure or a pterygoid implant placement to create enough bone to support a loaded prosthesis (see Chapters 13 to 15).

The buccolingual placement of an implant and the subsequent construction of the prosthesis will be an issue for anterior teeth in a dentition demonstrating bimaxillary protrusion. It is unlikely that an implant will be placed in the exact position of such a tooth, and little will be accomplished by preserving the natural tooth. It is this type of case that is best served by the use of a stent covered by a radiopaque material (barium sulfate) during computerized tomography[24] (see Chapter 3). The information gained from this procedure allows the team of dentists participating in treatment planning to relate the location and shape of the remaining alveolar process to the tooth position that is indicated for esthetics, lip support, and incisal occlusion.

These anterior dentitions are flared labially and have very thin buccal plates that are easily destroyed. As more cervical bone is lost, the residual ridge is located lingually to the optimal position for teeth, making restoration of implants awkward. It is particularly difficult for the edentulous candidate who requires a prosthesis that provides esthetics, phonetics, and cleansability. The horizontal distance from the labial surfaces of the teeth to the implants will be too wide and thus hard to clean. The problem becomes more complicated when the patient insists that any spacing be eliminated (Fig 1-15a). Therefore, it is helpful to establish this answer as early as possible to avoid disappointing the patient. Such patients frequently are best treated by removable prostheses, but many receive a fixed prosthesis when the implant can be properly inserted (Fig 1-15b).

The mandibular posterior region presents the formidable obstacle of the inferior alveolar nerve, the position of which is best discovered using three-dimensional radiography. The volume of bone occlusal to the nerve can be ascertained for both hopeless and questionable teeth; such a tooth may be considered strategic if for no other reason than the impossibility of implant placement.

A mandibular molar with compromised tooth structure should be evaluated relative to its possible restoration. Because a principal goal of treatment is to end the new restorative margin on sound tooth structure, a damaged tooth will be evaluated within the limitations of lengthening the clinical crown.[21] A tooth with fused roots or a long trunk is considered a better candidate for crown lengthening surgery than a tooth with a normal trunk length because it is necessary to reduce the periodontium to expose tooth structure without opening the furcation (Figs 1-16a to 1-16d). This becomes precarious as the apical region is approached, and dental implants are preferable. Bone removed in crown-lengthening surgery is permanently lost for implant purposes.

The periodontal prognosis of sectioned mandibular molars is favorable, but the incidence of endodontic and restorative complications dictates that the clinician proceed with caution.[25,26] It is considered to be more desirable for a short edentulous span to be coupled with a large distal root than with a mesial root, which is more difficult to restore. Clinical evidence suggests that success increases if greater control is exercised over this multidisciplinary project. A resultant failure rate of 5.6% compares closely with the reported failure rate of mandibular posterior implants.[17] Because both therapies are reported to have a similar effectiveness, the burden of decision making becomes one of individual considerations when the tooth is stable and in a good state of repair but is compromised periodontally.

The premature loss of mandibular first molars results in the mesial tipping of the second molars, and the proximal discrepancies of the cementoenamel junctions are reflected by an angular interproximal crest (See Volume I, Chapter 9). This radiographic hemiseptum is correctable by orthodontic uprighting if an inflammatory component has not been superimposed on it.[27]

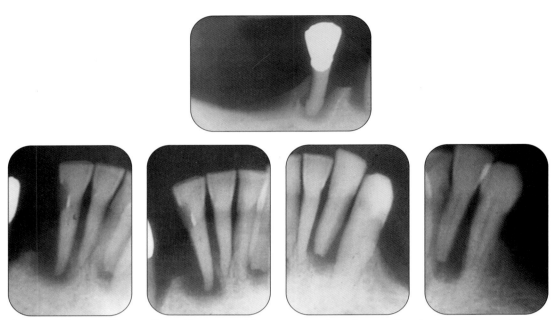

Fig 1-11a The mandibular radiographic survey evidences extreme loss of supporting structure. It is easy to make the decision to treat with dental implants.

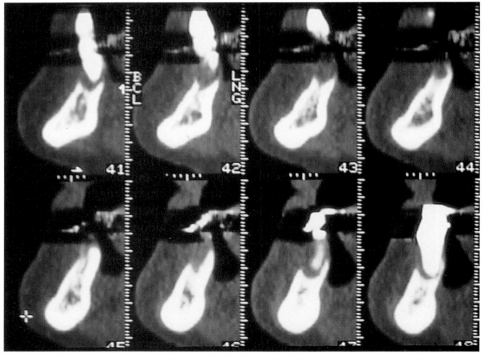

Fig 1-11b The CT scan confirms the periapical radiographs. There is a good volume of bone to support implants.

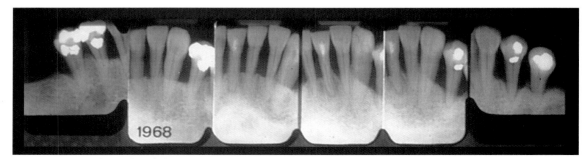

Fig 1-12a The radiographs of this patient provide an opportunity to observe the long-term successful treatment of periodontally compromised teeth. Treatment in 1968 included debridement, stabilization, pocket reduction by resection and regeneration procedures, and mucogingival surgery. Periodontal maintenance is provided with a 3-month periodicity.

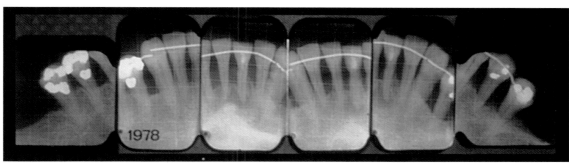

Fig 1-12b Radiographic survey made in 1978.

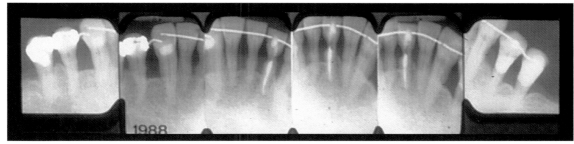

Fig 1-12c Radiographic survey made in 1988. All 10 teeth continue to be present and exhibit a better radiographic profile than they did in 1968.

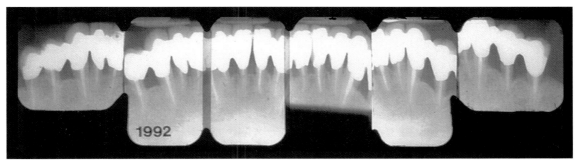

Fig 1-12d A fixed prosthesis was placed to upgrade esthetics.

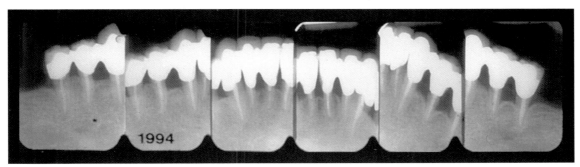

Fig 1-12e Radiographic survey made 28 years posttreatment (1994). Periodontally compromised teeth must not be extracted prematurely.

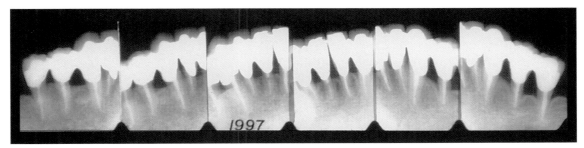

Fig 1-12f Radiographic survey made in 1997.

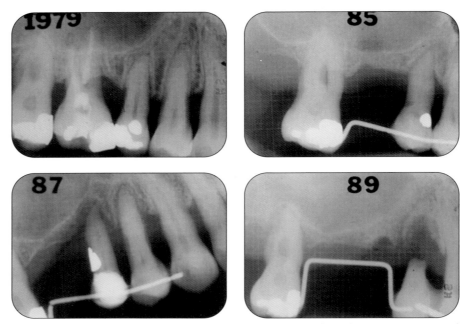

Fig 1-13 Refractory disease. The patient does not respond to traditional treatment as expected and continues to lose bone. It will not be possible to use implants without bone regeneration, and even then the crown-root ratio will be unfavorable.

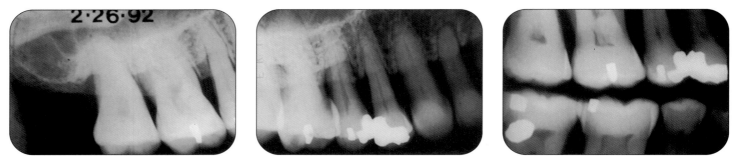

Fig 1-14a The periapical radiographs demonstrate advanced bone loss.

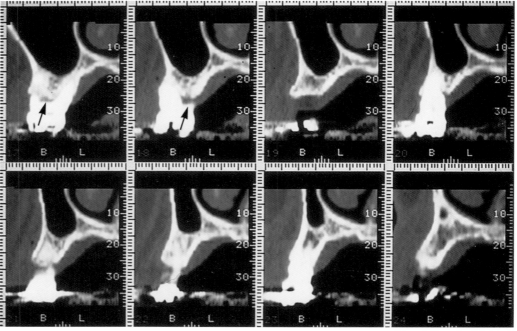

Fig 1-14b The findings in Fig 1-14a are confirmed by the CT scan. Note the loss of bone resulting from furcation invasion *(arrows)*. There will be little benefit from extracting the furcated molars because there is not enough bone to place an implant without an augmentation procedure. However, additional bone loss will increase the crown-root ratio in an area in which the patient can exert the most force. On balance, the teeth should be extracted before additional bone is lost.

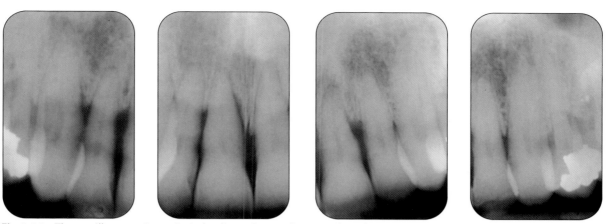

Fig 1-14c The maxillary anterior periapical radiographs reveal extreme bone loss.

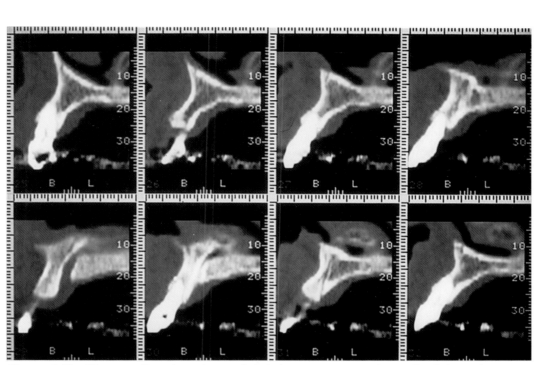

Fig 1-14d The CT scan confirms that only a small clinical root is present. Implants will only be used as a complete maxillary project. There is enough bone apical to the tooth apices to place implants. Therefore, there is no rush to change to implants immediately.

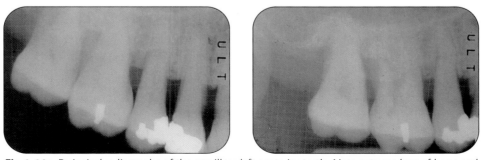

Fig 1-14e Periapical radiographs of the maxillary left posterior teeth. Note extreme loss of bone and furcation invasion.

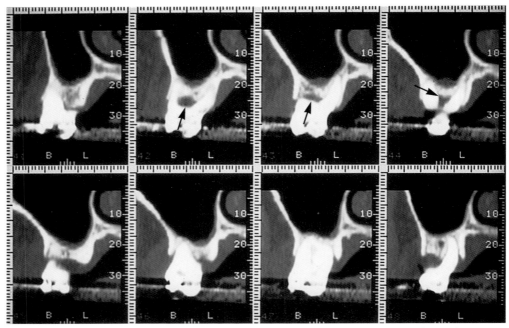

Fig 1-14f The findings are similar to those in Fig 1-14b, but the loss of bone is more advanced *(arrows)*.

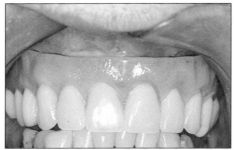

Fig 1-15a Complete maxillary prosthesis that compromises debridement procedures to satisfy esthetics and phonetics.

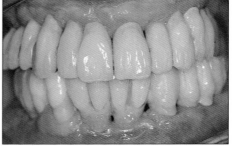

Fig 1-15b Screw-retained complete maxillary prosthesis. (Prosthetic dentistry by Dr Howard Hill.)

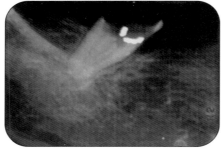

Fig 1-16a The mandibular molar has compromised tooth structure (1973).

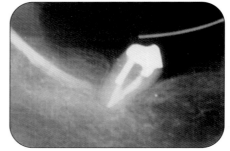

Fig 1-16b A cast post and core is cemented after crown-lengthening surgery.

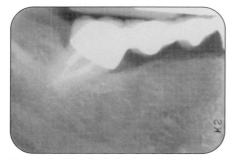

Fig 1-16c The final fixed partial denture is cemented in place.

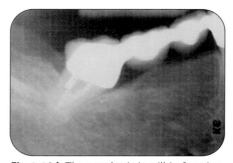

Fig 1-16d The prosthesis is still in function 23 years later. (Prosthetic dentistry by Dr Maurice Michaud.)

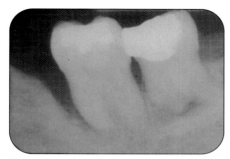

Fig 1-17a The mandibular molars have a poor prognosis and are to be extracted with simultaneous guided bone regeneration.

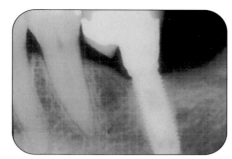

Fig 1-17b An implant is placed 10 months later. This is a difficult area for access, and the implant is positioned to allow for a small cantilever to enhance debridement.

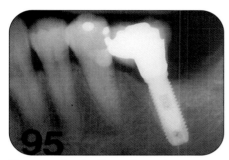

Fig 1-17c Postloading radiograph—3 years.

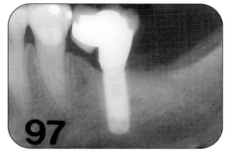

Fig 1-17d The 8-year postloading radiograph. Note that there is no loss of supporting bone after loading.

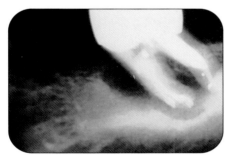

Fig 1-18a A hopeless molar is to be extracted immediately.

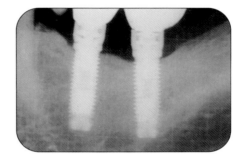

Fig 1-18b The molar is replaced with two implants.

When the angular crest predisposes the area to additional loss of supporting structures, periodontal regeneration has to be considered.[28] The disease may be so advanced, however, that extraction is the logical treatment, and guided bone regeneration is immediately implemented to prepare the area for future implants[29] (Figs 1-17 and 1-18). If the teeth are stable and the pattern of bone loss is treatable, the regenerative possibilities are considered. Tipped mandibular molars lose their contact points and a diminished embrasure space results, reducing the possibilities of root resection and prosthetic restoration. Successful regenerative treatment may resolve the inflammatory defect, but it will be necessary to perform ostectomy to create a flat edentulous ridge of bone[30] (see Chapter 3).

A very treatable osseous defect proximal to an edentulous region with implant treatment in the offing may suggest the occasion for considerable debate. Is it necessary to save this tooth and thus commit the patient to a significant surgical decision, or can it be added to the implant prosthesis by the use of a cantilever or another implant (Figs 1-19a to 1-19d)?

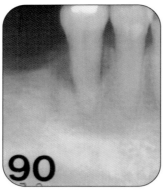

Fig 1-19a The mandibular first premolar has extensive loss of supporting bone and is a realistic candidate for periodontal regeneration. However, implants will be used to replace the missing teeth.

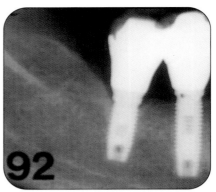

Fig 1-19b Two distal implants support a mesial cantilever to replace the extracted premolar. (Prosthetic dentistry by Dr Janice Conrad.)

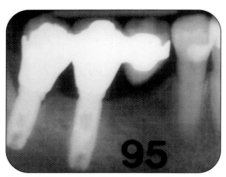

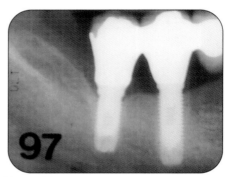

Figs 1-19c and 1-19d The prosthesis is shown 7 years later.

Conclusion

To answer the question of extraction timing and its effect on the successful future use of implants, the surgeon must take many factors into consideration, and the timing will vary within one dentition.

The decision to extract a specific tooth is important when contemplating a dental treatment plan. Figure 1-20 shows a dentition that requires dental implants to replace missing teeth in the maxillary left posterior and mandibular right posterior quadrants. The maxillary cuspid is in question. Retaining this tooth and performing crown-lengthening procedures to gain sound tooth structure for restorative margin placement will result in the removal of bone that could support a dental implant and simultaneously compromise the adjacent lateral incisor. It also would result in longer teeth in the final prosthesis, thus diminishing the esthetic result.

An implant treatment plan that does not recognize spatial limitations frequently results in problems greater than the edentulous space. The restorability of implants must be determined before they are installed.

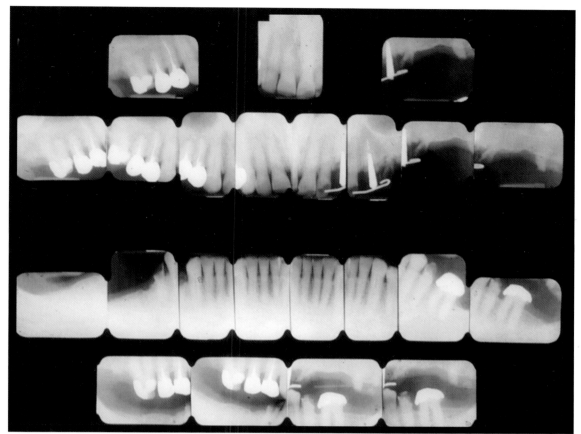

Fig 1-20a The pretreatment full-mouth radiographic survey reveals the need for tooth replacement in the maxillary left and mandibular right quadrants (1986). The maxillary left canine has a post and core restoration and caries. Crown-lengthening surgery will result in a compromised periodontium for the lateral incisor and reduce the vertical height of bone for future implants.

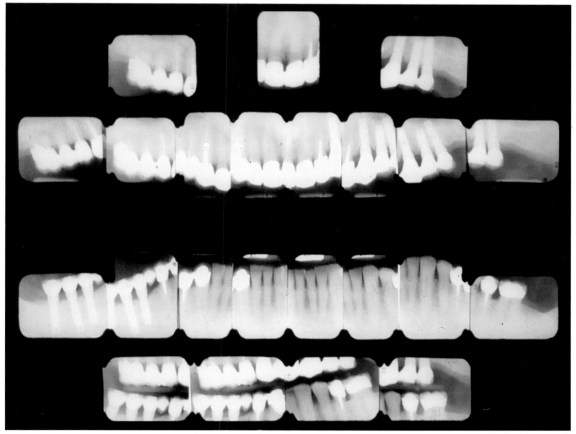

Fig 1-20b Posttreatment full-mouth radiographic survey (1989). Implant prostheses have replaced the missing teeth in the maxillary left and mandibular right quadrants.

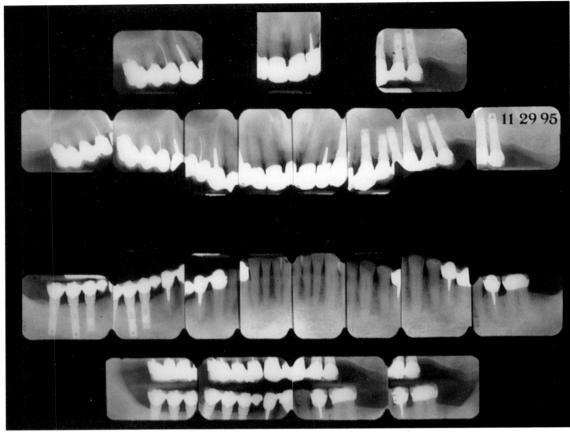

Fig 1-20c The follow-up full-mouth radiographic survey reveals complete stability of the implants and the bone level surrounding them (1995). (Prosthetic dentistry by Dr. Janice Conrad.)

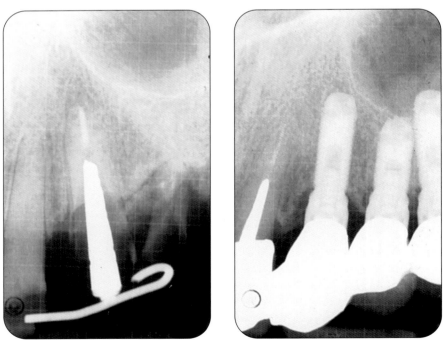

Fig 1-20d The maxillary left canine has been replaced by an implant.

References

1. Lewis S. Treatment planning: Teeth versus implants. Int J Periodont Rest Dent 1996;16(4):367–378.

2. Mellonig JT. Decalcified freeze-dried bone allograft as an implant material in human periodontal defects. Int J Periodont Rest Dent 1984;4(6):41–55.

3. Gottlow J, Nyman S, Lindhe J, Karring T, Wennström J. New attachment formation in the human periodontium by guided tissue regeneration. J Clin Periodontol 1986;13:604–616.

4. Bowers GM, Chadroff B, Carnevale R, Mellonig JT, Corio R, Emerson J, et al. Histologic evaluation of new attachment apparatus formation in humans. Part III. J Periodontol 1987;14:80–84.

5. McClain P, Schallhorn RG. Long term assessment of combined osseous composite grafting, root conditioning and guided tissue regeneration. Int J Periodont Rest Dent 1993;13:9–28.

6. Becker W, Becker B, Berg L, Samsam C. Clinical and volumetric analysis of three-wall intrabony defects following open flap debridement. J Periodontol 1986;57:277–285.

7. Amsterdam M. Periodontal prosthesis. In: Goldman H, Cohen DW (eds). Periodontal Therapy, ed 5. St Louis: Mosby, 1973:990.

8. Amsterdam M. Periodontal prosthesis: Twenty-five years in retrospect. Alpha Omegan 1974;67:29–31.

9. Nyman S, Ericsson I. The capacity of reduced periodontium to support fixed bridgework. J Clin Periodontol 1982;9:409–414.

10. Yulzari JC. Strategic extractions in periodontal prostheses. Int J Periodont Rest Dent 1982;2(6):51–66.

11. Skurow HM, Nevins M. The rationale of the preperiodontal provisional biologic trial restoration. Int J Periodont Rest Dent 1988; 8(1):9–29.

12. Nevins M. Interproximal periodontal disease: The embrasure as an etiologic factor. Int J Periodont Rest Dent 1982;2(6):9–27.

13. Jemt T, Lekholm U, Adell R. Osseointegrated implants in the treatment of partially edentulous jaws: A preliminary study on 876 consecutively placed fixtures. Int J Oral Maxillofac Implants 1989; 4:211–217.

14. Buser D, Weber HP, Brägger U, Balsiger C. Tissue integration of one-stage ITI implants: Three-year results of a longitudinal study with hollow cylinder and hollow screw implants. Int J Oral Maxillofac Implants 1991;6:405–412.

15. Jemt T, Lekholm U. Oral implant treatment in posterior partially edentulous jaws: A five-year follow-up report. Int J Oral Maxillofac Implants 1993;8:635–640.

16. Lekholm U, van Steenberghe D, Herrmann I, et al. Osseointegrated implants in the treatment of partially edentulous jaws: A prospective five-year multicenter study. Int J Oral Maxillofac Implants 1994; 9:627–635.

17. Nevins M, Langer B. The successful application of osseointegrated implants to the posterior jaw: A long-term retrospective study. Int J Oral Maxillofac Implants 1993;8:428–432.

18. Albrektsson T, Zarb GA, Worthington P, Eriksson AR. The long-term efficacy of currently used dental implants: A review and proposed criteria of success. Int J Oral Maxillofac Implants 1986;1:11–25.

19. Albrektsson T, Eriksson AR, Friberg B, et al. Histologic investigations on 33 retrieved Nobelpharma implants. J Clin Mater 1993;12:1–9.

20. Salama H, Rose LF, Salama M, Betts NJ. Immediate loading of bilaterally splinted titanium root-form implants in fixed prosthodontics—a technique reexamined: Two case reports. Int J Periodont Rest Dent 1995;15:345–362.

21. Wagenberg B, Eskow RN, Langer B. Exposing adequate tooth structure for restorative dentistry. Int J Periodont Rest Dent 1989; 9:323–333.

22. Nevins M, Langer B. The successful use of osseointegrated implants for the treatment of the recalcitrant periodontal patient. J Periodont Res 1995; 66:150–157.

23. Kramer GM. The case for ostectomy: A time-tested therapeutic modality in selected periodontal sites. Int J Periodont Rest Dent 1995;15:229–238.

24. Mecall RA, Rosenfeld AL. The influence of residual ridge resorption patterns on implant fixture placement and tooth position. Part II. Presurgical determination of prosthesis type and design. Int J Periodont Rest Dent 1992;12:33–51.

25. Langer B, Stein SD, Wagenberg B. An evaluation of root resections: A ten-year study. J Periodontol 1981;52:719–722.

26. Carnevale G, Di Febo G, Tonelli MP, Marin C, Fuzzi MA. Retrospective analysis of the periodontal-prosthetic treatment of molars with interradicular lesions. Int J Periodont Rest Dent 1991; 11:189–205.

27. Wise RJ, Kramer GM. Pre-determination of osseous changes associated with uprighting tipped molars by probing. Int J Periodont Rest Dent 1983;3(1):69–80.

28. Papanou PN, Wennström JL. The angular bone defect as an indicator of further alveolar bone loss. J Clin Periodontol 1991;18:317–322.

29. Nevins M, Mellonig JT. The advantages of localized ridge augmentation prior to implant placement: A staged event. Int J Periodont Rest Dent 1994;14:97–111.

30. Ochsenbein C. A primer for osseous surgery. Int J Periodont Rest Dent 1986;6(1):9–47.

CHAPTER 2

The Efficacy of Osseointegration for the Partially Edentulous Patient

Ulf Lekholm, DDS, PhD

The Brånemark implant system[1] (Nobel Biocare, Gothenburg, Sweden) was originally developed for use in edentulous patients, and so far several publications[2–6] have reported excellent long-term results of such treatment. During the past decade, the procedure has increasingly been used around the world in partially edentulous jaws also.[7–11] However, the outcome of the latter situation is not yet as well documented; it does not seem acceptable to extrapolate the success in edentulous jaws to partially edentulous arches. The only exception might be in Applegate-Kennedy class IV arches, where implants can be placed under conditions similar to those in edentulous jaws. In other locations, functional and biologic differences between the two situations might influence the treatment outcome. Consequently, it is important to specifically evaluate the implant results in partially edentulous jaws via separate long-term studies. It is not sufficient just to anticipate what the treatment outcome might be in these situations.

The aims of this chapter are to discuss the differences that exist in implant treatment for edentulous and partially edentulous jaws and to present some available long-term data on the efficacy of the Brånemark osseointegration technique when used in partially edentulous patients.

Differences in Implant Treatment for Edentulous and Partially Edentulous Jaws

Edentulous and partially edentulous jaws represent two completely different clinical environments, specifically regarding implant treatment. Beside the fact that teeth are either present or absent, implants are generally placed in the anterior regions of edentulous jaws, anterior to the maxillary sinuses or the mental foramina. In partially edentulous jaws, at least of Applegate-Kennedy classes I and II, they are located in the posterior areas. When comparing these two situations, the following differences regarding implant treatment are of interest: anatomic conditions, biomechanical aspects, and oral hygiene and microbiologic states.

Anatomic Conditions

It has been reported that the farther distal implants are placed within the alveolar process, the higher the risk that bone of poor quality will be engaged.[12,13] Furthermore, it has been shown that greater volumes of bone for implant placement can be found in the anterior regions of the jaws than in the posterior areas.[14] As long as the minimum volume of bone needed for implant placement is present, ie, 4 mm versus 7 mm,[15] a standard treatment protocol can still be carried out. Placing implants close to the maxillary sinus in partially edentulous jaws may, however, result in implant sites with very thin cortical bone layers, even if two layers are engaged, and bone volumes of poor density. Above the inferior alveolar nerve of the mandible, on the other hand, implants may be placed in areas of small bone volume, seldom engaging a second cortical layer.

From the standpoint of fixture stability, a reduced implant-to–cortical bone ratio has proven to provide less favorable retention of the implant after it has become osseointegrated.[16] It has also been shown[17] that implants placed in bone of poor quality, specifically type 4 bone, will have a higher rate of failure than those placed in denser bone, eg, type 1 and type 2 bone. Consequently, it seems less favorable, from an anatomic standpoint, to work with implants in partially edentulous jaws of at least Applegate-Kennedy classes I and II than in the anterior regions of edentulous patients.

Biomechanical Aspects

Reduced bone volumes mean that shorter implants have to be inserted. Several studies[17–19] have shown that the failure rate is higher when short implants are placed than when longer ones can be inserted.

Furthermore, prospective receptor areas with diminished bone volume permit only the placement of a few implants. The average number of implants reported for partially edentulous jaws is 2.6,[19] whereas for edentulous jaws the number is 5.2.[20] In the case of an implant failure, it is certainly an obvious difference if one implant of three is lost rather than one of five. This numerical variability of available implants has a direct effect on the clinical stability and function of the prostheses.

Implants in edentulous jaws will, in most instances, be placed in an arch-shaped position, as a result of the horseshoe shape of the jaws in the anterior regions. In the posterior areas, on the other hand, the implants are in general placed linearly, because the crest of the jaws has a comparable linear design. From a loading standpoint, the risk of creating unfavorable bending forces on the implants[21] is much higher if they are standing in a line with only one rotational axis. If, instead, several axes can be established, for example by placing the implants in an arch position as in edentulous jaws or by inserting at least three implants with somewhat divergent directions in partially edentulous arches, fewer bending forces will be transferred to the implants.[21] If only two implants are present, however, there will always be just one axis, which often is the case in posterior partial edentulousness.

With only two implants present there will also be a higher risk for mechanical complications.[9] Furthermore, the closer to the temporomandibular joints the implants are placed, the stronger the masticatory force on the implants, because of the hinge-joint situation. It has been shown by Laurell[22] and by Book et al[23] that the occlusal force in the molar region is approximately 40% greater than the load that can be exerted within the incisor region. Thus, from a biomechanical standpoint also, it seems that it would be less favorable to place implants in the posterior regions of partially edentulous jaws than in the anterior areas of edentulous patients.

Oral Hygiene and Microbiologic States

Several studies have indicated that in both jaw types it is possible to maintain an acceptably good level of oral hygiene.[24–26] Furthermore, it has been shown[26–28] that cocci and nonmotile rods dominate in plaque deposits in both situations. However, when the pathogens present were compared it was found that motile rods, together with spirochetes, amount to approximately 25% of the plaque in the partially edentulous jaw, whereas they constitute only 2% of plaque microflora in the edentulous arch. Thus, if teeth are still present when implants are placed, the pathogens seem capable of migrating from dental areas to the implant sites.

The significance of these data for the long-term outcome of implant treatment in partially edentulous jaws is currently not fully understood. It may, however, be a potential risk factor for peri-implant mucosal problems in the long term, specifically when considering the soft tissue attachment mechanism that exists at titanium implant surfaces.[29–31]

Consequently, at least theoretically, there seem to be several factors that may influence the possibility of successful treatment of partially edentulous jaws with osseointegrated implants. Still, the number of partially edentulous patients provided with Brånemark implants is rapidly increasing throughout the world today and currently accounts for about 50% of all jaws treated. Thus, it is of importance to analyze thoroughly the outcome of such treatment with separate long-term follow-up studies. Only then will it be possible to shed full light on the efficacy of the Brånemark technique for the partially edentulous patient.

Results in Partially Edentulous Jaws

The Brånemark procedure was used for the first time to treat a partially edentulous patient in 1968, when two fixtures were placed in a maxilla to support a two-unit fixed partial denture. The prosthesis is currently intact and functional. During the following 14 years, only another eight partially edentulous patients were provided with Brånemark implants by the team in Gothenburg. When the Brånemark procedure had its international breakthrough at the 1982 Toronto meeting, clinicians around the world were introduced to the system and began to use it to treat partially edentulous jaws. Consequently, there are no long-term follow-up studies currently available to present outcomes of the technique in partial edentulism based on observational periods much longer than 15 years.

The report with the longest follow-up time is the one by Lekholm et al,[32] presenting the first partially edentulous patients ever treated by the Brånemark team in Gothenburg, Sweden. However, this study is based on very few patients and a mixture of different prosthetic designs. It is thus not a relevant study to exemplify the outcome of the Brånemark technique in partial edentulism. Instead, three other articles[33–35] will be used to assess the current potential of the Brånemark technique in partially edentulous patients.

In the retrospective report by Nevins and Langer,[33] the outcome was based on the pooled patient materials of their two periodontal clinics. The study included a sufficiently large number of patients (n = 338), representing 200 mandibles and 193 maxillas. In these patients, 1,203 Brånemark system implants of various lengths and design were placed between January 1984 and September 1991. The implants were used to support 250 maxillary and 247 mandibular prostheses.

All clinical handling was performed according to the original Brånemark protocol,[1] but the fixed prostheses were of various designs, because some of them were constructed in combination with adjacent teeth and others were freestanding. Furthermore, in some instances, the occlusal material was porcelain and in others it was acrylic resin. Single-tooth restorations were also included.

In December 1992 the outcome was evaluated, meaning that a follow-up time of 1 to 8 years was presented in the data. The implant success rate was evaluated according to the criteria proposed by Albrektsson et al.[36] In all, 18% of the treated patients were withdrawn during the period, which is an acceptable figure for a long-term study performed at two different clinical centers.

The overall mean stability rates for the prostheses were 99.0% and 97.0% for the maxilla and mandible, respectively. The corresponding results regarding fixture survival rates were 95.2% and 95.5%, respectively, as means for the entire period. When the outcome of the subgroup representing 6 to 8 years was examined, it was observed that as many as 90.9% and 95.1% of the implants in maxillas and mandibles, respectively, were still functional.

These figures represent the longest follow-up data currently available, based on a sufficiently large number of consecutively treated and longitudinally documented patients with Brånemark implants. The outcome is very favorable and competes well with figures that have previously been presented for edentulous jaws[2] that were followed for the same length of time. Furthermore, the results also indicate that the Brånemark technique can be used at independent centers with a repeatedly successful outcome. However, the outcome is still somewhat limited because no information was given about jaw classification, jaw shape, bone quality, periodontal conditions, or marginal bone resorption during the follow-up periods. In addition, no mention was made about posttherapeutic complications.

In the report by Lekholm et al,[34] the research protocol was based on a multicenter approach and was carried out as a 5-year prospective follow-up study. Nine international centers were participating between July 1985 and April 1987, when 159 partially edentulous patients, 58% of them female, were treated. All arches belonged to Applegate-Kennedy classes I, II, and IV. A total of 68 maxillas and 91 mandibles were included. Examinations of jaw shape and bone qualities indicated that few extreme cases had been accepted into the study. Treated patients varied between 17 and 70 years of age (50% between 40 and 60 years).

Five hundred fifty-eight Brånemark fixtures of various lengths and diameters were inserted, using the standard protocol.[37] After a healing time of approximately 4 to 6 months, 154 of the patients were provided with 197 fixed prostheses, which were fabricated in the conventional way.[38] All constructions (76 maxillary and 121 mandibular) were freestanding from the natural dentition.

After having received the fixed partial dentures, the patients were examined annually to assess the following parameters:

1. Fixture survival
2. Prosthesis stability
3. Periodontal indices
4. Marginal bone resorption
5. Temporomandibular joint disorders
6. Complications

All examinations were performed according to standard techniques, as detailed elsewhere.[19] At the end of the 5-year follow-up period, the prostheses were also removed to check the individual implant stability, thereby making it possible to assess fixture success rather than implant survival, in accordance with the criteria of Albrektsson et al.[36]

To date, one 1-year presentation[19] and three 3-year reports[39–41] have been published. In the present chapter, the final 5-year outcome, originally reported by Lekholm et al[34] in 1994, will be reviewed. During the 5-year follow-up period, 27 patients (20%), representing a total of 116 fixtures and 33 restorations, dropped out for various reasons. A lifetable principle was used for the statistical analyses,[42] however, so that the withdrawn patients were still included in the published implant and prosthesis data.

The mean cumulative fixture success rate amounted to 93.3% for the entire group (92% for maxillary and 94.1% for mandibular jaws). Shorter fixtures were lost more often than longer ones, and wider implants showed the lowest failure rates. When a worst-case analysis was performed, ie, all failed and withdrawn implants were regarded as failures, 82.5% of the fixtures still survived after 5 years. No comparable figures have previously been presented regarding the outcome of implant treatment in partially edentulous jaws.

The mean cumulative prosthesis stability rate was 94.2% for both arches (94.4% for the maxilla and 94.1% for the mandible). All fixed prostheses were freestanding and were fabricated in either acrylic resin or porcelain. The condition of the temporomandibular joints, evaluated according to the Helkimo Index,[43] improved or was unchanged in as many as 81% of the treated patients. Consequently, for a majority of the patients, the osseointegrated fixed partial denture remained functional over the 5-year period without negatively influencing the status of the temporomandibular joint.

In general, the patients were capable of maintaining an acceptable level of cleanliness. Measurements were performed both on fixtures and on control teeth, and no statistically significant differences between the two locations were observed. The presence of plaque was low (0.4 ± 0.5 and 0.3 ± 0.5 for implants and teeth, respectively), as was the incidence of gingivitis (0.1 ± 0.5 and 0.1 ± 0.2 for implants and teeth, respectively). The probing depths were 3.2 ± 0.5 mm for implants and 2.3 ± 0.9 mm for teeth. Very small changes of the periodontal parameters took place over the research period.

The most commonly reported complications were related to acrylic resin fractures of the occlusal material of the prostheses. Loose anchorage components were the second-most-common problem observed. Fractures of fixtures were rare, whereas abutment screw fractures and gold screw fractures were reported infrequently. Few mucosal problems were found, once again indicating the prevalence of good oral hygiene. Except for paresthesia of the lower lip, which was reported in five instances after the first year and which was continuous in two patients 5 years later, few really severe complications occurred in the patient population. The study thus indicated that good treatment results could be obtained in partially edentulous jaws when the standard procedure of the oral implant technique ad modum Brånemark was used, even in a multicenter approach.

A discussion of the potential of the Brånemark implant technique in partially edentulous jaws must, of course, include results regarding single-tooth treatment. An early report was published by Jemt et al[44] in 1990 to show the adaptability of the Brånemark technique to the single-tooth situation. However, because the study, to a large extent, was based on development patients as well as on the first experience of just one clinic, the report is of limited value. No single-tooth patients were involved in the multicenter report presented by Lekholm et al[34] in 1994. Although such patients were included in Nevins and Langer's study,[33] no separate results were given.

Instead, the information is available from another multicenter report,[35] in which the outcome of 5 years of follow-up have been presented. Starting in 1987, seven international centers treated a total of 92 patients, who were 18 to 70 years of age at the time of implant placement. In all, 107 implants were included in the report, 88 in 78 maxillas and 19 in 15 mandibles. The study design was very much the same as that used by Lekholm et al,[34] and the treatment techniques followed conventional protocols.[45,46]

After 5 years of follow-up, the cumulative survival rate was 96.6% for implants and single crowns inserted in the maxillae and 100% for those in the mandibles. The overall soft tissue state was reported to be good, and very little marginal bone loss was observed during the 5-year follow-up period. Furthermore, very few complications were observed. Loosening of anchorage components was the most frequently reported problem. However, there appeared to be less loosening when gold locking screws were used than when titanium screws were employed. Only four crown fractures occurred after 5 years of follow-up. Thus, it was also possible to obtain a successful outcome for single-tooth situations, in selected patients, with the osseointegration method.

Conclusion

Based on the three reports reviewed,[33,34,35] use of the Brånemark implant procedure in partially edentulous patients, including in single-tooth situations, seems to provide treatment results similar to those found in edentulous jaws followed for the same length of time.[2] The efficacy of the standard protocol of the technique is good; consequently, the method can safely be recommended for use in partially edentulous arches. This holds true despite the previously presented, theoretically suggested, concerns regarding its use in posterior areas of partially edentulous jaws, at least from the perspective of 10 years of follow-up.

References

1. Brånemark P-I, Zarb GA, Albrektsson T (eds). Tissue-Integrated Prostheses: Osseointegration in Clinical Dentistry. Chicago: Quintessence, 1985.

2. Adell R, Eriksson B, Lekholm U, Brånemark P-I, Jemt T. A long-term follow-up study of osseointegrated implants in the treatment of the totally edentulous jaw. Int J Oral Maxillofac Implants 1990;5:347–358.

3. Jemt T, Chai J, Harnett, et al. A 5-year prospctive multicenter follow-up report on overdentures supported by osseointegrated implants. Int J Oral Maxillofac Implants 1996;11:291–298.

4. Friberg B, Nilson H, Olsson M, Palmquist C. MKII: The self-tapping Brånemark implant. 5-year results of a prospective 3-center study. Clin Oral Implants Res 1997;8:279–285.

5. van Steenberghe D, Quirynen M, Calberson L, Demand M. A prospective evaluation of the fate of 697 consecutive intraoral fixtures ad modum Brånemark in the rehabilitation of edentulism. J Head Neck Pathol 1987;6:53–58.

6. Zarb GA, Schmitt A. The longitudinal clinical effectiveness of osseointegrated dental implants. The Toronto study. Part I. Surgical results. J Prosthet Dent 1989;63:451–457.

7. Gunne J, Åstrand PO, Ahlén K, Olsson M. Implants in partially edentulous patients. A longitudinal study of bridges supported by both implants and natural teeth. Clin Oral Impl Res 1992;3:49–56.

8. Jemt T, Lekholm U, Adell R. Osseointegrated implants in the treatment of partially edentulous patients. A preliminary study on 876 consecutively installed fixtures. Int J Maxillofac Implants 1989;4:211–217.

9. Jemt T, Lekholm U. Oral implant treatment in posterior partially edentulous jaws. A 5-year follow-up report. Int J Oral Maxillofac Implants 1993;8:635–640.

10. Naert J, Quirynen M, van Steenberghe D, Darius P. A six-year prosthetic study of 509 consecutively inserted implants for the treatment of partial edentulism. J Prosthet Dent 1992;67:236–245.

11. van Steenberghe D, Sullivan D, Liström R, Balshi T, Henry P, Worthington P, Wahlström U. A retrospective multicenter evaluation of the survival rate of osseointegrated fixtures supporting bridges in the treatment of partial edentulism. J Prosthet Dent 1989;61:217–224.

12. von Wowern N. Variations in bone mass within the cortices of the mandible. Scand J Dent Res 1977;85:444–455.

13. von Wowern N. Variations in structure within the trabecular bone of the mandible. Scand J Dent Res 1977;85:613–622.

14. Cawood JI, Howell RA. A classification of the edentulous jaws. Int J Oral Maxillofac Surg 1988;17:232–236.

15. Lekholm U, Zarb GA. Patient selection. In Brånemark P-I, Zarb GA, Albrektsson T (eds). Tissue-Integrated Prostheses: Osseointegration in Clinical Dentistry. Chicago: Quintessence, 1985: 199–209.

16. Sennerby L, Thomsen P, Ericson L. A morphometrical and biomechanical comparison of titanium implants inserted in rabbit cortical and cancellous bone. Int J Oral Maxillofac Implants 1992;7:62–71.

17. Friberg B, Jemt T, Lekholm U. Early failures of 4641 consecutively installed Brånemark dental implants. I. A study from stage one surgery to installation of the completed prostheses. Int J Maxillofac Implants 1991;6:142–146.

18. Lekholm U. The Brånemark implant technique: A standardized procedure under continuous development. In: Laney WR, Tolman DE (eds). Tissue Integration in Oral, Orthopedic, and Maxillofacial Reconstruction. Chicago: Quintessence, 1992:194–199.

19. van Steenberghe D, Lekholm U, Bolender C, Folmer T, Henry P, Herrmann I, et al. The applicability of osseointegrated oral implants in the rehabilitation of partial edentulism. A prospective multicenter study on 558 fixtures. Int J Oral Maxillofac Implants 1990;5:272–281.

20. Aspe P, Ellen RP, Overall CM, Zarb GA. Microbiota and crevicular fluid collagenase activity in the osseointegrated dental implant sulcus. A comparison of sites in edentulous and partially edentulous patients. J Periodont Res 1989;24:96–105.

21. Rangert B, Jemt T, Jörneus L. Forces and moments on Brånemark implants. Int J Oral Maxillofac Implants 1989;4:241–247.

22. Laurell L. Occlusal forces and chewing ability in dentitions with cross-arch bridges. Swed Dent J 1985;suppl 26.

23. Book K, Karlsson S, Jemt T. Functional adaptation to full-arch fixed prosthesis supported by osseointegrated implants in the edentulous mandible. Clin Oral Impl Res 1992;3:17–21.

24. Adell R, Lekholm U, Rockler B, Brånemark P-I, Lindhe J, Ericsson I, Sbordone L. Marginal tissue reactions at osseointegrated titanium fixtures. I. A three year longitudinal prospective study. Int J Oral Maxillofac Surg 1986;15:39–52.

25. Lekholm U, Adell R, Lindhe J, et al. Marginal tissue reactions at osseointegrated titanium fixtures. II. A cross-sectional retrospective study. Int J Oral Maxillofac Surg 1986;15:53–61.

26. Quirynen M, Listgarten M. Distribution of bacterial morphotypes around natural teeth and titanium implants ad modum Brånemark. Clin Oral Impl Res 1990;1:8–12.

27. Lekholm U, Ericsson I, Adell R, Slots J. The condition of the soft tissues at tooth and fixture abutments supporting fixed bridges. A microbiological and histological study. J Clin Periodontol 1986;13:558–562.

28. Mombelli A, van Oosten M AC, Schurch E, Lang NP. The microbiota associated with successful or failing osseointegrated titanium implant. Oral Microbiol Immunol 1987;2:145–151.

29. Berglundh T, Lindhe J, Ericsson I, Marinello CP, Liljenberg B, Thomsen P. The soft tissue barrier at implants and teeth. Clin Oral Impl Res 1991;2:81–90.

30. Berglundh T, Lindhe J, Ericsson I, Marinello CP, Liljenberg B. Soft tissue reactions to de novo plaque formation on implants and teeth. An experimental study in the dog. Clin Oral Impl Res 1992;3:1–8.

31. Lindhe J, Berglundh T, Ericsson I, Liljenberg B, Marinello CP. Experimental breakdown of periimplant and periodontal tissue. A study in the beagle dog. Clin Oral Impl Res 1992;3:9–16.

32. Lekholm U, Jemt T, Adell R, Brånemark P-I. Fixture survival in partially edentulous jaws. A 10-year analysis. In: Worthington P, Brånemark P-I (eds). Advanced Osseointegration Surgery. Chicago: Quintessence, 1992:206–209.

33. Nevins M, Langer B. The successful application of osseointegrated implants to the posterior jaw: A long-term retrospective study. Int J Oral Maxillofac Implants 1993;8:428–432.

34. Lekholm U, van Steenberghe D, Herrmann I, Bolender C, Folmer T, Gunne J, et al. Osseointegrated implants in the treatment of partially edentulous jaws. A prospective 5-year multicenter study. Int J Oral Maxillofac Implants 1994;9:627–635.

35. Henry P, Laney W, Jemt T, et al. Osseointegrated implants for single-tooth replacement: A prospective 5-year multicenter study. Int J Oral Maxillofac Implants 1996;11:450–455.

36. Albrektsson T, Zarb GA, Worthington P, Eriksson RA. The long-term efficacy of currently used dental implants: A review and proposed criteria of success. Int J Oral Maxillofac Implants 1986;1:11–25.

37. Adell R, Lekholm U, Brånemark P-I. Surgical procedures. In: Brånemark P-I, Zarb GA, Albrektsson T (eds). Tissue-Integrated Prostheses: Osseointegration in Clinical Dentistry. Chicago: Quintessence, 1985:211–232.

38. Jemt T, Lindén B, Lekholm U. Failures and complications in 127 consecutively installed fixed partial prostheses supported by Brånemark implants. A study from prosthetic treatment up to the first annual check-up. Int J Oral Maxillofac Implants 1992;7:40–44.

39. Henry P, Tolman D, Bolender C. The applicability of osseointegrated implants in the treatment of partially edentulous patients. Three-year result of a prospective multicenter study. Quintessence Int 1993;24:123–129.

40. van Steenberghe D, Klinge B, Lindén U, Quirynen M, Herrmann I, Garpland C. Periodontal indices around natural and titanium abutments: A longitudinal multicenter study. J Periodontol 1993; 64:538–541.

41. Gunne J, Jemt T, Lindén B. Implant treatment in partially edentulous patients: A prosthetic report after 3 years. Int J Prosthodont 1994; 7:43–48.

42. Colton T. Longitudinal studies and the use of the lifetable. In: Colton T (ed). Statistics in Medicine. Boston: Little, Brown, 1974:241–249.

43. Helkimo P. Studies on function and dysfunction of the masticatory system. II. Svensk Tandläk Tidskr 1974;67:101–121.

44. Jemt T, Lekholm U, Gröndahl K. A three-year follow-up study of early single implant restorations ad modem Brånemark. Int J Periodont Rest Dent 1990;10:341–349.

45. Jemt T. Modified single and short-span restorations supported by osseointegrated fixtures in the partially edentulous jaw. J Prosthet Dent 1986;55:243–247.

46. Lekholm U, Jemt T. Principles for single tooth replacement. In: Albrektsson T, Zarb GA (eds). The Brånemark Osseointegrated Implant. Chicago: Quintessence, 1989:117–126.

Using Computerized Tomography to Develop Realistic Treatment Objectives for the Implant Team

Alan L. Rosenfeld, DDS
Richard A. Mecall, DDS, MS

CHAPTER 3

Defining the Team Concept in Implant Dentistry

When the concept of osseointegration was introduced internationally by Professor Per-Ingvar Brånemark in the early 1980s, few people appreciated the enormous impact this would have on the dental profession and its ability to offer permanent tooth replacement and improve the quality of life for orally debilitated patients worldwide. The resultant international, multicenter, scientific cooperation has been unprecedented in the field of dentistry. This singular achievement has inspired the profession and catalyzed a proliferation of implant manufacturers.

Because the delivery of implant-supported prostheses requires both surgical and prosthetic expertise, the emergence of an implant team vernacular has become professionally fashionable. Although the team concept suggests a greater likelihood of excellent patient care, too often this does not occur because the needs and concerns of the patient and the responsibilities of team members have not been clearly defined. In fact, some team members seem to assert greater dominance and suggest that their roles are of greater importance, usually at the expense of effective, interactive, multidisciplinary communication. This situation has often resulted in treatment failure caused by failure to satisfy the patient's needs, demands, and expectations.

Historical Development of the Team Concept

Hardware Development (1965 to 1987)

Brånemark is recognized as both the pioneer and father of osseointegration, and his vital microscopy laboratory investigations are legendary. These investigations first began in the early 1950s and culminated in landmark prospective clinical implant studies, which began in 1965.[1] The very nature of this period focused attention on implant performance standards, which were surgically driven. Rather than the means, it became the end to the delivery of patient care and was the benchmark of success. This period of development has been the galvanizing force driving modern implant dentistry.

The ugly legacy of implant failure and patient disfigurement was an enormous perceptual obstacle for Brånemark and his coworkers to overcome. For many years, the dental profession rebuked his ideas and refused to accept the Swedish research data. The perception of a metal screw penetrating the jaw bone was thought of as pure folly. So indelibly etched was this distasteful perception of implant failure in the minds of scientists and clinicians that nearly two decades of research had accumulated before public disclosure. The painful inertia that restrained Brånemark's disclosure delayed public introduction.

More than 15 years of scientific research preceded the landmark article by Brånemark and coworkers that introduced the concept of osseointegration to the profession.[2] Having clearly exceeded the criteria for implant success outlined in the National Institutes of Health Consensus Development Conference in 1978, the Swedish achievements were presented to North American academicians, clinicians, and scientists at the Toronto Conference in 1982.[3,4] Seventeen years of research preceded this conference. As a direct result of this conference, implant performance standards were defined by Albrektsson et al[5] in 1986 and have since become the clinical guidelines for measuring and comparing implant success.

Many people believed that the early implant prostheses, although functionally superior, had little cosmetic and esthetic appeal. Mechanical platforms secured to integrated implants were insufficient, in most cases, to satisfy patients' needs. In addition, these mechanical platforms usually failed to satisfy patients' esthetic and phonetic demands. As a result of the long developmental period, which defined a predictable surgical protocol leading to osseointegration of pure titanium implants, implant dentistry portrayed a surgical personality. This elevated the implant surgeon and the aura of surgery to a disproportionate level of importance on the implant team. In many instances, there was little regard for the prosthetic portion of treatment. The restorative dentist and laboratory technologist were saddled with the awesome and frustrating task of creating functional, esthetic, cosmetic, and phonetic prostheses to rest on implants that had little relationship to normal tooth position.

Prosthetic Component Development (1987 to 1991)

As a direct result of the failure to achieve predictable patient and professional satisfaction regarding esthetic and phonetic prostheses, a plethora of user-friendly components emerged. The profession was also seeking to define acceptable standards for patient care. The profession rapidly attempted to overcome surgical tunnel vision, which until this time had restricted artistic development. Although greatly benefiting from functionally secure prostheses, patients also wanted esthetic, cosmetic, and phonetic improvements. Simply put, patients were seeking improvement in the quality of their lives. The prosthetic component period was characterized by the development of clever, so-called user-friendly components designed to overcome the deficiencies of implant position and alignment.

The recurring nature of prosthetic deficiencies could not be consistently overcome by these new components alone. Component development was mistakenly thought of as a panacea to achieve more predictable esthetic and phonetic restorations. Failure to recognize the relationship between teeth and the alveolar process, as well as the postextraction resorptive patterns, led to implant placement incompatible with "optimal final tooth position." Implant position and size could rarely substitute for the lost tooth. Implant-prosthesis incompatibility was at the center of the problem. A failure on the surgeon's part to understand the sensitive relationship between the residual alveolar process, or ridge, and the optimal final tooth position continued to create difficulties for the dentist and laboratory technologist. The implant-supported prosthesis was replacing not merely lost tooth structure, but periodontium as well. Both tooth and alveolar bone influence function, speech, and facial appearance. What was missing from this treatment process was a method the restorative dentist could use to input clinically verified parameters that would guide the surgeon during implant placement.

Prosthetic-Guided Development (1990s)

Within a short time it became clear that prosthetic components, although enormously helpful, would not consistently offer simple solutions needed to overcome diagnostic treatment planning and surgical deficiencies. With the development of reformatted computerized tomographic (CT) radiography, it was now possible to visualize the residual jaw structure and assess implant-prosthesis compatibility. The profession now had a communicative vehicle to generate final prosthesis silhouettes on three-dimensional radiographs.

The roles and goals of the implant team could now become more clearly defined. For the first time, the implant team, in particular the restorative dentist, could predict the final prosthetic design, conduct confident patient consultation, determine fees, direct the surgical placement of implants, and consistently achieve patient satisfaction. The development of a diagnostically proactive team approach with well-defined roles was emerging, as were specific clinical treatment guidelines. The surgeon could be directed toward reconstructive surgery based on prosthetic and patient guidelines. Reconstruction of both hard and soft tissues could be three-dimensionally visualized and prosthetically generated with the singular purpose of satisfying patient demands. By understanding the patient's needs and concerns, and knowing how to translate this information into clear surgical and prosthetic directives, the team could accurately predict the prosthesis type and design more frequently.

This chapter is devoted to the development of presurgical implant diagnostics, treatment planning, and prosthetically directed implant placement. The CT scan becomes the implant team's communicative tool, because a clinically verified radiopaque template depicting optimal final tooth position can be generated. This information can be used to define the roles of all implant team members. This leads to synergistic communication and focuses the talents of the team to serve the needs of the patient more effectively. The implementation of these basic concepts enables the dental profession to harmoniously blend the science of osseointegration and the art of prosthetic dentistry to achieve consistently high standards of excellence in implant patient care.

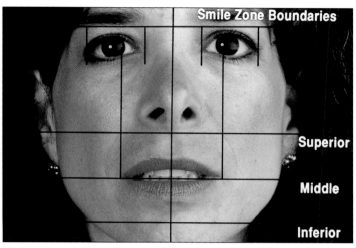

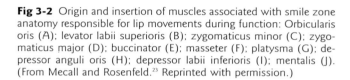

Fig 3-1 Boundaries and topographic anatomy of the smile zone in repose.

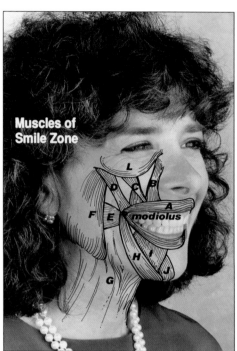

Fig 3-2 Origin and insertion of muscles associated with smile zone anatomy responsible for lip movements during function: Orbicularis oris (A); levator labii superioris (B); zygomaticus minor (C); zygomaticus major (D); buccinator (E); masseter (F); platysma (G); depressor anguli oris (H); depressor labii inferioris (I); mentalis (J). (From Mecall and Rosenfeld.[23] Reprinted with permission.)

Clinical Application of Normal Anatomy

The needs, concerns, and expectations of patients often exceed the mere restoration of oral function. It is therefore essential to have a clear understanding of smile zone and functional and skeletal anatomy for more effective treatment planning.

Topographic Anatomy Within the Smile Zone[6]

The smile zone comprises the lower third of the face and has been defined by its superior limit, which is bordered by a horizontal line drawn along the base of the nose. It is bordered inferiorly by a second horizontal line drawn along the base of the chin. The lateral limits of the smile zone are bordered bilaterally by vertical lines drawn from the pupils of the eyes to the corresponding lip commissures.

The smile zone can be further divided into superior, middle, and inferior thirds while in repose. The superior third of the smile zone comprises the alae of the nose, the nasolabial sulcus, and the philtrum. The middle third of the smile zone extends from the mucocutaneous border of the lower lip to one half the distance between it and the base of the chin. The lower one third of the smile zone is composed of the mandibular symphysis and associated musculature forming the chin (Fig 3-1).

Functional Anatomy of the Orofacial Musculature

The facial musculature associated with smile zone anatomy inserts directly into the skin. These muscles originate from the maxilla and mandible and insert into the upper and lower lips. The muscles of the smile zone are important not only for phonetics and facial expressions, but also for mastication and deglutition. These precise functions are the result of complex neuromusculature interactions that control lip movement.

Five muscle groups converge laterally to form the corners of the mouth. The convergence of the muscle groups forms the modiolus. The coordinated action of these muscle groups, along with the buccinator and orbicularis oris muscles, allows elevation, depression, retraction, protrusion, and compression of the lips. Buccinator function is associated with other perioral muscles and provides the lateral limits of the neutral zone, while the internal limits are established by the tongue. The concept of the neutral zone is important and is defined as that anatomic position where the summation of lingual force vectors from the buccinator and perioral muscles and the buccal force vectors of the tongue equal zero. It is in this spatial area that the teeth are located and are most stable. Violation of the neutral zone by prosthetic procedures may not only lead to occlusal instability but also affect phonetics and ultimately facial cosmetics. Implants placed in violation of the neutral zone can be the most difficult abnormality for the restorative dentist to modify and to which the patient must adapt (Fig 3-2).

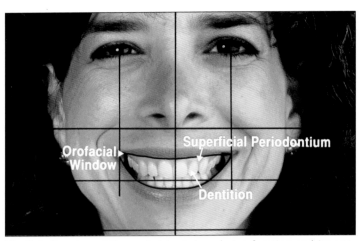
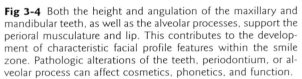

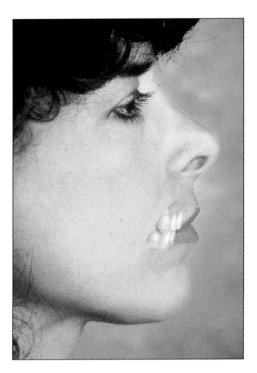

Fig 3-3 Opening of the orofacial window during function and its anatomic contents. These dimensions greatly influence the level of cosmetic commitment therapeutically.

Fig 3-4 Both the height and angulation of the maxillary and mandibular teeth, as well as the alveolar processes, support the perioral musculature and lip. This contributes to the development of characteristic facial profile features within the smile zone. Pathologic alterations of the teeth, periodontium, or alveolar process can affect cosmetics, phonetics, and function.

The smile is unique for each individual and is created by neuromuscular interaction of these muscle groups. As the smile expands, the dentition becomes more visible. There is great individual variance in the amount of dentition exposed during various lip movements. The opening of the orofacial window from a frontal view may reveal no teeth, a portion of the teeth, or the entire clinical portion of the teeth and superficial periodontium.

It must be recognized that, although these structures are visualized on expansion of the smile zone from a frontal view, it is the dentition and alveolar process that provide support to the perioral musculature, the vermilion portion of both lips, and the lip bodies. This is clearly seen in a profile view. In addition to providing support, the height and angulation of the alveolar process influence facial profile angles and facial esthetics. These variations are influenced by appositional growth of the mandibular condyles and growth within the sutures of the maxillae and palatine bones during development. This contributes to cosmetic individuality. For these reasons, knowledge of tooth size, shape, form, color, and periodontal and regional anatomy are essential when a pathologically altered smile is reconstructed.

The understanding of the functional anatomy of the orofacial musculature becomes critical when augmentation requirements are determined. Clinical evaluation to determine the augmentation needs of the deficient alveolar process or periodontium begins with the identification of the optimal final tooth position. Because the dentition provides support for the vermilion portion of the lips, it is critical to determine tooth length, tooth width, incisal edge position, and axial inclination to reestablish a lip position compatible with

esthetics, phonetics, and function. Although different methods have been described for determining proportional tooth width and length, great individual variation often exists. If available, prior facial photographs provide baseline information from which reconstructive treatment decisions can be made (Figs 3-3 and 3-4).

Skeletal Relationship: Normal Anatomy of the Maxilla and Mandible[7]

It is important to review bony anatomic features that influence the implant-prosthesis compatibility equation. Patterns of alveolar process resorption after tooth loss are greatly influenced by preexisting normal and pathologically altered anatomy.[8]

The supporting structures of the teeth are the maxilla and mandible. The maxilla is made up of right and left portions joined to the skull. It is cuboidal, consisting of a body and four processes: zygomatic, nasal, palatine, and alveolar. A hollow portion, the maxillary sinus, has particular relevance because it may be an anatomic limitation to implant placement and may not be easily modified. Important and reproducible anatomic landmarks include the incisive and canine fossae, canine eminence, maxillary tuberosity, and incisive canal (Fig 3-5). Each in its own way offers clues regarding prior tooth position in the dentate patient. These landmarks can also offer reference points with which to measure changes that occur following tooth loss.

The inferior portion of the maxilla consists of the alveolar process, which surrounds the teeth and is curved to con-

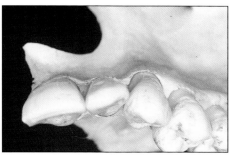

Fig 3-5 Dry skull specimen depicting important regional anatomic landmarks.

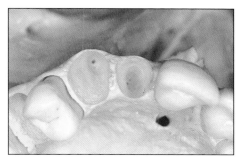

Fig 3-6 Dry skull specimen of the maxillary anterior segment. Note the thinness of the labial plate and the position of the apex of the alveolus as it relates to the body of the maxilla.

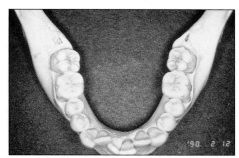

Fig 3-7 Dry skull specimen of the mandible. Note the more lingual position of the alveolar process and mandibular posterior teeth in relation to the body of the mandible. (From Mecall and Rosenfeld.[8] Reprinted with permission.)

form with the dental arch. It is critical to conceptualize the alveolar process, as well as individual root forms, in three dimensions. The shape and dimension of the alveolar process are influenced by tooth size and root form.

The alveolar process is composed of external and internal cortical bony plates. Although these bony plates are dense, consisting of compact bone, they are extremely thin. Cancellous bone is sandwiched between these thin cortical plates. The margins of the facial alveoli are frail, thin, and knife edged, whereas the palatal plate is thicker (Fig 3-6). The palatal bone becomes extremely thick over deeper portions of the process, brought about by a merging of alveolar process and palatal vault. This is noted throughout the arch, except for the area of the palatal roots of maxillary molars.

The mandible is horseshoe shaped, consisting of a body and two vertical portions called *rami*. Relevant external and surface landmarks include the incisive fossa, canine eminences, internal and external oblique ridges, and bilateral mental foramina. The position of the mental foramina is not consistent. The foramen is usually located at the apex of second premolars, equidistant superior-inferiorly as viewed laterally. The relevant internal surfaces include the mylohyoid ridge and sublingual and submaxillary fossae.

The bone quality of the mandible is not as cancellous as that of the maxilla. The facial cortical plate is as thick as at the lingual aspect except anteriorly, where the bone is extremely thin. Because the anterior teeth are tipped facially and the posterior teeth lingually, the alveolar process does not conform to the shape of the jaw body. The dental arch is therefore narrower than the mandibular arch. Despite the greater thickness of alveolar process in the mandible, tooth position plays an important role in post–tooth loss resorptive patterns (Fig 3-7). Similar to the maxilla, the mandible exhibits thin alveolar bone, composed of little cancellous tissue at the buccal surfaces of mandibular teeth. These features predispose the mandible to resorptive patterns not always favorable for implant placement.

The relationship of the mandibular canal and contents is of special importance. A thorough understanding of the course of the inferior alveolar nerve through the mandible and its relationship to the resorbed alveolar process is crucial for surgical safety and implant stability. Computerized tomography can be extremely helpful in assessing a suitable safe implant site.

The most critical anatomic determinants for implant placement are the maxillomandibular skeletal and alveolar process–alveoli relationships. Tooth size and form often predispose to underlying anatomic deformities, such as fenestration and dehiscence, that have little reparative potential because of the absence of cancellous bone. This general pattern is the most relevant factor in understanding resorptive patterns following tooth loss caused by simple extraction, periodontal disease, or tissue-bearing dental prostheses. An understanding of these issues will determine implant placement and its impact on emergence profile, esthetics, and phonetics.

The normal anatomic relationship between the tooth and alveolar process reveals an axial tooth position that is labial or buccal to the center of the alveolar process, often resulting in dehiscence or fenestration. Because almost all teeth exhibit thin cortical bone externally, reparative potential following extraction is compromised. This will result in a resorptive pattern that places the residual alveolar bone or ridge more lingual and apical to that in the normal periodontium. Therefore, the predictable sequela of tooth loss complicates implant-prosthesis compatibility.

An understanding of this relationship makes it apparent that even immediate implant placement into an alveolus has the potential to result in labial bone perforation or implant dehiscence. Attempts at implant alignment mimicking original tooth position often result in compromised buccal bone healing. The placement of an implant within the direct anatomic center of the ridge may lead to prosthetic difficulties that will alter cosmetics. These difficulties could include an incisally or labially placed screw access hole, thin or unsupported porcelain, and distortion of emergence profiles compatible with acceptable esthetics.

Some attempts to overcome these problems have been directed at implant design changes (eg, the conical implant) to eliminate coronal thread exposure in the event of soft tissue recession and to facilitate hygiene. Numerous user-friendly prosthetic components have also been developed either to cement final restorations, redirect screw hole positions, or create a restorative finish line at the level of the implant platform (eg, UCLA or single-tooth abutment).[9,10] With tooth loss and the onset of residual ridge atrophy, reduction in bone height and width makes surgical placement of implants more difficult. Incompatibility between the remaining ridge form and optimal prosthetic tooth position is accentuated.

The following points regarding the normal anatomy summarize the key issues affecting implant placement:

1. Axial tooth position is buccal to the anatomic center of the alveolar process.
2. Thin cortical bone results in compromised reparative potential following tooth loss.
3. Resorptive patterns result in available bone lingual and apical to the normal tooth position.
4. Original tooth position is a poor guide for implant placement.
5. Implants are not placed in bone previously occupied by the anatomic tooth root.
6. Normal anatomy aggravates implant-prosthesis incompatibility.

The Impact of Pathologic Changes of the Alveolar Process or Residual Ridge on Implant Placement

The greatest reduction of the residual ridge occurs in the early postextraction healing period, a time frame of 6 months to 2 years.[11] Clinical and cephalometric studies from the 1960s and early 1970s have demonstrated consistent results regarding the relationship between the time of extraction and the rate of bone loss measured.[12] Large variations occurred within samples studied. The anterior portion of the maxillary alveolar process has been shown to diminish by 85 mm^2, or 23%, in the first 6 months and an additional 32 mm^2, or 11%, in 5 years.[13]

Cephalometric study of the residual ridge in the posterior mandible has demonstrated a pattern of residual ridge resorption resulting in a more lingually located ridge crest.[14] This longitudinal analysis has indicated that resorption of the residual ridge occurs mainly from a buccal or labial direction. These resorptive patterns greatly alter the width and height of the residual ridge. In the past, tissue defects have been treated by conventional removable prosthetic techniques that position teeth on a denture base compatible with cosmetic, functional, and phonetic guidelines. Because the process of disuse atrophy is continuous, the need for modification of the denture base could be expected in future years.

The shape can be defined as the geometric form of the alveolar process or residual ridge. These forms may be rectangular, in which case the buccolingual width is similar in its inferior and superior horizontal dimensions. The ridge may be pyramidal, where the crestal horizontal dimension is narrower than the apical horizontal dimension. This is the most common geometric form. Finally, the ridge may be hourglass shaped. The hourglass form presents with constricture of the alveolar process or residual ridge. This occurs when the crestal and apical horizontal dimensions exceed the buccolingual constricture width.

Clinical manifestations of pathologic alterations are greatly influenced by the morphology of the underlying normal anatomy and position of the tooth in the alveolar process prior to extraction. The impact of ridge shape on implant placement may alter the sequence and type of augmentation necessary for implant-prosthesis compatibility.

Radiographic Techniques to Assess the Alveolar Process or Residual Ridge

In the past, dental implant treatment was dominated by the surgical specialist. Based solely on clinical guidelines, the well-intentioned restorative dentist could only provide limited information regarding proposed implant sites. Because the clinical information was deficient and inherently flawed, the surgeon was forced to make surgical decisions without accurate restorative guidelines, compromising implant location and axial position. Too frequently, the final tooth position was incompatible with implant placement. The restorative dentist and laboratory technologist were compelled to construct a final prosthesis that lacked proper form and function due to poor implant position. Worst of all, the so-called implant team failed to achieve consistent patient satisfaction.

The use of multiplanar reformatted computerized tomography has altered the clinical approach to implant diagnostics and treatment.[15,16] It has allowed the implant team to verify that a presurgically determined prosthetic plan is indeed compatible with the underlying maxillary and mandibular residual bony ridge. Computerized tomography has enabled the surgeon and restorative dentist to visualize cross-sectional images of the maxilla or mandible. There is a remarkable similarity between buccolingual histologic sections of the alveolar process and cross-sectional CT images.[17] These images are perpendicular to the long axis of the alveolar ridge and 95% accurate within 1 mm.[18,19]

Periapical radiographs are 50% accurate, while a panoramic radiograph is only 17% accurate.[20] Periapical and panoramic radiographs offer no information regarding the internal anatomy of the alveolar process or residual ridge. In addition, conventional dental radiographs do not permit accurate three-dimensional superimposition of a clinically

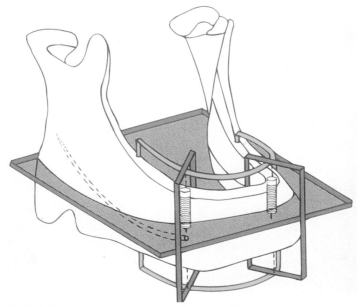

Fig 3-8 Composite representation of axial (red horizontal) plane and reformatted panoral (yellow linear) and cross-sectional (blue perpendicular) views of a typical CT scan for dental application. (Courtesy of Columbia Scientific, Inc.)

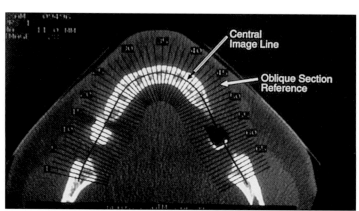

Fig 3-9 Axial images are reconstructed, and the central image line is drawn. The corresponding cross-sectional views are perpendicular to the central image line at specific intervals and can be numerically cross referenced.

verified radiopaque template, which can then be used as a surgical guide at the time of implant placement.

The computer program reconstructs data from the series of axial CT scans into a series of cross-sectional and panoramic CT reformations (Fig 3-8). An incremental series of tic marks alongside each view allows for precise correlation from one anatomic plane to the other. In addition, a corresponding millimeter scale for each view enables the dentist to calculate accurate measurements.

Computerized Tomography

The key to successful CT reformation is the complete absence of patient motion. The patient should be instructed to remain absolutely still during the scanning process. A gauze pad is placed between the patient's teeth to prevent jaw motion. The patient should refrain from swallowing, speaking, or moving the jaw during the examination.

The patient lies in the supine position on the table of the scanner. Sponge pads are placed bilaterally along the external surface of the patient's cheeks to reduce motion. The patient's head is oriented so that the occlusal surface of the template is parallel to the plane of the axial scan. A scout view is then completed in lateral view to confirm proper patient positioning and prescribe the upper and lower limits of the scan. This will enable the surgeon to more accurately relate the surgical template to the osteotomy site and associated vital structures.

Scan Interpretation

Four different images are produced by most CT software programs. The first image is a single axial view setup film, which is selected by the radiology technician to define the curvature of the alveolar process or residual ridge. Superimposed over the axial image is a curved line, which most represents the crest of the remaining bone. This is referred to as the *central image line*. It is important that the central image line intersect the crest of the bone because this represents the most accurate geometric pattern of the ridge crest.

Perpendicular to the central image line is a series of sequentially numbered lines extending along the central image line. These lines are called the *cross-sectional lines* and define the location of perpendicular images within the axial view. The spacing between these lines is variable. The number of millimeters between cross-sectional images is printed in the legend below the first axial image. This legend also includes information defining the number and type of pictures taken for the entire CT survey (Fig 3-9).

The Axial Composite Image

The axial images of the maxilla or mandible are often formatted differently. The maxilla and mandible are composed of sequential axial scans. Each axial image is numbered. The patient's right and left sides are identified as the film is viewed. Below each axial view is a millimeter scale for

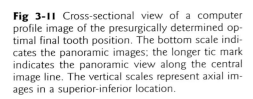

Fig 3-10 Panoramic view of a computer profile image. The vertical scales cross reference the axial images, while the horizontal scale cross references the cross-sectional images.

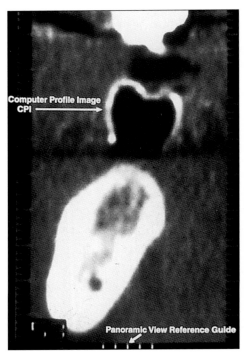

Fig 3-11 Cross-sectional view of a computer profile image of the presurgically determined optimal final tooth position. The bottom scale indicates the panoramic images; the longer tic mark indicates the panoramic view along the central image line. The vertical scales represent axial images in a superior-inferior location.

measurement purposes. The CT scans often have image size conversion factors. This means that all measurements must be multiplied by the conversion factor to coincide with the actual clinical measurements of the patient.

The axial images are utilized to determine the anatomic position of vital structures, such as the mandibular canal, mental foramen, floor of the nose, incisive foramen, incisive canal, and maxillary sinus. They are extremely useful in assessing tooth position and axial inclination of the roots of the teeth. The medullary portion of the alveolar process or residual ridge can also be evaluated from these views. The actual density of the bone is confirmed at the time of surgery.

Superimposed over certain axial views is the central image line with a corresponding cross-sectional reference scale. This allows the dentist to examine a localized area of the maxilla and mandible from a superior-inferior direction. In addition, the central image line defines the panoramic view; the center panoramic view coincides with the central image line.

Panoramic Views

Panorals are reformatted views included in each survey. The number of panoral images may vary, depending on the software format. All surveys will include at least one view along the central image line. Vertical and horizontal scales are located along the side and bottom of each panoramic view. The vertical tic marks indicate the corresponding axial image at that particular superior-inferior level. The lower or bottom tic mark indicates the corresponding cross-sectional image for evaluation. Both scales enable the dentist to ex-

amine horizontal (axial), panoramic (linear), and cross-sectional (perpendicular) views for any particular area, providing a three-dimensional perspective (Fig 3-10).

Cross-sectional Views

The cross-sectional views are numbered. The buccal surface of each view faces the left side and the lingual surface faces the right side. This is marked on the cross-sectional view of each series. A series of tic marks is positioned along the side of each cross-sectional image. These tic marks represent the position of each axial image. Therefore, tic mark No. 1 represents axial image No. 1. This allows the dentist to locate any anatomic structure on both views. The distance between these tic marks is dependent on the distance between the original axial CT slices. This distance between axial slices is indicated below the group of cross-sectional images. Along the bottom of each cross-sectional image is a series of tic marks representing the corresponding panoramic views (Fig 3-11).

The use of interactive CT data was first introduced in 1993.[21] This preoperative planning software (SIM/Plant, Columbia Scientific Inc, Columbia, MD), designated for the placement of dental implants, combines the accuracy of computerized tomographic (CT) imaging with the power of computer-aided design (CAD). SIM/Plant uses the actual CT scans and reformatted CT images combined with computer graphics to create a powerful preoperative planning tool for the placement of dental implants.[22] Reformatted CT images can be varied to locate important internal structures and inspect the anatomy of the alveolar ridge.

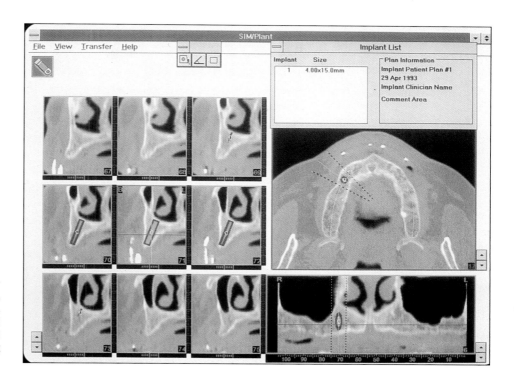

Fig 3-12 Computer monitor view of SIM/PLANT software, representing axial, panoral, and cross-sectional images, which when interactively manipulated result in simultaneous changes of all images. Note the silhouette of the barium-coated template and its relationship to the underlying bone and mandibular canal.

Once the implant is safely positioned on the CT reformation, bone quality can be assessed. The width and height of the bone at each proposed implant site can be evaluated. With these measurements, the proper length and diameter of the implants can be selected. The proposed implants can be modified, manipulated, and rotated into their correct orientation, consistent with optimal final tooth position and prostheses prediction. The implant position can be compared with neighboring CT images. By manipulating the gray scale, the relationship of the implant position to vital anatomic structures can be assessed. The entire series of CT reformations can be used interactively at the time of implant placement to serve as a surgical blueprint (Fig 3-12).

Solving the Fixture Compatibility Equation

$$\text{Optimal final tooth} = \frac{\begin{array}{l}\cdot\,\text{Clinical determinants}\\ +\,\text{Diagnostic waxup determinants}\end{array}}{\begin{array}{c}\text{Multiplanar reformatted computerized}\\ \text{tomography determinants}\end{array}}$$

It is important for the surgeon, restorative dentist, or dental laboratory technologist to predetermine this conceptual equation. There are three major determinants of the implant compatibility equation:

1. Diagnostic waxup determinants, which define the optimal final tooth position

2. Clinical determinants, which verify the provisional diagnostic waxup
3. Multiplanar reformatted computerized tomography determinants

Diagnostic Waxup Determinants

1. Physiologic occlusal vertical dimension
2. Maxillomandibular relationships
3. Tooth form
4. Embrasure determination for conventional or cantilevered ceramometal restoration

Because resorption of the alveolar process as a result of tooth loss or periodontal disease significantly limits the ability to place an implant in the exact axial position of the previous anatomic root, it is first necessary to identify the optimal tooth position and direct implant placement that is most compatible with this position. Determination of tooth position requires an evaluation of the physiologic occlusal vertical dimension and maxillomandibular relationship. These are important criteria for determining coronal form and its impact on a cosmetic, phonetic, and functional result. A provisional waxup or trial tooth setup provides the guidelines for determining the final prosthetic design.[20] It is the clinically tested diagnostic waxup that provides the baseline criteria for determining the optimal final tooth position (Fig 3-13). The relationship between the desired final tooth position and the impact of pathologic alterations on achieving this position can only be assessed presurgically with the use of reformatted computerized tomography.

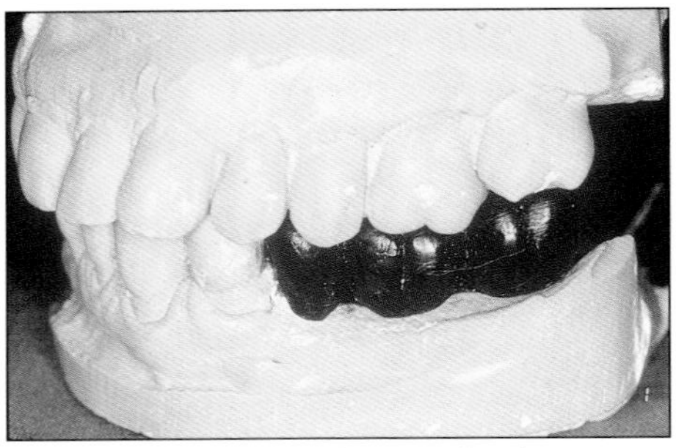

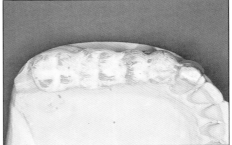

Fig 3-13 The diagnostic waxup has been completed. Both coronal form and embrasure space have been established for the optimal final tooth position. (From Mecall and Rosenfeld.[25] Reprinted with permission.)

Fig 3-14 A vacuum-formed template has been fabricated using the diagnostic waxup. The diagnostic template is evaluated clinically in an effort to verify the compatibility between the waxup determinants and the patient's clinical determinants. A radiopaque contrast medium has been applied to the template in the areas of proposed tooth replacement. (From Mecall and Rosenfeld.[25] Reprinted with permission.)

Clinical Determinants

The diagnostic waxup or trial tooth setup must be modified as it relates to oral musculature support, phonetics, and the ease of oral hygiene procedures. Because pathologic resorption of the ridge allows implant placement only in a position that is more lingual or palatal than the original tooth location, it may be difficult to provide lip support without modification of the prosthesis by labial or buccal cantilevering of the prosthetic tooth. The extent of this cantilever as it relates to the patient's ability to maintain adequate oral hygiene and biomechanical force distribution may require consideration of a different prosthetic design. Phonetics also can be altered by deviation of implant placement from the original tooth position. The most appropriate method of evaluating the effect of a prosthetic design on phonetics and oral musculature support is to construct an acrylic resin vacuum-formed template or trial tooth setup and evaluate it in the patient's mouth.

Once clinically tested, the provisional waxup or trial tooth setup allows the construction of a diagnostic template to create a computer profile image (CPI). The CPI enables the surgeon, restorative dentist, and laboratory technologist to transfer prosthetic information regarding the optimal final tooth position to a multiplanar reformatted computer tomography radiograph. The CPI now becomes the guideline or reference from which pathologic alterations of the resorbed alveolar or residual ridge can be evaluated. It provides a method for developing an optimal final tooth position

compatible with implant placement by predetermining the impact of bone resorption on the remaining residual ridge.

The computer profile image also allows the restorative dentist to verify presurgically that a prosthetic design of a given type is compatible with implant placement in the pathologically altered ridge. It eliminates the dilemma facing the restorative dentist whose final prosthesis design is often dictated by the surgeon's decision at the time of the implant placement.

Multiplanar Reformatted Computer Tomography Determinants

From a previously constructed diagnostic waxup, which has been clinically tested by parameters defining the optimal final tooth position, a vacuum-formed template is fabricated. This template is covered with a radiopaque contrast medium (Fig 3-14). A high-resolution CT scanner (eg, GE 9800, General Electric, Medical Systems, Inc, Milwaukee, WI) equipped with a dental software package is used to scan the patient while he or she wears the clinically tested diagnostic template. Axial views are generated. Reformatted computerized images are obtained in both panoramic and cross-sectional planes. It is important that the radiologist reconstruct axial images to include a central image line through the center of the crest of the residual ridge. Review of the reformatted radiographics shows profile images of the diagnostically waxed teeth in axial, cross-sectional, and panoramic views.

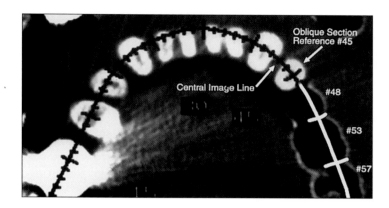

Fig 3-15 The axial view with corresponding computer profile image and central image line indicates that the mesiodistal centers of the proposed implant sites are reference Nos. 48, 53, and 57. Cross-sectional references are located, and analysis of computerized tomography determinants is initiated.

Developing a Computer Profile Image

Fabricating a Barium-Coated Template to Form a CPI Image

1. Maxillary and mandibular study models are obtained.
2. Casts are mounted at an accepted vertical dimension.
3. A clinically verified diagnostic waxup or trial tooth setup is obtained.
4. Optimal final tooth position is now ready to be analyzed by fabrication of a vacuum-formed template or trial acrylic resin tooth setup.
5. The Omnivac machine (Buffalo Dental Manufacturing, Syosset, NY) is used to press out the template, composed of .040-inch clear acrylic resin sheet material.
6. The template is trimmed to retain the entire tooth length.
7. A mixture of die hardener and barium sulfate is applied in a thin coating. This radiopaque material will form the silhouette on the scan.
8. A surgical guide template is constructed from a verified diagnostic waxup.
9. The template is trimmed from the lingual aspect; enough lingual surface is removed to be compatible with the implant compatible line. The remaining portion becomes the buccal angulation restriction during osteotomy preparation.

Analysis of the Proposed Implant Sites

Four radiographic variables play an important role in the predetermination of implant position as it relates to the computer profile image:

1. Vertical loss of the alveolar process or residual ridge
2. Horizontal loss of the alveolar process or residual ridge
3. Angle of the remaining alveolar process or residual ridge to the CPI
4. Vital anatomic structures and residual dental pathosis

Six sequential steps are involved in the analysis of any proposed implant site:

Step 1: Determining the Center of the Optimal Final Tooth Position

Analysis of the radiographic variables begins with the location of the center of the optimal final tooth position. From the axial images, the view depicting the central image line superimposed over the CPI is located. The axial image and cross-sectional reference line allow the implant team to accurately locate the mesiodistal center of each optimal tooth position as it relates to the underlying ridge. These positions can be verified by studying the panoramic views and comparing these mesiodistal distances with those on the diagnostic waxup (Fig 3-15).

If necessary, the variation from the actual size of the patient must be taken into consideration when the clinical accuracy of the image is evaluated. In addition, the positioning of the proposed implant site buccal or lingual to the central image line may affect the accuracy of mesiodistal distances when transferred to the clinical situation. For example, a central image line more lingual or palatal to the CPI may indicate a smaller mesiodistal dimension on the CT scan than actually exists in the patient's mouth. For this reason it is important that the central image line be placed along the crest of the residual ridge, rather than along the buccolingual center of the maxillary or mandibular basal bone. However, in patients exhibiting advanced resorption, the crest of the residual ridge and the center of the basal bone may be identical.

Step 2: Measuring the Vertical Loss of the Alveolar Process or Residual Ridge

Once the anatomic center of the optimal final tooth position has been located, cross-sectional images are analyzed. On the cross-sectional image representing the center of the desired final tooth position, a line AB (yellow) representing the long axis of the computer profile image is drawn. The greater-than-normal distance from the incisal edge or central fossa to the ridge represents the extent of hard and soft tissue that has been lost to disease. This includes loss of tooth structure, periodontium, and often basal bone.

Step 3: Determining the Anatomic Center of the Alveolar Process or Residual Ridge

A second line, CD (blue), drawn between the center of the ridge in its "widest upper horizontal and lower horizontal dimensions," represents the anatomic buccolingual center of the remaining ridge. A third line, ED (green), is drawn from the optimal screw access hole position to any point along line CD; this represents the implant compatible line. The maximum implant length is determined by calculating the distance from the crest of the residual ridge to the most apical position of the ridge along the implant compatible line.

Step 4: Measuring the Horizontal Loss of the Alveolar Process or Residual Ridge

The same cross-sectional image is used for assessment of horizontal resorption of the remaining ridge. A minimum of 5 mm of horizontal ridge width is needed for successful implant placement. Placement of a size-appropriate implant acetate overlay along the implant compatible line (ED) will allow verification that an implant can be placed along line ED for that CPI.

A size-appropriate implant acetate overlay allows the surgeon to evaluate more accurately the impact of horizontal resorptive patterns on implant placement. Placing the minified implant acetate overlay along line ED allows the surgeon to modify the surgical template accurately so that it can act as a guide during implant placement.

Step 5: Measuring the Angle of the Remaining Ridge to the CPI

The relationship of the angle of the remaining residual ridge to the computer profile image is important in determining the extent of buccolingual cantilevering of the final restoration. The distance from the labial surface to point H along line BH (red) represents the extent to which the prosthetic tooth will have to be cantilevered labially or buccally. The intersection of line ED and the red cervical line defines point H (Figs 3-16 to 3-18).

The *remaining ridge angle* can be defined as the angle formed by the intersection of the axial center of the optimal final tooth position (line AB) and the axial center of the remaining alveolar process or residual ridge (line CD). It is influenced by growth and development. In addition, it is significantly altered by pathologic resorption. A parallel relationship or small angle can impact on emergence profile or screw access hole location.

A large remaining ridge angle will create a significant disparity between the long axis of the ridge and the optimal final tooth position. Therefore, vertical resorption will lead to a disproportionately greater horizontal discrepancy. This will cause increased cantilever distances, leading to loading that may be detrimental to implant stability. It may also compromise accessibility for periodontal maintenance procedures by the patient. Finally, an increased remaining ridge angle will increase the need to reestablish support for the upper or lower lip. Bone or soft tissue augmentation often needs to be considered when a large ridge angle is present. This dictates that the alveolar process portion of the final prosthesis provide a greater proportion of lip support than the dentition aspect of the prosthesis. The incorporation of a prosthetic flange is often required to satisfy lip support requirements.

An increased remaining ridge angle can also be associated with a discrepancy between the alveolus and alveolar process. This occurs when the long axis of the tooth and alveolus are not parallel to the remaining alveolar process or body of the jaw. Tooth loss and ridge resorption in the presence of this nonparallel relationship will accentuate the disparity among the remaining ridge, the optimal final tooth position, and the horizontal distance needed to regain underlying physiologic support for the orofacial musculature. Unless the remaining ridge angle is small, any vertical resorption of the alveolar process will result in significant loss of horizontal width and alter cosmetics within the smile zone.

For the purpose of surgical reconstruction, the vertical and horizontal components of residual ridge resorption must be determined. Identification of vertical and horizontal resorption allows the team to plan augmentation needs presurgically, choose the most appropriate procedure, and sequence treatment.

Step 6: Locating the Vital Anatomic Structures and Residual Dental Pathosis

In the maxilla, positions of the maxillary sinus and nasal floor influence the length of implant placement. The cortical bone that lines these important anatomic structures also provides the opportunity to stabilize the implant in its apical region. The computer profile image makes it possible to precisely determine the implant length and the location of available cortical bone. Predetermination of this length enables the surgeon to avoid cortical bone perforation that could compromise implant stability. In addition, it avoids a potential downgrowth of epithelium from respiratory lining mucosa that could interfere with the integration process. Anatomic variances in the maxillary sinus or nasal floor may dictate the relocation of an implant site or the need for bone augmentation therapy.

The relationship of the incisive foramen to the computer profile image and the proposed implant site may also influence implant-prosthesis compatibility. The location of the incisive foramen anterior-posteriorly and its course superiorly may require relocation of a proposed implant site to avoid this vital structure. The CPI analysis will allow the implant team to assess accurately the impact of implant position changes on the final prosthetic design. The ability to evaluate the course of the incisive canal in relationship to the computer profile image may encourage the use of bone anterior to its position if compatible with the optimal final tooth position.

In the mandible, the positions of the mandibular canal and mental foramen in the superior-inferior and buccolingual directions greatly influence the utilization of a proposed implant site. Alteration of implant position or

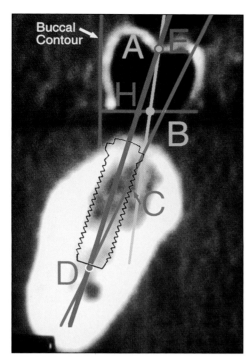

Fig 3-16 Cross-sectional section of a proposed implant site. The CPI analysis has been completed and an acetate overlay of an implant has been positioned along line ED to verify its compatibility with the computer profile image. Anatomic center of the CPI (line AB: yellow); anatomic center of the bone (line CD: blue); implant compatible line (line ED: green); extent of buccal cantilever (line HB: red).

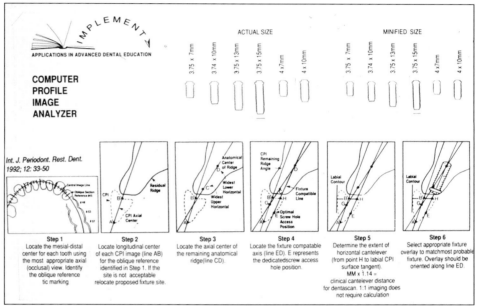

Fig 3-17 The computer profile image analyzer (with minified and actual size implants) allows presurgical verification of implant prosthesis compatibility. (Courtesy of IMPLEMENT, Park Ridge, IL.)

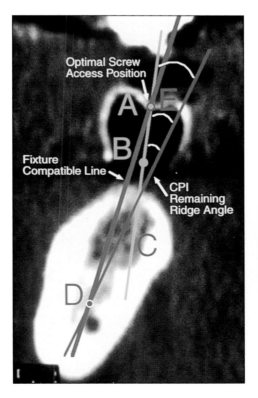

Fig 3-18a Because points A and E overlap, the template can be trimmed from the lingual aspect, corresponding to the intersection of the implant compatible line (ED, green) with the central occlusal surface.

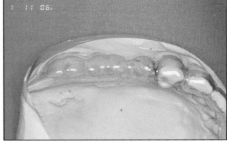

Fig 3-18b Template trimmed from the lingual aspect, which will serve as the surgical guide during osteotomy preparation.

angulation because of these vital structures should be verified with the computer profile image to ensure compatibility with a final prosthesis.

Frequently, residual dental pathosis in the region of a proposed implant site may alter plans for implant placement. Incomplete repair, resulting in fibrous healing, may dictate relocation of the proposed implant site. It is important that vital anatomic structures and residual dental pathosis be evaluated to assess the healing potential of the implant site for construction of the final prosthesis.

Analysis of radiographic variables as they relate to the computer profile image is important in the prediction of a final prosthesis type. The following are examples of these variables:

1. *Vertical bone loss.* The impact of vertical resorption of the residual ridge height is evaluated by measuring the distance from the incisal edge or central fossa of the computer profile image to the crest of the residual ridge along line AB. When optimal esthetics is a concern, this distance should not exceed 25% of the average crown length for that particular natural tooth. Distances greater than 25% imply that a significant portion of the periodontium requires replacement. Use of a fixed hybrid, clip-retained overdenture or spark-erosion prosthesis should be considered (Fig 3-19).

2. *Horizontal bone loss.* The effect of horizontal bone loss on final prosthetic design is best evaluated by measuring the horizontal distance from the implant compatible line at the CPI cervix (point H) to its most labial or buccal contour. With increased horizontal bone loss, the buccolingual center of the residual ridge is located more lingually in relation to the computer profile image. This requires the placement of an implant in a more lingual or palatal position. As the extent of cantilever increases, the patient's ability to perform effective daily plaque control procedures diminishes. This may also increase force moments that can potentially affect the dynamics of osseointegration and prosthetic components. It has been the authors' experience that cantilevers greater than 5 to 7 mm often require modification of the prosthetic design (Figs 3-20 to 3-22).

Prosthetic Designs

Using the CPI method of presurgical analysis can enable the implant team to predict a prosthesis type presurgically.[23] Four basic prosthetic designs have been used in the restoration of fully and partially edentulous patients.

Conventional Ceramometal Prosthesis

When horizontal and vertical ridge resorption are minimal, a conventional ceramometal restoration can be constructed.

The distance from the incisal edge or central fossa of the computer profile image to its cervix should not exceed 25% of the average crown length for that corresponding natural tooth, if optimal cosmetics are to be achieved.

When minimal horizontal resorption is observed, close proximity exists between the buccolingual center of the computer profile image and the implant compatible line. An emergence profile simulating that of the corresponding natural tooth can be achieved when the above-mentioned distance does not exceed one half the average anatomic buccolingual tooth dimension. Greater distances will lead to ridge-lapped labial or buccal contours. This diagnostic process enables precise calculation of the potential for a cantilevered prosthetic design.

Cantilevered Ceramometal Prosthesis

When the horizontal discrepancy between the optimal final tooth position and remaining ridge exceeds the previously mentioned distance, a buccolingual cantilevered prosthesis should be considered. Tooth length guidelines are the same as they are for the conventional ceramometal prosthesis. Although a large CPI-remaining ridge angle (intersections of lines AB and CD) is highly suggestive of the need for this prosthetic design, a precise calculation of the cantilevered distance is necessary to evaluate the effects of increased force moments and the compromise to oral hygiene maintenance. As mentioned earlier, a distance greater than 5 to 7 mm may dictate the need for consideration of another prosthetic design (Fig 3-23).

Fixed Hybrid Prosthesis

Vertical and horizontal resorptive patterns exceeding the established guidelines are evidence of the need to replace a significant portion of the periodontium in addition to the tooth. This requires the restoration of oral musculature support, compatible phonetics, and optimal cosmetics. This prosthesis usually requires a minimum of five integrated implants. When the needs for oral musculature support are considerable and cosmetics are compromised by the extent of sanitary design, the last category should be considered.

Clip-Retained Overdenture Prosthesis/ Spark-Erosion Prosthesis

When both horizontal and vertical ridge resorption are severe, a prosthetic design that allows for oral musculature support, phonetics, and cosmetics in the presence of limited implant site availability must be considered. This prosthesis requires a minimum of three to six integrated implants and follows traditional complete-denture prosthetic guidelines. The aspect of removability also simplifies oral hygiene maintenance for both the doctor and patient (Table 3-1).

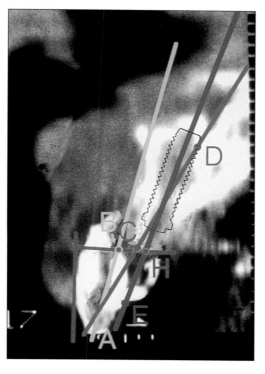

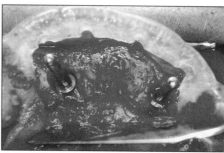

Fig 3-19 Preoperative analysis of DentaScan determinants. The acetate image analyzer overlay has been placed. The implant of vertical resorption is evaluated by measuring the distance from point A to the ridge crest along line AB (yellow). Horizontal resorptive patterns are evaluated by measuring the distance from point H to the labial contour of the profile image (red line). This measurement represents the extent of the cantilever buccally. When this distance is multiplied by the image correction factor, the exact distance of the cantilever in the final restoration, if an implant were placed along line ED, is known presurgically.

Fig 3-20 Surgical template with indicator pins in predetermined implant sites. The presurgical template has been adjusted so that the distance from the incisal edge to the lingual surface coincides with that measured on the CT scan (from points A to E). In addition, the template has been grooved in the exact mesiodistal center of the proposed final tooth position.

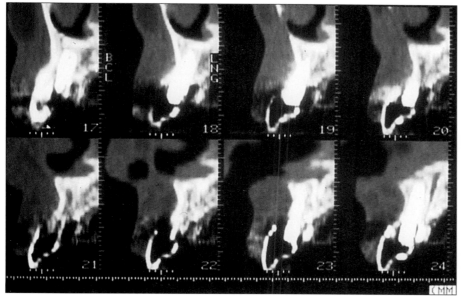

Fig 3-21 Postoperative CT scan with preoperative barium-coated diagnostic template inserted to compare actual implant placement position with previously planned position. Note the placement of the implant anterior to the incisive canal and compatible with the optimal final tooth position.

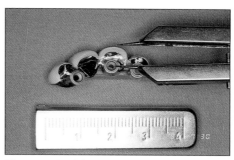

Fig 3-22 Final buccolingual cantilevered prosthesis. The extent of cantilever in the final prosthesis represents that which was predicted by the presurgical analysis.

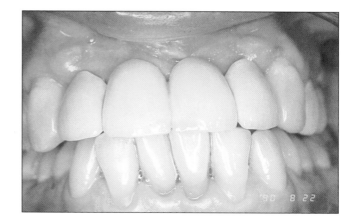

Fig 3-23 Final restoration. Buccal cantilevering was necessary to establish oral musculature support lost because of horizontal resorption of the residual ridge. Vertical resorptive patterns were not extensive and allowed construction of a final tooth form compatible with the length of the corresponding natural tooth.

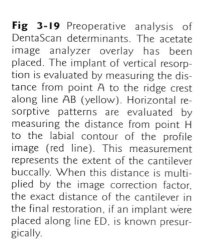

Table 3-1 Prosthesis predictor matrix

	Conventional ceramometal prosthesis	Cantilevered ceramometal prosthesis	Fixed hybrid prosthesis	Clip-retained overdenture prosthesis
Vertical resorption (distance from A to crest of residual ridge along line AB)	1. Minimal 2. Less than 25% deviation from a corresponding ideal tooth length	1. Minimal 2. Less than 25% deviation from ideal tooth length	1. Moderate 2. CPI to ridge crest length greater than 25% compared to a corresponding natural tooth (measured along line AB)	1. Advanced 2. Extensive distance CPI to ridge along line AB
Horizontal resorption (distance from H to labial surface along line BH)	1. Minimal 2. AB–ED distance should not exceed half of cervical buccolingual dimension for corresponding natural tooth	1. Minimal 2. Less than 5 to 7 mm between point H and labial surface along line BH	1. Moderate to advanced 2. Greater than 5 to 7 mm distance from H to labial surface along line BH	1. Advanced 2. Extensive distance from H to labial surface along line BH
CPI remaining ridge angle relationship (angle between lines AB and CD)	Minimal divergence between lines AB and CD	Minimal divergence between lines AB and CD	Moderate divergence between lines AB and CD	Maximal divergence between lines AB and CD
No. of implants	One or more	One or more	Five or six	Three or four

CPI = computer profile image.
See Fig 3-17 for illustration of points and lines on the CPI.

Prosthetic Predictor Modifiers

The prediction of a given prosthetic design must take into account the patient's expectations and needs. Predictor modifiers can be divided into facial anatomic features and unique patient preferences. Facial anatomic features such as lip length, lip width, and lip tonus may increase or decrease cosmetic challenges. A determination of the role these factors play should be made once a prosthetic type is predicted. Their influence may suggest that the clinician alter the predicted prosthetic plan. Finally, the ultimate decision regarding the construction of a predicted prosthetic design may be influenced by an individual patient's needs or expectations. The purpose of any prosthetic treatment is to satisfy the logical needs and emotional demands of the patient.

Conclusion

The goal of implant treatment is to restore form and function to the stomatognathic system. The ravages of caries, periodontal disease, trauma, and dentoalveolar atrophy not only upset this balance but also lead to significant cosmetic deformities. In the past, dentistry has relied solely on a prosthetic solution to these challenging problems. Results have fallen short of the ultimate goal because function may have been restored while form remained compromised.

The use of multiplanar reformatted computerized tomography and the generation of computer profile images have allowed the implant team to quantify the amount and type of tissue destruction caused by these diseases. The de-

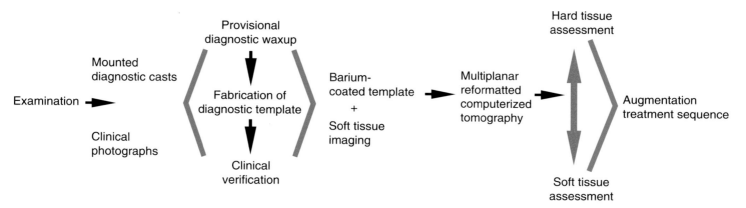

Fig 3-24 Typical investigative sequence used in determining augmentation requirement for proposed CPI of a particular prosthesis.

velopment of an optimal final tooth position as the reference point from which all other tissues of the alveolar process or residual ridge are reconstructed has enabled the implant team to determine presurgically the extent and type of augmentation procedures necessary to create harmony with the optimal final tooth position (Fig 3-24). The implant team can plan reconstructive procedures presurgically and determine the sequence of treatment most capable of predictably achieving its goals.

Most importantly, the development of a computer profile image has allowed the implant team to consult more effectively with the patient presurgically. Clarity in treatment goals and in required surgical or restorative procedures can be attained. Eliminating treatment uncertainty makes it easier to determine accurate patient fees, define the roles and responsibilities of the team members, and establish achievable treatment goals.

Computerized tomography becomes the communicative blueprint that allows the surgical-prosthetic decision-making analysis to focus on patient care. A CT study using a clinically verified barium-coated template can arm the implant team with the following information:

1. Anatomic limitations (vital structure)
2. Optimal final tooth position (interarch and intra-arch)
3. Accurate location of the implant site
4. Prediction of the screw access hole position
5. Prediction of the prosthesis type
6. Facilitation of implant team interaction and communication
7. Verification of the treatment objectives
8. Treatment sequencing
9. Treatment focused on the patient's needs and concerns

Acknowledgments

The authors wish to express their genuine appreciation to Lutheran General Hospital Media Services Department for its assistance in the preparation of the graphics for this chapter. In particular, our thanks to Todd Hochberg, medical photographer, for his production of slide material and computer graphics. Additionally, we would like to thank Janet Rosenfeld for her advice and assistance in the preparation of this chapter.

References

1. Brånemark P-I, Zarb G, Albrektsson T. Tissue-Integrated Prostheses: Osseointegration in Clinical Dentistry. Chicago: Quintessence, 1985.

2. Adell R, Lekholm U, Rockler B, Brånemark P-I. A 15-year study of osseointegrated implants in the treatment of the edentulous jaw. Int J Oral Surg 1981;10:387–416.

3. Schnitman PA, Schulman LB (eds). Dental implants: benefits and risks, an NIH Harvard consensus development conference. Washington D.C.: U.S. Dept of Health and Human Services, 1979:1–351.

4. Zarb G (ed). Proceedings of the Toronto conference on osseointegration in clinical dentistry. J Prosthet Dent 1983;49:6 and 50:1–3.

5. Albrektsson T, Zarb G, Worthington P, Eriksson AR. The long term efficacy of currently used dental implants: A review and proposed criteria for success. Int J Oral Maxillofac Implants 1986;1:11–25.

6. Renner PP. An Introduction to Dental Anatomy and Esthetics. Chicago: Quintessence, 1985.

7. Sicher H, DuBrul EL. Oral Anatomy. St. Louis: Mosby, 1970.

8. Mecall RA, Rosenfeld AL. The influence of residual ridge resorption patterns on fixture placement and tooth position. Part I. Int J Periodont Rest Dent 1991;11:8–23.

9. Kallus T, Henry P, Jemt T, et al. Clinical evaluation of angulated abutments for the Brånemark system: A pilot study. Int J Oral Maxillofac Implants 1990;5:39–45.

10. Lewis S, Beumer J, III, Hornberg P. The "UCLA" abutment. Int J Oral Maxillofac Implants 1988;3:183–189.

11. Tallgren A. Positional changes of complete dentures: A 7 year longitudinal study. Acta Odontol Scand 1969;27:539.

12. Tallgren A. The continuing reduction of residual alveolar ridges in complete denture wearers: A mixed longitudinal study covering 25 years. J Prosthet Dent 1972;27:120.

13. Carlsson GE, Bergman B, Hedegard B. Changes in contour of the maxillary alveolar process under immediate dentures. Acta Odontol Scand 1967;25:1.

14. Carlsson GE, Persson G. Morphological changes of the mandible after extraction and wearing of dentures: A longitudinal, clinical and x-ray cephalometric study covering 5 years. Odontol Rev 1967;18:27–54.

15. Schwarz MS, Rothman SLG, Rhodes ML, Chafetz N. Computed tomography. Part I. Preoperative assessment of the mandible for endosseous implant surgery. Int J Oral Maxillofac Implants 1987;2: 137–141.

16. Schwarz MS, Rothman SLG, Rhodes ML, Chafetz N. Computed tomography. Part II. Preoperative assessment of the maxilla for endosseous implant surgery. Int J Oral Maxillofac Implants 1987; 2:143–148.

17. Wheeler R. Textbook of Dental Anatomy and Physiology, 4th ed. Philadelphia: Saunders, 1965:336–338.

18. Williams MY, Mealey BL, Hallmon WW. The role of computerized tomography in dental implantology. Int J Oral Maxillofac Implants 1992;7:373–380.

19. Todd A, Gher M, et al. Interpretation of linear and computed tomograms in the assessment of implant recipient sites. J Periodontol 1993; 64:1243–1249.

20. Klinge B, Peterson A, Maly P. Location of the mandibular canal: Comparison of macroscopic findings, conventional radiography and computed tomography. Int J Oral Maxillofac Implants 1989;4: 327–332.

21. SIM/Plant for Windows. Columbia, MD: Columbia Scientific Incorporated.

22. Rosenfeld AL, Mecall RA. The use of interactive computed tomography to predict the esthetic and functional demands of implant supported prostheses. Compend Contin Educ Dent 1996;17:1161–1170.

23. Mecall RA, Rosenfeld AL. The influence of residual ridge resorption patterns on fixture placement and tooth position in the partially edentulous patient. Part III. Presurgical assessment of ridge augmentation requirements. Int J Periodont Rest Dent 1996;16:323–337.

24. Dawson PE. Evaluations, Diagnosis, and Treatment of Occlusal Problems. St. Louis: Mosby, 1989.

25. Mecall RA, Rosenfeld AL. The influence of residual ridge resorption patterns on fixture placement and tooth position. Part II. Presurgical determination of prosthesis type and design. Int J Periodont Rest Dent 1992;12:33–51.

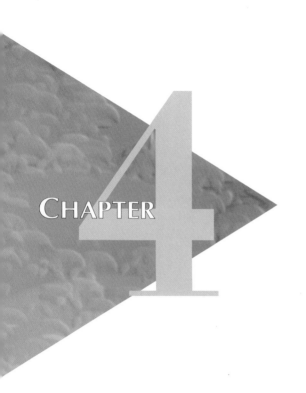

Biomechanical Interaction Between Implants and Teeth

Burton Langer, DMD, MSD
Bo Rangert, Mech Eng, PhD

The inception of osseointegration opened up a new vista in the world of implant therapy. With the exception of subperiosteal and mandibular staples, most implants were attached to adjacent teeth to gain support and stability. The osseointegrated implant was conceived and developed as an anchoring unit that created an attachment to the surrounding bone through the sharing of organic and inorganic elements. This fixation of bone to the implant was in a dynamic state of equilibrium, provided that the biologic metabolism was not violated.

Surgical determinants were well defined in the original recipe to ensure that the limits of bone healing would not be violated. With minor exceptions, the chances of obtaining a bone-implant interface without an intermediate connective tissue layer were extremely high. Coupled with this surgical phase was a complementary biomechanical counterpart developed to preserve the integration. Because the implants were well anchored to the bone, and had virtually no movement with the osseous structure, it could be hypothesized that, if united together within a precise framework, the implants would all function as one element and reciprocate with each other.

Minor discrepancies of fit, position within the dental arch, eccentricities of jaw movements, and the like were compensated by a system of abutments and gold cylinders with corresponding screws, all of which had gradations of flexibility and fatigue strength. This well-developed system was similar to an electric circuit fuse, in that there were protective screws that not only connected the prosthesis to the implants, but also shielded the bone by yielding before the forces destroyed the surrounding bone. Teeth were not necessary to stabilize the implants because they were stable enough on their own, and in most cases no teeth were available.

The early cases were uniform because they were mostly dedicated to the completely edentulous patient. However, a disparity in anchoring strength did exist between the maxilla and the mandible. The latter seemed to be more impervious to biomechanical overload because the bone between the mental foramina is most often denser than it is in other areas of the mouth, thus increasing the strength of anchorage. This allowed the placement of 15- to 20-mm-long cantilevers bilaterally on four to six implants.

The weaker bone in the maxilla, on the other hand, was impaired more easily by overload, induced by excessive cantilevers, parafunctional habits, or improperly designed or fitting frameworks. The diagnostic skill and technical abilities of the restorative dentist were most dramatically reflected in this arch. Although surgical expertise was necessary to obtain the first stage of osseointegration, it was the craftiness of the restoration that was crucial to its preservation.

Mixing Implants and Teeth

The application of principles of osseointegration in partially edentulous patients further complicated the diagnostic acuity of the implant team. For the first time, movable and nonmovable segments were combined. Teeth suspended by the periodontal ligament have a range of movement from around 50 µm in the normal periodontium[1] to tenths of a millimeter in compromised situations. Therefore, a new vision must be developed toward the admixture of teeth and implants, a different viewpoint than previously was conceived with other non-osseointegrated implants. This topic cannot be approached with tunnel vision or with a set of formulas and equations because it involves a multi-faceted problem.

To simplify the discussion, patients who are missing segments of teeth, in either the anterior or posterior portion of the mouth, are best treated with osseointegrated implants that are kept separate from the teeth. If the residual dentition is strong enough to stand by itself, implants are not necessary to give it support. Certainly, the osseointegrated implant per se does not need support from a tooth. If, however, the teeth are periodontally weak, the treatment plan must be reevaluated; this will be addressed later. Because factors such as the mobility and position of teeth are constantly changing, there is no predictable way to have a mechanical component correlate to the periodontal ligament of a tooth. The combination of freestanding segments of teeth and osseointegrated implants is therefore probably the most successful formula of treatment, irrespective of implant type.

Occlusion

The occlusion must also be viewed with a different perspective when teeth and implants are present in the same arch. The resilient apparatus of the teeth responds to load with an immediate deformation, as well as with a long-term reorganization among bone, periodontal ligament, and cementum. The osseointegrated implant does not have this accommodating system, and therefore tends to be the major load carrier when mixed in the same quadrant.[2] Consequently, the occlusal pattern and contacts should be carefully addressed, whether or not the supports are connected.

The natural mobility of the teeth should be considered when the occlusal contacts are established. Ideally, there should be a minimum of 50 μm of space between the implant-supported prosthesis and its opposing dentition, allowing the adjacent teeth to be loaded before the stiffer implant unit makes contact.[2] Clinical measurements would be required for qualifying its importance. In practice, most clinicians adjust occlusions in the same manner as they did when the arch was without implants, and a refined occlusal contact design is probably not necessary for the crossarch relationship.[3] However, it may possibly be helpful when teeth and implants are mixed in the same quadrant. Whatever the situation, clinical practice indicates that an important factor for reducing the possible overload of an implant restoration in a mixed situation is to eliminate lateral excursive contacts for this unit.[4]

The normal occlusal concepts of anterior guidance and canine protection, or group function if the latter is not obtainable, is a good starting point for reducing noncentric

contacts on the implants. Because the implant-bone interface lacks the resilient periodontal ligament and the surrounding bone is somewhat compressible, it seems logical to reduce lateral forces on the implants and transfer them to the teeth when possible. When these goals cannot be obtained, the insufficiency must be compensated for by the addition of more implants to overcome the potential for overload.

The alert clinician must always relate the dental profile of the patient to the quality and height of bone, the distribution of the implants, and the position and quality of the remaining teeth. There is a great variation in the anchoring capacity, depending on the number and precise placement of the implants,[4] and when optimized, the unit will balance normal and even certain hyperfunctional forces well. However, excessive forces over long periods of time, even at optimal implant placement, may prove destructive.

Connecting Implants to Teeth

The reasons for and experience with connecting teeth and implants are diverse, and there are only a few situations in which connections should be considered the treatment of choice. This conclusion differs from some other recommendations, where connection is advocated as the first alternative.[5,6] There is, however, a lack of long-term clinical studies supporting the feasibility of connection as a general approach. The difference between teeth, which have mobility, and implants, which are generally more rigid, requires that the clinician adopt a biomechanical perspective when combining the two.

A postulate has been presented that highlights the attractiveness of joining teeth to implants. Because there is an aspect of proprioception within the periodontal ligament, the advocates of this theory feel that the teeth will protect the implants from being overloaded.[7] However, this has not been clinically proven, and in reality, much of the feedback in the stomatognathic system resides within the muscles and ligaments of the temporomandibular articulation.[8] This is evidenced by the fact that tooth proprioception does not prevent patients from fracturing or traumatizing their natural dentition. Further research will be necessary to authenticate either side of this controversy.

Two problematic aspects of connection have been documented. First, a rigid structure is connected to a nonrigid structure, the more mobile of the two may act like a cantilever, increasing the load to the implant or its surrounding bone[4] (Fig 4-1). Second, if a nonrigid connector is employed rather than a solder joint, there is a tendency for teeth to intrude[9] (Fig 4-2). The potential for these complications must be evaluated during the treatment planning phase to determine if connection is worth the risk or ultimately necessary.

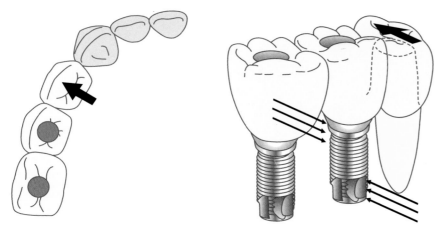

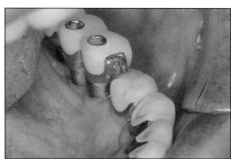

Fig 4-2 A movable connection between a multiple-implant unit and a separate tooth, or group of teeth, leads to a high susceptibility for intrusion. If the tooth is free to move away from the connector in the direction of the socket, it may not return completely to its original position, resulting in an orthodontic movement.

Fig 4-1 Two or more implants in a restoration form a stiffer unit than do adjacent teeth. A rigid connection between the teeth and the implant unit in such a situation, therefore, forces the implant unit to support the tooth or teeth and as a consequence be subjected to greater stress.

Biomechanical Aspects of Implant-Tooth Connection

Before different possibilities of connection are discussed in more detail, some fundamentals of a biomechanical nature will be discussed. Implants are stiffer in an axial direction than are teeth, even when built-in mobile elements are used,[10] and the flexibility of the periodontal ligament is unmatched by the mechanical system. On the other hand, many implants can, as single units, be considered flexible in bending and to various degrees compensate for the mobility of a tooth.[11] Different types of connectors should therefore be considered in relation to these mechanical properties of the implants, as well as to the reason for joining them to the teeth. The most rigid junction is the soldered fixed partial denture, which will transfer forces and moments in all directions, whereas different types of premanufactured attachments have various stress-breaking properties. The latter allows motion in predefined load directions, limiting the interaction between the supporting members.

The design and mechanical strength of the joint to the teeth are also crucial; a lack of firm contact may lead to intrusion of the teeth. The reasons for intrusion may vary, but if the tooth is free to move away from the connector in the direction of the socket, it may not return completely to its original position. The spring action must then originate from the ligament support only, and if this motion is counteracted by friction in the attachment, the tooth may be subjected to an orthodontic movement in its axial direction. A movable connection between a multiple-implant unit and a separate tooth or group of teeth, therefore, increases the susceptibility to intrusion. Even if the restoration is designed to counteract this phenomenon,[12] and works in some clinicians' hands, clinical experiences demonstrate that fracture of cement frequently occurs, making the intended function useless.[9] A disrupted cement bond may induce an orthodontic movement through contact friction, food accumulation, or plaque buildup.

Principles of Implant-Tooth Connection

There are three different options for joining implants and teeth: *(1)* one implant sharing the load with a tooth or teeth through rigid connection; *(2)* multiple implants supporting a tooth or teeth through stress-breaking attachment; and *(3)* multiple tooth abutments incorporated within long-span implant restorations. The reasons for the connection differ among these situations. In the one-implant–one-tooth situation, the purpose is to divide the load between the members. When a segment of multiple implants is connected to a tooth or teeth, it will provide support to the teeth. When teeth and implants are intermixed in a long-span restoration, the teeth will not contribute to the support of the prosthesis at all.

The case of connecting one implant to one tooth has proven viable in a 5-year prospective clinical study on 23 patients with partial prostheses in the posterior mandible, opposing complete dentures.[13] The inherent bending flexibility of the implant screw joint, which matches the axial mobility of a connected tooth,[11] seems to be a prerequisite for this result. An obvious advantage of this modality is that it may allow a fixed prosthesis where the anatomy will only allow the placement of one implant. The situation of joining a single implant to a healthy tooth or teeth to prevent rotation is only historically significant because the improved design of single implants allows them to be restored without loosening problems.

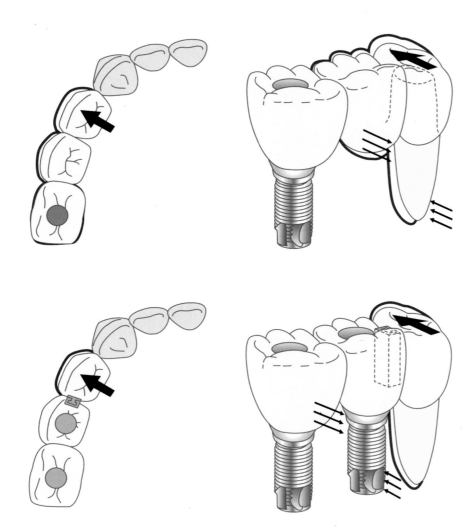

Fig 4-3 Rigid connection of one implant to one tooth has proven viable in some situations. Because the tooth is fully active in this arrangement, its good periodontal health is a prerequisite. Abnormal tooth mobility may lead to implant overload.

Fig 4-4 An alternative way of connecting implants to teeth, with the purpose of supporting the tooth or teeth, is to have a stress-breaking semiprecision attachment on the implant side. Potential problems include possible cement breakage and unpredictable long-term function of the attachment.

In this therapy, the connecting prosthesis should be rigidly attached to gain full support from the tooth (Fig 4-3); any stress-breaking characteristics of the attachment may induce play, leading to a less effective interaction. Because the tooth is fully active in this arrangement, its good periodontal health is a prerequisite, and abnormal tooth mobility may lead to implant overload. The dilemma of retrievability when rigid connection is used is still unanswerable, because the choices are either the use of a locking screw in the pontic or temporary cementation, both of which have inherent problems; locking screws often break, and temporary cementation may be too weak for long-term use.

It is important to distinguish the one-implant–one tooth connection (see Fig 4-3) from two or more implants connected to teeth (see Fig 4-1). The multiple-implant restoration will form a stiff unit that will not bend with the movement of the teeth. The rationale for connecting under these circumstances would be to support the tooth or teeth with the implant prosthesis. However, this design introduces the potential for overload because the coupling may act as an unsupported cantilever to the implants, resulting in elevated stresses to components and bone.

An alternative way of connecting one or multiple implants to teeth, with the purpose of supporting the teeth, is to include a semiprecision attachment on the implant side, eliminating bending of the implant[12] (Fig 4-4). Still, a number of potential problems with such an arrangement can be envisioned as a result of possible cement breakage and unpredictable function of the attachment.[8,9] The question is whether it is worth the trouble to maintain the clinical balance in this system for the benefit of preserving a questionable tooth. Because the predictability of the osseointegrated implants has been proven for both partial restorations[14] and complete arches, a more reliable treatment would most often be to extract the teeth in question.

In the final situation, natural teeth interspersed between multiple implants in long-span restorations (Fig 4-5) will not deliver any load support and will function merely as "living pontics." Because the functional deformation of a multiple-implant prosthesis is less than the natural mobility of a tooth, incorporation of teeth in such a restoration will render little risk for intrusion caused by relative motion. Clinical practice also indicates that this phenomenon, although present, is not a problem; it rarely occurs, and, when it does, it offers few clinical consequences. The deci-

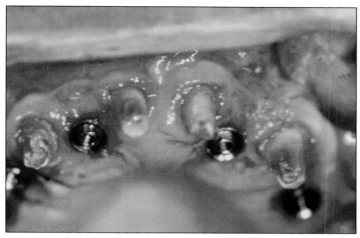

Fig 4-5 Natural teeth that are interspersed between multiple implants in long-span restorations will not deliver any load support and will function merely as living pontics.

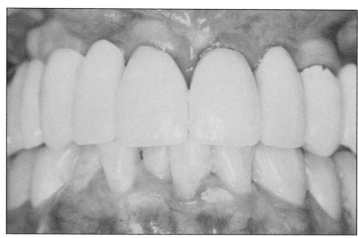

Fig 4-6 The decision whether to incorporate or to extract teeth interspersed between multiple implants should be based on the long-term predictability of the tooth conditions and the psychologic and esthetic requirements of the patient.

sion as to whether to incorporate or to extract teeth should, therefore, be based on concerns other than those derived from implant biomechanics. More relevant criteria are the long-term predictability of the tooth conditions and the psychologic and esthetic needs of the patient (Fig 4-6).

Summary

The use of teeth and implants in the same jaw segment calls for refined consideration of occlusion, whether they are connected or freestanding. Because the implant-supported part of the restoration has a tendency to carry a major share of the load, the quality of its anchorage is important for the longevity of the therapy.

The need for connection is very limited, and the freestanding implant therapy should be considered the first choice. Any rationale for connection should be thoroughly scrutinized; in most situations, such an analysis would reveal that a freestanding solution is to be preferred. Connection may be demonstrated to work in theory, but because it is biomechanically sensitive, it may lead to subsequent problems. Teeth may be left inactive, as living pontics, without much problem if they are healthy, and one implant might be rigidly combined with a strong tooth or teeth for a short-span restoration. Other than that, there seems to be little advantage to connecting teeth and implants.

References

1. Picton DCA. The effect of external forces on the periodontium. In: Melcher AH, Bowden WH (eds). Biology of the Periodontium. London: Academic Press, 1969:385.

2. Lundgren D, Laurell L. Biomechanical aspects of fixed bridgework supported by natural teeth and endosseous implants. Periodontology 2000 1994;4:23–30.

3. Richter E-J. In vivo vertical forces on implants. Int J Oral Maxillofac Implants 1995;10:99–108.

4. Rangert B, Krogh PHJ, Langer B, Van Roekel N. Bending overload and implant fracture. A retrospective clinical analysis. Int J Oral Maxillofac Implants 1995;10:326–334.

5. Kirch A, Ackermann KL. The IMZ osteointegrated implant system. Dent Clin North Am 1989;33:733–791.

6. Cavicchia F, Bravi F. Free-standing vs tooth-connected implant-supported fixed partial restorations: A comparative retrospective clinical study of prosthetic results. Int J Oral Maxillofac Implants 1994; 9:711–718.

7. Mühlbradt L, Mattes S, Möhlmann H, Ulrich R. Touch sensitivity of natural teeth and endosseous implants revealed by difference thresholds. Int J Oral Maxillofac Implants 1994;9:412–416.

8. Kay HB. Free-standing vs implant-tooth interconnected restorations: Understanding the prosthodontic perspective. Int J Periodont Rest Dent 1993;13:47–69.

9. Rieder C, Parel S. A survey of natural tooth abutment intrusion with implant-connected fixed partial dentures. Int J Periodont Rest Dent 1993;13:335–347.

10. Brunski J. Biomechanical factors affecting the bone-dental implant interface. Clin Mater 1992;10:153–201.

11. Rangert B, Gunne J, Glantz P-O, Svensson A. Vertical load distribution on a three-unit prosthesis supported by a natural tooth and a single Brånemark implant. An in vivo study. Clin Oral Implants Res 1995;6:40–46.

12. Cohen S, Ornstein J. The use of attachments in combination implant and natural-tooth fixed partial dentures: A technical report. Int J Oral Maxillofac Implants 1994;9:230–234.

13. Olsson M, Gunne J, Åstrand P, Borg K. Bridges supported by freestanding implants versus bridges supported by tooth and implant. A five-year prospective study. Clin Oral Implant Res 1995;6:114–121.

14. Lekholm U, van Steenberghe D, Herrmann I, Bolender C, Folmer T, Gunne J, et al. Osseointegrated implants in the treatment of partially edentulous jaws. A prospective 5-year multicenter study. Int J Oral Maxillofac Implants 1994;9:627–635.

Guided Bone Regeneration and Dental Implants

James T. Mellonig, DDS, MS
Myron Nevins, DDS

CHAPTER 5

Guided bone regeneration (GBR) is a reconstructive surgical procedure that evolved from the guided tissue regeneration (GTR) technique.[1,2] At one time, the terms *GTR* and *GBR* were used interchangeably. Currently, *GTR* is used to describe the treatment of osseous defects associated with natural teeth, and *GBR* is used specifically to denote the reconstruction of alveolar bone defects prior to or in association with the placement of dental implants. A barrier is used to isolate and create a protected space for the organizing blood clot and to prevent collapse caused by pressure from the tissue flap.[3–6] This allows the migration of osteoprogenitor cells into the space, resulting in new bone formation.[7] Although GBR is a relatively new procedure, the rationale for the technique is supported by a significant body of animal studies.[8–10]

Animal Studies

The principles of GBR were initially supported by studies in animals in which either a segment or a section of bone was surgically removed. The cut edges of the bone were then protected by placement of a plastic cage or joined by a plastic tube.[4,11] The test sites were isolated from the overlying connective tissue by the barriers, but the bone defects were not covered in the control sites. In experimental sites, where the barrier created a space, new bone filled the defects. Without a barrier, fibrous connective tissue was able to proliferate into the defect.

Dahlin et al[6] showed, in monkeys, complete healing of maxillary and mandibular bone defects associated with large periradicular defects and apicoectomies. In contrast, control defects showed varying degrees of connective tissue ingrowth. Dahlin et al[12] further described complete bone regeneration of critical-sized calvarial defects in rats with the use of the GBR technique. The most complete healing was found when expanded polytetrafluoroethylene membranes (e-PTFE) were placed on both the internal and external surfaces of the cranium, and autogenous bone was placed between the barrier membranes to maintain the space. The use of GBR to correct created calvarial defects in rabbits resulted in complete osseous bridging of the skull defects in the test specimens. In control specimens, fibrous connective tissue occupied the area of the skull defect.[13]

Animal studies also have indicated that the GBR technique can be applied to defects associated with the placement of dental endosseous implants. Dahlin et al[14] placed titanium-threaded implants in the tibias of rabbits in such a way as to produce dehiscence over the threads. Half of the implants received an e-PTFE membrane, the others did not. At retrieval, the test sites had a mean of 3.8 mm of bone formation in a coronoapical direction, while the control sites had a mean of 2.2 mm. Histologic analysis revealed osseointegration in the area of newly formed bone in the experimental sites.

In a similar study, defects were created in the jaws of dogs and implants were inserted so as to leave dehiscence defects.[15] Half of the dehiscence defects were covered with an e-PTFE membrane. Control sites were not covered. At 18 weeks, the mean midbuccal increase in bone height over the exposed threads was 1.3 mm, with bone-to-thread contact, in the covered sites, while the increase was 0.23 mm, with little or no contact, in control sites.

Likewise, the principles of GBR were applied in an attempt to generate bone to cover a subperiosteal implant.[16] Titanium frameworks were inserted on the tibias of rabbits, and half of the exposed implants were protected by an e-PTFE barrier. After 12 weeks, bone covered all test sites, whereas control sites were embedded in fibrous connective tissue.

Extraction-type circumferential defects were created in the mandibles of six dogs.[17] Hydroxyapatite(HA)-coated implants were inserted into the defects and covered with an e-PTFE barrier that was either fixed with a cover screw or placed over the top of the implant. Control sites received no barrier. Those sites treated with a barrier filled with new bone in contact with the implant surface. Control sites did not fill with appreciable amounts of new bone. More new bone formation was noted when the barrier was placed over the cover screw.

The same type of defect in monkeys was used by Gotfredsen et al[18] to evaluate the potential of GBR. Defects were treated with one of four different methods: e-PTFE alone, e-PTFE and porous hydroxyapatite particles (pHA), pHA alone, or no treatment. Results indicated that the GBR technique provides for healing of bone defects around implants and that pHA has no additional effect on bone healing.

Becker et al[19] evaluated the effect of GBR and growth factors around implants placed in immediate extraction defects. The results of their study supported the use of e-PTFE membranes, alone or with growth factors, as a potential method of promoting bone formation around implants. Currently, growth factors are only available for research purposes.

Lekholm et al[20] demonstrated in dogs that the maximum bone formation around oral implants is created if the barrier remains in place during the entire healing period. Another histologic study in the canine mandible demonstrated that bone regeneration in barrier-protected defects closely follows the pattern of normal bone growth and provides a suitable environment for bone development.[7] Early removal of the barrier results in less newly formed bone and an incomplete bone fill. Still another animal study confirmed that it is essential to avoid soft tissue dehiscence and barrier exposure if predictable results are to be obtained with GBR.

In addition, it appears that premature loading of the implant will result in less bone fill.[21] Implants were placed in 24 fresh extraction sites with buccal dehiscences in four dogs. Half the implants were augmented with e-PTFE barriers, which were removed at 3 months. Some of the implants were loaded for an additional 6 months, while others remained unloaded. Histologic analysis indicated that, at 3 months, new bone had formed under the barriers and in greater amounts than in defects without barriers. If left unloaded, the new bone matured and increased. Loaded barrier sites had significantly less bone than did unloaded

barrier sites. It was concluded that the newly formed bone under the barrier should be allowed extended healing periods prior to loading.

An additional study in dogs demonstrated that, after a 6-month healing period, new mandibular bone regenerated by the GBR technique responds to implant placement like nonregenerated bone. This newly formed bone is capable of bearing and sustaining a functional load.[22] The optimum time for loading bone regenerated with e-PTFE barriers has not been determined.

The ability to regenerate supracrestal bone or increase vertical alveolar ridge height has been investigated in animals. Jovanovic et al[23] placed titanium-reinforced e-PTFE barriers over implants in a supracrestal position. The results suggested that supracrestal bone regeneration is possible with the GBR technique. Jensen et al[24] also placed dental implants in a supracrestal position but supported the barrier with autogenous and allogeneic bone grafts. The barrier improved graft incorporation for vertical ridge augmentation and interface contact with the implant surface. Likewise, Lundgren et al[25] demonstrated that titanium domes placed on the skulls of rabbits can become completely filled with new bone, indicating that the use of a barrier with total occlusiveness, sufficient stiffness and stability, and reliable peripheral sealing will result in bone augmentation of spaces created beyond the skeletal envelope.

Animal studies provide the basis and rationale for the GBR procedure. They have indicated that:

1. The GBR procedure is capable of promoting new bone formation.
2. Bone defects, such as dehiscences, and fenestrations around dental implants, can be corrected by the GBR procedure.
3. Extraction-type circumferential defects can be corrected.
4. Vertical alveolar ridge augmentation is possible.
5. Bone grafts can improve new bone formation.
6. Newly formed bone will be in contact with both titanium and hydroxyapatite-coated implant surfaces.
7. Early barrier exposure complicates wound healing and limits new bone formation.
8. Premature loading of the implant may impair the new bone formed by the GBR procedure.

Procedure and Rationale

In the GBR technique, a cell-occlusive physical barrier or membrane is placed between the gingival connective tissue of the flap and the alveolar bone defect. The barrier is trimmed to shape and fitted over the bone defect so that the barrier completely covers and extends beyond the osseous defect margins by at least 2 mm, creating a space and preventing the connective tissue from occupying the defect. It also allows a blood clot to form and unimpeded healing within the bone compartment. Space creation is, therefore, critical because it allows cells in the isolated space to undergo amplifying cell division.[26]

Besides providing space, the physical barrier protects the blood clot by diverting mechanical stress that acts on the tissue flap during the critical early stages of wound healing.[27] Therefore, the barrier must be stabilized; the edges of barrier are tucked beneath the flap margins or miniscrews are used. Wound stabilization is critical, because micromovement of the barrier over the blood clot during initial wound healing directly influences cellular differentiation.[28] Movement of 10 to 20 μm during the early stages of osseous healing is enough to shift differentiation of mesenchymal cells from osteoblasts to fibroblasts.[29] Both creation of a space for bone ingrowth and stabilization of the wound are critical to success.[30] A nonbioabsorbable barrier is left in place until the second-stage or abutment surgery.

Besides space creation and wound stabilization, several other factors seem to influence the predictability of GBR[31]:

1. A barrier material of sufficient stiffness and/or barrier support to ensure the desired volume of the compartment
2. A healthy vascularized bone bed
3. Retention of the barrier in its submerged position
4. An appropriate amount of healing time, usually a minimum of 3 months of wound healing in the mandible and 6 months in the maxilla

Terminology

A defect may be either spacemaking or non-spacemaking. A naturally spacemaking defect is one that provides adequate support for the physical barrier to prevent collapse of the barrier into the osseous defect on wound closure. In large non-spacemaking osseous defects, there is insufficient support from the osseous walls to prevent collapse. Occasionally, spacemaking defects are referred to as *contained bone lesions*, while non-spacemaking defects are referred to as *noncontained lesions*.

Furthermore, the implant can be placed within or outside the envelope of bone. The envelope of bone is defined as the outer cortical alveolar plate that existed in health before any osseous destruction and/or resorption occurred. All large, noncontained, non-spacemaking defects and defects caused by implants placed outside the envelope of bone require bone augmentation grafts to support the barrier and to provide either a lattice network for osteoconduction or bone-inductive proteins for osteoinduction.[32,33] Mechanical support, such as fixation screws, is occasionally used to tent up the barrier with or without grafting materials.[1,34,35]

Applications for GBR Techniques

Since the advent of GBR in the late 1980s, a plethora of studies in humans have been published describing a wide variety of techniques and materials to treat osseous defects associated with dental implants.[22,31,34,36–44] These osseous defects, both the spacemaking and non-spacemaking, generally can be categorized as extraction site defects; dehiscences and fenestrations; localized alveolar ridge defects; and defects associated with peri-implantitis or the ailing or failing implant.[33,45] In addition, other variables of a technical or clinical nature, such as timing and location of implant placement, early exposure of the barrier, and type of bone grafting material, have been reported to play a role in regenerative outcomes.

Implants Placed in Extraction Sites

Initial observations with implants immediately placed in extraction sites and covered with an e-PTFE barrier suggested that both osseointegration and bone reconstruction could occur within the extraction site.[2,46] The advantage is that immediate implant placement combines the postextraction healing period with the integration phase and minimizes the time the patient must wear a removable or provisional appliance. The limitations of immediate placement are the occasional difficulties with implant insertion into the socket, the lack of sufficient bone at the inferior border of the socket to anchor the implant, and the inability to completely cover the barrier with soft tissue.

There are numerous reports on the successful implementation of this technique with titanium-threaded, titanium plasma-sprayed, hydroxyapatite-coated, and one-stage endosseous implants.[43,44,47–64] The composition of the barriers varies; an e-PTFE barrier has been used in the majority of the published reports.[43,44,46–53,55,56,61–64] Collagen,[57] Polyglactin 910,[51] polylactic acid,[65] Teflon,[54] fascia lata,[66] and autogenous gingival grafts[59] have been successfully used in a small number of cases.

The influence of the dimensions of the extraction socket on bone fill following GBR was evaluated by Gher et al.[62] Measurements were made to document the relationship of bone to implant at the time of implant placement and at the 6-month reentry. All implants were clinically osseointegrated at the 6-month reentry procedure (Figs 5-1a and 5-1b). Narrow bone defects showed complete bone fill, while wide defects showed partial bone fill. In addition, there was less bone fill in areas of thin or deficient cortical plates.

The influence of bone grafts on the healing of wide extraction site defects was then evaluated in humans.[63] Defects about hydroxyapatite-coated implants and plasma-sprayed implants were either grafted with decalcified (demineralized) freeze-dried bone allograft (DFDBA) or received no graft. Crestal bone apposition was noted at the most apical

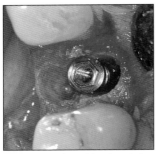

Fig 5-1a A dental implant is inserted into the fresh extraction site of a mandibular first premolar. The defect is within the envelope of bone and was treated with a Gore-Tex Augmentation Membrane (WL Gore, Flagstaff, AZ).

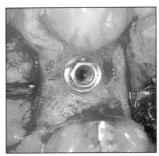

Fig 5-1b The area is reopened after 6 months and exhibits complete bone regeneration in the areas of voids.

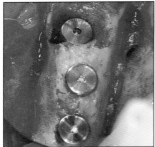

Fig 5-2a The mandibular first premolar is an excellent candidate for placement of an implant in a fresh extraction wound. This area was treated with a membrane and a mineralized freeze-dried bone allograft.

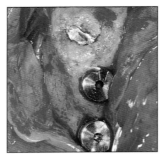

Fig 5-2b The site has been reopened and bone has formed over the cover screw. The regeneration of bone was successful.

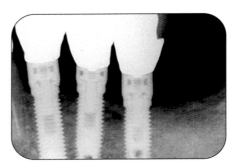

Fig 5-2c The posttreatment radiograph reveals complete bone anchorage.

part of the socket crest for sites treated with DFDBA, whereas crestal resorption was noted in the nongrafted group. Bone fill from the base of the deepest osseous defect was significantly greater for the grafted group than for the control group. Results of these studies indicated that wound healing of wide or extensive extraction site defects can be improved when a bone graft is placed in conjunction with GBR.

Therefore, in large non-spacemaking defects, DFDBA has been used to prevent collapse of the barrier membrane into the defect and to enhance new bone formation[44,48,50,52,56,57,63,64] (Figs 5-2a to 5-2c). Callan[48] reported on 61 patients in whom 126 implants were augmented with DFDBA and covered with an e-PTFE barrier. Eleven of the sites were fresh extraction sites, 59 were residual extraction sites, and five were impacted third molar sites. Clinical bone fill appeared to be 95% to 100%. The implants were followed for periods of 1 to 5½ years.

In a retrospective study, 66 implants with defects requiring treatment with GBR were placed in 47 patients.[44] In 89% of the cases, DFDBA was used. In this series, 14 implants were placed in fresh extraction sites. All of these implants were determined to be completely successful, as judged by the criteria of complete coverage of the implant's body with new bone.

In a prospective study, DFDBA and 63 e-PTFE barriers were used to treat bone defects associated with 110 implants, including nine implants inserted in fresh extraction sites.[56] The technique was considered successful if the exposed implant surfaces were at least 90% covered by new bone and not more than two threads were exposed. With these criteria, 61 of 63 (97%) of the cases were successful.

Landsberg et al[64] evaluated 32 implants placed in extraction sockets. A mixture of DFDBA and tetracycline was packed around the exposed implant parts. The implants were covered with e-PTFE barriers and removed at abutment connection. Biopsy specimens from regenerated bone consisted of particles of DFDBA in contact with newly formed or lamellar bone (Figs 5-3a to 5-3i). Likewise, case descriptions of one or two patients have reported that DFDBA has been successfully used in combination with GBR to augment bone around implants placed in fresh extraction sites.[50,52,53,57]

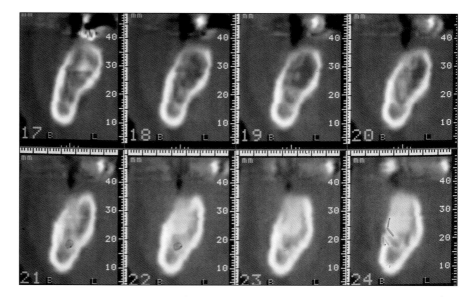

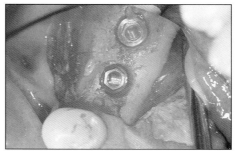

Fig 5-4f Computerized tomography scan made 6 months after guided bone regeneration procedures. The regenerated area can be identified immediately superior to the mental foramen, which precludes extension of the implant to preexisting bone. The mesial implant will only extend to grafted bone. The entire buccal wall appears to be reconstructed to the same height as native bone distal to it.

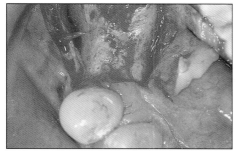

Fig 5-4g The surgical site is reentered to allow placement of implants. The bone is completely reconstructed and has significant vascularity.

Fig 5-4h Two implants are installed. The native bone is very cancellous and requires a 5-mm implant to be stable. The regenerated bone is very hard, resists drilling, and allows countersinking.

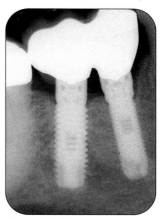

Fig 5-4i Three-year posttreatment radiograph.

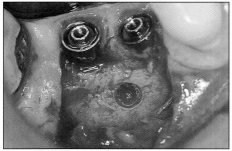

Fig 5-4j The patient allowed a bone biopsy specimen to be taken 3 years after the implants were loaded. The reflected buccal flap reveals an intact buccal wall of bone.

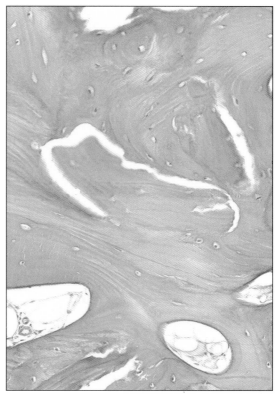

Fig 5-4k The biopsy specimen evidences mature, vital bone with concentric rings of haversian systems. Almost all lacunae are occupied by cells.

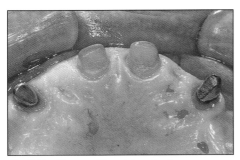

Fig 5-5a The maxillary lateral incisors were removed when the provisional prosthesis was inserted, but to allow the gingiva to heal over the extraction sites, implants were not placed.

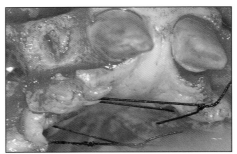

Fig 5-5b The implants are to be placed after 30 days. Clinical differentiation of osteoid and connective tissues is insignificant when the buccal plate is intact, but is difficult when the buccal plate is thin or partially damaged.

The problem associated with executing this procedure coincidental with extraction involves the likelihood of premature barrier exposure. The gingival tissue required to cover the extraction wound is frequently of insufficient dimension to obtain complete coverage of the barrier, despite innovative surgical techniques.[47] Barrier exposure may lessen the amount of bone augmentation achieved, but clinical experience suggests that this is only true when the barrier is mobile or has exposed margins. It is best, however, to keep it covered for the duration of the healing process.

The distinct advantage of immediately proceeding to regeneration can be related to an extraction vault that has been exposed as an acute wound. Extraction and removal of infected granulation tissue result in bony walls with multiple exposed marrow spaces and easy communication to the vascular and cellular elements associated with bone growth.

To obviate the barrier exposure, a 6-week period of wound healing is sometimes suggested to help create sufficient gingiva for complete wound coverage. This approach carries with it a significant liability: Following tooth extraction and initial clot formation, there is competition between connective tissue and bone to replace the clot.[83] This results in alveolar crestal resorption and fill of at least two thirds of the socket fundus with trabecular bone.[83,84] Unfortunately, the nature of the immature osseous tissue at 6 weeks is such that it will not support stable fixture placement and may be mistaken for soft tissue[85] (Figs 5-5a and 5-5b).

Another disturbing observation is cited by Carlsson et al,[86] who identified the loss of approximately one third of the vestibular plate of bone in the 1-month postextraction period. Of importance is that bone resorption began 1 week after extraction, resulting in considerable thinning of the original labial plate in the first 3 weeks and complete resorption of the original plate and only partial replacement after 5 or 6 weeks (Figs 5-6a to 5-6g). Therefore, reentering such an area at 3 to 6 weeks for any purpose other than to remove an exposed barrier is not recommended. One should not expect to find the vestibular plate of bone undisturbed

if nothing constructive is done at the time of extraction.

The maxillary anterior teeth frequently demonstrate prominent roots. Tooth loss and resorption of the buccal plate converts a potential rectangular ridge to an angulated spiny configuration that compromises implant positioning (Fig 5-7). Although 30 additional days of healing provides additional soft tissue coverage for barrier protection, it is a questionable trade-off when it causes the eventual bone morphology to be unsuitable for implant placement.

Because of the above-mentioned limitation, the authors have settled on a treatment of choice. When damage to the alveolar bone is so extensive after extraction that implant placement would compromise the prosthesis, the extraction site is treated with the combined approach of bone graft and physical barrier technique (Figs 5-8a to 5-8e). The bone graft functions as a space maintainer for the desired ridge morphology and provides osteoinduction and osteoconduction.[33] The physical barrier acts according to the principles of GBR.[1,2] The dental implant is placed after 6 to 10 months of wound healing, at which time there is sufficient osseous maturity to allow uncomplicated fixture placement.[85]

Delaying implant placement to attempt augmentation of the alveolar ridge at the time of tooth extraction is not without its disadvantages. Clinical experience suggests that only 75% of the sites treated by GBR can be covered completely with soft tissue. It may be that as many as 25% of these completely covered sites will experience soft tissue dehiscence, and thus barrier exposure, early in the course of wound healing.[44] Therefore, close and frequent monitoring of the patient is mandatory for successful results. In case of exposure, the barrier is left in place and cleansed with chlorhexidine until an edge of the barrier is exposed. Removal of the barrier at this point should not disturb wound healing because histologic evaluation of the healing extraction socket has indicated that osseous healing is well underway at this point.[83–85,87] If no exposure occurs, the barrier is left in place until placement of the fixture.

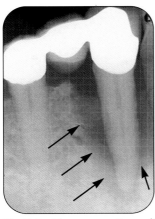

Fig 5-6a The preoperative radiograph demonstrates a periodontally compromised mandibular right canine *(arrows)*. The tooth was extracted without consideration of a regenerative procedure.

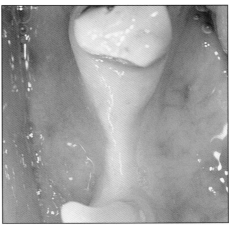

Fig 5-6b The healed edentulous ridge is too narrow to consider implant placement. The soft tissue is intact but taut and unable to cover a membrane. This is an example of ridge degeneration after extraction, which can be avoided by instituting guided bone regeneration procedures at the moment of extraction.

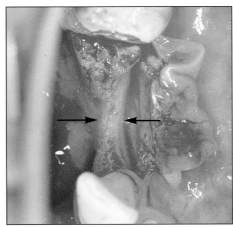

Fig 5-6c Reentry into this edentulous area reveals that the buccolingual width of bone is inadequate for implant placement *(arrows)*.

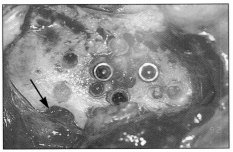

Fig 5-6d The surgical procedure has included decortication of the buccal plate and the use of Memfix screws to gain ridge enhancement. Note the mental foramen *(arrow)*. The decortication of the buccal plate allows the entities of the bone marrow spaces, including progenitor cells and vascularity, to access the area of regeneration.

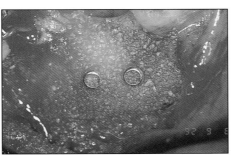

Fig 5-6e Mineralized freeze-dried bone allograft is packed to the surface of the screws.

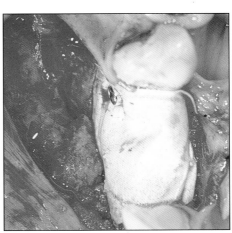

Fig 5-6f A Gore-Tex membrane is used to cover the previously described assembly and is held in place with a short Memfix screw.

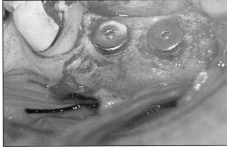

Fig 5-6g Two dental implants are placed in the regenerated ridge.

63

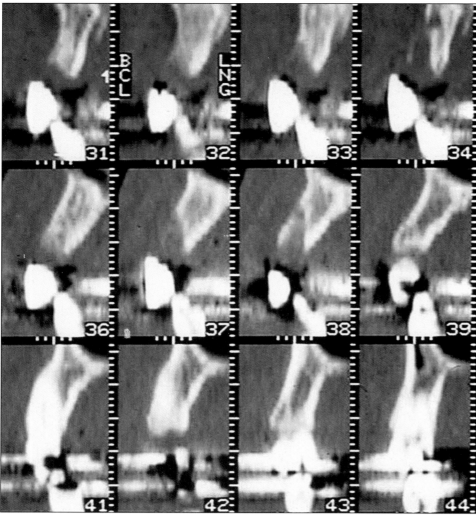

Fig 5-7 Computerized tomography scan made 30 days after extraction of prominent maxillary anterior teeth. Note the active resorption of the thin bone when there is no immediate regenerative effort (see Chapters 8, 9, 11, and 12).

The most important question to be considered is whether this new bone created by GBR can support loaded implants. To this end, a retrospective multicenter evaluation was initiated. Results revealed a remarkable record of success (Figs 5-9a to 5-9c). A failure rate of only 0.5% (2 of 349) was recorded for implants placed in a regenerated alveolar process and loaded for periods of up to 60 months.[88] This does not mean that every attempt to build bone will be successful or that all implants placed in this newly created bone were osseointegrated, but the results clearly address the issue of successful long-term loading.

O'Brien et al[89] reported on three cases in which the buccal plate of bone was destroyed after tooth extraction and successfully regenerated with the GBR technique. No bone graft was used in these naturally spacemaking defects, because the barrier appeared to be rigid enough to support itself and maintain a space into which new tissue could regenerate. The regenerated tissue was stable over a 2-year observation period.

With large ridge deformities that do not provide for natural spacemaking, some type of support for the barrier appears to be important. This support may consist of bone grafts, pins, or the combination of pins and bone grafts. Nevins and Mellonig[72] demonstrated the reconstruction of severely compromised non-spacemaking defects, using a combination of FDBA and an e-PTFE barrier to create a sufficient volume of bone to receive implants (see Figs 5-4 to 5-8). The use of FDBA provides a denser alveolar ridge than does DFDBA, which normally heals with corticocancellous bone with large marrow spaces.[90]

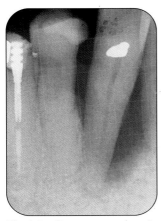

Fig 5-8a Pretreatment, there is extensive loss of the alveolar process and the tooth is mobile. Further retention jeopardizes the adjacent teeth.

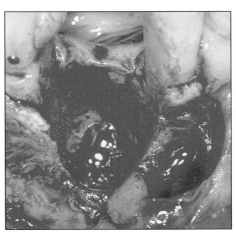

Fig 5-8b Extraction vault after degranulation. There is almost complete loss of the buccal plate, but there are some remnants still in place to help support the regenerative procedure. Now is the best time for regeneration. The marrow spaces are open and can contribute without mechanical perforation. Whatever bone remains can contribute to the regenerative process.

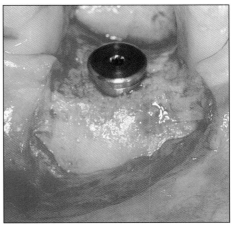

Fig 5-8c A dental implant is placed after 10 months. The regeneration was accomplished with mineralized freeze-dried bone allograft used in combination with a Gore-Tex Augmentation Membrane.

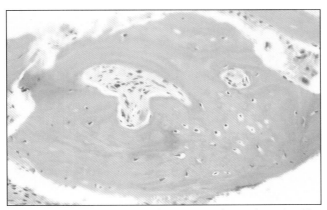

Fig 5-8d A trephine was used to prepare the implant site. The bone core demonstrates vital bone.

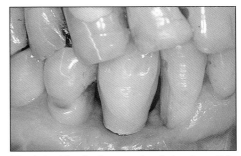

Fig 5-8e The final restoration is in place. It is loaded in occlusion and functions in lateral protrusive excursion.

The same authors demonstrated the successful reconstruction of alveolar bone destroyed by advanced periodontitis and endodontic failure.[35] Freeze-dried bone allograft, iliac cancellous bone, and marrow with GBR were used to reconstruct the alveolar ridge (Figs 5-10a to 5-10f). This treatment results in a sufficient bone volume to allow for uncompromised and esthetic implant placement. This outcome renders the GBR procedure as a staged event to be more than feasible and effective for the majority of patients.

Other types of graft material have been used. Several reports have indicated that the combination of DFDBA and GBR can augment a deficient alveolar ridge.[38,44,56] Likewise, collagen[1,2,43] and HA have been used successfully.[66] The principle of GBR combined with autogenous bone grafting can also be applied for localized ridge augmentation in a staged approach[35,91] (Figs 5-11a to 5-11d). Buser et al[91] used corticocancellous autogenous bone harvested from the retromolar area as a barrier-supporting device and an osteoconductive scaffold. The importance of proper placement of the barrier, its stabilization with miniscrews, and adequate wound closure to favorable results was emphasized. Furthermore, the authors indicated that primary soft tissue closure without barrier exposure is essential to prevent infection in the barrier site and to maintain the barrier function during the entire bone-healing period. Although early barrier removal may compromise results, it does not preclude successful alveolar ridge augmentation.[35,72]

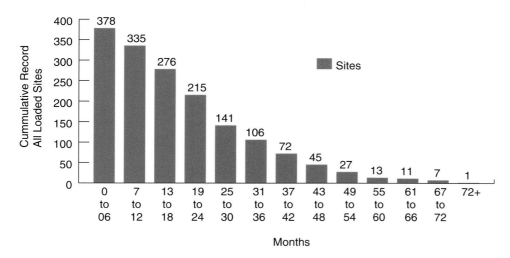

Fig 5-9a Implants placed in bone created by guided bone regeneration. Three hundred seventy-eight implants were included in the study. Eleven have been loaded for 5 years and 141 for 2 years.

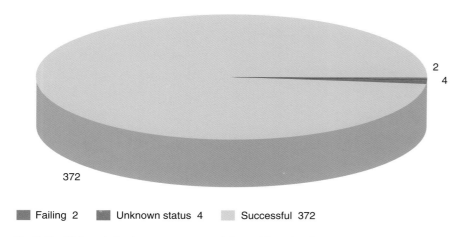

Failing 2   Unknown status 4   Successful 372

Fig 5-9b All but six implants are accounted for and functional.

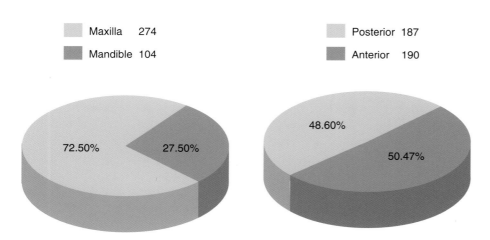

Maxilla   274   Posterior 187

Mandible 104   Anterior   190

Fig 5-9c Similar numbers of implants were placed in the anterior and posterior segments.

Figs 5-9a to 5-9c From Nevins M, Hanratty JJ, Nevins ML. Transfer of a gingival allograft between indentical twins. Int J Periodont Rest Dent 1991;11:25-32. Reprinted with permission.

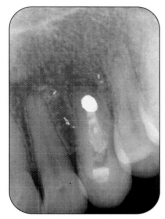

Fig 5-10a The maxillary left canine has undergone four apicoectomy procedures.

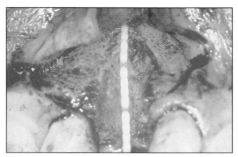

Fig 5-10b Surgical exposure reveals that no buccal plate is present.

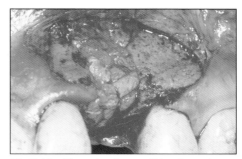

Fig 5-10c The extraction vault has been decorticated and packed with autogenous iliac crest bone.

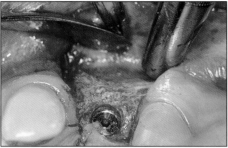

Fig 5-10d The area was treated with a dental implant after 1 year. Note the bone structure on the buccal surface that has been regenerated as a result of the combined use of a bone graft and a membrane. The membrane was removed after 2 months because of an exposure.

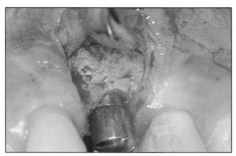

Fig 5-10e At the time of abutment placement, the buccal plate of bone appears identical to that at the time of implant placement, and the threads of the implant are completely covered.

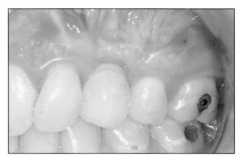

Fig 5-10f The final crown is in place. It functions in centric and lateral protrusive excursion. (Prosthesis by Dr Janice Conrad.)

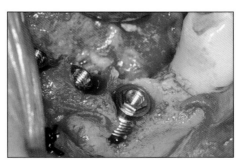

Fig 5-11a The buccal surface of the implant placed in an incomplete extraction wound is exposed and the threads are exposed.

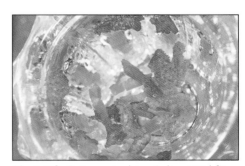

Fig 5-11b Autogenous bone is harvested from the twist drills during the drilling procedures.

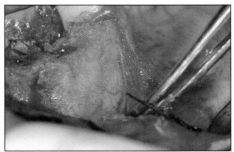

Fig 5-11c The bone is grafted over the exposed surface of the implant. The bone graft was covered with a Gore-Tex Augmentation Membrane.

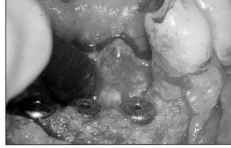

Fig 5-11d At the second-stage surgery, 5 months later, the exposed threads are completely covered with bone.

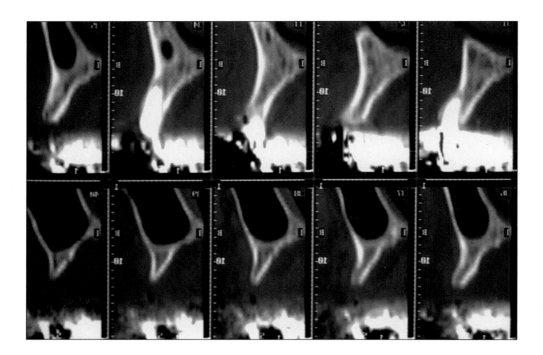

Fig 5-12a Computerized tomography reveals a narrow edentulous ridge in the maxillary premolar region. It is in the form of an isosceles triangle; this permits the expansion of the occlusal portion of bone and retains the wider base of bone to stabilize the implant.

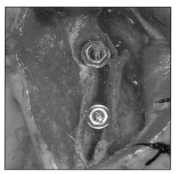

Fig 5-12b The cortical plates have been separated to create sufficient width for implant place-

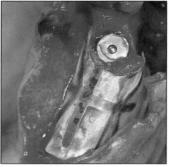

Fig 5-12c The split ridge, bone allograft, and implants are covered with a titanium-reinforced Gore-Tex membrane.

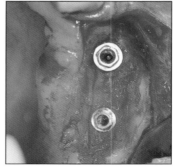

Fig 5-12d The second-stage surgery reveals mature bone filling the space between the cortical plates and in intimate contact with the implants.

Besides bone grafts, barrier-supporting devices such as miniscrews or pins are an alternative.[1,34,38,92] Buser et al[1,92] reported on several cases in which small fixation screws were used to support the barrier like a tent pole to secure the created space underneath the barrier and prevent collapse into the defect. Tension-free flaps and a healing period of 6 to 10 months were recommended to obtain a sufficient volume of bone for implant placement.

Likewise, absorbable orthodontic pins (polydioxanone) have been used to secure a space beneath the barrier.[34] Three defects treated with this technique were completely resolved, and implants were successfully placed in the augmented ridges. This type of pin should be used only with caution, because osteolytic lesions have been reported to result from use of biodegradable pins of polyglycolide or lactide-glycolide copolymer for internal fixation of a variety of orthopedic bone fractures.[93]

The combination of mechanical support and bone grafting is also used to augment large alveolar ridge defects. The combination of collagen, autogenous bone, FDBA, DFDBA with fixation pins, and GBR was reported to stabilize the blood clot beneath the barrier and provide additional scaffolding to ensure adequate space maintenance.[1,35,38,43,91]

A unique method for jawbone enlargement using an immediate implant placement has been reported.[94] Five patients with sufficient vertical ridge height but insufficient bone width for implant placement were treated with a split-ridge technique (Figs 5-12a to 5-12d). Implants were inserted between the two cortical plates and covered with an e-PTFE barrier. Biometric examination showed a gain in bone width, varying from 1.0 to 4.0 mm. Histologic evaluation showed regeneration of bone tissue between the two portions of the split crest.

The possibility for vertical ridge augmentation was investigated by Simion et al[95] (see Chapter 8). Five patients received 15 implants, which protruded 4 to 7 mm from the bone crest. Pure titanium miniscrews (1.3 × 10 mm) were positioned distally 3 to 4 mm from the bone level to evaluate osseointegration. The implants and the miniscrews were covered with a titanium-reinforced barrier of e-PTFE, and the flaps were sutured. The barriers were removed at stage 2 surgery after 9 months of healing. Measurements of biopsy specimens showed a gain in bone height of 3 to 4 mm. Histologic examination revealed that all retrieved miniscrews were in direct contact with bone. The results suggest that the placement of implants in a supracrestal position and treatment with GBR may result in vertical bone formation to the top of the implant cylinder and that the regenerated bone is able to be osseointegrated with pure titanium implants.

The successful treatment of a large, endodontically induced periradicular defect and soft tissue fenestration with combined endodontic therapy and GBR has been described.[96,97] The root apices were resected, retrograde alloy fillings were placed, defects were thoroughly debrided, and the exposed root surfaces were planed. Demineralized freeze-dried bone allograft was inserted into the periradicular defects and covered with an e-PTFE barrier. At 6 to 7 months, the barriers were removed. Complete bone regeneration resulted. Biopsy specimens from the grafted bone site exhibited mature lamellar bone.[96]

The results of the studies evaluating GBR for localized ridge augmentation indicate that:

1. Localized ridge augmentation with GBR is a predictable and successful technique for regenerating a sufficient volume of bone for implant placement.
2. The combination of GBR and autograft, GBR and allograft, and GBR and mechanical support are equally effective in reconstruction of lost bone in deficient alveolar ridges.
3. Extensive alveolar ridge defects may require the combination of mechanical support, grafting materials, and a barrier to produce satisfactory results.
4. The use of a barrier alone is effective in naturally spacemaking defects but may not provide adequate space in large osseous lesions or extensive ridge deformities.
5. Premature exposure of the barrier is a complicating factor but does not always result in poor ridge augmentation.
6. Large periradicular defects can be successfully treated with bone grafts used in combination with a barrier.

Failing Implants

A dental implant usually fails for one of two reasons, bacterial infection or occlusal trauma, and the condition is referred to as *peri-implantitis*. If the etiology cannot be corrected, the implant has failed and can no longer be considered as failing or ailing.

Microbiologic analysis of implants failing because of infection reveals a subgingival microbial flora in which spirochetes and motile rods average 42% of the total morphotypes, with a predominance of *Peptostreptococcus micros*, *Fusobacterium*, and gram-negative rods.[98] In contrast, implants failing because of a traumatogenic etiology usually have a problem related directly to the implant itself (mobility, fracture, or occlusal load). If the etiology is reversible, recovery is possible. Residual osseous defects may be treated with GBR.

Meffert and others have indicated that detoxification of the implant surface is important to the recovery process.[45,99–104] If the contaminated implant surface is coated with HA and is pitted, cracked, or exhibits a change in color, it is suggested that first the HA coating be removed with an ultrasonic instrument and then the implant be detoxified with citric acid (pH 1; 40% concentration) for 30 seconds to 1 minute. An HA-coated surface that is contaminated but does not exhibit visible surface alteration need only be treated with citric acid for no longer than 30 seconds. Longer treatment periods will adversely affect the calcium-phosphate ratios and the crystallinity of HA.[103] Titanium surfaces can be burnished with citric acid for 3 minutes or preferably with tetracycline (50 mg/mL) for 3 minutes.[45,99,100,102,103] Rinsing with chlorhexidine solution (0.12%) is also recommended.[98,99] However, the negative effects of chlorhexidine on fibroblasts may negate this detoxification method.[105,106]

Some studies in animals have supported the hypothesis that bone defects resulting from plaque-induced peri-implantitis can be treated with GBR,[10] while one study does not.[107] Guided bone regeneration procedures, used alone or combined with bone grafts, have been suggested as a means of regenerating lost osseous tissue in humans.[10,45,99,100,108,109]

The combination of GBR regenerative procedures and antimicrobial therapy may be a successful treatment approach for restoring the osseointegration of dental implants following bone loss caused by infection.[108] The defects, as well as the rough implant surfaces, were rinsed several times with 0.1% chlorhexidine solution, alternated with sterile saline solution. Clinical measurements confirmed the radiographic evidence of bone fill by demonstrating new tissue resistant to probing in close contact to the implant surface at the site of the previous defect. Chlorhexidine (0.12%) was also used in two cases to detoxify implants with severe peri-implantitis. Subsequently, e-PTFE barriers were adapted around the necks of the implants and flaps were sutured. The radiographic analysis 1 year after barrier removal revealed 2 to 4 mm of bone gain.

Ten implants with peri-implantitis and vertical bone loss were treated with GBR procedures following detoxification of the implant surface with an air-powder abrasive and a

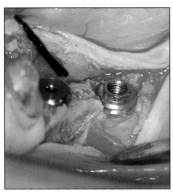

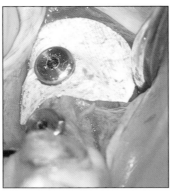

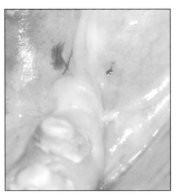

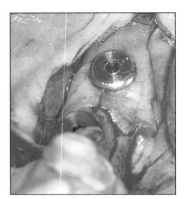

Fig 5-13a An implant is placed in a fresh extraction wound. There are proximal voids and exposed threads that must be covered with bone.

Fig 5-13b A Gore-Tex Augmentation Membrane is fitted and stabilized to cover all discrepancies. The proximal defects will be naturally space making within the envelope of bone.

Fig 5-13c The soft tissues have remained intact until second-stage surgery.

Fig 5-13d The area is reentered with the membrane in place.

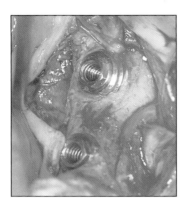

Fig 5-13e The membrane is removed. The proximal implant margins are covered by bone, but the threads remain exposed. The problem is considered to be one of space maintenance.

10% solution of chloramine-T.[10] The results showed a clinical reduction in probing depth and radiographic bone fill in seven of 10 peri-implant defects. Mellonig et al[109] reported on three cases of treatment of the failing implant. The defects were debrided and the implant surface was detoxified with tetracycline (50 mg/mL) for 3 minutes. Demineralized freeze-dried bone allograft was inserted into the osseous defects and covered with a barrier of e-PTFE in accordance with the principles of GBR. The barrier was removed 6 to 8 weeks after placement. Eight months to 1 year posttreatment, clinical, radiographic, and reentry documentation demonstrated that all sites had a substantial reduction in probing depth, a gain of clinical attachment, and bone fill adjacent to the implants.

Outcomes in this limited number of clinical case reports suggest that peri-implantitis is reversible. However, the application of the technique has yet to be proved predictable. The small number of reported failures makes it difficult to establish the boundaries of treatment and results that should be anticipated.

Barrier Exposure

It was first postulated by Becker and Becker[47] that the barrier should remain covered until retrieval at the abutment procedure to enhance bone formation adjacent to the implant. In a subsequent multicenter study, 49 implants in 49 patients were placed in immediate extraction sites and covered by e-PTFE barriers. Twenty of the barriers became exposed and were removed before stage 2 surgery. At the time of abutment connection, implants that remained covered until the abutment connection demonstrated significant bone fill and minimal implant thread exposure. Sites at which barriers were prematurely removed because of exposure showed less bone formation. The authors concluded that e-PTFE barriers will promote statistically significant amounts of bone around implants placed in fresh extraction sites. Retention of the barrier until the abutment-stage surgery improves the amount of bone promoted around implants but does not guarantee complete bone fill.

Others have also noted that exposure of the barrier material and subsequent inflammatory response requires premature removal of the barrier material.[62,63] Barrier exposure was associated with significantly smaller amounts of regenerated bone than was found at membrane-retained sites,[62,63,110,111] but the difference may not be significant when the clinical result is observed (Figs 5-13a to 5-13e). Histologic examination of newly formed tissue following barrier exposure shows the full range of wound healing: bone regeneration, connective tissue regeneration with intermittent bone regeneration, fibrous healing, and inflammatory granulation tissue formation.[61]

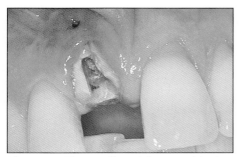

Fig 5-14a The maxillary right central incisor crown is missing. The fistula above the root will prevent coverage of a membrane.

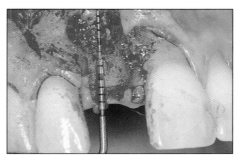

Fig 5-14b The extraction vault exhibits no buccal plate and a circular periapical bone defect.

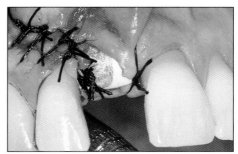

Fig 5-14c Treatment includes placement of mineralized freeze-dried bone allograft and a Gore-Tex regeneration membrane. It is not possible to cover the membrane, which was removed at 5 weeks.

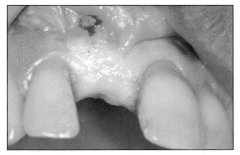

Fig 5-14d Edentulous ridge at second-stage surgery. There has been no gingival augmentation procedure.

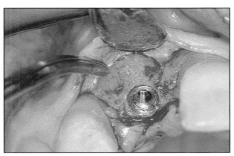

Fig 5-14e At second-stage surgery, the level of regenerated bone allows the implant to be placed near the approximating cementoenamel junctions. (Prosthesis by Dr James Stein.)

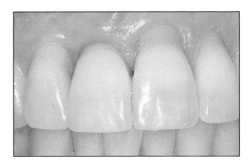

Fig 5-14f The final implant crown is in place. (Prosthesis by Dr James Stein.)

Further evidence for the significance of barrier exposure during wound healing was generated in a comparative study of the effectiveness of e-PTFE membranes with and without exposure during the healing period.[60] Two implants were placed in each of five patients. One implant was placed 30 to 40 days after tooth extraction to ensure complete coverage of the barrier by soft tissue. The other implant was inserted immediately after tooth extraction so as to leave the barrier exposed. Exposed barriers were removed 30 to 45 days after placement. At sites with no exposure, there was 97% bone fill, and four of five sites demonstrated complete remission of the bone defect. At sites with exposed barriers, there was only 42% bone fill; all sites had incomplete bone fill.

Although these studies strongly indicate that complete wound closure over the barrier is extremely important, premature exposure of the barrier does not always preclude success. As reported in one series of case reports, 18 of 63 barriers were prematurely removed because of exposure. All but two of these sites were considered to be successful[44] (Figs 5-14a to 5-14f).

Simion et al[112] examined the possibility that oral bacteria could migrate through the occlusive portion of e-PTFE barriers and demonstrated that contaminated barriers exhibit partial penetration of the bacteria through the barrier within 2 to 3 weeks. After 4 weeks of exposure, complete bacterial penetration and contamination of the inner surface takes place. If the external surface of the barrier is mechanically debrided with the aid of chlorhexidine, complete invasion of bacteria and initial colonization of the barrier's inner surface may be modified.[113] A relatively simple flora, consisting mainly of cocci and short rods, was found in bacterial deposits forming under the influence of chlorhexidine; in untreated specimens, it was possible to observe a more mature and complex plaque, composed of mostly filamentous bacteria.[113] Therefore, after a period of 4 weeks, prematurely exposed barriers should probably be removed to prevent bacterial infection of the underlying regenerating tissue.

Although evidence indicates that premature exposure may have a deleterious influence on bone fill, this does not mean that sites with an exposed barrier cannot attain complete bone fill.[35,44,56,72,79] The lack of primary closure or premature exposure of the barrier does not necessarily affect the regenerative result if a regimen of close follow-up and diligent oral hygiene is followed.[79]

Bioresorbable Barriers

There are limited reports on bioresorbable barriers and GBR.[51,65,114,115,116] Lundgren et al[65] reported on the use of a bioresorbable barrier in four patients with six implant exposures after placement. Four of the defects were non-spacemaking and required autogenous bone chips for support. At the abutment connection, 6 to 7 months after surgery, complete bone fill was found in four defects (two with and two without bone chips) and partial fill in two defects with bone chips. The results suggest that a bioresorbable barrier, composed of polylactic acid, may be used for GBR. It is strongly emphasized that in particular situations related to defect morphology, the barrier needs separate support to prevent its collapse into the bone defect or onto the implant surface.

A study in dogs evaluated the use of a bioresorbable barrier in accordance with the principles of GBR.[117] Non-spacemaking dehiscence-type defects were surgically created in the mandibles of dogs. Root-form threaded titanium implants were inserted. The osseous defects randomly received treatment with a bioresorbable barrier composed of a copolymer of lactide and glycolide, an e-PTFE barrier, or no barrier. Clinical and histologic results after 3½ months of wound healing indicated that exposed threads were covered with bone when treated with an e-PTFE barrier but only minimally covered when treated with the bioresorbable barrier or the control. The results imply that the mechanical properties of bioresorbable barriers are incapable of creating and maintaining a secluded space to promote bone formation and prevent soft tissue ingrowth. A follow-up study using a similar methodology demonstrated that the use of DFDBA as support for the bioresorbable barrier substantially improved clinical and histologic results[118] (Figs 5-15a to 5-15f).

The advantage of a bioresorbable barrier is that the second-stage surgical procedure can be limited to the implant placement or abutment connection, thus avoiding the need for barrier removal. However, the early bioresorption and/or lack of stiffness of these barriers appears to be a significant mechanical limitation because barriers must possess a certain stiffness to prevent them from collapsing into the defect and to allow a defined period of undisturbed wound healing.[7,119] Because the bioresorbable barriers do not have space-maintaining properties for bone augmentation, bone grafts are needed to support the barrier in non-spacemaking defects. Future bioresorbable materials may overcome these disadvantages, but the need to reenter the area surgically for implant placement neutralizes the advantage of using a bioresorbable barrier for GBR.

Bone Graft Materials for GBR

In the majority of studies regarding implants in fresh extraction sites, implants with osseous dehiscence or fenestration defects, and localized ridge augmentations, autogenous or allogeneic bone grafts are used in non-spacemaking situations. However, the freeze-dried allografts are used most often.

Bone Autografts

Particulate autogenous bone, harvested intraorally from the surgical area in which the regenerative procedure is performed, has been recommended as a graft material to help support the barrier[65] (see Figs 5-10 and 5-11). Autogenous cortical blocks from the mandibular symphysis or retromolar area have also been recommended[85,120–122] (see Chapter 15). The popularity of autogenous grafts is based on the possibility of maintenance of cellular viability,[123] but this depends on the rapid revascularization of the autograft, which in turn depends on the thickness of the graft.[124] The more dense (cortical) and thicker the autograft, the less the possibility of revascularization and the greater the possibility of cell death.[124,125]

Besides being technically demanding and time consuming, autografts from the mandibular symphysis or retromolar area pose the possibility of neurosensory disturbances.[126] It is frequently difficult to obtain a sufficient quantity and quality of autogenous bone from other intraoral donor sites to fill large or multiple osseous defects.[125] The additional surgical site for graft procurement and patient morbidity are other limitations of autografts.

Bone Allografts

Freeze-dried bone allografts are available in sufficient quantities, can be maintained on the shelf until ready for use, are resorbed and replaced by host bone, and can induce new bone formation.[32] The potential of FDBA to enhance new bone in intraoral alveolar sites has been demonstrated in field tests.[127–129] The antigenicity of FDBA in intraoral osseous defects was determined by microcytotoxicity assays in both animals and humans.[130,131] Results indicated that there was markedly less humoral and cell-mediated immune response to FDBA than to a fresh bone allograft.[130] At no time could any specific donor anti-HLA antibodies be detected in any patient.[131] These conclusions are consistent with the long history of clinical safety associated with FDBA.

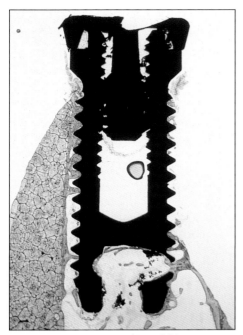

Fig 5-15a Non-spacemaking dehiscence-type defect treated only with flap replacement (control).

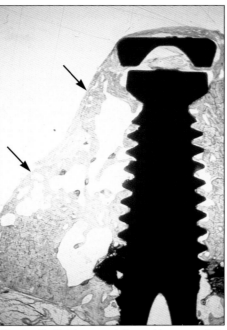

Fig 5-15b Dehiscence defect with exposed titanium implant threads treated with guided bone regeneration with an e-PTFE barrier. New bone formation *(arrows)*.

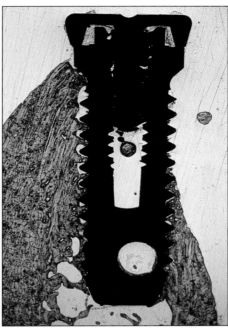

Fig 5-15c Dehiscence defect treated with a bioresorbable barrier demonstrating minimal new bone formation over previously exposed titanium implant threads.

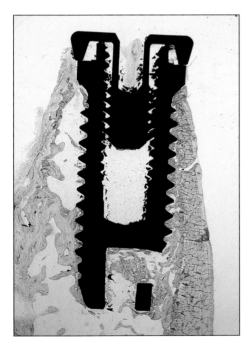

Fig 5-15d Dehiscence defect treated with a bioresorbable barrier and decalcified freeze-dried bone allograft. Extensive new bone formation, equal to that observed with a non-bioresorbable barrier, can be noted.

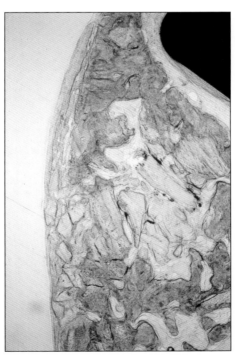

Fig 5-15e Dehiscence defect treated with an e-PTFE barrier and decalcified freeze-dried bone allograft. Extensive new bone formation can be noted on and about the previously exposed implant.

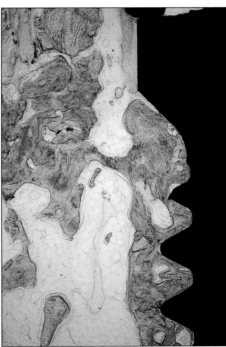

Fig 5-15f Note the intimate contact of new bone with consecutive implant threads.

Numerous experiments in animals have indicated that demineralization of a cortical bone graft induces new bone formation and greatly enhances its osteogenic potential.[132–134] This type of bone allograft, as commercially available from a tissue bank, is known as *DFDBA*. Demineralization with hydrochloric acid exposes the bone-inductive proteins located in the bone matrix.[135,136] These proteins are collectively called *bone morphogenetic protein* (BMP).[137] They are composed of a group of acidic polypeptides that have been cloned and sequenced.[138] Bone morphogenetic protein stimulates the formation of new bone by osteoinduction.[139] The demineralized graft induces host cells to differentiate into osteoblasts,[140] whereas FDBA functions by osteoconduction as it affords a scaffold for new bone formation. However, a few researchers have questioned the osteogenic potential of DFDBA.[141–143]

The healing sequence of DFDBA has been identified as a sequential developmental cascade.[144] The cascade includes activation and migration of undifferentiated mesenchymal cells by chemotaxis; anchorage-dependent cell attachment to the bone matrix via fibronectin; mitosis and proliferation of mesenchymal cells; differentiation of cartilage; mineralization of the cartilage; vascular invasion and chondrolysis; differentiation of osteoblasts and deposition of bone matrix; and finally mineralization of bone and differentiation of hemopoietic marrow in the newly developed ossicle. Therefore, new bone formed from a graft of DFDBA will result in corticocancellous bone with hematopoietic marrow. This type of bone may not be of a sufficient density to allow implant placement but may be suitable for growth around implants that have already been placed.

Because FDBA heals by osteoconduction, the cortical bone particles take a long time to be resorbed and replaced by new host bone.[145] The end result is a healed graft site composed mainly of cortical bone. For this reason, FDBA is preferred for localized ridge augmentation and for other defects in which implants are to be placed.

Another study in humans compared the ability of autogenous bone and DFDBA to enhance bone formation around dental implants placed in recent extraction sites.[146] The histologic results demonstrated that GBR techniques are capable of producing new bone osseointegrated with titanium implants. Among the graft materials, autogenous bone provided the densest and greatest amount of new bone, but DFDBA also improved bone regeneration compared to the barrier alone after 6 months of healing.

Safety of Bone Allografts

The possible transmission of infectious diseases by the transplantation of contaminated tissue is an overriding concern of clinicians and patients alike. Viral, bacterial, and fungal infections have been transmitted via a variety of tissue allografts, such as bone, skin, cornea, heart valves, whole organs, blood, and semen.[147,148] Human immunodeficiency virus (HIV), hepatitis B virus (HBV), hepatitis C virus (HCV), bacterial infection, and the prion responsible for Creutzfeldt-Jakob disease (CJD) are the most widely discussed agents and form the basis for concern in the dental and medical communities and the media.[149] Over the past decade, improvements in donor-screening criteria, such as excluding potential donors with infection and those with behaviors risky for HIV-1 and hepatitis infection, and the introduction of new donor blood tests, have greatly reduced the risk of transmission of HIV and hepatitis and have nearly eliminated the risk of transmission of CJD.

It is important to recognize that not all allografts are alike, and they cannot be considered as a unit when safety is discussed. There are several types of bone allografts: fresh-frozen, FDBA, and DFDBA. It is estimated that 500,000 bone allograft procedures are performed in the United States annually. Approximately 200,000 of these are for dental purposes. To date, no incidents of disease transfer from FDBA or DFDBA have been reported over the 25-year history of these materials. However, the concern of a potential risk for disease transmission unrealistically persists.

Procurement and Processing

More than 85% of the allografts implanted are processed by six tissue banks in the United States.[150] This fact alone provides some measure of safety. The first step in the procurement of allogeneic bone involves the selection of an acceptable donor. The development of exclusionary criteria for donor procurement has provided a significant degree of safety for the transplantation of disease-free allografts of all types. It is calculated that the chance of obtaining a fresh or frozen bone allograft from an HIV-infected donor whom screening techniques failed to exclude is one in 1.67 million.[151] Donors from high-risk groups are excluded by medical and social screening. Unless reliable information regarding previous hospitalizations, blood transfusions, serious illnesses, and lifestyle can be ascertained, the donor must be regarded as unacceptable.

Donors are screened by HIV antibody and antigen testing. An autopsy is sometimes performed to rule out occult disease, such as carcinoma. Special lymph node studies beyond those usually performed at autopsy are accomplished. Such studies are performed to recognize changes characteristic of early HIV infection and provide another opportunity to exclude individuals with morphologic nodal changes typical of nonspecific infection (eg, bacterial, viral, parasitic, fungal, and chronic infection or drug abuse). Blood cultures are done to rule out bacterial contamination. Serologic tests for syphilis and all types of hepatitis are performed. Follow-up studies of grafts from the same donor are done. A third of the donors are concomitant donors of vital organs such as heart, kidneys, and liver. With the exception of fresh bone allografts, months usually pass between procurement and the clinical use of a processed bone allograft. If a vital organ recipient were identified as being HIV seropositive or as having AIDS or another related illness, the bone from the donor would not be released for clinical use.

To ensure sterile material, bone allografts are procured in a sterile manner, usually within 12 hours of death of the donor. After this period, there is a significant increase in the incidence of bacterial contamination. If bacterially contaminated, the bone is subjected to secondary means of sterilization. Irradiation and ethylene oxide are currently used as end-stage sterilizing agents. Although the use of irradiation is controversial,[152–159] it is generally agreed that doses higher than 2.0 to 2.5 megarads of gamma irradiation are destructive to new bone formation.[156]

Ethylene oxide, a powerful alkylating agent, also has significant deleterious effects on bone induction.[157,158] An ethylene oxide sterilization procedure of sufficient dose to kill spores will render a bone allograft incapable of inducing new bone formation. Furthermore, residual levels of ethylene oxide will cause morphologic changes in fibroblasts cocultured with the allograft.[158]

Although the processing of a freeze-dried bone allograft varies from tissue bank to tissue bank, it usually includes the following steps:

1. Cortical bone is harvested in a sterile manner. Long bones are the source for mineralized freeze-dried bone allograft and demineralized or decalcified freeze-dried bone allograft. The cortical bone is harvested because it has been found to be less antigenic than cancellous bone.[159] Because the bone-inductive proteins are located in the bone matrix,[160,161] and because cortical bone has more bone matrix than cancellous bone, cortical bone is the material of choice.

2. All soft tissue is removed from the bones. Cortical bone is rough cut to a particle size ranging from 500 μm to 5 mm and subjected to repeated washings to remove the bone marrow. This fragmentation increases the efficiency of defatting bone and subsequent decalcification, if the bone is to be demineralized.

3. The graft is then immersed in 99+% ethanol for 1 hour to remove fat that may inhibit osteogenesis.[162] Viral infectivity is undetectable within 1 minute of treatment with 70% ethanol.[163] This procedure may be repeated at various stages during processing.

4. Bones are frozen in liquid nitrogen for 1 or 2 weeks to interrupt the degradation process. During this time, the results from bacterial cultures, serologic tests, and antibody and antigen tests are analyzed. If contamination is found, the bones are discarded or, more likely, sterilized by irradiation or ethylene oxide.

5. Sterile graft material free of infectious agents is now freeze dried. Freeze drying is a process in which dehydration is achieved by removing water directly from the frozen state to vapor state and by sublimination.[164] Freeze drying removes more than 95% of the moisture content from the bone. Although freeze drying kills all cells (the bone lacunae become empty spaces), it facilitates long-term storage.

6. The cortical bone is ground and sieved to a particle size of approximately 250 to 750 μm. Particle sizes within this range have been shown to promote osteogenesis.[165,166] Particles smaller than 125 μm are quickly engulfed by multinucleated foreign-body giant cells.[165]

7. If the bone allograft is to be decalcified, it is immersed in 0.6 N hydrochloric acid. Demineralization removes the calcium and exposes the BMP. This step is not necessary if FDBA is the desired end product. Cortical FDBA has the same amount of BMP as does DFDBA, but the calcium must be biologically removed over a long period of time before induction can take place.

8. The bone is washed in a sodium phosphate buffer to remove residual acid. Repeated washings with various solutions are frequently done throughout the processing.

9. If the bone is demineralized, it is freeze dried again. Some banks arrange the processing steps so that only a single freeze-drying cycle is necessary.

10. The graft material is vacuum sealed in vials to protect against contamination and degradation of the material and to permit storage at room temperature for an indefinite period of time.

Disease Transmission

Human Immunodeficiency Virus

Laboratory tests for the detection of HIV are mandatory for the screening of bone allograft donors. An enzyme-linked immunosorbant assay (ELISA) has been used as the standard test to detect the presence of HIV antibody.[167] The major disadvantage to the ELISA test is that there may be a prolonged period of time between infection with the virus and seroconversion with subsequent development of antibodies to HIV. Based on blood bank data, the chance of a patient's having a negative reaction to the ELISA antibody test and yet being a carrier of HIV has been estimated at 1 in 40,000 to 1 in 153,000.[168,169] Another test that is now used for HIV screening is based on polymerase chain reaction (PCR) technology. The PCR test is extremely accurate in the detection of donors who are HIV carriers.[170] The PCR test provides the most reliable screen possible.

There are four known cases of HIV transmission from a fresh bone allograft donor.[171] There has never been a reported case of disease transfer from FDBA or DFDBA, both of which are viewed as posing less risk for viral transmission than large, unprocessed fresh-frozen osteochondral allografts. This perceived reduction in risk is attributed to an expectation that the chemical agents used in the processing, such as ethanol and hydrochloric acid, have a virucidal effect on tissue-borne HIV.

The ability of chemical agents to inactivate HIV under clinical and laboratory conditions is well known.[163,172] Exposure of 7 to 10 logs of infectious viral dose to alcohol at 70% concentration inactivated HIV to below detectable levels within 1 minute.[163] It has been demonstrated that ethanol will completely penetrate cortical bone (5.5 × 2.5 cm) within 15 minutes following introduction of this virucidal agent.[173] Further evidence of the effectiveness of chemical decontamination was gathered through a study in monkeys.[174] Bone contaminated with the simian immunodeficiency virus (SIV) was either processed with ethanol or frozen before implantation. All monkeys receiving unprocessed frozen bone allograft tested positive for SIV within 2 weeks. No animal receiving ethanol-treated bone became infected with SIV.

Furthermore, exposure of HIV to a low pH, such as that obtained with 0.6 N hydrochloric acid, will inactivate the virus.[172,175] Strongly acidic solutions have been shown to disrupt the phosphodiester bonds of nucleic acids.[176] It has been demonstrated that HIV, HBV, HCV, cytomegalic virus, and the polio virus can be inactivated by the demineralization process used to prepare DFDBA. Reports indicated that freezing[177] and freeze drying[178] may also reduce the infectivity of HIV.

Additional evidence that FDBA and DFDBA are safe for human implantation is provided by a study in which bone free of HIV and bone contaminated with HIV were tested for viral activity.[179] Both spiked bone and infected bone were treated with a virucidal agent and demineralization. Replication of viable HIV could not be demonstrated after treatment. Even if an HIV-infected donor could escape detection by the various exclusionary techniques, processing with a virucidal agent such as ethanol, hydrochloric acid, or other suitable chemical agents will render the bone allograft safe for human implantation. The probability that a particular brand of DFDBA contains HIV has been calculated to be one in 2.8 billion.[180]

Hepatitis

Hepatitis A is spread by person-to-person contact, and is highly unlikely to be transmitted in tissues.[181] In addition, hepatitis A is usually a mild subclinical illness and is unlikely to result in a chronic carrier state. Patients who have a history of hepatitis A are eliminated as allograft donors.

Hepatitis B is almost always transmitted by blood, blood products, and semen. Screening is mandatory. The standard test for hepatitis B is hepatitis B surface antigen test (HBsAG). As with HIV, there is a window of approximately 6 weeks between infection and development of the antibody. However, combined with the fact that acute hepatitis B infection is an easily recognizable condition, screening of donors by blood testing, history, and physical examination provides a very sensitive evaluation. A test for the presence of antibody to hepatitis B surface antigen (anti-HBs) is also performed, because the level of this antibody begins to peak at about 6 months after infection.[182] An additional test is used for antibody to hepatitis B core antigen (anti-HBc), which can be found in all but the earliest phases of HBV infection, is detectable in more than 95% of HBsAG-positive donors, and may be the only marker for hepatitis B infection.[183]

Hepatitis C (non-A, non-B hepatitis) is the chief cause of posttransfusion hepatitis.[181] Screening is mandatory. The standard test is antibody to hepatitis C virus (anti-HCV). The introduction of PCR in testing for HCV has improved screening methods.[184] Alcohol will inactivate HCV because it is a lipid-containing virus.[149]

Syphilis

Syphilis, caused by the spirochete *Treponema pallidum*, is not known to be transmissible in bone or soft tissue. The causative agent is sensitive to antibiotics, heat, and drying. Tissue banks test for syphilis mostly because blood banks have historically tested for syphilis.[167] The tests generally used include the rapid plasma reagin test, the Venereal Disease Research Laboratory test, and the fluorescent treponemal antibody absorption test.

Bacterial Infection

Bacterial infection was reported in 7% of a series of 303 applications of small freeze-dried bone allografts.[185] Twelve of the 21 infections were minor infections characterized by local wound erythema. Therefore, the overall incidence was 4%. The most commonly isolated organism was *Staphylococcus epidermidis*. Cultures from only one of 11 patients who had positive wound cultures showed the same bacterium that had been cultured postoperatively from the allograft.[185] The allograft infection rate compares favorably with the 4% infection rate reported for autogenous bone grafts.[186]

Creutzfeldt-Jakob Disease

Creutzfeldt-Jakob disease is a slow, progressive encephalopathy. It is caused by a prion, a novel self-replication protein, and is the smallest known infectious particle.[187] In the United States and Europe, the estimated crude annual incidence is one case in 1 million.[188] The principle routes of disease transmission are through infected neurologic tissue such as dura mater, pituitary growth hormone, and cornea.[147] Bone is not known to have transmitted CJD. The exclusion of donors with a past medical history of neurologic disease or surgery renders the possibility of CJD disease transfer with a bone allograft to the realm of academic interest only.

Conclusion

Although there is much concern about the risk of disease transfer with FDBA and DFDBA, these concerns are unfounded. There has never been a case of disease transfer with FDBA of DFDBA in the 25-year history of these materials. Exclusionary techniques and chemical processing of the allogeneic bone render freeze-dried bone allografts safe for human use.

References

1. Buser D, Bragger U, Lang NP, Nyman S. Regeneration and enlargement of jawbone using guided tissue regeneration. Clin Oral Implants Res 1990;1:22–32.

2. Nyman S, Lang NP, Buser D, Bragger U. Bone regeneration adjacent to titanium dental implants using guided tissue regeneration: A report of two cases. Int J Oral Maxillofac Implants 1990;5:9–14.

3. Murray C, Holden R, Roachlau W. Experimental and clinical study of new growth of bone in a cavity. Am J Surg 1957;95:385–387.

4. Melcher AH, Dreyer CY. Protection of the blood clot in healing circumscribed bone defects. J Bone Joint Surg 1962;44B:424–430.

5. Boyne PJ. Regeneration of alveolar bone beneath cellulose acetate filter implants [abstract]. J Dent Res 1964;43:827.

6. Dahlin C, Gottlow J, Linde A, Nyman S. Healing of maxillary and mandibular bone defects using a membrane technique. An experimental study in monkeys. Scand J Plast Reconstr Surg 1990;24:13–19.

7. Schenk RK, Buser D, Hardwick WR, Dahlin C. Healing pattern of bone regeneration in membrane-protected defects. A histologic study in the canine mandible. Int J Oral Maxillofac Implants 1994;9:13–29.

8. Linde A, Alberius P, Dahlin C, Bjurstam K, Sundin Y. Osteopromotion: A soft-tissue exclusion principle using a membrane for bone healing and bone neogenesis. J Periodontol 1993;64:1116–1128.

9. Kenney EB, Jovanovic SA. Osteopromotion as an adjunct to osseointegration. Int J Prosthodont 1993;6:131–136.

10. Jovanovic SA, Kenney EB, Carranza FA Jr, Donath K. The regenerative potential of plaque-induced peri-implant bone defects treated by a submerged membrane technique: An experimental study. Int J Oral Maxillofac Implants 1993;8:13–18.

11. Dahlin C, Linde A, Gottlow J, Nyman S. Healing of bone defects by guided tissue regeneration. Plast Reconstr Surg 1988;81:672–676.

12. Dahlin C, Alberius P, Linde A. Osteopromotion for cranioplasty: An experimental study in rats using a membrane technique. J Neurosurg 1991;74:487–491.

13. Hammerle CHF, Schmid J, Olah AJ, Lang NP. Osseous healing of experimentally created defects in the calvaria of rabbits using guided bone regeneration. A pilot study. Clin Oral Implants Res 1992;3:144–147.

14. Dahlin C, Sennerby L, Lekholm U, Linde A, Nyman S. Generation of new bone around titanium implants using a membrane technique: An experimental study in rabbits. Int J Oral Maxillofac Implants 1989;4:19–25.

15. Becker W, Becker BE, Handelsman M, Celletti R, Ochsenbein C, Hardwick R, Langer B. Bone formation at dehisced dental implant sites treated with implant augmentation material: A pilot study in dogs. Int J Periodont Rest Dent 1990:10:93–102.

16. Hjørting-Hansen E, Helbo M, Aaboe M, Gotfredsen K, Pinhold EM. Osseointegration of subperiosteal implant via guided tissue regeneration. Clin Oral Implants Res 1995;6:149–154.

17. Caudill R, Meffert R. Histologic analysis of the osseointegration of endosseous implants in simulated extraction sockets with and without ePTFE barriers. I. Preliminary findings. Int J Periodont Rest Dent 1991;11:207–214.

18. Gotfredsen K, Warrer K, Hjørting-Hansen E, Karring T. Effect of membranes and porous hydroxyapatite on healing in bone defects around titanium dental implants. An experimental study in monkeys. Clin Oral Implants Res 1991;2:172–178.

19. Becker W, Lynch SE, Lekholm U, Becker BE, Caffesse R, Donath K, Sanchez R. A comparison of ePTFE membranes alone or in combination with platelet-derived growth factors and insulin-like growth factor-1 or demineralized freeze-dried bone in promoting bone formation around immediate extraction socket implants. J Periodontol 1992;63:929–940.

20. Lekholm U, Becker W, Dahlin C, Becker B, Donath K, Morrison E. The role of early versus late removal of GTAM membranes on bone formation at oral implants placed into immediate extraction sockets. Clin Oral Implants Res 1993;4:121–129.

21. Becker W, Lekholm U, Dahlin C, Becker B, Donath K. The effect of clinical loading on bone regenerated by GTAM barriers: A study in dogs. Int J Oral Maxillofac Implants 1994;9:305–313.

22. Buser D, Ruskin J, Higginbottom F, Hardwick R, Dahlin C, Schenk RK. Osseointegration of titanium implants in bone regenerated in membrane-protected defects: A histologic study in the canine mandible. Int J Oral Maxillofac Implants 1995;10:666–681.

23. Jovanovic SA, Schenk RK, Orsini M, Kenney EG. Supracrestal bone formation around dental implants: An experimental dog study. Int J Oral Maxillofac Implants 1995;10:21–23.

24. Jensen OT, Greer RO, Johnson L, Kassebaum D. Vertical guided bone-graft augmentation in a new canine mandibular model. Int J Oral Maxillofac Implants 1995;10:335–344.

25. Lundgren D, Lundgren AK, Sennerby L, Nyman S. Augmentation of intramembraneous bone beyond the skeletal envelope using an occlusive titanium barrier. Clin Oral Implants Res 1995;6:67–72.

26. Iglhaut J, Aukhil I, Simpson D, et al. Progenitor cell kinetics during experimental guided tissue regeneration procedure. J Periodont Res 1988;23:107–117.

27. Selvig K, Nilvéus R, Fitzmorris L, et al. Scanelectron microscopic observations of cell population and bacterial contamination of membranes used for guided periodontal tissue regeneration in humans. J Periodontol 1990;61:515–520.

28. Phillips JH. Effects of fixation on endochondral and endomembraneous graft survival: A bone is a bone is a bone. In: Holmes RE (ed). Bone Grafting. III. Biology and Application for Maxillofacial Indications. San Diego, CA: 1988.

29. Hjørting-Hansen E, Worsaae N, Lemons J. Histologic response after implantation of porous hydroxyapatite ceramic in humans. Int J Oral Maxillofac Implants 1990;5:255–263.

30. Haney JM, Nilveus RE, McMillan PJ, Wikesjö UME. Periodontal repair in dogs: Expanded polytetrafluoroethylene barrier membranes support wound stabilization and enhance bone regeneration. J Periodontol 1993;64:883–890.

31. Jovanovic SA, Nevins M. Bone formation utilizing titanium reinforced barrier membranes. Int J Periodont Rest Dent 1995;15:57–69.

32. Mellonig JT. Autogenous and allogeneic bone grafts in periodontal therapy. Crit Rev Oral Biol 1992;3:333–352.

33. Mellonig JT, Nevins M. Guided bone regeneration of bone defects associated with implants: An evidence-based outcome assessment. Int J Periodont Rest Dent 1995;15:168–185.

34. Becker W, Becker BE, McGuire MK. Localized ridge augmentation using absorbable pins and ePTFE barrier membranes: A new surgical technique. Case reports. Int J Periodont Rest Dent 1994;14:49–61.

35. Nevins M, Mellonig JT. The advantages of localized ridge augmentation prior to implant placement: A staged event. Int J Periodont Rest Dent 1994;14:97–111.

36. Dahlin C, Andersson L, Linde A. Bone augmentation at fenestrated implants by an osteopromotive membrane technique. A controlled clinical study. Clin Oral Implants Res 1991;2:159–165.

37. Gelb DA. Immediate implant surgery: Three-year retrospective evaluation of 50 consecutive cases. Int J Oral Maxillofac Implants 1993;8:388–399.

38. Fugazzotto PA. Ridge augmentation with titanium screws and guided tissue regeneration: Technique and report of a case. Int J Oral Maxillofac Implants 1993;8:335–339.

39. Hurzeler MB, Quinones CR, Strub JR. Advanced surgical and prosthetic management of the anterior single tooth osseointegrated implant: A case presentation. Pract Periodontics Aesthet Dent 1994;6:13–21.

40. Bahat O. Surgical planning. J Calif Dent Assoc 1992;May:31–46.

41. Bahat O, Fontanesi RV, Preston J. Reconstruction of the hard and soft tissues for optimal placement of osseointegrated implants. Int J Periodont Rest Dent 1993;13:255–275.

42. Buser D, Hirt H-P, Dula K, Berthold H. Guided bone regeneration-technique/implant dentistry. Schweiz Monatsschr Zahnmed 1992;102:1491–1501.

43. Jovanovic SA, Spiekermann H, Richter E-J, Koseoglu M. Guided tissue regeneration around titanium dental implants. In: Laney WR, Tolman DE (eds). Tissue Integration in Oral, Orthopedic & Maxillofacial Reconstruction. Proceedings of the Second International Congress on Tissue Integration in Oral, Orthopedic, and Maxillofacial Reconstruction. Chicago: Quintessence, 1992:208–215.

44. Mellonig JT, Triplett RG. Guided tissue regeneration and endosseous dental implants. Int J Periodont Rest Dent 1993;13:109–119.

45. Meffert RM. Treatment of the ailing, failing implant. J Calif Dent Assoc 1992;20:42–45.

46. Lazzara RJ. Immediate implant placement into extraction sites: Surgical and restorative advantages. Int J Periodont Rest Dent 1989;9:333–344.

47. Becker W, Becker B. Guided tissue regeneration for implants placed into extraction sockets and for implant dehiscences: Surgical techniques and case reports. Int J Periodont Rest Dent 1990;10:377–391.

48. Callan DP. Use of human freeze-dried demineralized bone prior to implantation. Part I. Pract Periodontics Aesthet Dent 1990;2:14–18.

49. Wachtel HC, Langford A, Bernimoulin J, Reichart P. Guided bone regeneration next to osseointegrated implants in humans. Int J Oral Maxillofac Implants 1991;6:127–135.

50. Sevor J, Meffert R, Block C. The immediate placement of dental implants into fresh maxillary extraction sites. Pract Periodontics Aesthet Dent 1991;3:55–59.

51. Balshi T, Hernandez R, Cutler R, Hertzog C. Treatment of osseous defects using Vicryl mesh (Polyglactin 910) and the Brånemark implant: A case report. Int J Oral Maxillofac Implants 1991;6:87–91.

52. Wilson TG. Guided tissue regeneration around dental implants in immediate and recent extraction sites: Initial observations. Int J Periodont Rest Dent 1992;12:185–194.

53. Cochran DL, Douglas HB. Augmentation of osseous tissue around nonsubmerged endosseous dental implants. Int J Periodont Rest Dent 1993;13:507–519.

54. Novaes AB Jr, Novaes AB. Bone formation over a TiAl6V4 (ImZ) implant placed into an extraction socket in association with membrane therapy (Gingiflex). Clin Oral Implants Res 1993;4:106–110.

55. Knox R, Lee K, Meffert R. Placement of hydroxyapatite-coated endosseous implants in fresh extraction sites: A case report. Int J Periodont Rest Dent 1993;13:245–253.

56. Rominger JW, Triplett RG. The use of guided tissue regeneration to improve implant osseointegration. J Oral Maxillofac Surg 1994; 52:106–112.

57. Cosci F, Cosci R. Guided bone regeneration for implant placement using absorbable collagen membranes: Case presentation. Pract Periodontics Aesthet Dent 1994;6:35–41.

58. Becker W, Dahlin C, Becker BE, Lekholm U, van Steenberghe D, Higuchi K, Kultje C. The use of ePTFE barrier membranes for bone promotion around titanium implants placed into extraction sockets: A prospective multicenter study. Int J Oral Maxillofac Implants 1994;9:31–40.

59. Evian CI, Cutler S. Autogenous gingival grafts as epithelial barriers for immediate implants: Case reports. J Periodontol 1994;65:201–210.

60. Simion M, Baldoni M, Rossi P, Zaffe D. A comparative study of the effectiveness of ePTFE membranes with and without early exposure during the healing period. Int J Periodont Rest Dent 1994;14:167–180.

61. Augthun M, Yildirim M, Spiekermann H, Biesterfeld S. Healing of bone defects in combination with immediate implants using the membrane technique. Int J Oral Maxillofac Implants 1995;10:421–428.

62. Gher ME, Quintero G, Sandifer JB, Tabacco M, Richardson AC. Combined dental implant and guided tissue regeneration therapy in humans. Int J Periodont Rest Dent 1994;14:333–347.

63. Gher ME, Quintero G, Assad D, Monaco E, Richardson AC. Bone grafting and guided bone regeneration for immediate dental implants in humans. J Periodontol 1994;65:881–891.

64. Landsberg C, Grosskopf A, Weinreb M. Clinical and biologic observations of demineralized freeze-dried bone allograft in augmentation procedures around dental implants. Int J Oral Maxillofac Implants 1994;9:586–592.

65. Lundgren D, Sennerby L, Falk H, Fribert B, Nyman S. The use of a new bioresorbable barrier for guided bone regeneration in connection with implant installation. Clin Oral Implants Res 1994;5:177–184.

66. Callan DP, Rohrer MD. Use of bovine-derived hydroxyapatite in the treatment of edentulous ridge defects: A human clinical and histologic case report. J Periodontol 1993;64:575–582.

67. Adele R, Lekholm U, Rockler B, Brånemark PI. A 15-year study of osseointegrated implants in the treatment of edentulous jaws. Int J Oral Maxillofac Surg 1981;10:387–416.

68. Dahlin C, Lekholm U, Linde A. Membrane induced bone augmentation at titanium implants. Int J Periodont Rest Dent 1991; 11:273–282.

69. Dahlin C, Lekholm U, Becker W, Becker B, Higuchi K, Callans A, van Steenberghe D. Treatment of fenestration and dehiscence bone defects around oral implants using the guided tissue regeneration technique: A prospective multicenter study. Int J Oral Maxillofac Implants 1995;10:312–318.

70. Jovanovic SA, Spiekermann H, Richter EJ. Bone regeneration around titanium dental implants in dehisced defect sites: A clinical study. Int J Oral Maxillofac Implants 1992;7:233–245.

71. Shanaman RH. The use of guided tissue regeneration to facilitate ideal prosthetic placement of implants. Int J Periodont Rest Dent 1992;12:257–265.

72. Nevins M, Mellonig J. Enhancement of the damaged edentulous ridge to receive dental implants: A combination of allograft and the Gore-Tex membrane. Int J Periodont Rest Dent 1992;12:97–111.

73. Fugazzotto PA. Bone regeneration over a poorly-positioned implant to correct an esthetic deformity: A case report. J Periodontol 1993; 64:1088–1091.

74. Israelson H, Plemons JM. Dental implants, regenerative techniques, and periodontal plastic surgery to restore maxillary anterior esthetics. Int J Oral Maxillofac Implants 1993;8:555–561.

75. Andersson B, Odman P, Widmark G, Waas A. Anterior tooth replacement with implants in patients with a narrow alveolar ridge form. A clinical study using guided tissue regeneration. Clin Oral Implants Res 1993;4:90–98.

76. Farris NJ, Meffert RM. Guided tissue regeneration around dental implants: Three case reports. Pract Periodontics Aesthet Dent 1993; 5:59–63.

77. Vlassis JM, Wetzel AC, Caffesse RG. Guided bone regeneration at a fenestrated dental implant: Histologic assessment of a case report. Int J Oral Maxillofac Implants 1993;8:447–451.

78. Mattout P, Nowzari H, Mattout C. Clinical evaluation of guided bone regeneration at exposed parts of Brånemark dental implants with and without bone allograft. Clin Oral Implants Res 1995;6:189–195.

79. Shanaman RH. A retrospective study of 237 consecutive sites. Int J Periodont Rest Dent 1994;14:293–301.

80. Sevor JJ, Meffert RM, Cassingham RJ. Regeneration of dehisced alveolar bone adjacent to endosseous dental implants utilizing a resorbable collagen membrane: Clinical and histologic results. Int J Periodont Rest Dent 1993;13:71–83.

81. Jones JK, Triplett RG. The relationship of cigarette smoking to impaired intraoral wound healing: A review of evidence and implications for patient care. J Oral Maxillofac Surg 1992;50:237–239.

82. Hurzeler MB, Quinones CR. Installation of endosseous oral implants with guided tissue regeneration. Pract Periodontics Aesthet Dent 1991;3:21–29.

83. Amler MH, Johnston PL, Salman I. Histochemical investigation of human alveolar socket healing in undisturbed extraction wounds. J Am Dent Assoc 1960;61:32–44.

84. Pietrovski J, Massler M. Ridge remolding after tooth remodeling in rats. J Dent Res 1967;46:222–231.

85. Evian CI, Rosenberg ES, Coslet JG, Corth H. The osteogenic activity of bone removed from healing extraction sockets in humans. J Periodontol 1982;53:81–85.

86. Carlsson GE, Thilander H, Hedegard G. Histologic changes in the upper alveolar process after extractions with or without insertion of an immediate full denture. Acta Odontol Scand 1967;25:1–31.

87. Gugliernotti MB, Cabrini RL. Alveolar wound healing and ridge remodeling after tooth extraction in the rat. J Oral Maxillofac Surg 1985;43:359–364.

88. Nevins M, Mellonig JT, Clem DS, Reiser G, Buser DA. Implants in Degenerated Bone: Long-term survival. Int J Periodont Rest Dent 1998;18:35-45.

89. O'Brien TP, Hinrichs JE, Schaffer EM. The prevention of localized ridge deformities using guided tissue regeneration. J Periodontol 1994; 65:17–24.

90. Mellonig JT, Bowers GM, Cotton W. Comparison of bone graft materials. II. New bone formation with autografts and allografts: A histologic evaluation. J Periodontol 1981;52:297–302.

91. Buser D, Dula K, Belser U, Hirt H-P, Berthold H. Localized ridge augmentation using guided bone regeneration. II. Surgical procedure in the mandible. Int J Periodont Rest Dent 1995;15:11–29.

92. Buser D, Dula K, Belser U, Hirt H-P, Berthold H. Localized ridge augmentation using guided bone regeneration. I. Surgical procedure in the maxilla. Int J Periodont Rest Dent 1993;13:29–45.

93. Bostman O. Osteolytic changes accompanying degradation of absorbable fracture fixation implants. J Bone Joint Surg 1991; 73:679–682.

94. Simion M, Baldoni M, Zaffe D. Jawbone enlargement using immediate implant placement associated with a split-crest technique and guided tissue regeneration. Int J Periodont Rest Dent 1992; 12:463–473.

95. Simion M, Trisi P, Piattelli A. Vertical ridge augmentation using a membrane technique associated with osseointegrated implants. Int J Periodont Rest Dent 1994;14:497–511.

96. Pinto VS, Zuolo ML, Mellonig JT. Guided bone regeneration in the treatment of a large periapical lesion: A case report. Pract Periodontics Aesthet Dent 1995;7:76–82.

97. Tseng C, Chen Y, Huang C, Bowers G. Correction of a large periradicular lesion and mucosal defect using combined endodontic and periodontal therapy: A case report. Int J Periodont Rest Dent 1995;15:377–383.

98. Rosenberg ES, Torosian JP, Slots J. Microbial differences in two clinically distinct types of failures of osseointegrated implants. Clin Oral Implants Res 1991;2:135–144.

99. Meffert RM. Treatment of failing dental implants. Curr Opin Dent 1992;2:109–114.

100. Meffert RM. How to treat ailing and failing implants. Implant Dent 1992;1:25–33.

101. Wittrig EE, Zablotsky MH, Layman DL, Meffert RM. Fibroblastic growth and attachment of hydroxyapatite-coated titanium surfaces following the use of various detoxification modalities. Part I. Noncontaminated hydroxyapatite. Implant Dent 1992;1:189–194.

102. Zablotsky M, Meffert R, Mills O, Burgess A, Lancaster D. The macroscopic, microscopic and spectrometric effects of various chemotherapeutic agents on the plasma-sprayed hydroxyapatite-coated implant surface. Clin Oral Implants Res 1992;3:189–198.

103. Zablotsky M, Meffert R, Caudill R, Evans G. Histological and clinical comparisons of guided tissue regeneration on dehisced hydroxyapatite-coated and titanium endosseous implant surfaces: A pilot study. Int J Oral Maxillofac Implants 1991;6:294–303.

104. Hammerle C, Fourmousis I, Winker J, Weigel C, Bragger U, Lang N. Successful bone fill in late peri-implant defects using guided tissue regeneration. A short communication. J Periodontol 1995;66:303–308.

105. Veksler A, Kayrouz G, Newman M. Reduction of salivary bacteria by pre-procedural rinses with chlorhexidine 0.12%. J Periodontol 1991; 62:649–651.

106. Cline N, Layman D. The effects of chlorhexidine on the attachment and growth of cultured human periodontal cells. J Periodontol 1992; 63:598–602.

107. Grunder U, Hurzeler MB, Schupbach P, Strub JR. Treatment of ligature-induced peri-implantitis using guided tissue regeneration: A clinical and histologic study in the beagle dog. Int J Oral Maxillofac Implants 1993;8:282–293.

108. Lehmann B, Bragger U, Hammerle C, Fourmousis I, Lang N. Treatment of an early implant failure according to the principles of guided tissue regeneration (GTR). Clin Oral Implants Res 1992; 3:42–48.

109. Mellonig J, Griffiths G, Mathys E, Spitznagel J. Treatment of the failing implant: Case reports. Int J Periodont Rest Dent 1995; 15:385–395.

110. Sander L, Karring T. New attachment and bone formation in periodontal defects following treatment of submerged roots with guided tissue regeneration. J Clin Periodontol 1995;22:295–299.

111. Nowzari H, Matian F, Slots J. Periodontal pathogens on polytetrafluoroethylene membrane for guided tissue inhibit healing. J Clin Periodontol 1995;22:469–474.

112. Simion M, Trisi P, Maglione M, Piattelli A. A preliminary report on a method for studying the permeability of an expanded polytetrafluoroethylene membrane to bacteria in vitro: A scanning electron microscopic and histological study. J Periodontol 1994;65:755–761.

113. Simion M, Trisi P, Maglione M, Piattelli A. Bacterial penetration in vitro through a GTAM membrane with and without topical chlorhexidine application. J Clin Periodontol 1995;22:321–331.

114. Lundgren D, Nyman S, Mathissen T, Isaksson S, Klinge B. Guided bone regeneration of cranial defects, using biodegradable barriers: An experimental pilot study in the rabbit. J Craniomaxillofac Surg 1992;20:257–260.

115. Lang NP, Bragger U, Walther D, Beamer B, Kornman KS. Ligature-induced peri-implant infection in cynomolgus monkeys. I. Clinical and radiographic findings. Clin Oral Implants Res 1993;4:2–11.

116. Sandberg E, Dahlin C, Linde A. Bone regeneration by the osteopromotion technique using bioabsorbable membranes: An experimental study in rats. J Oral Maxillofac Surg 1993;51:1106–1114.

117. Mellonig J, Nevins M, Sanchez R. Evaluation of a bioabsorbable physical barrier for guided bone regeneration. Part I. Material alone. Int J Periodont Rest Dent 1998;18:129–137.

118. Mellonig J, Nevins M, Sanchez R. Evaluation of a bioabsorbable physical barrier in guided bone regeneration. Part II. Material and a bone replacement graft. Int J Periodont Rest Dent 1998;18:139–149.

119. Schenk RK. Bone regeneration: Biologic basis. In: Buser D, Dahlin C, Schenk RK (eds). Guided Bone Regeneration in Implant Dentistry. Chicago: Quintessence, 1994:49–100.

120. Jensen J, Sindet-Pedersen S. Autogenous mandibular bone grafts and osseointegrated implants for reconstruction of the severely atrophied maxilla. A preliminary report. J Oral Maxillofac Surg 1991; 49:1277–1287.

121. Misch CM, Misch CE, Resnik R, Ismail Y. Reconstruction of maxillary alveolar defects with mandibular symphysis grafts for dental implants: A preliminary procedural report. Int J Oral Maxillofac Implants 1992;7:360–366.

122. Friberg B. Bone augmentation at single-tooth implants using mandibular grafts: A one-stage surgical procedure. Int J Periodont Rest Dent 1995;15:437–445.

123. Goldberg V, Stevenson S. Natural history of autografts and allografts. Clin Orthop 1987;225:7–16.

124. Kusiak J, Zins J, Whitaker L. The early revascularization of membraneous bone. Plast Reconstr Surg 1985;76:510–514.

125. Marx RE. The science of reconstruction. In: Bell WH (ed). Modern Practice in Orthognathic and Reconstructive Surgery. Philadelphia: Saunders, 1992:1449–1452.

126. Misch CM. Ridge augmentation using mandibular ramus bone grafts for placement of dental implants: Presentation of a technique. Pract Periodontics Aesthet Dent 1996;8:127–135.

127. Mellonig J, Bowers G, Bright R, Lawrence J. Clinical evaluation of freeze-dried bone allograft in periodontal osseous defects. J Periodontol 1976;47:125–129.

128. Sepe W, Bowers G, Lawrence J, Friedlaender G, Koch R. Clinical evaluation of freeze-dried bone allografts in periodontal osseous defects. J Periodontol 1978;49:9–14.

129. Sanders J, Sepe W, Bowers G, et al. Clinical evaluation of freeze-dried bone allograft in periodontal osseous defects. III. Composite freeze-dried bone allografts with and without autogenous bone grafts. J Periodontol 1983;54:1–8.

130. Turner DW, Mellonig JT. Antigenicity of freeze-dried bone allograft in periodontal osseous defects. J Periodont Res 1981;16:89–99.

131. Quattlebaum JB, Mellonig JT, Hensel NF. Antigenicity of freeze-dried cortical bone allograft in human periodontal osseous defects. J Periodontol 1988;59:394–397.

132. Chalmers J, Gray D, Rush J. Observations on the induction of bone in soft tissue. J Bone Joint Surg 1975;57:36–41.

133. Koskinen E, Ryoppy S, Linkholm T. Osteoinduction and osteogenesis in implants of allogeneic bone matrix. Clin Orthop 1972;87:116–131.

134. Urist MR. Bone formation by autoinduction. Science 1965; 150:893–899.

135. Urist MR, Dowell TA. Inductive substratum for osteogenesis in pellets of particulate bone matrix. Clin Orthop 1970;61:61–78.

136. Urist MR, Dowell TA, Hay PH, Strates BS. Inductive substrates for bone formation. Clin Orthop 1968;59:59–96.

137. Urist M, Strates B. Bone morphogenetic protein. J Dent Res 1971; 50;1392–1406.

138. Wozney J, Rosen V, Celeste A, Mitsock L, Whitters M, Kritz R, et al. Novel regulators of bone formation: Molecular ions and activities. Science 1988;242:1528–1534.

139. Urist M, Strates B. Bone formation in implants of partially and wholly demineralized bone matrix. Clin Orthop 1970;71:271–278.

140. Harakas N. Demineralized bone matrix induced osteogenesis. Clin Orthop 1984;188:239–251.

141. Becker W, Becker B, Caffesse R. A comparison of demineralized freeze-dried bone and autogenous bone to induce bone formation in human extraction sockets. J Periodontol 1994;65:1128–1133.

142. Becker W, Urist M, Tucker L, Becker B, Ochsenbein C. Human demineralized freeze-dried bone: Inadequate induced bone formation in athymic mice. A preliminary report. J Periodontol 1995;66:822–828.

143. Becker W, Schenk R, Higuchi K, Lekholm U, Becker BE. Variations in bone regeneration adjacent to implants augmented with barrier membranes alone or with demineralized freeze-dried bone or autologous grafts: A study in dogs. Int J Oral Maxillofac Implants 1995; 10:143–154.

144. Ripamonti U, Reddi H. Growth and morphogenetic factors in bone induction: Role of osteogenin and related bone morphogenetic proteins in craniofacial and periodontal bone repair. Clin Rev Oral Biol Med 1992;3:1–14.

145. Heiple K, Chase S, Herndon C. A comparative study of the healing process following different types of bone transportation. J Bone Joint Surg 1963;45:1593–1599.

146. Simion M, Dahlin C, Trisi P, Piattelli A. Qualitative and quantitative comparative study on different filling materials used in bone tissue regeneration: A controlled clinical study. Int J Periodont Rest Dent 1994;14:199–215.

147. Gottesdiener KM. Transplanted infections: Donor-to-host transmission with the allograft. Ann Intern Med 1989;110:1001–1010.

148. Kayaiga R, Miller WV, Gudino MDL. Tissue transplant transmitted infections. Transfusion 1991;31:277–284.

149. Eastlund T. Infectious disease transmission through tissue transplantation: Reducing the risk through donor selection. J Transplant Coordination 1991;1:23–30.

150. Buck BE, Malinin TL. Human bone and tissue allografts. Clin Orthop 1994;303:8–17.

151. Buck BE, Malinin T, Brown MD. Bone transplantation and human immunodeficiency virus. Clin Orthop 1989;240:129–136.

152. Wientroub S, Reddi AH. Influence of irradiation on the osteoinductive potential of demineralized bone matrix. Calcif Tissue Int 1988;42:255–260.

153. Munting E, Wilmart J, Wijne A, Hennebert P, Delloye C. Effect of sterilization on osteoinduction. Comparison of five methods in demineralized bone matrix gelatin. Acta Orthop Scand 1988;59:34–38.

154. Schwarz N, Heinz R, Schiesser A, et al. Irradiation-sterilization of rat bone matrix gelatin. Acta Orthop Scand 1988;59:165–167.

155. Conway B, Tomford WW, Mankin HJ, Hirsch MS, Schooley RT. Radiosensitivity of HIV-1 potential application to sterilization of bone allografts. AIDS 1991;5:608–609.

156. Forsell JH. Irradiation of musculoskeletal tissues. In: Tomford WW (ed). Musculoskeletal Tissue Banking. New York: Raven Press, 1993:149–180.

157. Aspenberg P, Johnsson E, Thorngren K. Dose-dependent reduction of bone inductive properties by ethylene oxide. J Bone Joint Surg 1992;72:1036–1037.

158. Zislis T, Martin SA, Cerbas E, Heath JR, Mansfield JL, Hollinger JO. A scanning electron microscopic study of in vivo toxicity of ethylene oxide sterilized bone repair materials. J Oral Implant 1989;1:41–46.

159. Friedlaender G, Strong M, Sell K. Studies on the antigenicity of bone. I. Freeze-dried and deep frozen bone allografts in rabbits. J Bone Joint Surg 1976;58:854–858.

160. Urist M, Iwata H. Preservation and biodegradation of bone morphogenetic property of bone matrix. J Theor Biol 1973;38:155–167.

161. Urist M, Jurist J, Dubuc D, Strates B. Quantitation of new bone formation in intramuscular implants of bone matrix in rabbits. Clin Orthop 1970;68:279–293.

162. Aspenberg P, Thoren K. Lipid extraction enhances bank bone incorporation. Acta Orthop Scand 1990;61:546–548.

163. Resnick L, Veren K, Salahuddin S, Tondreau S, Markhan P. Stability and inactivation of HTLV-III/LAV under clinical and laboratory environments. JAMA 1986;255:1887–1891.

164. Flosdorf EW, Hyatt GW. The preservation of bone grafts by freeze-drying. Surgery 1952;31:716–719.

165. Mellonig JT, Levey R. The effect of different particle sizes of freeze-dried bone allograft on bone growth. J Dent Res 1984;63:222.

166. Fucini SE, Quintero G, Gher ME, Black BS, Richardson RC. Small versus large particles of demineralized freeze-dried bone allograft in human intrabony periodontal defects. J Periodontol 1993; 64:844–847.

167. Tomford WW. Surgical bone banking. In: Tomford WW (ed). Musculoskeletal Tissue Banking. New York: Raven Press, 1993:19–60.

168. Cummings PD, Wallace EL, Schorr JB, et al. Exposure of patients to human immunodeficiency virus through the transfusion of blood products that test antibody-negative. N Engl J Med 1989; 321:941–946.

169. Ward JW, Holmberg SD, Allen JR, et al. Transmission of human immunodeficiency virus (HIV) by blood transfusions screen as negative for HIV antibody. N Engl J Med 1988;318:473–478.

170. Wolinsky SM, Rinaldo CR, Kwok S, et al. Human immunodeficiency virus type 1 (HIV-1) infection a median of 18 months before a diagnostic Western blot. Ann Intern Med 1989;111:961–972.

171. Simonds RJ, Holmberg SD, Hurwitz R, Coleman T, et al. Transmission of human immunodeficiency virus Type 1 from a seronegative organ and tissue donor. N Engl J Med 1992; 326:726–732.

172. Martin LS, McDougal JS, Loskoski SL. Disinfection and inactivation of the human T lymphotropic virus Type III/lymphadenopathy associated virus. J Infect Dis 1985;152:400–403.

173. Prewett AB, O'Leary R, Harrell J. Kinetic evaluation of the penetration of ethanol solutions containing virucidal agents through mid-diaphylseal cortical bone. Osteotech Tech Report. Shrewsbury, NJ: Osteotech, 1991.

174. Prewett AB, Cook SD, Manrique A. Simian immunodeficiency virus (human HIV-II) transmission in allograft bone procedures. Presented at the 12th Annual Meeting, Mid-America Orthopaedic Association, Bermuda, 1994.

175. Ongradi J, Ceccheini-Neilli L, Pistello M, Specter S, Bendinelli M. Acid sensitivity of cell-free associated HIV-1: Clinical implications. AIDS Res Human Retrovirus 1990;12:1433–1436.

176. Vodicka P, Hemminki K. Phosphodiester cleavage in apurinic dinucleotides. Chem Biol Interact 1988;68:153–164.

177. Buch BE, Resnick L, Shah SM, Malinin T. Human immunodeficiency virus cultured from bone. Implications for transplantation. Clin Orthop 1990;251:249–253.

178. Quinnan GV, Wells MA, Wittek AE, et al. Inactivation of human T-cell lymphotropic virus, Type III by heat, chemicals, and irradiation. Transfusion 1986;26:481–483.

179. Mellonig JT, Prewett AB, Moyer MP. HIV inactivation in a bone allograft. J Periodontol 1992;63:979–983.

180. Russo R, Scarborough N. Inactivation of viruses in demineralized bone matrix. Presented at the FDA Workshop on Tissue for Transplantation and Reproductive Tissue. Bethesda, MD, 20–21 Jun 1995.

181. Tomford WW. Cadaver donor musculoskeletal tissue banking. In: Tomford WW (ed). Musculoskeletal Tissue Banking. New York: Raven Press, 1993:61–148.

182. Hollinger FB. Specific and surrogate screening tests for hepatitis. In: Menitov HE (ed). American Association of Blood Banks. Arlington, VA: American Association of Blood Banks, 1987:69–86.

183. Dodd RY, Popovsky MA. Members of the scientific sections coordinating committee: Antibodies to hepatitis B core antigen and the infectivity of the blood supply. Transfusion 1991;31:433–449.

184. Cha TA, Kilberg J, Irvine B, et al. Use of a signature nucleotide sequence of the hepatitis C virus for the detection of viral RNA in human serum and plasma. J Clin Microbiol 1991;29:2528–2534.

185. Tomford WW, Starkweather RJ, Goldman MH. A study of the clinical incidence of infection in the use of banked allograft bone. J Bone Joint Surg 1981;63:244–248.

186. Cruse PJE. Incidence of wound infection on the surgical services. Surg Clin North Am 1975;55:1269–1275.

187. Puisner SB, Scott M, Foster D, et al. Transgenetic studies implicate interactions between homologous PrP isoforms in scrapies prion replication. Cell 1990;60:673–686.

188. Brown P, Preece MA, Will RG. "Friendly fire" in medicine: Hormones, homografts, and Creutzfeldt-Jakob disease. Lancet 1992;340:24–27.

Use of Guided Bone Regeneration to Facilitate Ideal Prosthetic Placement of Implants

Richard H. Shanaman, DDS

The ultimate goal in implant prosthetics is to replace a missing tooth or teeth with a prosthesis that appears natural in form, size, position, proportion, function, and color. Gingival esthetics is critical as well. Ideally, patients should have a mucogingival complex that has an adequate band of healthy, pink, tightly bound keratinized gingiva that blends smoothly into the alveolar mucosa without the facial depressions often observed with loss of the labial plate after extraction. There should be no evidence of hyperplasia or inflammation, and the gingival sulcus should be shallow and not bleed with slight provocation. Gingival margins should be knifelike and symmetric, and interdental papillae should be tucked neatly into the interproximal embrasures so that no "black triangles" exist.

The crown should have a natural emergence profile, without creating shoulders or ridge lap contours that are difficult to maintain. There should be no dark gingival appearance from the implant at the gingival margin.

The ideal is not always possible to obtain, but guided bone regeneration (GBR) provides the opportunity to achieve the ideal in numerous situations. When normal bone and gingival contours can be maintained or regenerated, it is often possible to reach the ultimate goal (Figs 6-1a and 6-1b).

Indications

An adequate height of interproximal bone is a prerequisite for placing an implant and regenerating bone to cover its threads, providing for normal facial contours, and achieving acceptable gingival contours. Thin or varying heights of

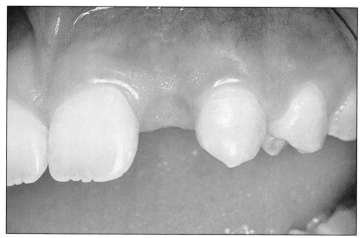

Fig 6-1a The lateral incisors are congenitally missing.

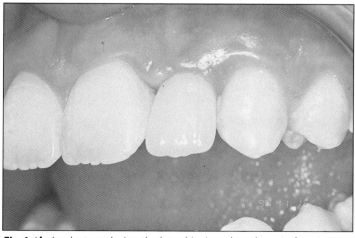

Fig 6-1b Implants replacing the lateral incisors have been in function 2.5 years.

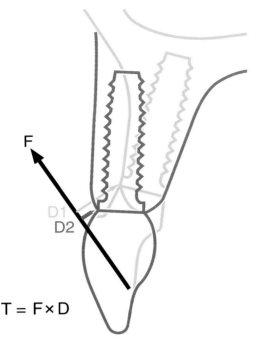

$$T = F \times D$$

Fig 6-2a Torque (T) = resultant force (F) × distance (D). The torque increases as the crest of the ridge and the implant are located more apically.

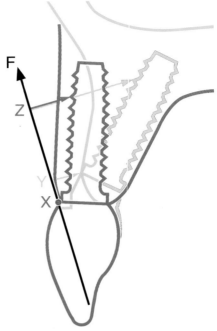

Fig 6-2b As the fixture is angled to the center of the ridge, the resultant force (F) becomes more inclined, which exaggerates the torque with a more apically located ridge and implants.

interproximal bone could lead to an unacceptable esthetic result and would best be handled with a staged approach recommended by Nevins and Mellonig.[1] In this approach, GBR is completed first, and the implant is placed after 6 to 10 months. If necessary, additional gingival or bone regeneration could be accomplished.

Prior to the development of guided bone regeneration techniques, it had been traditional for implant placement to be determined by the quantity and shape of the alveolar ridge. Thus, bone determined the position, angulation, and ultimately the possibility for osseointegrated implants.

Because the greatest reduction of alveolar bone occurs in the first 6 months to 2 years after extraction of the teeth, ideal prosthetic placement of implants was impossible for most patients before GBR. Carlsson and Persson[2] demonstrated that approximately one third of the vestibular plate of bone is lost in the first month after extraction in the maxillary alveolar process. They noted bone resorption 1 week after extractions, resulting in considerable thinning of the original labial plate in the first 3 weeks. This process accounts for the very common depression of the facial contours in areas of tooth loss. In the prosthetic replacement of these teeth, a ridge lap design for the pontic or crown was required to provide adequate facial contours. These techniques made daily maintenance much more difficult for the patient and still did not always achieve ideal prosthetic outcomes.

To help solve this problem, Lazzara[3] suggested placing implants immediately in the extraction site to allow bone to regenerate in the area and help preserve normal ridge contours. In these cases, however, the tooth is typically positioned labially or buccally to the anatomic center of the alveolar process.

Consequently, if the implant is placed in an optimum position for restoration, even with immediate fixture placement, a fenestration or dehiscence is likely to develop. Mecall and Rosenfeld[4,5] noted that the typical resorptive pattern after extraction places alveolar bone at a position that is more lingual-palatal and apical than that of the normal periodontium.

Therefore, if the long axis of an implant is directed in the anatomic center of the ridge, the screw access hole would often emerge from the labial aspect. The fixture in this situation would have been placed so that the occlusal forces on the implant would be in a lateral direction, which is the least tolerated force[6] (Figs 6-2a and 6-2b). It has been demonstrated clinically in humans and in animal studies that nonaxially loaded implants do not produce adverse osseous changes. However, such forces can produce loosening and failure of the prosthetic components.[7,8,9]

Many times GBR is the therapy of choice to overcome the problems of insufficient crest width, restoration of bone over dehiscences and fenestrations associated with prosthetically guided implant placement, and voids between the implant and surrounding bony walls encountered during immediate fixture placement in extraction sockets.

Predictability

Dahlin et al[10] treated the mandibles of rats using expanded polytetrafluoroethylene (e-PTFE) membranes as barriers. In the control sites, where no barriers were used, connective tissue filled the defect. In the experimental sites, where the

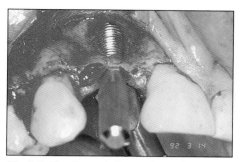

Fig 6-3 The fixture is in good prosthetic position but has a fenestration defect.

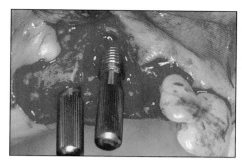

Fig 6-4a The fixtures are secured apically.

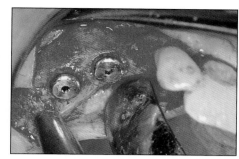

Fig 6-4b Regeneration has occurred over the dehiscence.

e-PTFE membrane created and protected a space, new bone filled the space. This study was followed by one in which implants were placed in rabbit tibias.[11] The threads of the implants were deliberately exposed, creating a dehiscence-type defect. The experimental side was covered with an e-PTFE membrane, while on the control side no barrier was placed. In the test sites, new bone covered the threads. Minimal new bone formation was noted in the control sites. Histologic evaluation demonstrated direct contact of bone and implant. Similar results were observed in dogs; significantly more regeneration of bone occurred where the barrier had been utilized than in the control sites.[12,13]

The consensus reached by these studies was that GBR utilizing barrier materials can be accomplished predictably to help solve the problems of insufficient ridges for implant placement. Subsequently, clinical studies and case reports of barrier techniques used with dental implants in humans began to appear in the literature.

Factors Critical to Success

There are numerous variations and techniques used in GBR. Some common factors, however, seem to be of paramount importance for successful results.

Stability of the Implant

For osseointegration to occur, the implant must be placed in a sufficient amount of bone to provide rigid stability during healing.

In fenestration-type defects, stability is easily attained because the fixture can be securely supported, apically and coronally. If the bone is of very poor quality, such as type III or IV, it is important to place a sufficiently long fixture to access the dense cortical bone at the sinus or nasal floor[14] (Figs 6-3 and 6-4), or use a wide-diameter fixture capable of engaging the buccal and lingual cortical walls.[15,16,17] One can also use osteotomes for preparation of the osteotomy site.

These instruments will compress the bone trabeculae both laterally and apically, producing much denser walls for implant stabilization.

It is possible, but technically very difficult, to place an implant with adequate stability when most or all of the length of the implant is dehisced. It is crucial in such cases that a significant portion of the fixture be kept within the bony ridge and as much of the circumference as possible be covered by bone (Figs 6-5a to 6-5c). The delivery of the implant is facilitated by holding a titanium instrument, such as a periosteal elevator, securely against the fixture, providing the necessary support of the fourth "wall."

If an adequate amount of the fixture length is not secured in bone so that a majority of the circumference is covered by bone, the implant will not be stable enough to allow osseointegration (Fig 6-6).

Unimpeded Healing

The barrier material must be sufficiently cell occlusive to prevent any invasion of fibrous connective tissue into the area to be regenerated with new bone. This allows unimpeded ingrowth of angioblasts and osteogenic cells from the bone marrow, which establish early bone formation.

In membrane-protected defects, bone regeneration takes place under the membrane, while, in control sites, the tissue tends to collapse into the defect and the defect fills primarily with connective tissue.[18] It was demonstrated that bone healing occurs progressively from the bony margins. If the membrane is not left in place for a sufficient time, areas of the defect most remote from the bony margins may still be at risk for filling with connective tissue, because bone would not have formed in that area yet.

It is also important for the membrane to extend a few millimeters onto healthy, uninvolved bone to prevent leakage of soft tissue under the membrane and into the defect, possibly interfering with the regenerative process. Should the fibrous connective tissue invade the intended site of bone regeneration, it could prevent or reduce the amount of bone formation.[19]

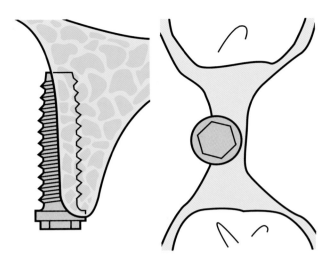

Fig 6-5a The widest diameter of the fixture is within bone.

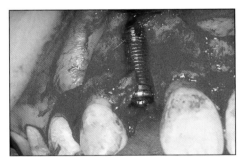

Fig 6-5b The fixture exhibits a dehiscence along its entire length.

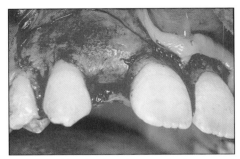

Fig 6-5c The implant is completely covered with new bone.

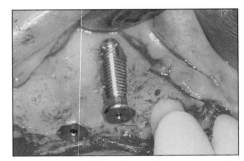

Fig 6-6 Most of the widest diameter of the fixture is not within the bony housing. Although there was some subsequent regeneration of labial bone, osseointegration did not occur, and the fixture was removed.

Preparation of the Surgical Site

After the flaps have been reflected, large curettes are used to remove all granulation tissue and residual connective tissue fibers attached to the bone. If any pathosis is present, meticulous debridement of the area with ultrasonic instruments and curettes must be accomplished.

Quite often the area requiring regeneration has a very dense cortical plate and is not well vascularized. Because the greatest potential source of osteogenic cells is the bone marrow, it is necessary to perform decortication. Small holes are drilled through the cortical plate into the underlying marrow spaces with small (No. ½ to No. 2) round burs. This will permit rapid ingrowth of vascular channels and osteoprecursor cells found in the bone marrow stroma and endosteum. These holes are made in areas of anticipated vascularity.[20,21]

Protection and Stabilization of the Clot

The organization of the clot with invading vascular sprouts and osteoprecursor cells is the basis for new bone forma-tion. Therefore, the clot that forms between the bone and membrane must be protected by diverting functional and mechanical stresses on the mucogingival flap that might otherwise jeopardize clot adhesion.[22,23] Phillips et al[24] noted that the micromovement during early phases of wound healing directly influences cellular differentiation. Movement of only 10 to 20 μm during early stages of fracture healing is enough to divert the differentiation of mesenchymal cells into fibroblasts instead of osteoblasts.

Because the membrane is an important factor in stability of the clot, it must be positioned so that there is no movement during healing. Stabilization is achieved by careful shaping and contouring of the material, tucking the material under the periosteum, and good flap closure[25] (Figs 6-7a to 6-7c). Some surgeons have used cover screws and miniscrews to aid in this process.[12,26] Because the outer portion of the e-PTFE membrane has an open microstructure, this area is rapidly infiltrated with fibroblasts, which help in membrane stabilization. This process can be so effective that it is often necessary to remove the membrane with sharp dissection at the time of second-stage surgery because of its integration with the tissue.

It is also important that no pressure be applied to the membrane by the patient or by the provisional prosthesis.

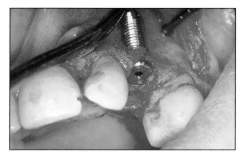

Fig 6-7a The fixture exhibits a severe dehiscence.

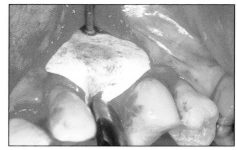

Fig 6-7b The barrier membrane significantly overlaps the defect margins to provide the membrane with stability.

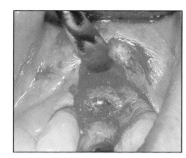

Fig 6-7c The fixture is completely covered with new bone 8 months later.

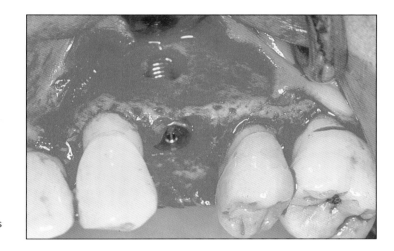

Fig 6-8 An implant is in place after extraction of the fractured root. This is a naturally spacemaking defect.

Adequate Space

Adequate space must be provided for clot formation, which leads to eventual bony regeneration. Some defects where implants would be placed within the bony housing are naturally spacemaking (Fig 6-8), but there are many situations in which this is not the case (see Figs 6-3a and 6-4b). In these situations, bone replacement grafts have been used to provide space and a lattice network for osteoinduction or osteoconduction of new bone.[27]

Autogenous bone, the material of choice, can be harvested orally or from areas such as the iliac crest with a cutdown procedure or a Westerman Jensen biopsy needle. This, however, adds an additional oral site and increases surgical pain. Significant amounts of autogenous bone can often be obtained during preparation of the fixture sites. Osseous coagulum can be harvested during any necessary osseous reshaping and is easily collected with a bone trap (available from Quality Aspirators, Duncanville, TX). Bone can also be retrieved from the tuberosity and retromolar regions with chisels and rongeurs or from the chin with trephine burs.

It is not uncommon for insufficient quantities of intraoral autogenous bone to be readily available or for patients to object to harvesting of bone from areas such as the chin or the iliac crest. In these situations, bone allografts can be used to help maintain the space necessary for regeneration.

Studies by Mellonig et al[28,29] demonstrated that bone allografts can be used successfully to regenerate bone and compare favorably with autogenous bone. A number of case reports and retrospective studies concerning ridge regeneration and coverage of dehisced or fenestrated implants attest to the clinical effectiveness of both demineralized freeze-dried bone allografts (DFDBA) and mineralized freeze-dried bone allograft (FDBA).[13,24,25]

It has been the experience of the author that in cases where fixtures are covered by very thin cortical bone (less than 1 mm) the threads were found to be exposed at second-stage surgery. The explanation for this phenomenon may be that the thin cortical plate that originally covered the threads resorbed, allowing soft tissue to contact the implant, thus preventing osteogenesis. A similar situation has also been noted occasionally when demineralized freeze-dried bone allograft is used under the membrane to correct a bony defect around a fixture in the maxillary anterior region (Figs 6-9a to 6-9c). This type of graft may resorb too quickly, allowing the material to collapse against the implant before new bone has formed. The use of a space-maintaining membrane such as the Gore-Tex Regenerative Material Titanium-Reinforced Configurations (WL Gore, Flagstaff, AZ) may eliminate this problem. Since the resorbable barriers such as Bio-Gide (Osteohealth, Shirley, NY) have no spacemaking ability, use of these will require some type of graft material.

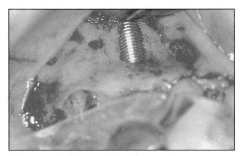

Fig 6-9a A fixture with a fenestration was covered with DFDBA and GTAM.

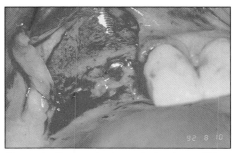

Fig 6-9b Six months later, the implant still has the fenestration at reentry. This time it was covered with FDBA and GTAM.

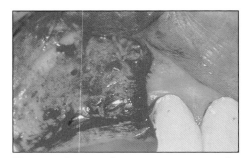

Fig 6-9c At second-stage surgery, 4 months later, the implant is completely covered with new bone.

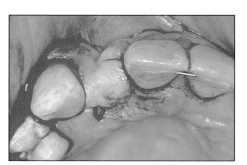

Fig 6-10a A partial-thickness dissection is started at the palatal aspect, and the flap ends with a full-thickness dissection at the occlusolabial line angle of the ridge.

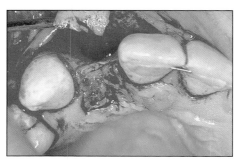

Fig 6-10b The combination partial- and full-thickness flap is raised. The remaining partial-thickness flap is still in place and will be reflected palatally.

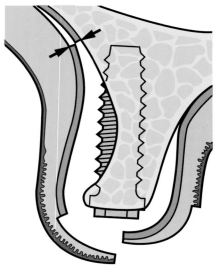

Fig 6-10c The combination partial- and full-thickness flaps are raised (*arrows*). Sharp dissection through the periosteum and the undermining sharp dissection.

Prevention of Infection

If infection is allowed to occur in the newly forming granulation tissue, it will stop osteogenesis immediately and may result in a greater loss of bone than that of the original defect. Therefore, it is recommended that clinicians prescribe systemic antibiotic regimens, such as amoxicillin, to begin 2 hours before the time of surgery and to be continued for the next week to 10 days. If primary closure is not obtained, some clinicians will have the patient continue with doxycycline, 100 mg per day, until the membrane is removed. This ideally occurs at a minimum of 8 weeks, depending on defect size.

Soft Tissue Coverage

Presently there is some controversy about the need for complete primary closure over the membrane. Some believe that it is critical to establish and maintain soft tissue coverage, and others think that closure is not a factor. If the flap can be designed to ensure adequate tissue mobility to attain primary closure over the regenerative materials, this will greatly facilitate postoperative care, minimize complications, and maximize the predictability of the procedure. Flap design must be carefully planned and provide adequate access for proper debridement and membrane adaptation, as well as tension-free soft tissue closure.

Various flap design modifications have been developed to help obtain such closure. The rotation of pedicle flaps from palatal or buccal tissue can help to achieve passive primary closure.[32] Others have described a combination of partial- and full-thickness flap dissections that begins palatally as a partial-thickness incision and extends to the buccal aspect as a full-thickness flap[33,34] (Figs 6-10a and 6-10b). Vertical or divergent oblique releasing incisions can be extended well beyond the mucogingival junction into the buccal turn of the vestibule to provide significant mobilization of soft tissue to cover the barrier membrane. Undermining sharp dissection through the periosteum can provide further mobilization (Fig 6-10c). The use of apically divergent releasing incisions provides more tissue in a mesiodistal direction as the flap is brought coronally.

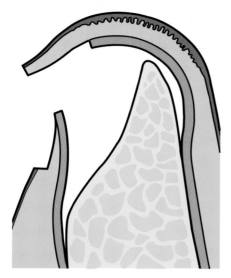

Fig 6-11a Combination of partial- and full-thickness flaps. A supraperiosteal incision is begun near the mucobuccal fold and moves coronally to the mucogingival junction, where the periosteum is incised and the remainder of the flap is full thickness.

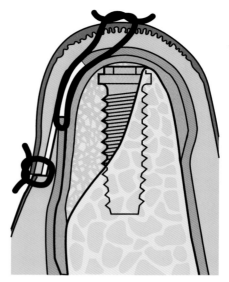

Fig 6-11b The elasticity of the mucosa, freed from its periosteum, allows closure over the membrane without tension.

When the flaps are sutured in position, a combination of a vertical mattresslike sutures on the labial flap and an interrupted approach on the palatal flap enables the connective tissue surface of the palatal flap to be brought under the labial flap. It is critical not to create tension on the flaps because this would cause ischemia and the primary closure would be lost.

Buser et al[35] described a variation of this technique for the mandible. The flap begins with a superperiosteal incision on the buccal aspect, near the mucobuccal fold, and is continued coronally to the mucogingival junction. At this point, a full mucoperiosteal flap is raised to the lingual. Closure of these flaps is achieved with mattress and interrupted suturing techniques[35] (Figs 6-11a and 6-11b).

Careful flap design and execution can help prevent excessive pressure on the membrane, which would reduce space and compromise the blood supply, possibly leading to flap necrosis and exposure of the membrane.

Wound Healing

Because of compelling negative data, the simultaneous approach to implant placement and regeneration is not recommended for those patients who smoke.

Smoking may have significant deleterious effects on wound healing. Jones and Triplett[36] reported complications with simultaneous implant placement and regeneration in 80% of patients who smoked. Complications were reported in only 10% of the nonsmokers.

In another retrospective study, Bain and Moy[37] followed 2,179 implants consecutively placed between 1984 and 1990. Utilizing implant removal or more than 50% radiographic bone loss as criteria for failure, they found that smokers had a significantly higher rate of failure (11.28%) than did nonsmokers (4.76%).

In an unpublished study, carried out in the author's private practice between 1986 and 1992, 599 fixtures were placed consecutively in 168 patients. For 202 of these fixtures, regeneration was accomplished with barrier membranes. The number of failures requiring removal of the fixtures was noted to be significantly higher in smokers (14.0%) than in nonsmokers (2.4%). The overall failure rate was 3.5%.

Conclusion

The regeneration of bone around implants with favorable bone and soft tissue contours can be a predictable result if certain factors are addressed. Successful outcomes will result from good compliance by the patient and precise surgical execution with attention to details such as design of the flap and atraumatic handling of tissue; maintenance of space between the implant and membrane; stabilization of the membrane, and therefore the clot; prevention of infection; and provision of protection for immature granulation tissue. The concepts of guided bone regeneration greatly expand the clinical avenues open to the clinician to integrate functional implant placement with esthetics.

References

1. Nevins M, Mellonig JT. The advantages of localized ridge augmentation prior to implant placement: A staged event. Int J Periodont Rest Dent 1994;14:97–111.

2. Carlsson GE, Persson G. Morphologic changes of the mandible after extraction and wearing of dentures. A longitudinal, clinical, and x-ray cephalometric study covering 5 years. Odontol Rev 1967;18:27–54.

3. Lazzara R. Immediate implant placement into extraction sites: Surgical and restorative advantages. Int J Periodont Rest Dent 1989;9:333–344.

4. Mecall RA, Rosenfeld AL. The influence of residual ridge resorption patterns on implant fixture placement and tooth position. Part I. Int J Periodont Rest Dent 1991;11:9–24.

5. Mecall RA, Rosenfeld AL. The influence of residual ridge resorption patterns on implant fixture placement and tooth position. Part II. Presurgical determination of prosthesis type and design. Int J Periodont Rest Dent 1992;12:33–51.

6. Weinberg LA, Kruger B. Clinical utilization of nonrotational capability in osseointegrated prostheses: A technical note. Int J Oral Maxillofac Implants 1994;9:326–332.

7. Gelb DA, Lazarra RJ. Hierarchy of objectives in implant placement to maximize esthetics: Use of preangulated abutments. Int J Periodont Rest Dent 1993;13:277–287.

8. Sakaguchi RL, Borgersen SE. Nonlinear contact analysis of preload in dental implant screws. Int J Oral Maxillofac Implants 1995;10:295-302.

9. Celletti R, Pameijer CH, Bracchetti G, Donath K, Persichetti G, Visani I. Histologic Evaluation of Osseointegrated Implants Restored in Nonaxial Functional Occlusion With Preangled Abutments. Int J Periodont Rest Dent 1995;15:563–574.

10. Dahlin C, Linde A, Gottlow J, Nyman S. Healing of bone defects by guided tissue regeneration. Plast Reconstr Surg 1988;81:672–676.

11. Dahlin C, Sennerby L, Lekholm U, Linde A, Nyman S. Generation of new bone around titanium implants using a membrane technique: An experimental study in rabbits. Int J Oral Maxillofac Implants 1989;4:19–25.

12. Becker W, Becker BE, Handelsman M, Celletti R, Ochsenbein C, Hardwick R, Langer B. Bone formation at dehisced dental implant sites treated with implant augmentation material: A pilot study in dogs. Int J Periodont Rest Dent 1990;10:93–102.

13. Caudill RF, Meffert RM. Histologic analysis of the osseointegration of endosseous implants in simulated extraction sockets with and without e-PTFE barriers. Part I. Preliminary findings. Int J Periodont Rest Dent 1991;11:207–215.

14. Langer B, Sullivan DY. Osseointegration: Its impact on the interrelationship of periodontics and restorative dentistry. Int J Periodont Rest Dent 1989;9:85–105.

15. Graves SL, et al. Wide diameter implants: Indications, considerations and preliminary results over a two-year period. Aust Prosthodont J 1994;8:31–37.

16. Langer B, Langer L, Herrmann I, Jorneus L. The wide fixture: A solution for special bone situations and a rescue for the compromised implant. Part I. Int J Oral Maxillofac Implants 1993;8:400–408.

17. Lazzara RJ. Criteria for implant selection: surgical and prosthetic considerations. Pract Periodontics Aesthet Dent 1994;6:55–62.

18. Schenk RK, Buser D, Hardwick WR, Dahlin C. Healing pattern of bone regeneration in membrane-protected defects. Int J Oral Maxillofac Implants 1994;9:13–29.

19. Mellonig JT, Triplett RG. Guided tissue regeneration and endosseous dental implants. Int J Periodont Rest Dent 1993;13:109–119.

20. Schenk RK. Bone regeneration: Biologic basis. In: Buser D, Dahlin C, Schenk RK (eds). Guided Bone Regeneration in Implant Dentistry. Chicago: Quintessence, 1994:49–100.

21. Cohen ES. Atlas of Cosmetic and Reconstructive Periodontal Surgery, ed 2. Philadelphia: Lea & Febiger, 1994:285–321.

22. Selvig KA, Nilvéus RE, Fitzmorris L, Kersten B, Khorsandi SS. Scanning electron microscopic observations of cell population and bacterial contamination of membranes used for guided periodontal tissue regeneration in humans. J Periodontol 1990;61:515–520.

23. Wikesjö UME, Nilvéus R. Periodontal repair in dogs: Effect of wound stabilization on healing. J Periodontol 1990;61:719–724.

24. Phillips RW, Jendresen MD, Klooster J, McNiel C, Preston J, Schallhorn R. Report of the Committee on Scientific Investigation of the American Academy of Restorative Dentistry. J Prosthet Dent 1990;64:74–110.

25. Shanaman RH. The use of guided tissue regeneration to facilitate ideal prosthetic placement of implants. Int J Periodont Rest Dent 1992;12:257–265.

26. Buser D, Brägger U, Lang NP, Nyman S. Regeneration and enlargement of jaw bone using guided tissue regeneration. Clin Oral Implants Res 1990;1:22–32.

27. Mellonig JT. Autogenous and allogeneic bone grafts in periodontal therapy. Crit Rev Oral Biol Med 1992;3:333–352.

28. Mellonig JT, Bowers GM, Baily R. Comparison of bone graft materials. Part I. New bone formation with autografts and allografts determined by strontium-85. J Periodontol 1981;52:291–296.

29. Mellonig JT, Bowers GM, Cotton W. Comparison of bone graft materials. Part II. New bone formation with autografts and allografts: A histological evaluation. J Periodontol 1981;52:297–302.

30. Hempton TJ, Fugazzotto PA. Ridge augmentation utilizing guided tissue regeneration, titanium screws, freeze-dried bone, and tricalcium phosphate: Clinical report. Implant Dent 1994;3:35–37.

31. Shanaman RH. A retrospective study of 237 sites treated consecutively with guided tissue regeneration. Int J Periodont Rest Dent 1994;14:293–301.

32. Becker W, Becker B. Guided tissue regeneration for implants placed into extraction sockets and for implant dehiscences: Surgical techniques and case reports. Int J Periodont Rest Dent 1990;10:377–391.

33. Buser D, Dula K, Belser U, Hirt H-P, Berthold H. Localized ridge augmentation using guided bone regeneration. I. Surgical procedure in the maxilla. Int J Periodont Rest Dent 1993;13:29–45.

34. Langer B, Langer L. The overlapped flap: A surgical modification for implant fixture installation. Int J Periodont Rest Dent 1990;10:209–215.

35. Buser D, Dula K, Belser UC, Hirt H-P, Berthold H. Localized ridge augmentation using guided bone regeneration. II. Surgical procedure in the mandible. Int J Periodont Rest Dent 1995;15:3–40.

36. Jones JK, Triplett RG. The relationship of cigarette smoking to impaired intraoral wound healing: A review of evidence and implications for patient care. J Oral Maxillofac Surg 1992;50:237–239.

37. Bain CA, Moy PK. The association between the failure of dental implants and cigarette smoking. Int J Oral Maxillofac Implants 1993;8:609–615.

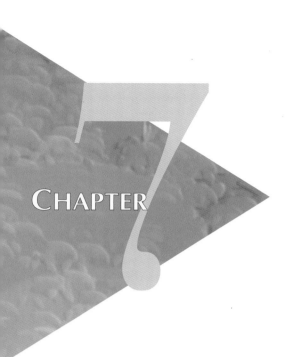

CHAPTER 7

Protected Space Development for Bone Formation Using Reinforced Barrier Membranes

Sascha A. Jovanovic, DDS, MS

The treatment of compromised edentulous alveolar ridges with bone reconstructive techniques is a challenging goal in preprosthetic surgery. Improved understanding of the biologic principle of guided bone regeneration (GBR) and continued innovations of the surgical technique have resulted in significant amounts of new bone.[1-7] These advances have extended the indications for implant placement to sites previously thought unsuitable, and have resulted in the successful augmentation of localized bone defects before and during implant placement. This affords the clinician new opportunities to correct hard and soft tissue defects resulting from trauma, endodontic failure, periodontal failure, or long-term denture use.[3-5,7]

The principle of GBR is based on early studies, which introduced the protected space theory, ie, that exclusion of connective tissue from the wound area will result in new bone formation.[8-12] The membrane technique compartmentalizes wound healing by excluding undesirable cell populations and accommodating the mitosis and chemotaxis of osteoprogenitor cells.[1-7,13] In this manner, the membrane is used as a mechanical barrier to create a protected space for the organizing blood clot and to prevent collapse of the space due to the pressure of the soft tissue flap. The result is the migration of bone-forming elements into this space.[13]

Clinical and experimental observations[1-7,13] have shown that new bone formation is enhanced by *(1)* a healthy, vascularized bone base; *(2)* a large protected space under the membrane; *(3)* full soft tissue coverage of the membrane site during the complete healing period; and *(4)* a minimum healing period of 7 months. The most common reasons for clinical failure in regenerative bone sites appear to be the collapse of the membrane toward the defect (Figs 7-1a to 7-1c), unrealistic expectation of the biological regenerative capacity of a bony defect, and premature membrane exposure through the soft tissue.[3,5] The occurrences of soft tissue perforations, unsatifactory bone regeneration, and

membrane collapse have decreased as a result of the improvement of surgical techniques, better understanding of the biologic tissue reaction to membrane application, and experience with the technique.[5,14]

Protected Space Development

The creation of a large protected space under the membrane is a prime determinant of the achievable volume of new bone. The main reason for membrane collapse seems to be soft tissue pressure, especially in defects that do not demonstrate natural spacemaking form, and with membranes that do not have the rigidity to maintain space.[3,5,13] Clinical studies have demonstrated successful application of bone autografts and allografts for support of the membrane and to supplement spacemaking.[3-6] The addition of an autograft usually requires another surgical site as a donor source. If the intraoral availability is limited, it is necessary to access an extraoral surgical site for donor material. This increases the cost of the procedure and the morbidity for the patient. Therefore, freeze-dried bone allografts are often used as substitutes for autogenous bone; however, unsubstantiated fear of disease transfer may limit their use.

Reinforced Barrier Membranes

Reinforced membranes are able to maintain a protected space without the addition of graft material.[13,15-17] An expanded polytetrafluoroethylene (e-PTFE) membrane reinforced with thin titanium mesh has been evaluated for treatment of bone and implant defects (Figs 7-2a to 7-2d).[18-20] The titanium is encased in two layers of e-PTFE (WL Gore, Flagstaff, AZ).

Figs 7-1 to 7-c Cross-sectional views of implant exposure. A significant circumference of the implant is outside of the bony housing.

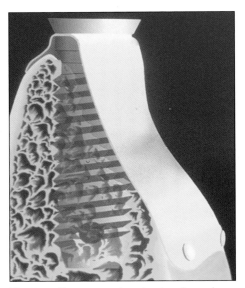

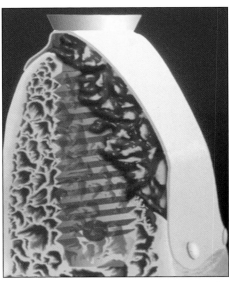

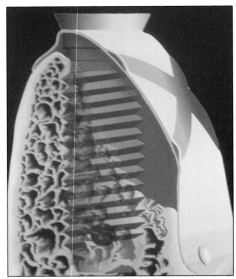

Fig 7-1a If no supporting structure is used underneath a standard nonresorbable membrane, the membrane collapses toward the implant.

Fig 7-1b A bone graft is used to support the membrane, stabilize the blood clot, and supplement spacemaking activities.

Fig 7-1c A significant protected space filled with a hematoma is developed between the implant surface and the inner part of the titanium-reinforced membrane.

Figs 7-2a to 7-2d Results of an experimental study evaluating vertical bone formation in the beagle dog. (From Jovanovic et al.[19] Reprinted with permission.)

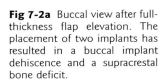

Fig 7-2a Buccal view after full-thickness flap elevation. The placement of two implants has resulted in a buccal implant dehiscence and a supracrestal bone deficit.

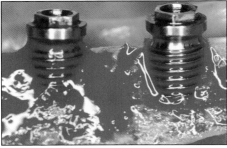

Fig 7-2b The space under the membrane was filled with peripheral blood from the animal and bleeding from the local bone surface. Note the blood clot formation and the shaping of the titanium-reinforced membrane.

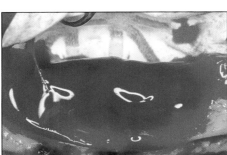

Fig 7-2c Buccal view after 6 months of submerged healing and the removal of the titanium-reinforced membrane. The supracrestal deficit is completely filled with bone tissue after a superficial soft tissue layer is removed.

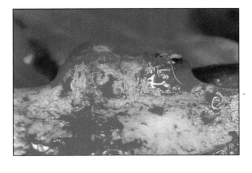

Fig 7-2d Buccolingual section of a titanium-reinforced site. The site showed good space maintenance at the completion of an uneventful healing period and good vertical and horizontal bone fill. Note the overgrowth of bone superior to the implant rim. (Ground section; surface staining with toluidine blue and basic fuchsin; original magnification ×2.5.)

The reinforced membrane, with its individual struts, can be bent to achieve the desired form and adaptation for the defect morphology (see Figs 7-3b and 7-5c). The membrane is trimmed in a normal fashion so that the stiffer portion with the titanium mesh covers the defect and the flexible portion overlaps the edge of the bone on the periphery of the defect by approximately 4 mm. The corners of the material are rounded to allow close adaptation of the membrane to the periphery of the bone defect and to prevent flap perforation.[9] The material is then stabilized with cover screws or fixation screws.

Placement of Reinforced Membranes

Presurgical evaluation includes radiographic surveys and clinical examinations to determine the degree of ridge resorption.[21] The patient is provided with detailed information about the risks and benefits of the reconstructive membrane therapy.

The surgical care and execution are similar for most patients. The patient is premedicated with an antibiotic regimen, and the mouth is rinsed prior to surgery with 0.12% chlorhexidine for 1 minute. The regimen is continued up to 1 week after surgery.

The preferred flap design in the maxilla is a crestal incision placed slightly on the palatal side of the crest (see Fig 7-3b), and in the mandible it is a split-to-full–thickness buccal or crestal incision[5,14] (see Fig 7-4a). Vertical releasing incisions are used to enhance flap elasticity. They are placed at a reasonable distance from the anticipated edge of the membrane and are usually at the distal line angles of the adjacent teeth. The mucoperiosteal flaps are elevated so as to preserve the periosteum. All soft tissue remnants are removed from the bone surface (see Fig 7-3a).

Intramarrow penetration is performed with small-diameter drills, used under copious irrigation with sterile saline (see Fig 7-5b), to achieve a bleeding bone surface. This enhances the access of blood vessels and bone-forming progenitor cells to the defect site. The bone marrow is the source of cells that contribute to angiogenesis and osteogenesis.[22,23] It also is the source for various growth factors.[24] Because of the critical role the local tissue bed plays in any regenerative procedure, it should be handled with care.

If implant placement is planned, it is performed using the standardized technique described by Adell et al,[25] except that screw tapping is usually eliminated. The use of a membrane to correct osseous deformities associated with the dental implant is indicated when the implant (1) has good primary stability and (2) is placed in an optimal prosthetic position. If a patient presents with an extremely narrow, compromised edentulous ridge, and implant placement is determined to be unrealistic, the patient is treated in two stages; a reconstructive membrane procedure precedes implant placement (see Figs 7-5a to 7-5h).[4,5]

The following protocol is suggested for the application of reinforced nonresorbable membranes:

1. If implant exposure is moderate (eg, dehiscence < 8 mm in height), or if a moderate spacemaking defect (a defect that provides membrane support) is present, a nonreinforced membrane with bone graft or reinforced membrane without bone graft materials can be chosen.
2. If implant exposure is large (eg, dehiscence > 8 mm in height), and the defect is either spacemaking or non-spacemaking, a reinforced membrane can be applied without bone graft materials. (Figs 7-3 and 7-4).
3. Larger implant exposures and those that are outside of the bony housing are usually non-spacemaking bone defects. These may be treated with a reinforced membrane supported by a bone graft.

Primary flap closure with no tension is essential and of utmost importance. The periosteum is released at the base of the flap, and connected internally with the vertical incisions by cutbacks. Closure of the flap is achieved with horizontal and interrupted sutures.[5,14] The patient is then discharged from the dental office with appropriate analgesics and cold packs. The sutures are removed 2 to 3 weeks after surgery, and no removable prosthesis is used for as long as possible (a minimum of 3 weeks). The removable prosthesis is then carefully adjusted and relined to prevent trauma to the augmented site. Fixed provisional restorations can be placed immediately after surgery as long as no pressure is applied to the surgical sight. The patient is observed frequently during the first 6 weeks, and monthly thereafter.

Length of Healing Period and Removal of the Membrane

At present, the length of time needed to regenerate peri-implant defects covered with barrier membranes is unknown and is probably patient and site dependent. Clinical and experimental results suggest a minimum healing period of (1) 7 months for the combination of an autograft and a membrane[26]; (2) 8 months for the membrane alone[13,19]; and (3) 9 months for the combination of a membrane and an allograft.[6]

Clinical studies have demonstrated that, after a healing period of 7 to 12 months, titanium-reinforced membranes are retained in proper position under the soft tissue with very few membrane-reinforced sites showing collapse of a titanium strut.[18,19] Some force is required to separate the titanium-reinforced membranes from the surface of the bone. The regenerated tissue under the reinforced membranes appears to be a hard, bonelike structure with a superficial soft tissue layer of up to 3 mm (see Figs 7-5a to 7-5i). The fibrous layer is left in place around most implants, but an assessment can be made of the thickness by incising the layer with a scalpel down to bone. It is advisable to overdevelop the space underneath the membrane by bending it into the desired shape, to anticipate the development of a superficial soft tissue layer over the regenerated bone.

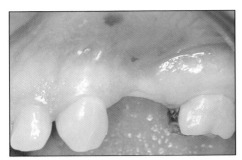

Fig 7-3a A partially edentulous space, located in the upper left jaw, with moderate horizontal and vertical loss of tissue.

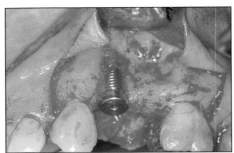

Fig 7-3b After careful elevation of a large mucoperiosteal flap, a 13-mm standard Brånemark implant (Nobel Biocare, Gothenburg, Sweden) is placed in the optimal position, resulting in a superficially dehisced implant surface. Perforations are made in the cortical plate to achieve a bleeding bone surface.

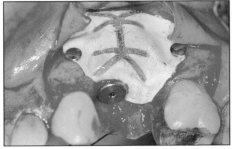

Fig 7-3c A titanium-reinforced membrane is bent to achieve the desired form, trimmed, and then secured with the cover screw and two fixation pins. Note the development of the large space between the implant and the membrane, resulting in good stabilization of the blood clot, and the intimate adaptation of the membrane margin to the underlying bone. No bone graft is placed.

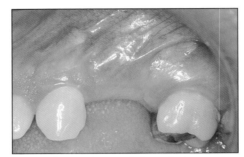

Fig 7-3d Buccal view of the soft tissues after an uneventful healing period of 7 months.

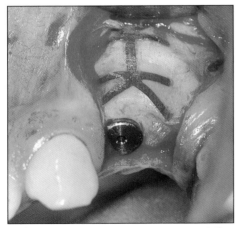

Fig 7-3e Elevation of a mucoperiosteal flap demonstrates an intact titanium-reinforced membrane with no evidence of a collapsed space or a titanium strut.

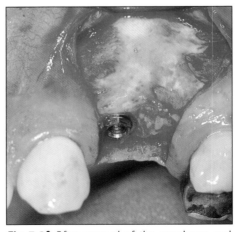

Fig 7-3f After removal of the membrane and the fixation pins, a combination of new bone and a superficial soft tissue layer is visible.

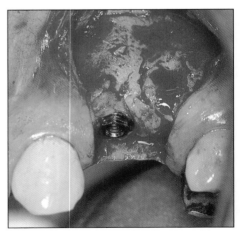

Fig 7-3g Excision of the soft tissue layer reveals complete closure of the buccal dehiscence and localized ridge augmentation with new bone.

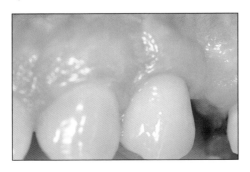

Fig 7-3h The 1-year clinical evaluation reveals healthy peri-implant tissues and the final restoration in place. (Prosthetic dentistry by Dr G. Farina.)

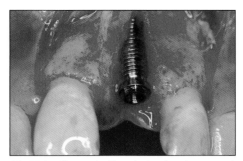

Fig 7-4a A remote flap design has been used in the anterior maxilla of a 30-year-old woman 2 months after extraction of a central incisor. The large residual bone defect after extraction is visible. A 15-mm standard Brånemark implant has been placed in the ideal prosthetic position, and a dehiscence is evident over 13 mm of the implant surface. The buccal implant surface is within the housing of the bone.

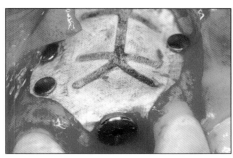

Fig 7-4b A large titanium-reinforced membrane without a bone graft is used to treat the dehisced anterior implant. Careful attention has been given to the development of a blood clot in the space between the implant and the membrane. The membrane is stabilized with three pins, resulting in a close adaptation of the periphery of the membrane to the bone surface.

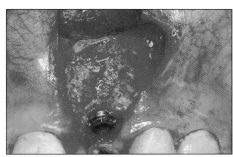

Fig 7-4c A full-thickness flap is elevated, and the membrane is removed after 8 months of uneventful healing. The previous defect is regenerated with newly formed bone.

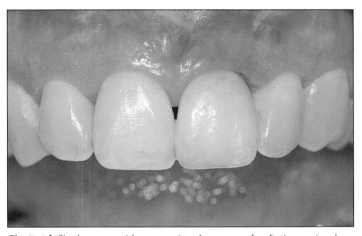

Fig 7-4d Final crown with appropriate harmony of soft tissues in place after 3 years. (Prosthetic dentistry by Dr Hugo Albera.)

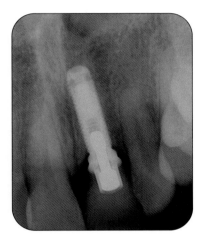

Fig 7-4e A periapical radiograph 3 years after implant placement demonstrates normal bone structures around the implant.

Indications for Reinforced Membranes

The use of titanium-reinforced barrier membranes appears to be indicated for the treatment of dehisced implants and localized ridge deficiencies with a variety of non-spacemaintaining defects. The main advantage of a titanium-reinforced membrane is its ability to maintain a large protected space between the membrane and the bone surface without the addition of a supportive device.

Jovanovic and Nevins[19] treated patients with the titanium-reinforced membrane design and reported that significant new bone was formed. These results are comparable to the bone gain reported in previous clinical trials evaluating treatment of dehisced implant sites and localized ridge defects.[3,5] Five titanium-reinforced membranes were used, without a filling material, around dehisced implant sites and one localized ridge defect. The reentry procedures revealed successful treatment of large implant and bone defects with a titanium-reinforced membrane alone. New

bone formation with a superficial soft tissue layer was noted in all five of these sites.

Other titanium-reinforced membrane sites were additionally treated with bone grafts.[19] One membrane site was augmented with an autograft and the other membrane site with a freeze-dried bone allograft. Both sites achieved complete fill of the defects with new bone and a superficial soft tissue layer. No residual defects were noted, resulting in an average change of implant exposure of 8.2 ± 2.3 mm for sites with buccal dehiscences and between 5 and 6 mm of ridge enlargement in localized bone defects. This finding is in agreement with those of previous studies, which have demonstrated that combined treatment with a membrane and an autograft or allograft results in complete bone regeneration.[26] The amount of bone formation was somewhat greater in the sites treated with a bone graft and a titanium-reinforced membrane than in those treated with a titanium-reinforced membrane alone. This was attributed to the presence of a thicker soft tissue layer underneath titanium-reinforced membranes placed without graft material.[19]

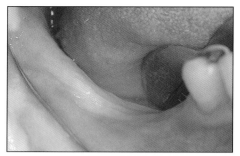

Fig 7-5a A severely resorbed posterior mandible is evident in a 40-year-old woman. Note the severe loss of the vertical bone component, which prevents predictable implant placement.

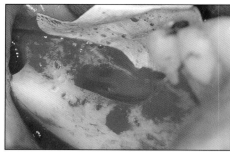

Fig 7-5b A crestal incision extending from the mesial of the premolar to the retromolar area, allows for the elevation of a mucoperiosteal flap. After a large intraosseous defect and the bone surface are cleaned, bone is harvested from the retromolar area with an 8-mm trephine (Hu-Friedy, Chicago, IL). Note the stabilization of a large titanium-reinforced membrane on the lingual with two fixation pins developing a secluded space for the bone graft.

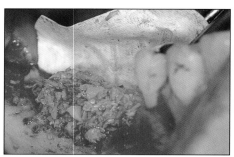

Fig 7-5c The cortical bone blocks are particulated (Quetin bone mill, Leimen, Germany) and condensed into the bone defect and in a supracrestal position.

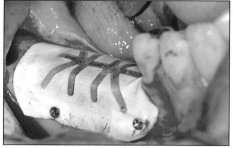

Fig 7-5d The titanium-reinforced membrane is bent and trimmed into shape and secured with fixation screws (Osteomed, Dallas, TX) to the buccal bone surface. Note the new anticipated level of the bone crest.

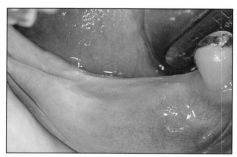

Fig 7-5e An uneventful healing results in healthy soft tissues in a new vertical position. No prostheses are used by the patient in this period.

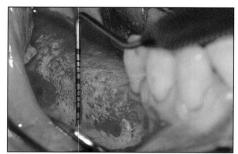

Fig 7-5f After a healing period of 9 months the tissues are reopened and the membrane removed. Note the vertical bone augmentation and the healthy vascularized new bone surface.

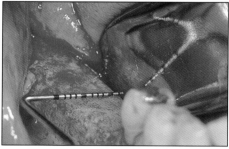

Fig 7-5g Note the horizontal bone augmentation and the healthy vascularized new bone crest of 8 mm.

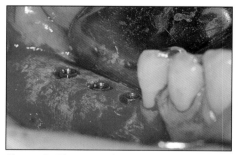

Fig 7-5h Three standard Brånemark implants of 13-mm length can be placed in the ideal vertical and horizontal prosthetic position.

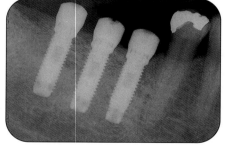

Fig 7-5i A periapical radiograph taken at the time of abutment connection 5 months later shows the normal trabeculation of the newly regenerated bone and the maintenance of the vertical bone height.

Simion et al[18] and Jovanovic et al[20] presented clinical and experimental results of the treatment of critical-sized non-spacemaking defects around supracrestal implant defects for vertical ridge augmentation. The implants were covered with a titanium-reinforced membrane alone and demonstrated 3 to 4 mm of clinical gain and 2 to 6 mm of histometric gain in a supracrestal direction.

The clinical observation of the presence of a thin fibrous layer between the membrane and the newly formed bone has been reported.[3,5,18,19] The soft tissue oriented toward the membrane site is composed of loose connective tissue with thin collagen fibers. The soft tissue oriented toward the bone surface is well vascularized with active bone formation.[13]

The use of reinforced membranes has limitations. Increased stiffness can make precise adaptation of the membrane to the bone surface more difficult and soft tissue closure difficult.[18,19] In addition, the stiffness can result in a large space of such a volume that it cannot be completely obliterated by a blood clot or be completely populated with osteoprogenitor cells.[20] Furthermore, exposure of reinforced membranes (without bone grafts) through the soft tissues results in limited bone formation.

The following techniques are recommended to limit these clinical and biologic complications:

1. Precise trimming and fixation of the flexible portion of the membrane barrier[18,19]
2. Placement of a bone graft to support the membrane to take advantage of its potential osteogenic properties, and to decrease the overall volume of space[19]
3. Careful bone preparation to achieve a bleeding surface[22–24]

A rate-limiting parameter of bone formation may be the volume of bone to be replaced.

Conclusion

The use of a reinforced membrane as a barrier results in significant formation of new bone in both large non-space-making implant dehiscences and localized large bone defects. The modification and reinforcement of membranes provides rigidity for significant space development without the need for a supportive device. The regenerated tissue under the reinforced membrane appears to have the quality of bone structure with a superficial fibrous layer. This fibrous layer is more pronounced in sites that are treated with a membrane alone than in sites in which a bone graft is combined with a membrane. Larger defects are treated with a reinforced membrane supported completely, or in part, by a bone graft.

The positive clinical results achieved have been attributed to careful management of the flap; preparation of the bone bed; maintenance of a large space between the defect and the inner surface of the membrane; stabilization of the blood clot and the membrane; and an undisturbed submerged healing period of 7 to 12 months. Clinical results over the last four years demonstrate that the use of a reinforced membrane seems a viable alternative for the clinical treatment of non-spacemaking implant and bone defects. Further clinical and experimental investigations are recommended to optimize the clinical management of complex reconstruction sites.

References

1. Dahlin C, Linde A, Gottlow J, Nyman S. Healing of bone defects by guided tissue regeneration. Plast Reconstr Surg 1988;81:672–676.

2. Dahlin C, Sennerby L, Lekholm U, et al. Generation of new bone around titanium implants using a membrane technique: An experimental study in rabbits. Int J Oral Maxillofac Implants 1989;4:19–25.

3. Jovanovic SA, Spiekermann H, Richter EJ. Bone regeneration on titanium dental implants with dehisced defect sites. A clinical study. Int J Oral Maxillofac Implants 1992;7:233–245.

4. Nevins M, Mellonig JT. The advantages of localized ridge augmentation prior to implant placement: A staged event. Int J Periodont Rest Dent 1994;4:97–111.

5. Buser D, Dula K, Belser U, et al. Localized ridge augmentation using guided bone regeneration. In: Buser D, Dahlin C, Schenk RK (eds). Guided Bone Regeneration in Implant Dentistry. Chicago: Quintessence, 1994:188–233.

6. Simion M, Dahlin C, Trisi P, Piatelli A. Qualitative and quantitative comparative study on different filling materials used in bone tissue regeneration: A controlled clinical study. Int J Periodont Rest Dent 1994;14:199–215.

7. Becker W, Dahlin C, Becker BE, et al. The use of ePTFE barrier membranes for bone formation around titanium implants placed into extraction sockets. A prospective multicenter study. Int J Oral Maxillofac Implants 1994;9:31–40.

8. Murray G, Holden R, Roschlau W. Experimental and clinical study of new growth of bone in a cavity. Am J Surg 1957;93:385.

9. Melcher AH, Dreyer CJ. Protection of the blood clot in healing circumscribed bone defects. J Bone Joint Surg 1962;44B:424.

10. Boyne PJ. Regeneration of alveolar bone beneath cellulose acetate filter implants. J Dent Res 1964;43:827.

11. Vargerik K, Ousterhout DK. Clinical and experimental bone formation. Adv Plast Reconstr Surg 1987;4:95.

12. Boyne PJ. The restoration of resected mandibles in children without the use of bone grafts. J Head Neck Surg 1983;6:626–631.

13. Schenk RK, Buser D, Hardwick WR, Dahlin C. Healing pattern of bone regeneration in membrane-protected defects: A histologic study in the canine mandible. Int J Oral Maxillofac Implants 1994;9:13–29.

14. Jovanovic SA, Buser D. Guided bone regeneration in dehiscence defects and delayed extraction sockets. In: Buser D, Dahlin C, Schenk RK (eds). Guided Bone Regeneration in Implant Dentistry. Chicago: Quintessence, 1994:155–188.

15. Linde A, Thoren C, Dahlin C, Sandberg E. Creation of new bone by an osteopromotive membrane technique: An experimental study in rats. J Oral Maxillofac Surg 1993;51:892–889.

16. Schmid J, Hammerle CHF, Stich H, Lang NP. Supraplant, a novel implant system based on the principle of guided bone regeneration. A preliminary study in the rabbit. Clin Oral Implants Res 1991;2:199–202.

17. Boyne PJ. Restoration of osseous defects in maxillofacial casualties. J Am Dent Assoc 1969;78:767.

18. Simion M, Baldoni M, Zaffe D. Vertical bone formation utilizing guided tissue regeneration. Int J Periodont Rest Dent 1994;14:497–512.

19. Jovanovic SA, Nevins M. Bone formation utilizing titanium-reinforced barrier membranes. Int J Periodont Rest Dent 1995;15:57–69.

20. Jovanovic SA, Schenk RK, Orsini M, Kenney EB. Supracrestal bone formation around dental implants. Int J Oral Maxillofac Implants 1995;1:23–32.

21. Mecall RA, Rosenfeld AL. The influence of residual ridge resorption patterns on implant fixture placement and tooth position. Int J Periodont Rest Dent 1991;11:19.

22. Wlodarski KH. Properties and origin of osteoblasts. Clin Orthop 1990;252:276.

23. Beresford JN. Osteogenic stem cells and the stromal system of bone and marrow. Clin Orthop 1989;240:270.

24. Mizuno K, Nineo K, Tachibana T, et al. The osteogenic potential of fracture haematoma. Subperiosteal and intramuscular transplantation of the haematoma. J Bone Joint Surg 1990;72:822.

25. Adell R, Lekholm U, Rockler B, Brånemark PI. A 15-year study of osseointegrated implants in the treatment of the edentulous jaw. Int J Oral Surg 1981;10:387–416.

26. Buser D, Dula K, Belser UC, Hirt HP, Berthold H. Localized ridge augmentation using guided bone regeneration. II. Surgical procedure in the mandible. Int J Periodont Rest Dent 1995;15:11–29.

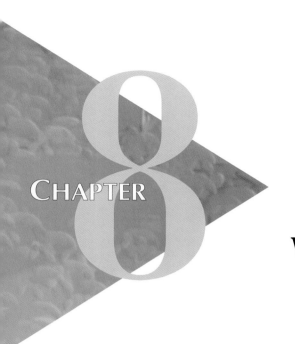

CHAPTER 8

Guided Bone Regeneration for Vertical Ridge Augmentation Associated With Osseointegrated Implants

Massimo Simion, MD, DDS
Paolo Trisi, DDS
Adriano Piattelli, MD, DDS

Guided bone regeneration (GBR) techniques have been used successfully in the last few years to treat bone defects around osseointegrated implants or to augment severely resorbed jaw bones prior to implant placement.[1–7] Barrier membranes are placed over bone defects to create a secluded space between the bone and the membrane. The space created can be populated only by osteoprogenitor cells from the adjacent bone tissue, allowing bone to regenerate in the defects.

The biologic mechanisms and histologic features of guided bone regeneration have been investigated extensively in animal studies.[8–11] Schenk et al[10] have described the sequence and pattern of bone regeneration in membrane-protected defects in foxhound dogs. The histologic evaluation showed that the sequence of events that leads to bone regeneration progresses through a series of maturation steps, which closely resemble the pattern of bone regeneration and growth. Moreover, the study showed, once more, that the test sites treated with a membrane exhibit significantly better bone healing than do control sites without a membrane.

One of the most frequent reasons for failure of bone regeneration with the membrane techniques is the collapse of the membrane toward the surface of the bone in non-space-making defects, as a result of the pressure of the overlying soft tissues.[3,4] To solve this problem, clinicians and researchers have investigated the placement of different grafting materials under the membrane to prevent its collapse. Moreover, some grafting materials are considered to be osteoconductive because of their ability to act as a scaffold for bone regeneration.[11] In some cases, they are thought to be osteoinductive for the possibility of transferring both vital cells with osteogenic capacity and stimulating factors incorporated in the bone matrix.[12]

Among grafting materials, the most widely used in association with GBR are autogenous bone and human demineralized freeze-dried bone (DFDB). The use of autogenous bone graft particles stabilized with supporting miniscrews has been proposed for width augmentation of limited-extension ridges.[2–4] The advantages of autogenous bone grafts are their biocompatibility, their long-lasting space-maintaining ability, and their possibility of being completely resorbed and substituted with the normal turnover of bone. The disadvantages are the limited availability in the oral surgical sites and the necessity of extraoral donor sources for major augmentations.

Bone Regeneration in a Human Implant Model: The Harvest Cover Screw

Methods and Materials

Simion et al[13] presented a new technique to compare, in a human model, the histologic characteristics of different grafting materials after 6 months of healing. In the study, five totally edentulous patients were treated with osseointegrated implants. Each patient received five titanium implants (Nobel Biocare, Gothenburg, Sweden), positioned into delayed postextraction sockets, placed according to the standard procedure described by Adell et al[14] (Fig 8-1). Modified commercially pure titanium cover screws were used to cover the implants after placement. The modified cover screws, termed *harvest cover screws* (HCSs), were basket shaped to allow formation of tissue on top and into the hollow of the basket (Figs 8-2 and 8-3).

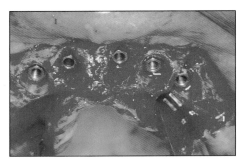

Fig 8-1 Each patient received five titanium implants positioned into delayed postextraction sockets, according to the standard procedure.

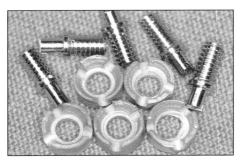

Fig 8-2 The harvest cover screws are pure titanium baskets, shown with the corresponding fixation screws.

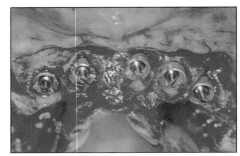

Fig 8-3 The HCSs are positioned in the implant sites. Angular bone defects of different sizes are present around the implants covered with the HCSs.

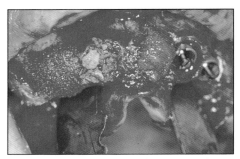

Fig 8-4 Three different grafting materials are positioned over the defects and the HCSs in a randomized distribution. Two HCSs are not grafted and are considered the control sites.

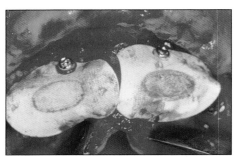

Fig 8-5 Two GTAM membranes have been positioned to cover all but one HCS. The latter received no graft and no membrane and was considered the untreated control.

Each patient was treated with different grafting materials, randomly distributed in each site. One site received autogenous bone chips, collected from the adjacent areas of the same surgical site with bone forceps and covered with a Gore-Tex Augmentation Material (GTAM) membrane (WL Gore, Flagstaff, AZ). The second site was filled with human cortical demineralized freeze-dried bone (Musculoskeletal Transplant Foundation, Holmoel, NJ), rehydrated in sterile saline for 30 minutes before placement, and covered with a GTAM membrane. The third site was treated with Grafton (Musculoskeletal Transplant Foundation), a form of DFDB prepared in a gel solution, which was injected into the site and covered with a GTAM membrane. The fourth site received only the membrane without any grafting material, and the fifth site received no membrane or grafts and served as the control (Figs 8-4 and 8-5).

After a healing period of 6 months, all the HCSs were removed, and small biopsy specimens were taken from the regenerating tissues adherent to the titanium surfaces. The biopsy specimens were fixed and processed for histologic analysis.

Results

Of the 25 implants and HCSs placed, 23 remained covered by the gingival tissues for the entire healing period. Two sites showed an early exposure, and the membrane was prematurely removed because of the purulent inflammation of the adjacent tissues.

At the second-stage surgery, the 23 unexposed implant sites showed healthy gingival tissue. The membranes adhered to the underlying newly formed tissue, and no signs of inflammation were present (Fig 8-6).

The histologic findings showed a wide variability in the quality and quantity of newly formed bone among all the groups, but it was evident that new bone formed over the HCSs in the membrane-treated sites. The overall images of the autogenous bone grafted specimens showed denser bone formation and a greater amount of bone formation (Fig 8-7a). The implanted autogenous bone chips were completely integrated with the newly formed bone; in fact, polygonal areas of the old bone were surrounded by new bone, which was more intensely stained with basic fuchsin (Fig 8-7b). In some cases, the bone was in direct contact with the membrane (Fig 8-7c). In other cases it was separated by a dense fibrous tissue with scattered fibroblasts and fibrocytes.

Sites treated with demineralized freeze-dried bone showed a variable degree of new bone formation (Fig 8-8a). In some specimens, progressive remineralization was evident in most of the demineralized particles. The mechanism of remineralization was "acellular mineral deposition," as described by Yamashita and Takagi.[15] Small, rounded mineralized bodies arose inside the demineralized bone matrix, gradually increasing in size and fusing with one another (Figs 8-8b and 8-8c). In areas where this fusion was more advanced, the zones of tissue that were not yet mineralized were small. In some of the remineralized areas, large osteocytes were present inside the lacunae, and, occasionally, an osteoblastic rim

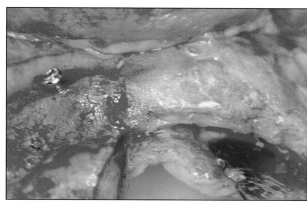

Fig 8-6 At the reentry, after 6 months, the membranes appear to be adherent to underlying tissues, and no signs of inflammation are present.

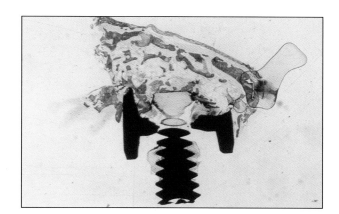

Fig 8-7a An overall image of an autogenous bone graft–treated specimen reveals that the space between the membrane and the chamber is filled with bone trabeculae. (Original magnification ×6.)

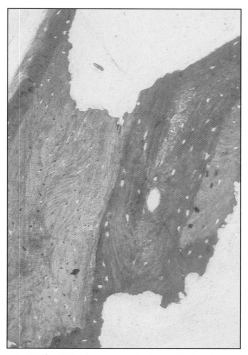

Fig 8-7b At higher magnification, the implanted autogenous bone chips appear to be completely integrated with the newly formed bone. (Original magnification ×100.)

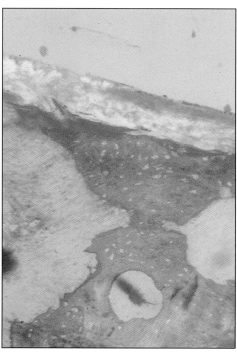

Fig 8-7c The newly formed bone is in direct contact with the membrane. (Original magnification ×200.)

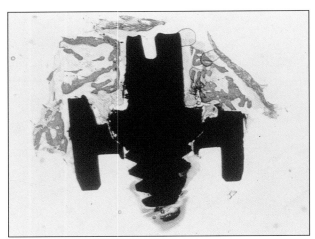

Fig 8-8a In this specimen, treated with human demineralized freeze-dried bone, progressive remineralization is evident in most of the demineralized particles. (Original magnification ×6.)

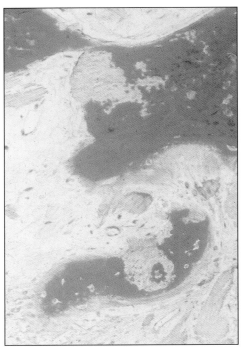

Fig 8-8b Higher magnification of newly formed tissue under the membrane treated with DFDB reveals that small, rounded, and confluent mineralized bodies are present inside the demineralized bone matrix. (Original magnification ×200.)

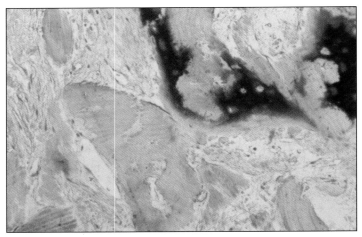

Fig 8-8c Von Kossa histochemical staining for mineralized tissues reveals the presence of areas of mineralization inside the DFDB particles. (Original magnification ×200.)

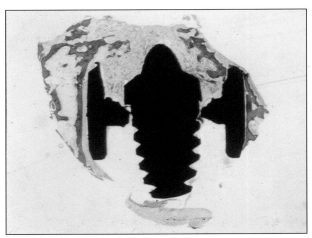

Fig 8-8d In this specimen, bone filling and DFDB substitution with bone is incomplete. In this case, 6 months of healing were not sufficient to achieve a complete substitution. (Original magnification ×8.)

surrounded one side of the bone particles, encasing the DFDB in newly formed bone. This process was particularly evident in some specimens, whereas others showed a lesser degree of new bone formation (Fig 8-8d).

The Grafton-treated specimens showed bone regeneration characteristics similar to those of sites treated with DFDB powder (Figs 8-9a to 8-9c).

The control group that was treated with only the membrane exhibited less bone formation than did the grafted groups, as a result of the tendency of the membrane to col-lapse toward the HCS (Fig 8-10). The control group that was treated with no membrane and no graft showed an absence of any bone formation around or inside the HCSs. Only fibrous connective tissue completely surrounded the HCS (Figs 8-11a and 8-11b).

Most of the test specimens showed areas of direct contact between the newly formed bone and the HCS titanium surface (Figs 8-12a and 8-12b), but, although a histomorphometric analysis was not possible, it was evident that the percentage of direct bone-titanium contact was quite low.

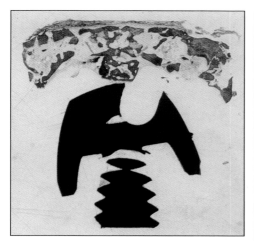

Fig 8-9a A harvest cover screw treated with Grafton shows histologic bone features similar to those of HCSs treated with DFDB. (Original magnification ×6.) (Fig 8-9 from Simion et al.[13] Reprinted with permission.)

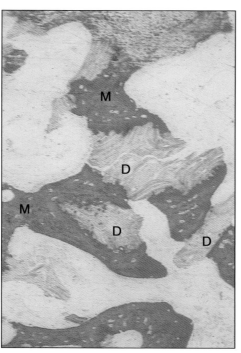

Fig 8-9b Demineralized bone particles (D) are embedded in the structures of newly formed bone (M). Grafton seems to act as a scaffold for the ingrowth of bone. (Original magnification ×100.)

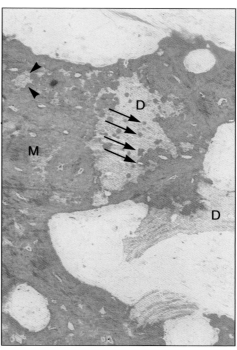

Fig 8-9c Higher magnification reveals that the mechanism of remineralization, in demineralized particles (D), proceeds as acellular mineral deposition. Small, rounded mineralized bodies (*arrows*) arise inside demineralized bone matrix, gradually increasing in size and fusing with one another, thus regenerating bone (M). In areas where this fusion is more advanced, the zones that are not yet mineralized are small (*arrowheads*). (Original magnification ×200.)

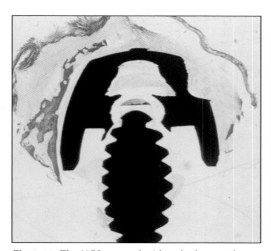

Fig 8-10 The HCSs treated with only the membrane show less bone than the grafted group, as a result of the tendency of the membrane to collapse toward the HCS in the former group. Note the bone growth over the coronal portion of the chamber. (Original magnification ×10.) (From Simion et al.[13] Reprinted with permission.)

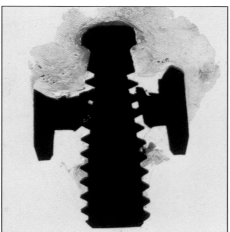

Fig 8-11a In the control group, which received no graft and no membrane, no bone is detectable, and dense connective tissue completely surrounds the HCS. (Original magnification ×10.) (Fig 8-11 from Simion et al.[13] Reprinted with permission.)

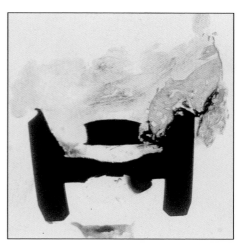

Fig 8-11b In only one specimen in the control group, a small bridge of bone has colonized the superior part of the harvest chamber. (Original magnification ×10.)

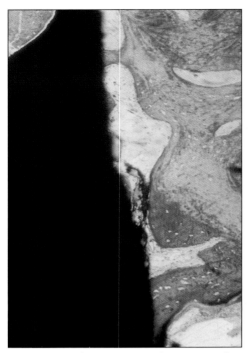 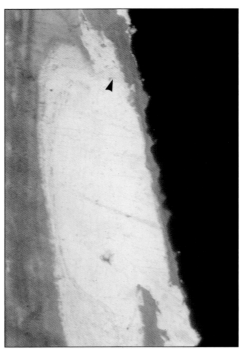

Fig 8-12a In this specimen, a direct contact between the newly formed bone and the titanium is present. (Original magnification ×100.) (Fig 8-12 from Simion et al.[13] Reprinted with permission.)

Fig 8-12b The histologic specimen reveals that in some areas bone detached from the titanium surface during the retrieval surgery (*arrowhead*). In other areas, bone still adheres to the titanium surface. (Original magnification ×200.)

Discussion

The investigation clearly demonstrated that all the grafting materials tested had a positive effect on bone regeneration. One explanation for this positive effect could be the long-lasting space-maintaining effect. This is in accordance with a previous study by Dahlin et al,[16] who reported that the amount of newly formed bone is determined and limited by the space available between the membrane and the surface of the defect. Histologic observations from the HCSs study by Simion et al[13] showed evidence of the tendency of GTAM membranes used alone to collapse toward the defect and the HCS, thereby reducing the space for new bone formation. In contrast, the specimens from the grafted groups had a wider space under the membranes and, therefore, a larger amount of new bone formation. This demonstrated that the membrane was effectively supported by both the autologous and the DFDB grafts.

Besides the ability to maintain an adequate space under the membrane, the transplanted autogenous bone chips may be able to integrate with the newly formed bone, acting as a scaffold for bone formation and reducing the amount of new bone formation required to achieve complete regeneration. Osteoconductive capacity could also be attributed to DFDB; in fact, histologic observations have shown the ability of DFDB to be completely encased by the new bone.

Another explanation for the positive effect of grafting materials is their osteoinductive activity. Burwell[17] demonstrated that the necrosis of autogenous red marrow grafts may liberate substances capable of inducing primitive marrow cells to differentiate to osteoblasts. Moreover, Urist et al[18,19] suggested that demineralization of bone grafts exposes the bone-inductive proteins located in bone matrix and thus enhances their osteogenic potential.

Questions that remain unanswered are whether the demineralized bone particles have the ability to be completely resorbed and substituted with host bone and the time required to achieve a complete substitution. After 6 months of healing, all the DFDB specimens in the HCSs study showed an incomplete substitution of the demineralized particles. A report from Simion et al[20] has evaluated the histologic and histochemical characteristics of bone regenerated with DFDB associated with an expanded polytetrafluoroethylene (e-PTFE) membrane around a human implant retrieved after 4 years of loading. The implant, retrieved because of the fracture of the cast-gold post and core, was clinically stable at the removal. At low magnification, the peri-implant bone showed that, most likely, the implant was in contact with vital bone at almost all of the titanium interface (Fig 8-13a). The bone surrounding the implant was, in the regenerated portion, compact with a limited amount of medullary spaces or wide haversian canals. In some limited areas, the interosteonic spaces, usually occupied by interstitial lamellae, were occupied by traces of residual particles of DFDB partially remineralized and embedded in the normal bone (Figs 8-13b and 8-13c).

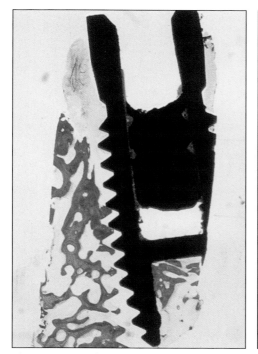

Fig 8-13a Histologic overview of an implant treated with DFDB and a GTAM and retrieved after 4 years of loading. The implant was accidentally displaced from the bone during the retrieval procedure. However, the peri-implant bone indicates that, most likely, the implant is in contact with vital bone at almost all of the titanium interface. (Original magnification ×6.)

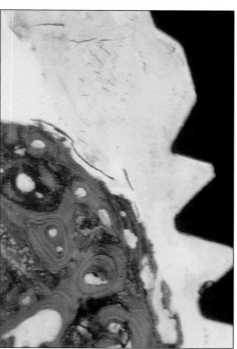

Fig 8-13b In some of the regenerated areas, the interosteonic spaces are occupied by traces of residual particles of DFDB that has been partially remineralized and embedded in the normal bone. (Original magnification ×100.)

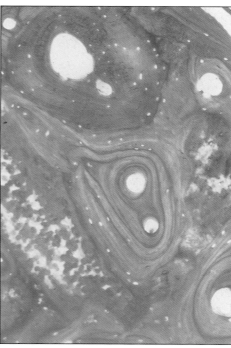

Fig 8-13c Higher magnification of partially remineralized residual DFDB. (Original magnification ×200.)

Conclusion

Histologic and histochemical observations have shown that DFDB particles can be resorbed and substituted with vital newly formed bone, but the rate of resorption is very slow and not complete after 4 years. However, the load-bearing capacity and the characteristics of the bone regenerated with the membrane technique used in association with DFDB seems to be similar to those of normal bone.

Vertical Ridge Augmentation Using Titanium-reinforced Membranes

Methods and Materials

On the basis of the experience acquired with the harvest chambers, a study protocol was designed to evaluate the possibility of obtaining vertical augmentation of atrophic edentulous ridges in six patients.[21] The surgical protocol included the use of a new type of e-PTFE membrane reinforced with a pure titanium structure (TR GTAM, WL Gore, Flagstaff, AZ).

The TR GTAM membranes can be bent and shaped, and maintain the desired form because of the titanium mesh. This characteristic allows the creation and preservation of sufficient space between the membrane and the bone defect. Therefore, regeneration could also be obtained in situations where the anatomy of the defect is not naturally spacemaking.

The surgical technique is shown in Figs 8-14a to 8-14g. A full-thickness crestal incision was made, within the keratinized gingiva, from the distal aspect of the last residual tooth to the distal end of the edentulous ridge. The incision was extended intrasulcularly and anteriorly to the mesial aspect of the adjacent tooth. Vertical releasing incisions were made at the mesiobuccal and mesiopalatal line angles and at the distal aspect of the crestal incision.

The buccal and palatal flaps were widely reflected with a periosteal elevator (Pritchard 1-2, Hu-Friedy, Chicago, IL) so as to gain sufficient access for implant and membrane placement. Care was taken not to damage the palatine arteries and the mental nerve in severely resorbed maxillas and mandibles. The flaps were gently handled to minimize soft tissue trauma and to avoid flap perforations. Once exposed, the cortical bone was curetted with a back-action chisel to remove all residual connective tissue and the periosteum.

The implant surgery was performed according to the standard procedure described by Adell et al,[14] except for some details. The recipient sites were not pretapped to

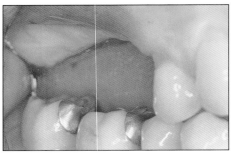

Fig 8-14a Implant sites selected in the study had to have sufficient bone width (greater than 6 mm). Furthermore, the top of the edentulous ridge had to be at least 4 to 5 mm lower than the gingival margin of the residual natural teeth, and the interarch space had to be too wide to be compatible with an esthetic and functional fixed prosthetic rehabilitation. (Fig 8-14 from Simion et al.[21] Reprinted with permission.)

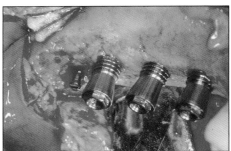

Fig 8-14b Three conical Brånemark implants have been inserted in the maxilla. The implants have been left so that they protrude 6 to 7 mm from the bone crest. A pure titanium miniscrew, protruding 3 mm from the bone level, is visible in the third molar region.

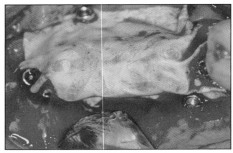

Fig 8-14c The TR GTAM membrane has been positioned in the surgical site and has been fixed to the bone with five Memfix fixation screws.

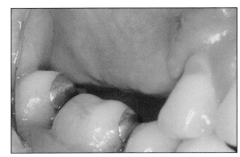

Fig 8-14d The healing was uneventful and no dehiscences of the membrane occurred. The vertical augmentation of the edentulous ridge is evident.

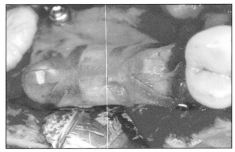

Fig 8-14e At the membrane removal after 9 months, the membrane and the fixation screws have been found in proper position. There are no clinical signs of inflammation.

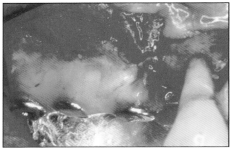

Fig 8-14f The membrane has been gently dissected from the underlying newly formed tissue. On the surface, whitish and scarcely bleeding soft tissue was present.

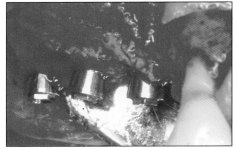

Fig 8-14g The soft tissue has been scraped away with curettes until the newly formed hard bone is evident. A maximum of 3 to 4 mm of bone has been regenerated.

improve primary stability, and the implants were left to protrude 4 to 7 mm from the bone crest. Therefore, the countersink was not used.

A pure titanium miniscrew (1.3 mm in diameter and 10 mm in length) was positioned distally to the implants in each surgical site to serve as a "tent pole" for the membrane. The miniscrews were also left to protrude from the bone level for 3 to 4 mm (Fig 8-14b). Before the membrane was placed, the cortical bone was perforated with a round bur to expose the cancellous bone and encourage bleeding.

The titanium structures of GTAM membranes were bent with pliers to obtain a proper shape of the membrane. The external portion of the membrane was trimmed with scis-

sors to extend at least 4 to 5 mm beyond the defect margins. The membranes were tried in and reshaped several times until a close adaptation to the underlying bone and to the implants was achieved.

Once positioned in the surgical site, the membranes were fixed to the bone with three to five Memfix fixation screws (Straumann, Cambridge, MA).[2-4] The fixation screws were applied at the mesiobuccal and mesiopalatal, as well as at the distal, edges of the membranes to achieve optimal stabilization (Fig 8-14c). Where the augmentation material was next to natural teeth, 2 mm of crestal bone was left uncovered to prevent interference with the healing process of the periodontal tissues.

Releasing incisions in the periosteum at the base of the buccal flaps were made to enhance the elasticity of the flaps and to achieve a tension-free adaptation at closure. Closure was achieved with alternating vertical mattress sutures and interrupted sutures.

Patients were not allowed to wear any partial denture on the surgical site until the stage 2 surgery to avoid any pressure on the wound area. Chemical plaque control with chlorhexidine (0.12% solution twice a day) was instituted for 15 days. The sutures were removed after 10 days, after topical application of 0.2% chlorhexidine gel (Corsodyl Gel) for 2 minutes to reduce bacterial contamination of the wound. Following suture removal, the patients were regularly checked once a week for the first month and, then, once a month until the stage 2 surgery.

Membranes were removed at the stage 2 surgery after 9 months of healing. After removal of the membrane, the pure titanium miniscrews were removed with a small trephine in such a way that a small biopsy specimen of preexisting and newly formed tissue was collected from each site. The specimens were processed for histologic examinations.

Results

Only one patient developed an abscess involving the entire surgical site after 1 month of healing. The membrane was removed, and, at the reopening after 9 months, no signs of bone regeneration were evident. In the remaining five patients participating in the study, no dehiscence of the membranes occurred during the entire healing period (Fig 8-14d).

At the membrane removal after 9 months, all the membranes and the fixation screws were found to be in proper position, and there were no clinical signs of inflammation (Fig 8-14e). The fixation screws were removed with the proper screwdriver, and the membranes were gently dissected from the underlying newly formed tissue. At the surface, whitish and scarcely bleeding soft tissue was present at all the sites (Fig 8-14f). The soft tissue was scraped away with curettes until the newly formed hard bone was evident (Fig 8-14g).

The biometric measurements showed a gain in bone height varying from 3 to 4 mm. Histologic examination of bone biopsy specimen revealed that all the retrieved miniscrews were in direct contact with bone. Nevertheless, the most coronal portions of the screws were over the crestal level of the bone, immersed in a dense fibrous tissue (Figs 8-15a to 8-15c). The histomorphometric analysis of the percentage of bone contact gave a mean value of 42.5% + 3.6% for five of the six examined miniscrews. In the remaining miniscrew, which was positioned in the tuberosity of the maxilla, only the 21.6% of the surface was in contact with bone. The portion of the miniscrews surrounded by supracrestal connective tissue had a mean value of 2.2 + 0.46 mm. This tissue consisted of densely packed collagen fibers with few cells and few blood vessels.

Discussion

In this study in the human, the possibility of circumferential bone formation in a vertical direction from flat cortical bone surfaces was verified around titanium implants. The results clearly demonstrated that, with the surgical protocol described, it is possible to obtain up to 4 mm of vertical augmentation of jawbone with a high degree of predictability. On the other hand, this investigation failed to demonstrate vertical bone regeneration over that limit. In fact, the most coronal part of the implants, left protruding more than 4 mm from the bone crest, was always surrounded by dense fibrous tissue. The apical portion of the bone in contact with the screws showed an advanced stage of bone maturation, while the most coronal bone showed bone-forming activity (Fig 8-15d). This observation substantiates the hypothesis that bone regeneration was still in progress at the time of membrane removal after 9 months.

Different hypotheses offer potential explanations for the the absence of complete bone regeneration over the 4-mm limit.

1. The adaptation of a flat membrane to a three-dimensional, curved anatomic shape caused different amounts of folds at the borders of the membrane. The folds may act as spots of "leakage," partially reducing the mechanical barrier effect of the membrane. Such spots of leakage could be of limited effect when a small volume of bone has to be regenerated, but might hinder complete bone regeneration when considerable vertical augmentation is required. From this point of view, the e-PTFE membrane could be considered as capable of retarding the penetration of connective tissue long enough to allow the vertical regeneration of a maximum of 3 to 4 mm of bone.

2. The large blood clot under the membrane could undergo a certain amount of shrinkage during the early stage of healing, thus reducing the amount of bone regeneration. In this case, the use of some filling material, able to stabilize the blood clot, could be helpful in augmenting the formation of new bone. This hypothesis is in accordance with previous studies[13] that have shown that the amount of bone regeneration is greater when grafting materials are used under the membranes.

3. The blood supply in the most coronal portion of the space, secluded under the membrane, could be insufficient to allow osteogenic activity.

4. A longer period of time might be necessary to achieve complete bone regeneration up to the internal surface of the membrane. This statement is supported by the histologic finding in this study of bone-forming activity in the most coronal portion of bone regenerated around the titanium miniscrews. This finding demonstrated that the bone regeneration was still in progress after 9 months, at the time of membrane removal.

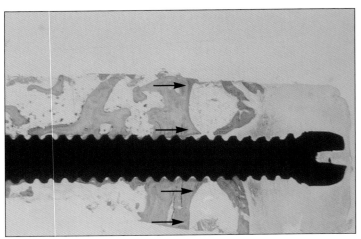

Fig 8-15a Histologic section of the retrieved miniscrew in site 47 (patient 1). The old bone is distinguishable, because it has a lower staining affinity for basic fuchsin. Level of the preexisting bone (*arrows*). (Original magnification ×10.) (Fig 8-15 from Simion et al.[21] Reprinted with permission.)

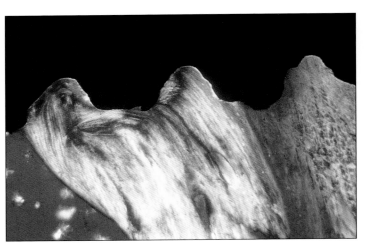

Fig 8-15b Higher magnification of the specimen in Fig 8-15a. The regenerated bone is in direct contact with the titanium surface. Polarized light microscopy reveals a bone pattern of spongious bone of lamellar type. (Original magnification ×100.)

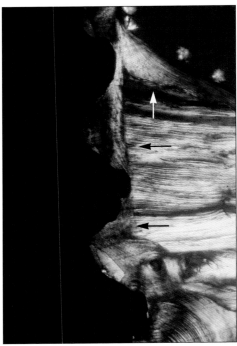

Fig 8-15c Higher magnification of the specimen in Fig 8-15a. Polarized light microscopy reveals that the lamellae present in the preexisting bone have a different direction from the lamellae in the new bone (*arrows*). Osseointegration is evident. (Original magnification ×100.)

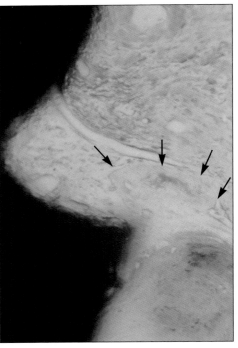

Fig 8-15d Bone formation activity is present at the top of the regenerating bone around the miniscrew (site 37, patient 1). Islands of osteoid tissue, with ongoing intramembranous ossification, are visible (*arrows*). (Original magnification ×100.)

Conclusion

The results of this study suggest that the placement of membranes around implants protruding 3 to 4 mm from the top of resorbed bone surfaces may result in vertical bone regeneration up to the top of the implant cylinder and that the regenerated bone is able to "osseointegrate" pure titanium implants. Further research is needed to evaluate the load-bearing capability and the long-term results of the newly formed bone.

In a recent study,[22] the effect on vertical bone regeneration of the addition of DFDBA or autogenous bone chips to the same membrane technique was investigated.

Twenty partially edentulous patients with vertical jaw bone deficiencies were selected for this study. The patients were divided into two groups of 10. The 10 patients in Group A received a total of 26 Brånemark implants in 10 surgical sites. The 10 patients of Group B received a total of 32 implants in 12 surgical sites.

Fifty-two out of 58 placed implants (22 in Group A and 30 in Group B) extended 1.5 to 7.5 mm superior to the bone crest. Pure titanium miniscrews (1.3 × 10 mm) were

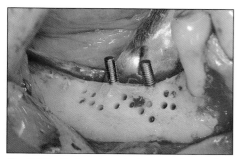

Fig 8-16a A staged surgical approach was chosen. Two commercially pure titanium pins were placed 5 mm above the bone crest to support the reinforced membrane. Multiple perforations were made in the cortical bone plate to favor bleeding and stimulate bone repair.

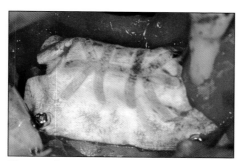

Fig 8-16b Autogenous bone particles, collected from the chin, were positioned over the bone crest and a titanium-reinforced membrane was stabilized with Memfix screws.

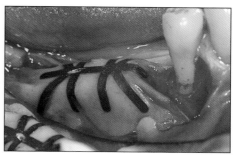

Fig 8-16c After flap elevation at the second-stage surgery, the membrane demonstrated good space maintenance and ridge contour.

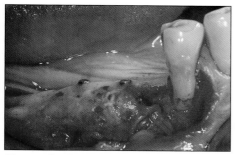

Fig 8-16d After the membrane removal, the regenerated bone is visible under a thin layer of soft tissue. The titanium pins are almost completely embedded in new bone.

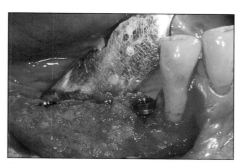

Fig 8-16e Three Brånemark implants have been positioned with a standard technique. One of the pins was removed and analyzed for histomorphometric evaluation.

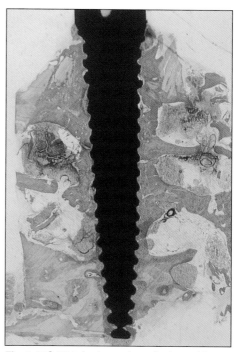

Fig 8-16f Histologic section of a bone biopsy from a site treated with autogenous bone chips. The preexisting cortical bone plate is still distinguishable at 3 mm from the apex of the titanium pin. The regenerated bone extends up to the top of the pin and shows a high rate of direct contact with the titanium surface. (Basic fuchsin; original magnification ×12).

positioned distally to the implants protruding 3 to 7 mm from the bone crest. Titanium-reinforced e-PTFE membranes were used to cover the implants. Before complete membrane fixation, DFDBA particles were condensed under the membrane in Group A, and autogenous bone chips were used in Group B (Figs 8-16a to 8-16e).

At re-entry, after 7 to 11 months, the membranes were removed and small biopsies, which encompassed the miniscrews, were collected from 11 sites. The clinical measurements from Group A demonstrated a mean vertical bone gain of 3.1 mm (SD = 0.9, range 1 to 5 mm) with a mean percentage of bone gain of 124% (SD = 46.6). The measurements from Group B showed a mean vertical bone gain of 5.02 mm (SD = 2.3, range 1 to 8.5 mm) with a mean percentage of bone gain of 95% (SD = 26.8).

Histomorphometric analysis clearly demonstrated a direct correlation between the density of the preexisting bone and the density of the regenerated bone. The mean percentage of new bone-titanium contact was from 39.1% to 63.2% depending on the quality of the native bone (Fig 8-16f). Both the clinical and histologic results from this study indicated that vertical ridge augmentation procedures, using DFDBA or autogenous bone particles in addition to the membrane technique, can be considered predictable in humans.

References

1. Becker W, Becker BE. Guided tissue regeneration for implants placed into extraction sockets and for implant dehiscences: Surgical techniques and case reports. Int J Periodont Rest Dent 1990;10:377–392.

2. Buser D, Brägger U, Lang NP, Nyman S. Regeneration and enlargement of jaw bone using guided tissue regeneration. Clin Oral Implants Res 1990;1:22–32.

3. Dahlin C, Andersson L, Lindhe A. Bone augmentation at fenestrated implants by an osteopromotive membrane technique. A controlled clinical study. Clin Oral Implants Res 1991;2:159–165.

4. Buser D, Dula K. Localized ridge augmentation using guided bone regeneration. I. Surgical procedure in the maxilla. Int J Periodont Rest Dent 1993;13:13.

5. Nevins M, Mellonig JT. Enhancement of the damaged edentulous ridge to receive dental implants: A combination of allograft and the Gore-Tex membrane. Int J Periodont Rest Dent 1992;12:12.

6. Jovanovic S, Spiekermann H, Richter EJ. Bone regeneration on titanium dental implants with dehisced defect sites. A clinical study. Int J Oral Maxillofac Implants 1992;7:233.

7. Simion M, Baldoni M, Zaffe D. Jawbone enlargement using immediate implant placement associated with a split-crest technique and guided tissue regeneration. Int J Periodont Rest Dent 1992;12:463–473.

8. Dahlin C, Sennerby L, Lekholm U, et al. Generation of new bone around titanium implants using a membrane technique: An experimental study in rabbits. Int J Oral Maxillofac Implants 1989;4:19.

9. Becker W, Becker B, Handelsman M, et al. Bone formation at dehiscent dental implant sites treated with implant augmentation material: A pilot study in dogs. Int J Periodont Rest Dent 1990;10:93.

10. Schenk RK, Buser D, Hardwick WR, Dahlin C. Healing pattern of bone regeneration in membrane protected defects. A histologic study in the canine mandible. Int J Oral Maxillofac Implants 1994;9:13–29.

11. Schenk RK. Bone regeneration: Biologic basis. In: Buser D, Dahlin C, Schenk RK (eds). Guided Bone Regeneration in Implant Dentistry. Chicago: Quintessence, 1994:49–100.

12. Cushing M. Autogenous red marrow grafts: Potential for induction of osteogenesis. J Periodontol 1969;40:492–497.

13. Simion M, Dahlin C, Trisi P, Piattelli A. Qualitative and quantitative comparative study on different filling materials used in bone tissue regeneration: A controlled clinical study. Int J Periodont Rest Dent 1994;14:199-215.

14. Adell R, Lekholm U, Brånemark PI. Surgical procedures. In: Brånemark P-I, Zarb G, Albrektsson T (eds). Tissue-Integrated Prostheses: Osseointegration in Clinical Dentistry. Chicago: Quintessence, 1985:199.

15. Yamashita K, Takagi T. Ultrastructural observation of calcification preceding new bone formation induced by demineralized bone matrix gelatin. Acta Anat Basel 1992:143:261–267.

16. Dahlin C, Alberius P, Linde A. Osteopromotion for cranioplasty. An experimental study in rats using a membrane technique. J Neurosurg 1991;74:487–491.

17. Burwell RG. Studies in the transplantation of bone. VII. The fresh composite homograft autograft of cancellous bone. J Bone Joint Surg 1964;46B:110.

18. Urist MR. Bone formation by autoinduction. Science 1965;150:893–899.

19. Urist MR, Dowel TA, Hay PH, Strates BS. Inductive substrates for bone formation. Clin Orthop 1968;59:59–96.

20. Simion M, Trisi P, Piattelli A. Guided bone regeneration with e-PTFE membrane associated with DFDB graft: Histological and histochemical analysis in an human implant retrieved after 4 years of loading. Int J Periodont Rest Dent 1996;16:339–347.

21. Simion M, Trisi P, Piattelli A. Vertical ridge augmentation using a membrane technique associated with osseointegrated implants. Int J Periodont Rest Dent 1994;14:497–511.

22. Simion M, Jovanovic SA, Trisi P, Scarano A, Piattelli A. Vertical ridge augmentation around dental implants using a membrane technique and bone auto or allografts in humans. Int J Periodont Rest Dent 1998;18:9–23.

CHAPTER 9

The Placement of Maxillary Anterior Implants

Myron Nevins, DDS
James M. Stein, DMD

Osseointegration had been clearly demonstrated to be an efficacious treatment for the edentulous maxilla, but the application of this science to the partially dentate maxilla has captured the imagination of both the professional and the layperson.[1–5] Dentistry is seldom as interesting to the patient as when the esthetic zone is encountered.

Perhaps the most important factor to consider when contemplating the use of implant dentistry in the maxillary anterior segment is the vertical height of the alveolar process and its relationship to the proposed position of the final restoration. In addition, it is necessary to allot the correct mesiodistal space for each tooth. When the height of bone is correct and the horizontal width appropriate for a tooth or teeth to be replaced in the absence of meaningful bone concavities, the optimum placement of implants then can be achieved by establishing the proposed position of the labial surface of the tooth to be supported by the implant (Figs 9-1a to 9-1f) (see Chapter 3).

Clinical Examination

The pathosis resulting in tooth loss is a major determinant of the healed edentulous ridge of bone. An inadequate ridge form or size in combination with a reduced quantity of keratinized gingiva will diminish the esthetics of an implant restoration. The failure to intercept and reconstruct such defects prior to surgical placement of the fixture is a recipe for eventual esthetic disappointment. These problems are magnified by the presence of a high smile line or malaligned dentition.

The clinical and radiographic examinations may contraindicate implant dentistry and indicate that a conventional removable or fixed partial denture is the alternative of choice. Periapical radiographs are essential for establishing the prognosis of the teeth adjacent to a proposed implant site, but offer limited information regarding the edentulous volume of bone necessary to support a properly placed implant. The size and shape of the available bone architecture of the edentulous area are best imaged by a tomographic section and can be further confirmed by soft tissue sounding.[6–10] The use of a radiopaque stent in combination with computerized tomography (CT) has the potential to forecast the ideal position of the restoration in relation to the prevailing bone crest (Fig 9-2). It cannot, however, offer a clear solution to the management of soft tissue that is so necessary for an optimum restoration.

The Submergence Profile of Implants

Clinical experience has identified an end point goal for single-fixture placement that results in osseointegration and an ideal implant-gingiva complex. The submergence profile of implants is the vertical discrepancy between the occlusal surface of the implant and the peaks of the bony septae proximal to the adjacent teeth. The most pleasing esthetic results occur when this discrepancy is minimal.

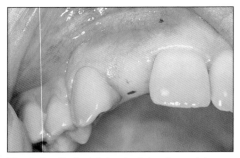

Fig 9-1a A dental implant is planned to replace the maxillary right lateral incisor. There is an abundant, healthy frame of keratinized gin-

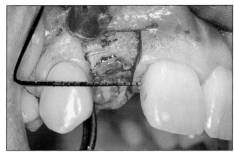

Fig 9-1b A trapezoidal incision is made so as to preserve the approximating interdental papillae. The mesiodistal space is appropriate for tooth replacement. The bone is wide buccolingually; there is no buccal concavity. The vertical height is 2 to 3 mm apical to approximating CEJs.

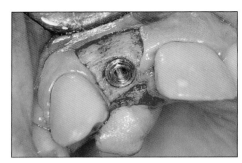

Fig 9-1c The implant is placed with the potential for ideal restoration. The shoulder of the implant is coincident with the level of bone.

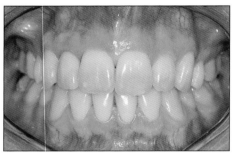

Fig 9-1d The final restoration is in place and is inconspicuous with the anterior dentition.

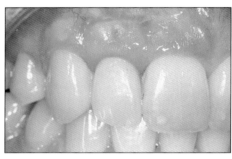

Fig 9-1e The interdental papillae are complete. (Courtesy of Dr George Biron.)

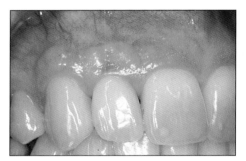

Fig 9-1f After 6 years, the result is stable.

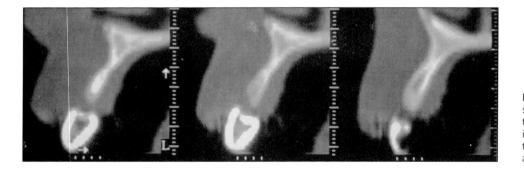

Fig 9-2 A stent coated with radiopaque barium sulfate is inserted before the CT scan to identify the desired position for the implant crown. This is related to the alveolar process and helps establish the esthetic prognosis before surgery. It also addresses the possibility of an implant.

The first 1 mm of cementum apical to the cementoenamel junction (CEJ) on the proximal surfaces of teeth is populated by transeptal fibers. It would thus follow that the edentulous osseous ridge cannot be closer than 1 mm to an imaginary line joining the bordering cementoenamel junctions. It is realistic to assume that at least 1 mm of bone will have been inadvertently sacrificed by the trauma of tooth loss. Therefore, the optimum practical linear starting point for the osseous level after tooth loss would be 2 to 3 mm apical to the adjacent cementoenamel junctions (Figs 9-1 and 9-3). Because this would be the best-case scenario, the shoulder of the implant would be positioned 2 to 3 mm

apically to the adjoining cementoenamel junctions and, therefore, would provide ample vertical space for the implant abutment.

The void to be occupied by gingiva in this scenario is minimal, and expectations optimistic for the result to include complete esthetic interdental papillae. It appears that the soft tissues surrounding implants follow similar dimensional patterns as they do with teeth, in that the biologic width hypothesis of 3 mm is readily accomplished, resulting in a healthy, firmly attached gingiva.

The surgical flap is best elevated for first- and second-stage implant surgery by the reflection of a trapezoidal flap

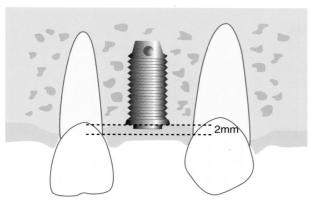

Fig 9-3 The vertical height of bone is approximately 2 mm apical to an imaginary line connecting the approximating cementoenamel junctions.

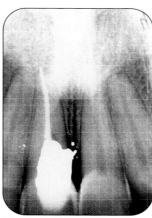

Fig 9-4a The pretreatment radiograph reveals a poor proximal restoration with interproximal bone loss.

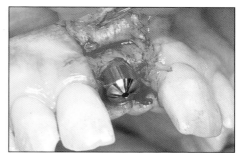

Fig 9-4b A healing abutment is attached at second-stage surgery. The implant is in the proper position to be restored but is somewhat (4 to 5 mm) apical to the ideal position, as reflected by the vertical bone height.

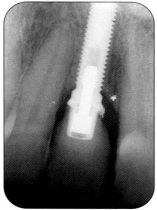

Fig 9-4c The posttreatment radiograph reveals 4 to 5 mm loss of bone from approximate cementoenamel junctions.

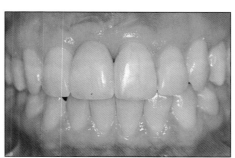

Fig 9-4d The final crown is in place. There is a slight loss of interdental papilla, but this reaches the limit of gingival framing for the crown. (Courtesy of Dr Edith Segal.)

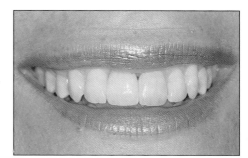

Fig 9-4e The smile line framed by the lips is agreeable to the patient, but the tip of the papilla is missing.

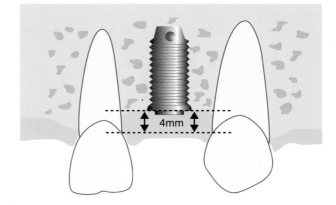

Fig 9-4f The vertical height of bone is 4 mm apical to approximating CEJs.

that does not include the approximating papillae (see Figs 9-1a to 9-1f). The apical extension, or base, is the largest side of the trapezoid, although space limitations may preclude this approach. Preservation of the papillae is an important factor in creating the gingival frames for the final implant restoration.

When osseous levels demonstrate greater than 2 to 3 mm of vertical loss, a soft tissue compromise emerges as a significant factor; the suggested solution involves placing excessive restorative materials subgingivally. A vertical level of bone 4 to 6 mm apical to adjacent cementoenamel junctions can be restored successfully but introduces small compromises unless the abutments and crown extend subgingivally (Figs 9-4a to 9-4f). Any further loss of bone would only be compensated for by undesirably deep subgingival placement of restorative components (Figs 9-5a to

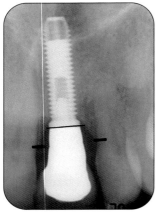

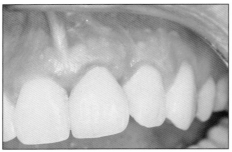

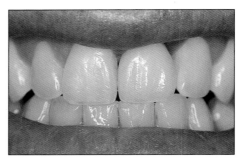

Fig 9-5a The posttreatment radiograph of a single-incision implant with the bone level 6 mm apical to approximating CEJs.

Fig 9-5b The final crown is in place. It is now difficult to match the gingival framing of the natural tooth and not extend substantially subgingivally.

Fig 9-5c The smile line.

9-5c). The patient should be prepared for a longer crown or the possibility of periodic problems, including the loss of support for adjacent teeth. This treatment decision is subject to question, in view of the complications encountered in periodontally compromised patients when restorative margins are placed excessively subgingivally and the paucity of clinical data substantiating this practice with implants.

The previous examples indicate that maximizing bone volume is an important component of creating an ideal esthetic restoration. A single implant placed too far apically at the time of extraction will result in restorative complications. Even following a successful regeneration procedure, the restoration may be larger than neighboring teeth and/or extend too far subgingivally (Figs 9-6a to 9-6g). This can result in an inflammatory reaction and fistulation and can necessitate additional surgery to reposition the gingival margin apically (Figs 9-7a and 9-7b). The placement of implant shoulders beyond 5 mm apical to the cementoenamel junction should be avoided, especially in the esthetic zone, even in patients with a relatively low smile line.

The problem leading to extraction can result in various forms of destruction of the edentulous area and seriously influences the decision whether to place an implant at the moment of extraction or resort to a staged approach, which offers the opportunity to achieve maximum predictability. Because the implant is not inserted until the results of guided bone regeneration are achieved, the clinician knows the exact level of bone and the limitations to be expected (Figs 9-8a to 9-8f).

A clinical decision that needs to be reconsidered is the replacement of exfoliated teeth in the adolescent patient. The likelihood of root resorption and ankylosis following reimplantation is significant; they lead to difficult surgical removal of teeth in young adulthood that is accompanied by compromised extraction vaults (Figs 9-9a to 9-9c). It may be preferable to prosthetically replace the missing tooth, rather than to reimplant it, and to consider implants after the individual's growth and development are complete, as determined by radiographic analysis of joint maturation and physical examination.

When not treated orthodontically, impacted canines contribute to premature loss of lateral incisors (Figs 9-10a to 9-10b). Special attention is demanded by the decision to replace a single maxillary incisor with an implant prosthesis. It is frequently better to reconstruct the missing bone before the decision to use an implant is made, because its placement is critical to the final esthetic result. The proper vertical height of bone is mandatory, and there must be sufficient width of bone available to avoid the incisive canal when a central incisor is absent (Fig 9-10c). It is necessary to preserve the papillae to maximize esthetics.

It is necessary to continually consider the merits of the traditional fixed partial denture and remember that an implant may not be the best answer to replace missing anterior teeth (Figs 9-11a and 9-11b). The state of repair of adjoining teeth that would be proposed abutments should be considered; it is far more realistic to develop a soft tissue pontic area than to construct bone vertically to implement ideal implant placement.

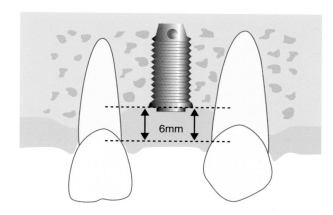

Fig 9-6a The vertical height of bone is 6 mm apical to the approximating CEJs.

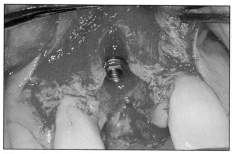

Fig 9-6b An implant is placed in an extraction socket of a tooth that was ankylosed and lost the buccal plate to root resorption.

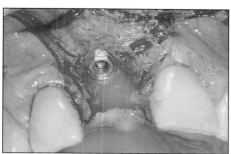

Fig 9-6c Guided bone regeneration has been accomplished with a bone allograft and an expanded polytetrafluoroethylene barrier membrane. The implant is now completely encased in bone but it is located too far apically.

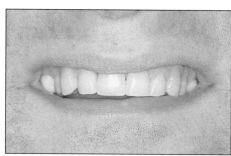

Fig 9-6d This patient has the perfect smile for this restoration. Esthetics is not a problem.

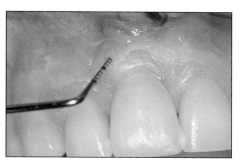

Fig 9-6e A fistula has developed after 2 years.

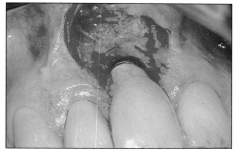

Fig 9-6f The gingiva is opened to gain access and investigate the problem. There is no bone loss but the restorative materials extend too far subgingivally.

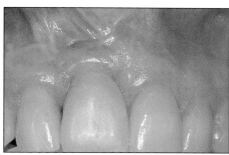

Fig 9-6g The tissue has been repositioned further apically, and less ceramic surface is located subgingivally. The crown is now longer and only acceptable because of the patient's drooping lip.

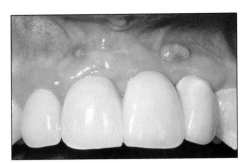

Fig 9-7a Fistulas are present above the prosthesis, which has apparently normal-length crowns. This patient has been treated elsewhere and seeks a solution to this problem.

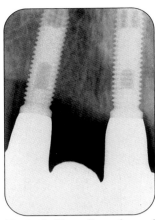

Fig 9-7b The radiograph reveals that elongated crowns extend farther below the gingiva than is indicated clinically in Fig 9-7a. A conventional fixed prosthesis would have been an excellent alternative.

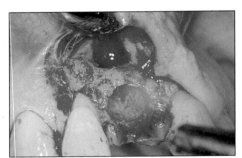

Fig 9-8a Endodontic failure and extraction of the maxillary central incisor have preceded well-planned, precise implant placement. It would be difficult to place an implant in a precise position to be restored.

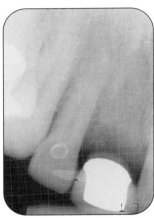

Fig 9-8b The old crown is connected to the adjacent teeth by resin composite bonding. The healing bone is radiographically homogeneous; the healed extracted area is well blended.

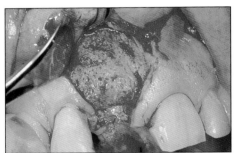

Fig 9-8c This area is reopened after successful guided bone regeneration. The flap is trapezoidal to preserve the interdental papillae. This is the perfect time to place a dental implant because the periodontist is aware of the final bone height after regeneration.

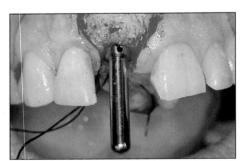

Fig 9-8d The drilling position is tested with an indicator. The vertical bone height should predispose to a fine esthetic result.

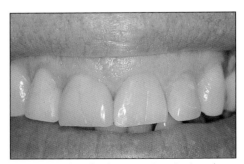

Fig 9-8e The final restoration is in place, framed by the smile line.

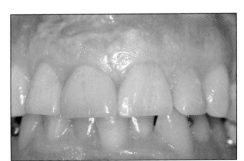

Fig 9-8f The final restoration is well framed by the gingiva, and the gold standard of inconspicuousness has been achieved.

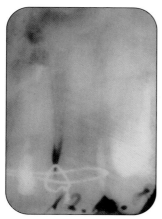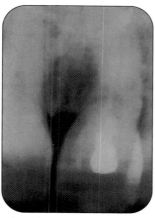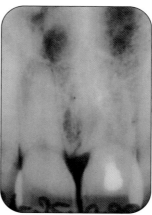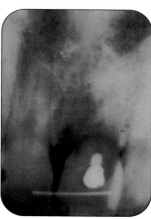

Fig 9-9a An avulsed tooth was reimplanted and splinted in 1982. The short-term prognosis was good, but severe root resorption is evident by 1994. The short-term gain resulted in marginal bone loss and long-term compromise for the placement of a dental implant.

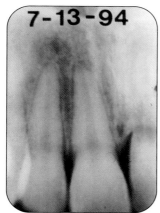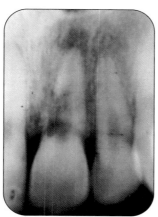

Fig 9-9b Root resorption is apparent on the reimplanted central incisor.

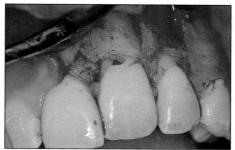

Fig 9-9c The root resorption extends apical to the CEJ on the buccal surface and involves the proximal bone on the mesial surface. This tooth is ankylosed, and it will be difficult to extract it without damaging its bony housing. Note that the ankylosed tooth did not continue to erupt and that the bone level is adversely affected.

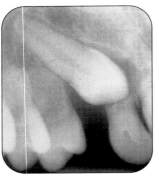
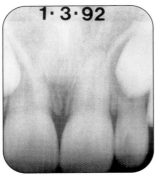
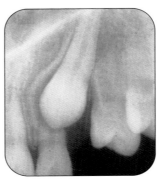

Fig 9-10a The impacted maxillary canines have destroyed the roots of the lateral incisors.

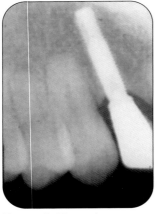
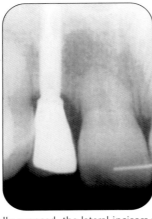
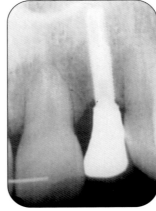
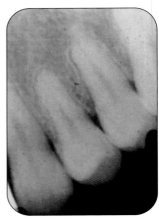

Fig 9-10b The canines were surgically exposed, the lateral incisors were extracted, and the canines were orthodontically positioned in place. The lateral incisors were replaced with implants.

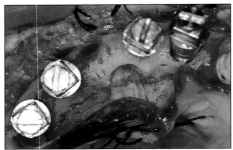

Fig 9-10c A large incisive canal compromises the position of central incisor implants. This important factor must be considered when the prosthesis is planned.

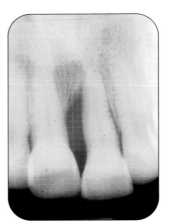
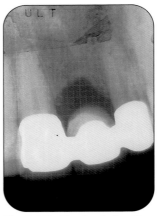

Fig 9-11a The left central incisor is to be extracted, but the vertical loss of bone is too extensive to allow placement of an implant.

Fig 9-11b The tooth is effectively replaced by a traditional fixed partial denture after the pontic area is augmented with soft tissue grafting.

Regeneration of the Maxillary Anterior Region

Extraction Wounds

An important consideration in the timing of implant insertion is the phase of osseous healing after extraction (Figs 9-12a to 9-12e). The examination of a tomographic scan taken 30 days after extraction of the maxillary incisors reveals the healing process. Early resorption of up to 30% of the buccal plate has been previously recorded,[11] lending credence to the value of initiating guided bone regeneration at the time of extraction, because the loss of buccal plate results in a deformed, narrow edentulous ridge that is not receptive to proper implant placement.[12] The regenerative procedure can be considered prophylactic when implants are considered to replace prominent roots.

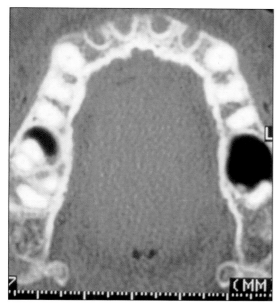

Fig 9-12a Computerized tomography scan made 30 days after the extraction of four prominent maxillary incisors. The buccal plate of bone is being resorbed.

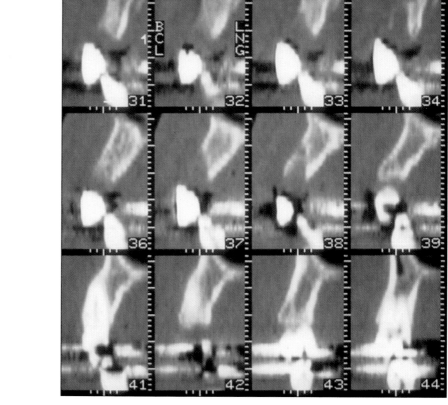

Fig 9-12b Sagittal sections of Fig 9-12a. Note the loss of the buccal plate to resorption and the resultant angular edentulous ridge.

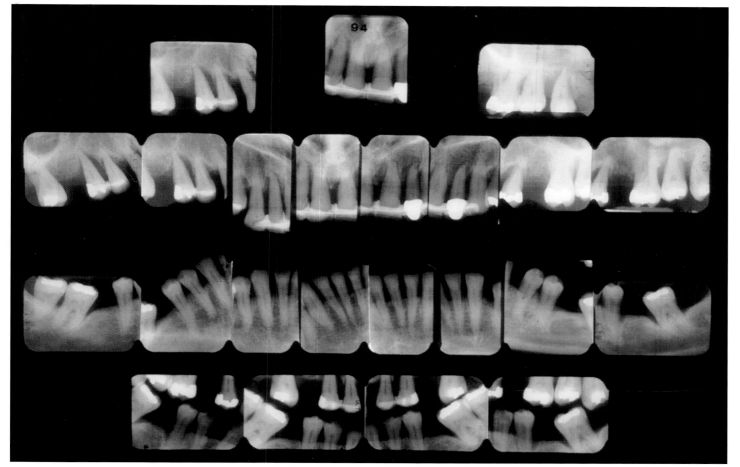

Fig 9-12c There is extensive loss of bone in the maxilla, and the teeth are to be extracted. The maxilla will be committed to guided bone regeneration at the time of extraction to protect the fragile buccal plates and allow for a rectangular ridge for implant placement.

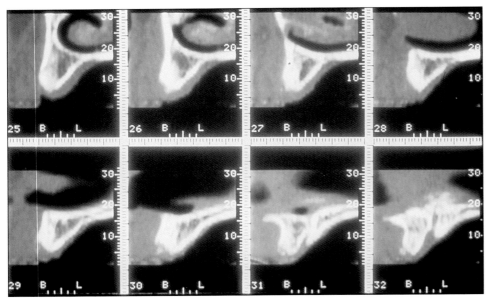

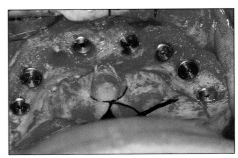

Fig 9-12d Computerized tomography scan made 6 months after the guided bone regeneration procedure. Compare the rectangular bone section with buccal plate preservation to the angular bone sections in Fig 9-12b.

Fig 9-12e Implants are installed 9 months after the extractions and regenerative procedures. The alveolar process is of ample width, as shown in Fig 9-12d.

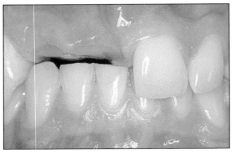

Fig 9-13a The maxillary right incisors are missing; there is a Bolton Index deficiency that results in too much mesiodistal space for two pontics and too much vertical overbite for a resin-bonded prosthesis.

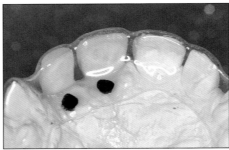

Fig 9-13b The missing teeth are waxed on a cast to share the prediction for the final crowns with the patient. A stent is constructed to direct surgical placement. Note the diastemata.

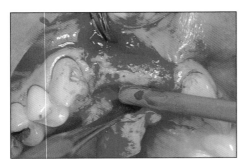

Fig 9-13c The height of the edentulous ridge is good, but the buccal plate has been lost to trauma. The implants will be placed in the area of the cingula.

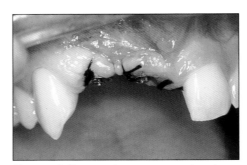

Fig 9-13d At second-stage surgery, there is no gingival frame or papilla between the incisors.

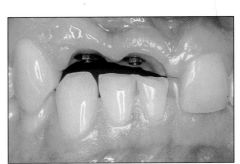

Fig 9-13e The gingival frame is developed with the use of provisional crowns, placed to encourage guided gingival growth. Note the interdental papilla that is evident here, but was missing in Fig 9-13a.

Guided Gingival Growth

Missing teeth combined with a Bolton deficiency require a multidisciplinary diagnostic exercise to achieve a well-directed implant treatment plan (Figs 9-13a to 9-13e). When orthodontics is considered ill advised because it would disrupt an otherwise sound dentition, and a conventional fixed prosthesis is contraindicated because the mesiodistal width of the prosthesis would violate a reasonable height-to-width ratio of the teeth, implants offer a conclusive solution (Fig 9-13a). The demonstration of a tooth-colored waxup of the proposed prosthesis is helpful for both the clinician and the patient (Fig 9-13b). The vertical height of bone in a dentition with multiple diastemas is the dictating factor for the possibility of reconstructing missing interdental papillae (Fig 9-13c). It is here that "guided gingival growth" (GGG) is attempted to provide the necessary esthetic correction (Figs 9-13d and 9-13e).

Guided gingival growth may be defined as the nonsurgical controlled genesis of circumabutment gingival tissues after abutment connection and throughout the provisional phase.[13] The term *control* implies the ability to influence directly the height and the form of the soft tissue papillae and the cervicofacial framing gingiva.

The minimal dimension of the connective tissue fibers, the junctional epithelium, and the sulcular depth for teeth is approximately 3 mm.[13–15] A minimal vertical discrepancy between the proximal cementoenamel junctions and the fixture head allows the subgingival peri-implant tissues to be developed to approach this same dimension. At second-stage surgery, the careful preservation of the interproximal papillae and placement of a titanium abutment provide the scaffold to encourage guided gingival growth.

For anterior teeth, there is a difference in height between the midfacial cervical zone and the interproximal papillae that must be preserved to generate an inconspicuous final restoration. The provisional acrylic resin restoration is screw retained to the transepithelial abutment, the cervical portion adapted so as to leave unveneered titanium circumferentially exposed wherever GGG is desired. This technique is a short-term inconvenience for patients with high smile lines but guides the growth of the interdental papillae to at least the height of 3 mm.

Placement of a titanium abutment at least 1 mm taller than the desired level is suggested to increase the height of a bordering papilla. The cervical design of the provisional restoration will be the precursor to the anticipated guided gingival growth. Every effort should be made, in conceiving and constructing the gingival portion of the provisional restoration, to generate a natural soft tissue outline. Once the desired gingival migration has been accomplished, that area of exposed titanium will be covered by extending the margin of the provisional restoration, precluding further GGG. During the 6- to 8-week healing phase, this migration should be observed at 2-week intervals. Addition, subtraction, or contour alterations of the provisional crown are performed as needed to effect the result.

The porous surface of acrylic resin that exists at the acrylic resin–gingival interface is a challenge to a plaque-controlled and inflammation-free healing. It may be necessary to debride and polish the exposed head surfaces of the transitional and/or provisional prosthesis at 2-week interval visits, because the greatest GGG has been observed on smooth and clean titanium surfaces. The aberrant use of interdental cleansing devices has the potential to disrupt the papillary growth.

The Provisional Restoration

The role of the provisional restoration is not limited to maintaining the position of the adjacent teeth and opposing dentition.[16] Imprecision may destabilize arch form, compromise occlusal stability, and prove detrimental to the health of the peri-implant hard and soft tissues. The provisional restoration must promote, and not deter, local healing at the second-stage surgery and abutment delivery. The ideal gingival architecture of the edentulous ridge between the first- and second-stage surgery would possess a flat surface and papillae that blend with the neighboring teeth without structural or esthetic defects.

The second-stage surgical procedure should be minimally invasive and simply enucleate the layer of tissues covering the fixture head to attach a titanium transepithelial abutment that would be incorporated with the provisional restoration. This manipulation should be accomplished without damage to the adjoining papillae and circumimplant tissues. However, this simple and ideal scenario rarely occurs. Too often, the anatomic incongruities mentioned earlier are the norm. Some deficit in the surrounding gingival form is usually present after second-stage surgery. Therefore, there exists the need to restore, improve, or modify the gingival topography to complement the esthetic final prosthesis. Most GGG is accomplished in the initial 10 weeks after abutment connection, although it has been observed to continue for longer periods of time.

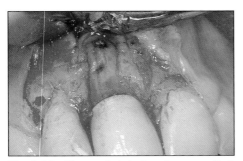

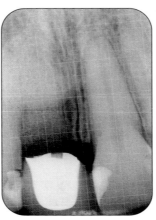

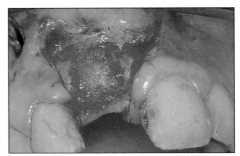

Fig 9-14a The central incisor has a vertical root fracture.

Fig 9-14b The extraction socket is still visible after 9 months. It is unlikely that the guided bone regeneration procedure has been successful.

Fig 9-14c The edentulous ridge is reopened. The bone graft has not integrated. An implant should not be used.

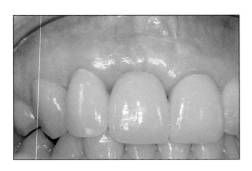

Fig 9-14d The central incisor is supplied in a three-unit fixed partial denture. (Courtesy of Dr John Machell.)

Challenges to the Successful Use of Implants

Failure of Guided Bone Regeneration

The growth of new bone is viewed as successful when it is homogeneous with preexisting bone radiographically and clinically. If it is possible to distinguish the outline of an extraction wound or the graft material after 6 months of observation, it is unlikely that new bone has formed. The successful regeneration of a decimated edentulous area is radiographically predictable but not completely confirmed until clinical investigation (Figs 9-14a to 9-14d). The decision to use implants is predicated on the volume of bone regeneration that occurs. Although guided bone regeneration has had many successes, it does not always prove successful.[17–23] Failure occurs, and it is necessary to recognize the problems rather than forge ahead and compound the failure by placing a dental implant. A three-unit ceramometal prosthesis is then the preferable treatment.

Narrow Buccolingual Ridge

The next problem that challenges the successful use of dental implants is a narrow width of bone buccolingually. This deficiency can be addressed by using a small-diameter implant, by splitting the ridge and separating the cortical plates, or by adding to the buccal plate with a bone graft (Figs 9-15 to 9-17). This is a problem frequently encountered when teeth are congenitally missing and the alveolar process has not widened sufficiently to accommodate the roots of the permanent teeth.

Implants of a smaller diameter are a good solution to replace lateral incisors when the angulation of placement can be readily restored (Figs 9-15a to 9-15d). Even if the goal of bicortical stabilization is not realized in this region, the bone quality is good and one implant seems to successfully replace a single tooth. A significant concavity in the apical area of the edentulous ridge would result in excessive angulation of the implant placement and guided bone regeneration.

The small-diameter implant is not used when the positioning would be incorrect. The narrow ridge is then treated by bone splitting[24,25] (Figs 9-16a and 9-16b) (see Chapter 12)

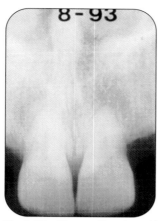
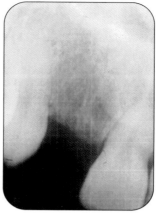
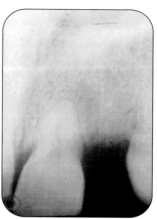

Fig 9-15a The maxillary lateral incisors are missing. There appears to be good vertical bone available, but the patient resists a CT scan to investigate the horizontal bone dimension.

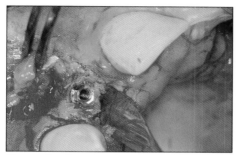

Fig 9-15b There is only enough bone to place a 3-mm implant, but it can be placed in an easily restored position.

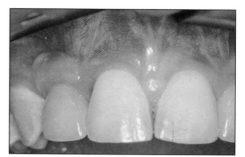

Fig 9-15c The final restoration is well framed by the gingiva.

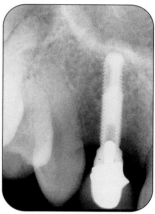

Fig 9-15d Final radiograph. Note the bicortical stabilization.

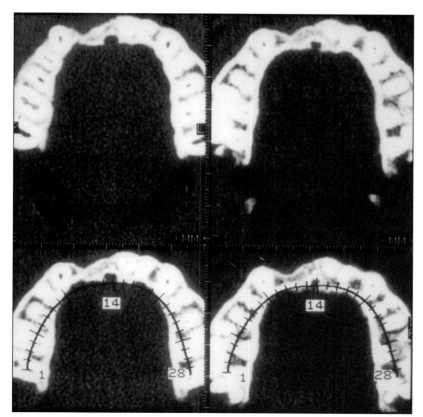

Fig 9-16a The anterior maxilla is narrow. It is also located too far lingually for an implant to be properly restored.

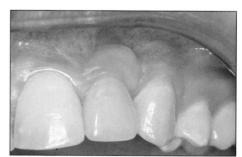

Fig 9-15e The final implant crown in place for the maxillary left lateral incisor.

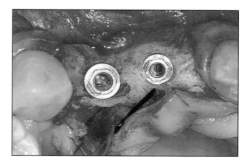

Fig 9-16b The edentulous ridge has been split to separate the cortical plates by moving the buccal plate further buccally to accept a 3.75-mm implant. A smaller diameter implant is used to replace the central incisor and to avoid an encounter with the incisive canal.

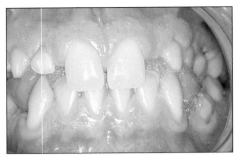

Fig 9-17a The multiple congenitally missing teeth are complicated by the fact that the alveolar process did not continue to form to accommodate the eruption of permanent teeth. The result is an exaggerated vertical space.

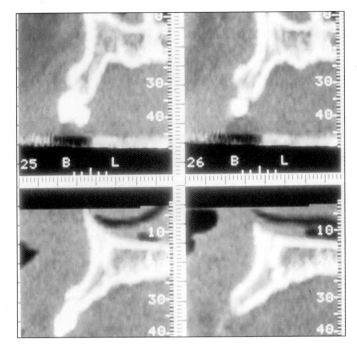

Fig 9-17b The sagittal CT sections reveal the buccal concavities.

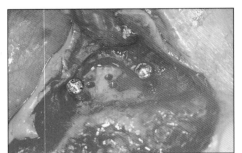

Fig 9-17c The buccal concavity is prepared for bone regeneration to allow implants to be placed in bone. Stainless steel screws are inserted horizontally to support a bone allograft and a membrane.

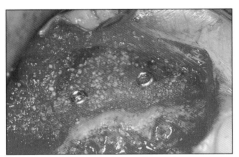

Fig 9-17d The bone graft is placed around the screws.

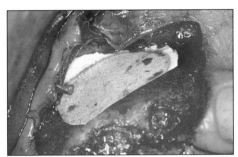

Fig 9-17e The membrane is placed to cover the assembly.

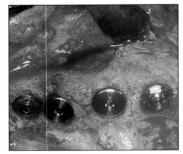

Fig 9-17f Posttreatment result. The staged approach allows the placement of implants in positions that are easily restored and coincidentally in bone. The concavity is now a convexity in the incisor-canine region.

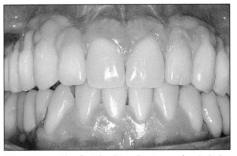

Fig 9-17g The finished implant prosthesis is in place. Pink ceramics provide the vertical space filler to adjust the void caused by the absence of eruption of permanent teeth. It is constructed so that interproximal brushes easily fit between the ceramics and the gingiva. (Courtesy of Dr Kenneth Malament.)

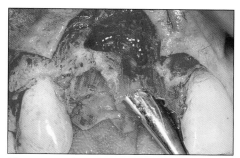

Fig 9-18a The maxillary right incisors have been extracted after failure of endodontic treatment. There is no buccal plate remaining for the central incisor. The edentulous ridge should be committed to guided bone regeneration before implants are considered. Immediate placement is contraindicated.

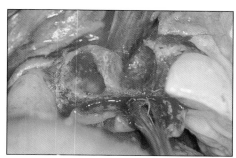

Fig 9-18b Occlusal view of the noncontained extraction vaults.

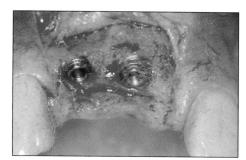

Fig 9-18c The reconstructed area is shown at the time of the delivery of implants, 10 months later.

or bone onlay grafts to widen the recipient site. The onlay grafting can be accomplished with autogenous block grafts from the chin or iliac crest (see Chapter 15) or with particulate bone reinforced with stainless steel pins and a Gore-Tex Augmentation Membrane (WL Gore, Flagstaff, AZ) (Figs 9-17a to 9-17g).

The most effective treatment of the narrow edentulous ridge is to prevent it from happening. This is best accomplished by intercepting the problem and providing regenerative treatment at the time of extraction[19] (Figs 9-18a to 9-18c).

High Smile Line

The patient with a high smile line presents the ultimate challenge. This is especially true when there is a demand for a fixed restoration, when there are insufficient natural teeth to serve as abutments for a conventional prosthesis, and when the loss of the incisor teeth has resulted in an apical position of the alveolar process. The horizontal width of the residual bone and the size and location of the incisive canal may leave little choice but to place the implants where there is sufficient bone to support them rather than in the optimal mesiodistal position for prosthetic treatment

(Figs 9-19a to 9-19f). Because this type of case is best restored by a hybrid prosthesis, the solution will be a variable of the artistic skills of the prosthodontist and the technician. The possibility of guided gingival growth is outdistanced by the residual level of bone and the stated desire to avoid substantial subgingival extension of a prosthesis.

Conclusion

Initial identification of the diagnostic factors that result in a positive submergence profile, coupled with a lucid treatment sequence, will result in excellent function and esthetics. Some of the limitations described in this chapter offer impediments to the development of the final prosthesis and must be considered in the planning stage. Proper development of a provisional restoration to gain guide gingival growth enhances the natural appearance. Dental implants provide excellent solutions for the replacement of missing maxillary anterior teeth. This fact should stimulate all dentists to consider this alternative for patients, from adolescents to young adults to mature adults.

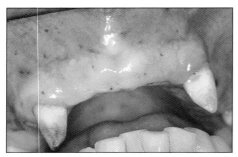

Fig 9-19a All four incisors are missing. It will not be necessary to frame a single crown to fit with adjacent natural teeth.

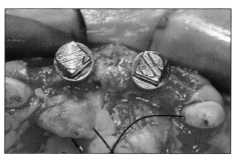

Fig 9-19b Implant placement is determined by bone volume and a large incisive canal that preclude the central incisor positions. The ridge becomes too narrow toward the lateral incisor regions.

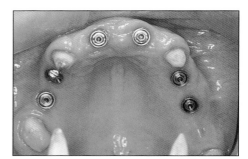

Fig 9-19c Maxilla after second-stage surgery. There will be one freestanding prosthesis for the left premolar and another for the right premolar implants. The three natural teeth are to be restored with single crowns, and the two incisor implants have a freestanding prosthesis.

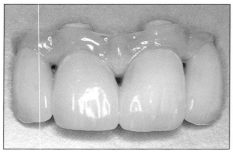

Fig 9-19d The incisor prosthesis has been constructed with pink ceramics to allow the length of the anterior teeth to be of appropriate size for the esthetic scheme. Note the natural appearance of the small interdental spaces to emulate the patient's previous fixed restoration.

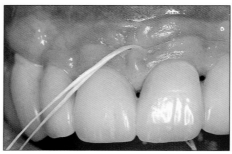

Fig 9-19e The final prosthesis is in place. The patient is capable of easily removing plaque from the prosthesis.

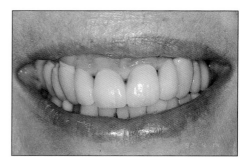

Fig 9-19f The high smile line mandates the use of pink ceramics to provide satisfactory esthetics.

References

1. Jemt T, Lekholm U, Adell R. Osseointegrated implants in the treatment of partially edentulous jaws: A preliminary study on 876 consecutively placed fixtures. Int J Oral Maxillofac Implants 1989; 4:211–217.

2. Buser D, Weber HP, Brägger U, Balsiger C. Tissue integration of one-stage ITI implants: Three year results of a longitudinal study with hollow cylinder and hollow screw implants. Int J Oral Maxillofac Implants 1991;6:405–412.

3. Weber HP, Buser D, Fiorellini J, Williams R. Radiographic evaluation of crestal bone levels adjacent to nonsubmerged titanium implants. Clin Oral Impl Res 1992;2:181–188.

4. Jemt T, Lekholm U. Oral implant treatment in posterior partially edentulous jaws: A five-year follow-up report. Int J Oral Maxillofac Implants 1993;8:635–640.

5. Lekholm U, van Steenberghe D, Herrmann I, et al. Osseointegrated implants in the treatment of partially edentulous jaws: A prospective five-year multicenter study. Int J Oral Maxillofac Implants 1994; 9:627–635.

6. Stella J, Tharanon WA. A precise radiographic method to determine the location of the inferior alveolar canal in the posterior edentulous mandible: Implications for dental implants. Part 2. Clinical application. Int J Oral Maxillofac Implants 1990;5:23–29.

7. Quirynen M, Lamoral Y, Dekeyser C, et al. C.T. scan standard reconstruction technique for reliable jaw bone volume determination. Int J Oral Maxillofac Implants 1990;5:384–389.

8. Mecall RA, Rosenfeld AL. Barium-coated surgical stents and computer assisted tomography in the preoperative assessment of dental implant patients. Int J Periodont Rest Dent 1991;12:53–62.

9. Williams M, Mealey B, Hallmon W. The role of computerized tomography in dental implantology. Int J Oral Maxillofac Implants 1992;7:373–380.

10. Todd A, Gher M, Quitero G, Richardson A. Interpretation of linear and computer tomograms in the assessment of implant recipient sites. J Periodontol 1993;64:1243–1249.

11. Carlsson GE, Thalander H, Hedegard G. Histologic changes in the upper alveolar process after extractions with or without insertion of an immediate full denture. Acta Odontol Scand 1967;25:1–31.

12. Stein J, Nevins M. The use of guided gingival growth to frame the single maxillary anterior implant prosthesis. Accepted for publication, Int J Periodont Rest Dent (in press).

13. Gargiulo AW, Wentz FM, Orban BJ. Dimensions and relations of the dentogingival junction in humans. J Periodontol 1961;32:261.

14. Maynard JG, Wilson RD. Physiologic dimensions of the periodontium fundamental to successful restorative dentistry. J Periodontol 1979; 50:170–174.

15. Nevins M, Skurow HM. The intracrevicular margin, the biologic width, and the maintenance of the gingival margin. Int J Periodont Rest Dent 1984;4(3):31–50.

16. Skurow HM, Nevins M. The rationale of the preprosthetic provisional biologic trial restoration. Int J Periodont Rest Dent 1988;8(1):9–30.

17. Buser D, Brägger U, Lang NP, Nyman S. Regeneration and enlargement of jawbone using guided tissue regeneration. Clin Oral Impl Res 1990;1:22–32.

18. Buser D, Dula K, Belser U, Hirt H-P, Berthold H. Localized ridge augmentation using guided bone regeneration. I. Surgical procedure in the maxilla. Int J Periodont Rest Dent 1993;13:29–45.

19. Nevins M, Mellonig JT. The advantages of localized ridge augmentation prior to implant placement: A staged event. Int J Periodont Rest Dent 1994;14:97–111.

20. Andersson B, Odman P, Widmark G, Waas A. Anterior tooth replacement with implants in patients with a narrow alveolar ridge form: A clinical study using guided tissue regeneration. Clin Oral Impl Res 1993;4:90–98.

21. Mellonig JT, Triplett RG. Guided tissue regeneration and endosseous dental implants. Int J Periodont Rest Dent 1993;13:109–119.

22. Buser D, Dula K, Belser UC, Hirt H-P, Berthold H. Localized ridge augmentation using guided bone regeneration. II. Surgical procedure in the mandible. Int J Periodont Rest Dent 1995;15:11–29.

23. Mellonig JT, Nevins M. Guided bone regeneration of bone defects associated with implants: An evidence-based outcome assessment. Int J Periodont Rest Dent 1995;15:169–185.

24. Simion M, Baldoni M, Zaffe D. Jawbone enlargement using immediate implant placement associated with a split-crest technique and guided tissue regeneration. Int J Periodont Rest Dent 1992; 12:463–474.

25. Buser D, Dula K, Belser U, Hirt HP, Berthold H. Localized ridge augmentation using guided bone regeneration. II. Surgical procedure in the mandible. Int J Periodont Rest Dent 1995;15:11–29.

CHAPTER 10

The Placement of Mandibular Anterior Implants

Myron Nevins, DDS

The efficacy of treating the edentulous mandible with implants is well established. Therefore the patient who presents with advanced periodontal disease, including mobile and displaced teeth, may be the best candidate to immediately proceed to implant therapy.[1-8] The mandibular anterior teeth are often crowded, resulting in inadequate room for the replacement of a single tooth with a single implant (Fig 10-1). Treatment decisions about whether to treat or replace the incisor teeth are influenced by the maxillomandibular relationship, the vertical overbite, embrasure spaces, and the state of repair of the teeth. In the absence of anatomic obstacles, long implants provide considerable stability, and two implants can easily supply four incisors.

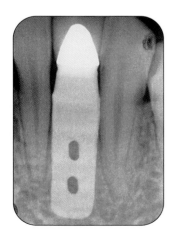

Fig 10-1 A dental implant is too large to replace a single missing mandibular incisor. This 16-year-old patient now has periodontally compromised adjacent teeth and a difficult prognosis.

Obstacles to Implant Placement

Mesiodistal Discrepancies

Ideally, a minimal mesiodistal dimension of 7 mm should be available (Fig 10-2) to allow a dental implant to be placed and restored in a cleansable, esthetic fashion. However, the average central incisor is 5 mm wide mesiodistally, and the average lateral incisor is 6.5 mm wide mesiodistally.[9] This space is reduced in the presence of crowding.

A single intrabony defect involving one incisor might lead to extraction and replacement with a conventional fixed prosthesis. Lack of embrasure space frequently precludes complete-coverage restorations, and a deep overbite and thin teeth eliminate the resin-bonded restoration from consideration. Orthodontic tooth movement in combination with the extraction of the periodontally compromised incisor is not valid if the adjacent teeth would be moved out of bone and into a defect for the purpose of closing space and opening an embrasure. Periodontal regeneration is the better treatment when the defect offers a predictable prognosis[10-13] (Figs 10-2 and 10-3).

The replacement of two incisors by two implants is seldom possible because of the minimal mesiodistal space available. Each implant is approximately 4 mm in diameter, and there should be 2-mm embrasures between the implants and between the implants and the remaining teeth. This requires 14 mm of mesiodistal space, 12.6 mm if 3.2-mm implants are selected. Compared to the average width of uncrowded central and lateral incisors, even 12 mm is a stretch. If

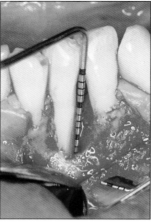

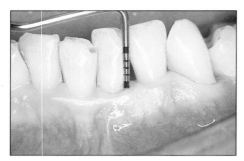

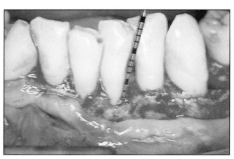

Fig 10-2a The 10-mm probing depth on the distal surface of the left central incisor is accompanied by crowded incisors and no potential for an embrasure to permit the construction of a conventional fixed prosthesis. The deep overbite and resultant thin incisal edges eliminate the possibility of a resin-bonded prosthesis.

Fig 10-2b There is a deep un-contained osseous defect. It will be impossible to orthodontically move the lateral incisor mesially to open the limited incisor-canine embrasure. Implant placement will be precarious because of the vertical loss of bone. The optimal treatment would be the regeneration of the lost periodontium.

Fig 10-2c Periodontal regeneration is clinically evident at the reopening of the region after 1 year. Treatment consisted of the use of a bone allograft in combination with a Gore-Tex interproximal membrane (WL Gore, Flagstaff, AZ).

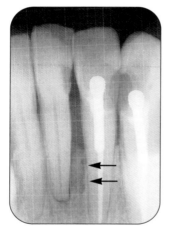

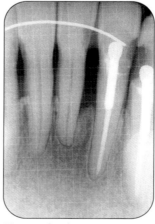

Fig 10-3a Presurgical radiograph. Note the deep defect on the distal surface of the left central incisor (*arrows*).

Fig 10-3b Three-year postsurgical radiograph. The damaged crest has been regenerated.

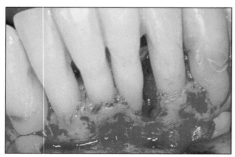

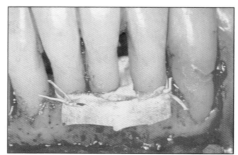

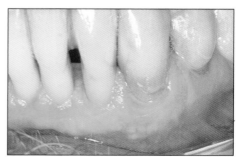

Fig 10-3c The osseous defect is found between the left mandibular incisors.

Fig 10-3d The osseous defect is covered with a Gore-Tex anterior interproximal membrane.

Fig 10-3e Four years after surgery, there is minimal probing depth.

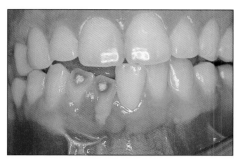

Fig 10-4a Both right incisors were treated endodontically when the patient was hospitalized after an automobile accident. Both teeth are mobile and severely periodontally compromised.

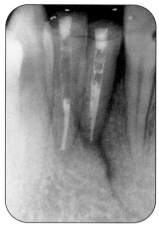

Fig 10-4b The traumatic fracture of the alveolar process is evident in the radiograph.

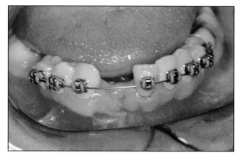

Fig 10-4c The extraction of both incisors provides too much mesiodistal space for one incisor and too little space for two incisors. Orthodontic tooth movement is used to close the space so that one incisor will be sufficient.

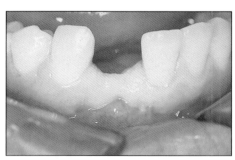

Fig 10-4d The space can now be restored with a single implant and one tooth.

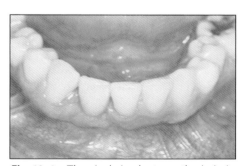

Fig 10-4e The single-implant prosthesis is in place. (Courtesy of Dr Jeffrey Dornbush.)

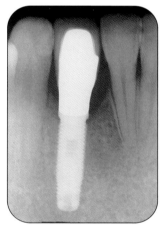

Fig 10-4f Radiographic image of the loaded implant in place.

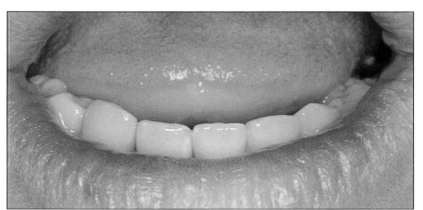

Fig 10-4g At maximal visibility with an exaggerated smile, the restoration is most esthetic.

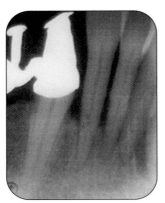
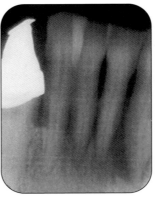
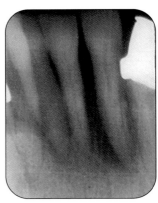

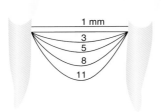

Fig 10-5a Vertical levels of bone loss. Loss of 1 to 3 mm is of little consequence in determining the implant site, but greater than 5 mm requires careful consideration of the proximal bone on the canines.

Fig 10-5b The pretreatment radiographs reveal advanced vertical loss of bone (1991).

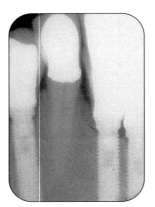
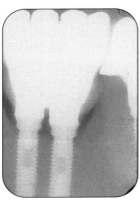
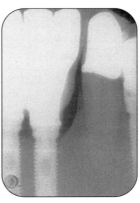

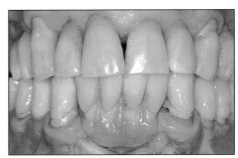

Fig 10-5c The loaded implants were carefully placed so as not to encroach on the mesial supporting bone of the canines and to provide an embrasure between them (1995).

Fig 10-5d The final prosthesis in place. Note the use of pink ceramics to allow the appearance of shorter teeth. (Courtesy of Dr James Stein.)

crowding exists, orthodontic reduction of the edentulous space should be considered so that one implant and one crown will solve the problem (Figs 10-4a to 10-4g). This is considered to be a conservative solution compared to constructing a fixed prosthesis with the preparation of the mandibular canines and incisors.

Vertical Discrepancies

The replacement of four compromised mandibular incisors in the presence of periodontally sound canines is an interesting project, in that the loss of alveolar process will be far more extensive for the incisors. It is almost impossible to place implants in the lateral incisor sites without encroaching on the central incisor area or compromising the mesial bone support of the canines. It is therefore necessary to consider the replacement of the four incisor teeth relative to the level of bone loss in the area (Fig 10-5a). When the loss of bone is less than 5 mm, there will be little danger of an angular lid of bone in a small space between the canine and the implant. Conversely, a discrepancy of bone greater than 5 mm between the alveolar housing of the canine and the

area of the extracted incisors will produce a result that is difficult to debride unless this is taken into account before the implants are placed. If so, the implants are placed in a position between the lateral and central incisors, permitting cleansable embrasures throughout the region (Figs 10-5b to 10-5d). The implant prosthesis is developed similarly to that for a hybrid case.

The placement of dental implants at the time of the extraction of the four incisors can be an expedient procedure, but the crowding of the incisors will compromise the positions of the implants[14,15] (Figs 10-6a to 10-6d). This procedure should be limited to those cases where there is not a deep vertical discrepancy. It is impossible to place and restore an implant that is placed in the extraction site of a tooth in buccal version, so the two implants will occupy the spaces of the other three teeth. An implant in the site of a lateral incisor with sufficient embrasure room from the canine will also use most of the central incisor site. The extraction vaults can then be committed to regenerative procedures to ensure osseointegration. It is suggested that the procedure of choice be a staged approach. One should extract the incisors and allow time for healing before the implants are placed (see Figs 10-7a to 10-7d).

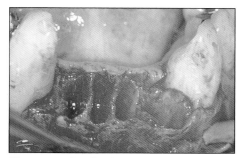

Fig 10-6a The alveolar process is shown after the extraction of the four mandibular incisors. It is impossible to place an implant in the position of the labially placed left lateral incisor. It is necessary to provide an interproximal embrasure next to the right canine.

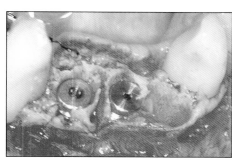

Fig 10-6b Bone loss is horizontal from canine to canine. Note that the implant on the right occupies the space of both incisors.

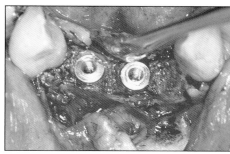

Fig 10-6c Second-stage surgery reveals complete bone regeneration. This was accomplished with bone allograft and a Gore-Tex Augmentation Membrane.

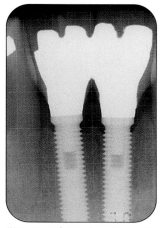

Fig 10-6d Final radiograph, taken 2 years after loading.

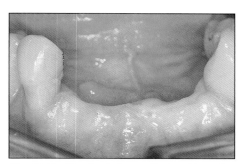

Fig 10-7a The healed mandibular ridge after extraction.

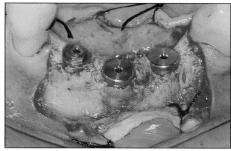

Fig 10-7b The implants can be placed in optimal positions after the extraction wounds have healed. Compare to Fig 10-6b.

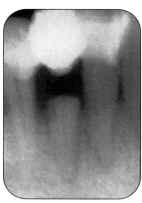
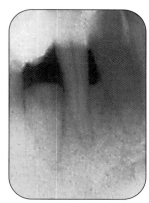
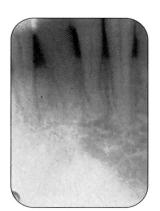
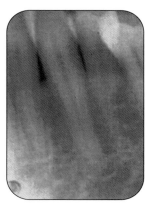

Fig 10-7c Pretreatment radiographs of mandibular anterior teeth. Treatment was precipitated by the fractured right canine.

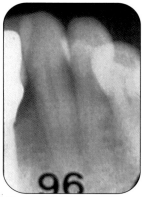
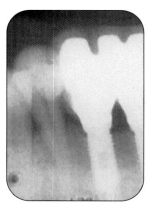
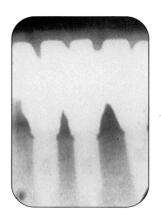
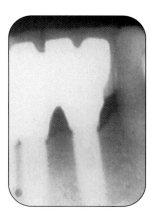

Fig 10-7d Posttreatment radiographs.

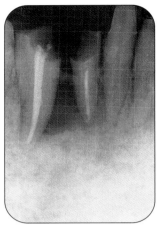

Fig 10-8a Radiograph of the mandibular right canine and lateral incisor. Loss of the interdental septum is complete.

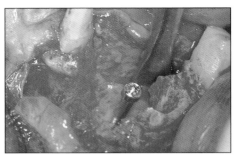

Fig 10-8b The extraction vault is shown after removal of the two teeth and the infected granulation tissue. Note the loss of both the buccal and lingual plates. A stainless steel pin is used to support the bone graft.

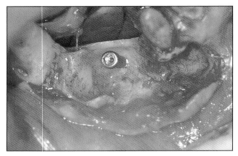

Fig 10-8c Occlusal view of the extraction site. The area is decorticated to ensure exposure of the marrow spaces.

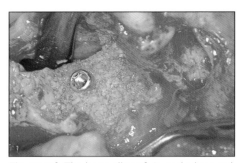

Fig 10-8d The bone allograft is packed around the pin and fills the void.

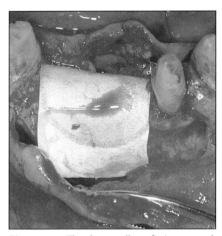

Fig 10-8e The bone allograft is covered with a Gore-Tex Augmentation Membrane.

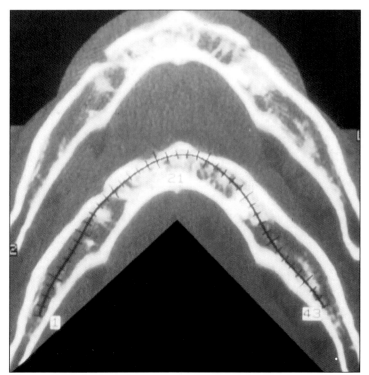

Fig 10-8f The horizontal computerized tomography (CT) images demonstrate the regeneration of the damaged mandible.

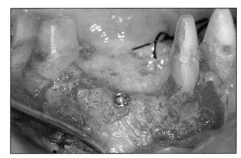

Fig 10-8g The buccal flap is reflected to remove the screw after 8 months. Note the regeneration of bone to the relationship of the pin and the graft at the time of surgery (see Figs 10-8b and c).

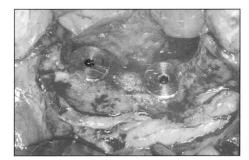

Fig 10-8h The implants are shown at second-stage surgery.

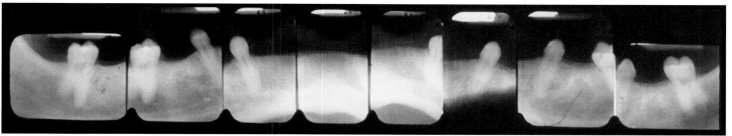

Fig 10-9a The mandibular radiographic series reveals partial anodontia.

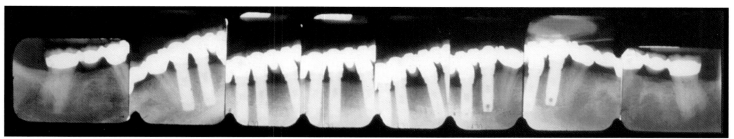

Fig 10-9b Posttreatment radiographic series. Fixed prostheses were constructed for the posterior teeth, and an implant prosthesis was fabricated to replace the anterior teeth.

In the event of severe loss of bone involving two or more mandibular anterior teeth, guided bone regeneration procedures should be initiated before implant placement.[15,16] After the extraction of hopeless teeth and the removal of all granulation tissue, the bone deformity is assessed for the potential for reconstruction (Figs 10-8a to 10-8h). If the defect is contained and the peripheral bone walls are in place for most of the vertical depth, the prognosis will be good for regeneration of the edentulous ridge. If the buccal wall is missing, the prognosis is less favorable; if the buccal and lingual walls are compromised, the prognosis becomes questionable.

It may be beneficial to use a stainless steel pin to support the bone graft and to tent the membrane, as well as to stabilize the blood clot and initiate hard tissue regeneration.[17] With this type of procedure, there must be complete soft tissue closure over the membrane, and the area must be allowed to heal for a significant period of time, perhaps 6 to 8 months, before implant placement is considered. The regeneration of new bone can be confirmed by computerized tomography and surgical exposure. The screw is then removed, and the implants are placed.

Buccolingual Discrepancies

The next issue is the presence of a narrow buccolingual dimension of bone. The edentulous mandible, or the partially edentulous patient with multiple missing teeth where proximity to adjacent teeth can be avoided, is treated by reduction of a small amount of the narrow crest. This procedure may also be necessary for patients when teeth are congenitally missing. The alveolar ridge normally expands to accommodate the eruption of the permanent dentition, but this does not occur in partial anodontia, especially if multiple teeth are missing (Figs 10-9a to 10-9d). The knifelike surface of bone is not critical to containing implants in this region and can be reduced in conjunction with implant placement, assuming that the body of the mandible is of sufficient size.

Another possibility is to use the split-ridge technique to increase the volume of bone and allow implants to be correctly placed within the confines of preexisting bone.[18,19] The ideal candidate for ridge splitting is identified on a sagittal radiographic image as having the shape of an isosceles triangle with a base at the apical margin and min-

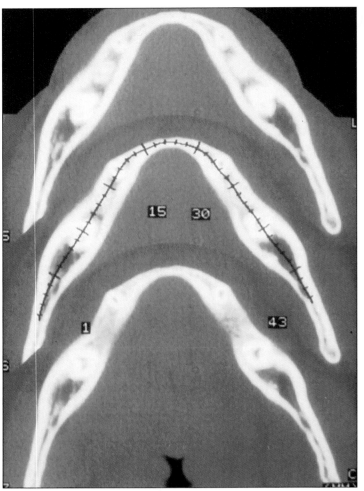

Fig 10-9c Horizontal cuts from the computerized tomography scan. Note the narrow bone in the anterior region where permanent teeth are congenitally missing. The alveolar process never widened because there was no eruption of teeth to accommodate.

imal occlusal width of at least 3 mm. It is difficult to split a rectangular ridge and maintain continuity (Figs 10-10a to 10-10e). The initial gingival incision is made toward the palate or lingually to prevent membrane exposure and healing problems. The occlusal cortical bone is first cut with a non-crosscutting fissure bur to a depth of 2 mm to bypass the cortical lid. A thin chisel with a sharp, beveled cutting edge is then introduced to a depth of 6 mm, providing sufficient width to allow engagement of larger, 10-mm monobeveled chisels. The bevel faces the buccal plate, which is expanded buccally to result in a width of approximately 6 or 7 mm. The length of the longest beveled chisel is 10 mm, but it is important to maintain some portion of the most apical bone in one piece to fix the implant. The surgeon must not countersink the buccal plate or attempt to tap these sites because it is crucial to maintain complete attachment of the buccal plate and its blood supply. Self-tapping implants with a circumference of 3.75 mm are used if possible, and smaller diameter implants are substituted when necessary. The trough is then filled with autogenous or allograft bone and covered with a barrier membrane to promote the growth of bone. Others have reported using only a membrane or nothing, but this is a complicated procedure, and use of both approaches is suggested.[18,19]

Autogeneous bone blocks can be used to predictably increase the width of a narrow edentulous ridge (Figs 10-11a to 10-11f). They can be harvested from the chin or from the ramus area of the mandible, and are stabilized with surgical screws. Particulate bone, autograft, or allograft is added at the periphery of the block to accomplish a smooth result for implant placement.

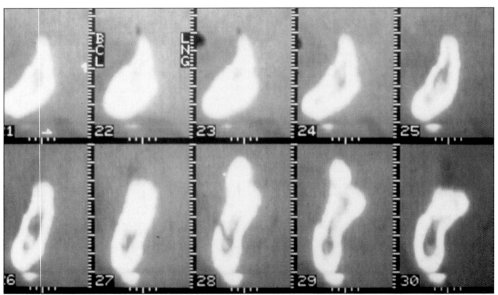

Fig 10-9d Sagittal sections from the CT scan. There is a generous volume of bone in the body of the mandible, but the alveolar process presents as a narrow band of bone.

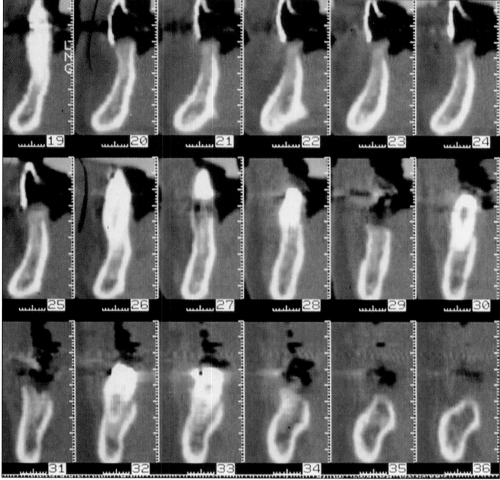

Fig 10-10a Presurgical CT scan taken with a radiopaque stent in place. The relationship of the stent to the bone is ideal, except that the bone is very narrow.

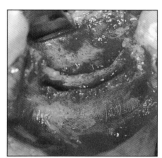

Fig 10-10b The bone has been split to increase the horizontal distance between the cortical plates and allow implant placement.

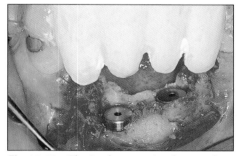

Fig 10-10c The implants are in place, and an autogenous bone graft fills the void. The stent is used to show their position.

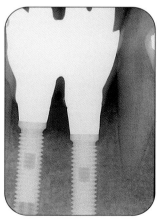

Fig 10-10d Final radiograph.

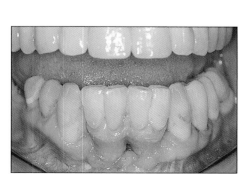

Fig 10-10e Final implant prosthesis. (Courtesy of Dr Howard Hill.)

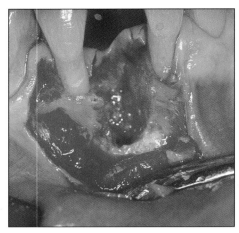

Fig 10-11a The buccal wall of bone has been lost to periodontal disease.

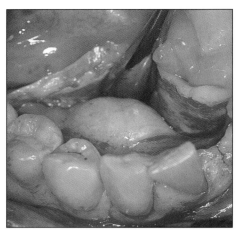

Fig 10-11b The block bone graft will be harvested from the mandibular torus.

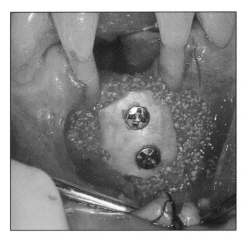

Fig 10-11c The graft is held in place by two surgical screws and surrounded by bone chips and bone allograft.

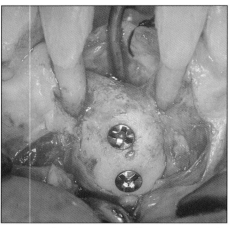

Fig 10-11d The regenerated bone is now ready to receive an implant (buccal view).

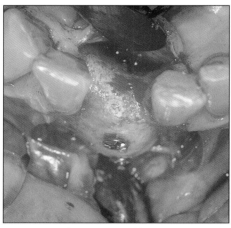

Fig 10-11e The regenerated bone is now ready to receive an implant (occlusal view).

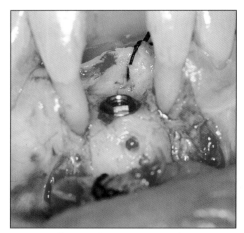

Fig 10-11f A single implant is in place.

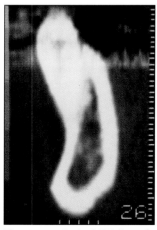

Fig 10-12a Sagittal CT view of a mandibular anterior tooth in a patient with bimaxillary protrusion.

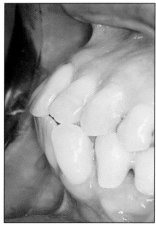

Fig 10-12b Clinical view of the dentition in Fig 10-12a.

Occlusal Discrepancies

The patient with bimaxillary protrusion may be better treated with conventional restorations. The teeth are not placed in the center of the alveolar process and are tilted far buccally to articulate with the maxillary incisors. Their awkward positioning is manageable but prevents an implant from occupying the same location the tooth previously occupied (Figs 10-12a and 10-12b). It is likely that an implant will be placed in a lingual or palatal position with this occlusal relationship.

Conclusion

The mandibular anterior sextant has been the subject of substantial long-term retrospective investigation and has emerged as a most suitable site for the successful loading of dental implants. The mandibular incisor region routinely demonstrates crowding with the mesiodistal space between the canines limited. It is critical to plan for embrasure space, with the result that the implants are placed in a space previously cohabited by the central and lateral incisors. This situation is frequently accentuated by the vertical bone loss due to periodontal disease or trauma.

References

1. Adell R, Lekholm U, Rockler B, Brånemark P-I. A 15-year study of osseointegrated implants in the treatment of the edentulous jaw. Int J Oral Surg 1981;10:387–416.

2. Brånemark P-I. Introduction to osseointegration. In: Brånemark P-I, Zarb GA, Albrektsson T (eds). Tissue-Integrated Prostheses: Osseointegration in Clinical Dentistry. Chicago: Quintessence, 1985:11–76.

3. Albrektsson T, Zarb GA, Worthington P, Eriksson AR. The long-term efficacy of currently used dental implants: A review and proposed criteria of success. Int J Oral Maxillofac Implants 1986:11–25.

4. Albrektsson T, Dahl E, Enbom L, Engevall S, Engquist B, Eriksson AR, et al. Osseointegrated implants: A Swedish multicenter study of 8139 consecutively inserted Nobelpharma implants. J Periodontol 1988;59:287–296.

5. Jemt J, Lekholm U, Adell R. Osseointegrated implants in the treatment of partially edentulous patients: A preliminary study on 876 consecutively placed fixtures. Int J Oral Maxillofac Implants 1989; 4:211–217.

6. Buser D, Weber HP, Brägger U, Balsiger C. Tissue integration of one-stage ITI implants: Three year results of a longitudinal study with hollow cylinder and hollow screw implants. Int J Oral Maxillofac Implants 1991;6:405–412.

7. Anderson B, Odman P, Widmark G, Waas A. Anterior tooth replacement with implants in patients with a narrow alveolar ridge form: A clinical study using guided tissue regeneration. Clin Oral Implants Res 1993;4:90–98.

8. Lekholm U, van Steenberghe D, Herrmann I, et al. Osseointegrated implants in the treatment of partially edentulous jaws: A prospective five year multicenter study. Int J Oral Maxillofac Implants 1994;9:627–635.

9. Ash MM. Wheeler's Dental Anatomy, Physiology and Occlusion. Philadelphia: Saunders, 1984;138–153.

10. Mellonig JT. Decalcified freeze-dried bone allograft as an implant material in human periodontal defects. Int J Periodont Rest Dent 1984;4:41–55.

11. Bowers GM, Chadroff B, Carnevale R, Mellonig J, Corn J, Emerson J. Histologic evaluation of new attachment apparatus formation in humans. Part III. J Periodontol 1989;60:683–693.

12. McClain PK, Shallhorn RG. Long-term assessment of combined osseous composite grafting, root conditioning and guided tissue regeneration. Int J Periodont Rest Dent 1993;13:9–27.

13. Cortellini P, Bowers GM. Periodontal regeneration of intrabony defects: An evidence-based treatment approach. Int J Periodont Rest Dent 1995;15:128–145.

14. Lazzara RJ. Immediate implant placement into extraction sites: Surgical and restorative advantages. Int J Periodont Rest Dent 1989; 9:333–344.

15. Mellonig JT, Nevins M. Guided bone regeneration of bone defects associated with implants: An evidence-based outcome assessment. Int J Periodont Rest Dent 1995;15:168–185.

16. Nevins M, Mellonig JT. The advantages of localized ridge augmentation prior to implant placement: A staged event. Int J Periodont Rest Dent 1994;14:97–111.

17. Buser D, Dala K, Belser U, Hirt HP, Berthold H. Localized ridge augmentation using guided bone regeneration. I. Surgical procedures in the maxilla. Int J Periodont Rest Dent 1993;13:29–45.

18. Simion M, Baldoni M, Zaffer D. Jawbone enlargement using immediate implant placement associated with a split-crest technique and guided tissue regeneration. Int J Periodont Rest Dent 1992; 12:463–474.

19. Sciproni A, Bruschi GB, Calesini G. The edentulous ridge expansion technique: A five year study. Int J Periodont Rest Dent 1994; 14:451–459.

The Placement of Mandibular Posterior Implants

Myron Nevins, DDS

The use of dental implants to replace teeth in the posterior mandible has become a predictable standard of care[1-6] (Fig 11-1). With the most formidable obstacle being the inferior alveolar nerve (Figs 11-2 and 11-3), implant decisions are dependent on information provided by computerized tomography (CT), including nerve location and the volume of bone superficial to the nerve[8-13] (Figs 11-4 and 11-5). The information provided can also help the clinician to ascertain both hopeless and questionable teeth, or may lead the clinician to consider a tooth strategic, if for no other reason than the impossibility of implant placement.

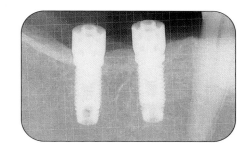

Fig 11-1a Successful placement of dental implants in the posterior mandibular region requires three-dimensional location of the inferior alveolar nerve.

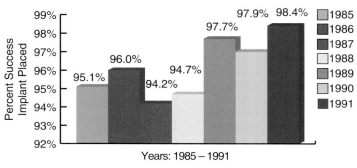

Fig 11-1b An account of 551 consecutive implants placed in the posterior mandible by two periodontists from 1985 to 1991. The success rate was 95.5%. (From Nevins and Langer.[5] Reprinted with permission.)

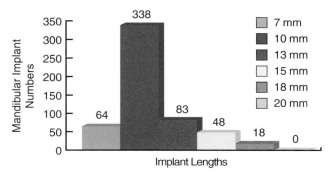

Fig 11-1c The majority of implants were 10 mm with few long implants. This is to be expected because of the anatomic obstacle of the inferior alveolar nerve. (From Nevins and Langer.[5] Reprinted with permission.)

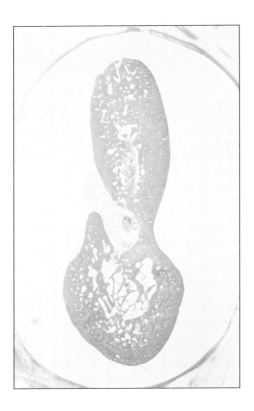

Fig 11-2 Histologic cross section of the mental foramen area. The position of the mental foramen limits the bone available for implant placement. It is rarely possible to place an implant lateral to the nerve. (From Gher and Richardson.[7] Reprinted with permission.)

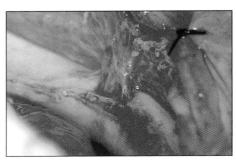

Fig 11-3 Isolation of the mental bundle following blunt dissection. It may be located on the occlusal surface of the mandible in atrophic cases.

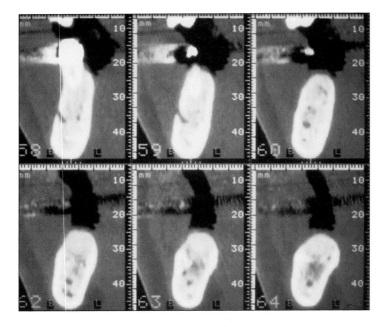

Fig 11-4 Computerized tomography permits the clinician to quantify bone volume and identify vital structures. The inferior alveolar nerve is usually apical to the mental foramen.

Obstacles to Implant Placement

Mental Foramen and Inferior Alveolar Nerve

The anatomic shape of the mandible and the position of the inferior alveolar nerve and mental foramen influence many treatment plans (Figs 11-6a to 11-6c). Three-dimensional radiographs usually demonstrate that the mental foramen is positioned superior to the trunk of the nerve. In those instances where the location of the nerve is difficult to establish, its position can be ascertained by measuring from the lower border of the mandible to the position of the nerve at the sagittal cut that includes the mental foramen. This measurement is transferred to other cuts, starting at the lower border of the mandible, to estimate the approximate location of the canal.

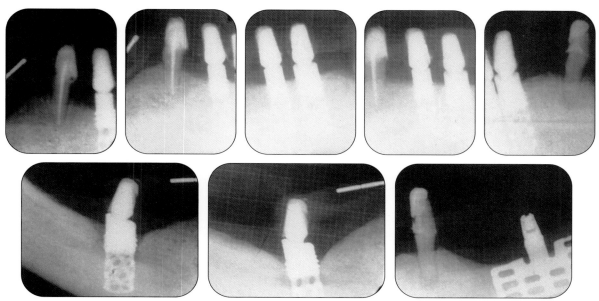

Fig 11-5a Dental implants have violated the nerve bilaterally. Two-dimensional radiographs are insufficient to treat mandibles where the nerve is close to the surface.

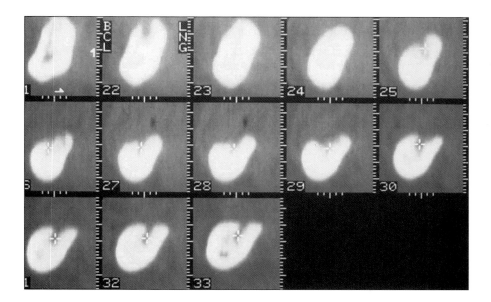

Fig 11-5b The CT scan demonstrates that the posterior implant was placed directly into the canal.

The surgical approach to the patient with limited bone height above the mental foramen should be cautious. Local anesthesia is administered only by infiltration to allow the patient to respond to possible encroachments before permanent damage occurs. The surgeon may also elect to locate the mental foramen and nerve with blunt dissection as a precise clinical measure of bone height available (Fig 11-6b). It is best to be conservative and measure from the crest of the edentulous area to the top of the foramen.

As the inferior alveolar nerve courses through the mandible, its position will dictate implant placement. The nerve enters the mandible lingual to the ramus, where local anesthesia is deposited for a mandibular block, and gradu-

ally traverses the body of the mandible until it exits buccally in the mental foramen. Another consideration in the posterior mandible is bone quality. When the bone is dense, the implant should not be closer than 2 mm to a vital nerve structure. There is no recorded evidence that a longer implant will be more successful in this region, and extending deeper into very soft bone only increases the risk of nerve damage (Figs 11-7a and 11-7b). Implants placed in this geographic location cannot achieve bicortical stabilization unless there is transposition of the nerve (Figs 11-8a and 11-8b). Therefore, countersinking may be inappropriate because it damages what little surface cortical bone exists, and should be minimized (see Fig 11-6c). The

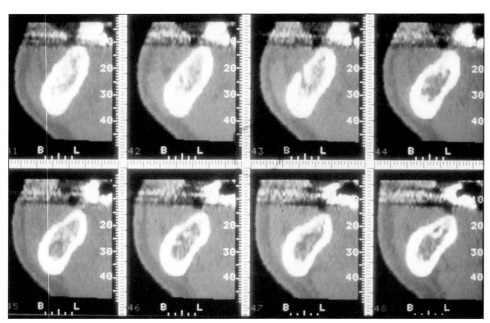

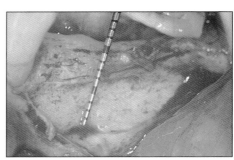

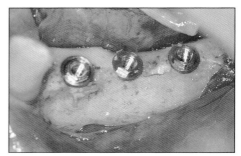

Fig 11-6b Clinical identification of the mental nerve allows the practitioner to measure precisely its position relative to the osseous crest. It is then compared to the CT scan (Fig 11-6a). All mandibular posterior implants are placed using only infiltration local anesthesia.

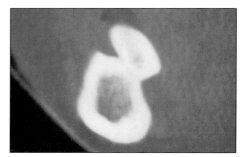

Fig 11-6a CT scan demonstrating the inferior alveolar nerve and mental foramen. The mental foramen is located in the upper half of the mandible. There is only about 11 mm of bone superior to the estimated location of the nerve.

Fig 11-6c Implant placement following clinical identification of the mental foramen. Damage to vital nerve structure has been avoided.

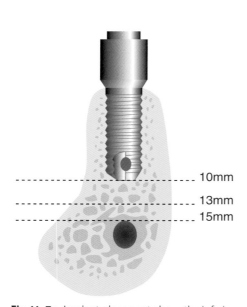

10mm

13mm

15mm

Fig 11-7a Implant placement above the inferior alveolar nerve. There is no evidence that additional implant length will increase the success rate in a patient with poorer bone quality. Therefore, there is no value to coming close to the nerve position.

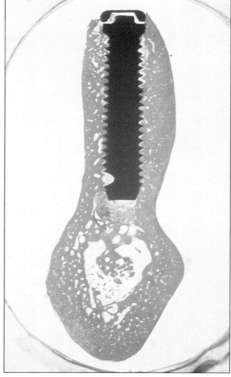

Fig 11-7b Histologic cross section of an implant encroaching on the inferior alveolar nerve. A shorter implant would be sufficient. (From Gher and Richardson.[13] Reprinted with permission.)

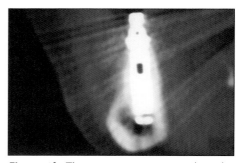

Fig 11-8a This patient had resective surgery to remove an ameloblastoma and then a rib graft to reconstruct the mandible. The inferior alveolar nerve resides in the recess between the graft and the body of the mandible.

Fig 11-8b The nerve was transposed at the time of implant delivery to prevent paresthesia. (From Rugge et al.[15] Reprinted with permission.)

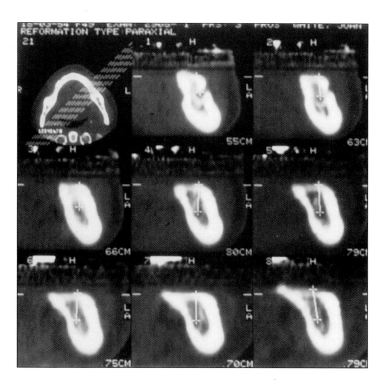

Fig 11-9a The inferior alveolar nerve is in mid-mandible. There is enough bone for 7-mm implants above and distal to the foramen. The first premolar was replaced with an 18-mm implant at the time of extraction.

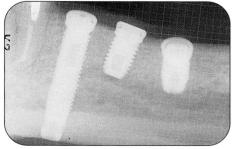

Fig 11-9b The position of the inferior alveolar nerve in this patient forces the surgeon to utilize an angular approach to prevent paresthesia (1988).

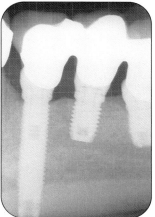

Fig 11-9c Radiograph taken 8 years after functional loading (1996).

placement of an additional implant is a reflection of the cancellous bone in the posterior mandible and is frequently contemplated as a failsafe and for purposes of force distribution (see Fig 11-6c).

The treatment of a patient with limited vertical bone height above the inferior alveolar nerve may include placement of the implants in a buccolingual or linguobuccal direction to avoid confrontation with the nerve. In most cases, these implants will be of minimal length but will engage the opposite cortical wall with their apical extension (Figs 11-9a to 11-9c). When the inferior alveolar nerve is located near the crest, implants are contraindicated or the patient must undergo nerve transposition[14,15] (see Figs 11-8a and 11-8b). The location of the nerve in the body of the mandible makes it very risky to try to bypass it laterally during the drilling procedure. This is true particularly in the presence of a mandible with a narrow waist.

Shape of the Mandible

When the inferior alveolar nerve and mental foramen do not have a role in treatment planning, the shape of the mandible may become the dominating factor. This is especially true in a patient with a skeletal Class II, division I malocclusion, when the mandible is smaller than the maxilla. The bucco-occlusal line angle of the mandibular posterior teeth does not articulate with the central fossa of the maxillary posterior teeth in centric relation, as it does in the convenience position of centric occlusion. However, the shape of the mandible and the canal position may dictate implant placement in a less than ideal position. These problems are coincident with special occlusal decisions for this jaw size discrepancy. If the mandible slants to the lingual, ideal implant placement may not be possible, and it is critical to plan the implant placement with the occlusal scheme as a determinant (Figs 11-10a to 11-10c).

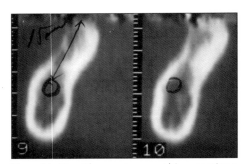

Fig 11-10a These topographic sections demonstrate the angular morphology of the mandible. The position of the inferior alveolar nerve influences treatment planning decisions, in that the implant will be placed in the area of maximum bone height, that is, lingual to the optimal occlusal position.

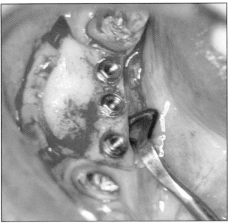

Fig 11-10b The implants are placed in a position that permits restoration with a fixed partial denture. The implants are slightly lingual to the ideal position.

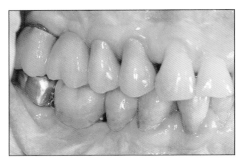

Fig 11-10c The final three-unit fixed partial denture prosthesis has restored the posterior occlusion. (Courtesy of Dr Jeffrey Dornbush.)

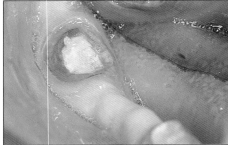

Fig 11-11a This mandibular molar has fused, short roots and was originally slated for extraction.

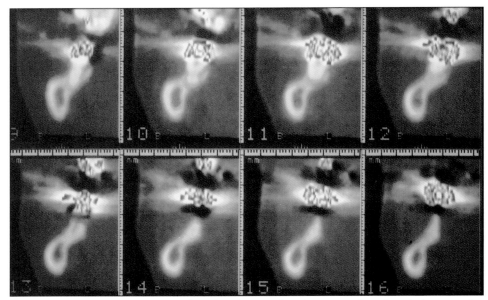

Fig 11-11c The sagittal sections confirm that the use of implants to replace the missing posterior teeth is precluded by a thin, knife-edged bony crest.

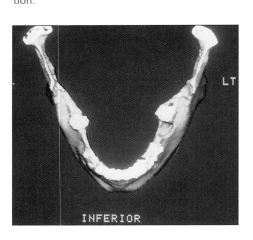

Fig 11-11b The reformatted three-dimensional view presented by the CT scan reveals a thin, knifelike edentulous ridge and forces reconsideration of the molar as an abutment tooth.

The thin, knife-edged mandibular posterior edentulous ridge has long been identified as an obstacle in the construction of removable partial dentures. The prevalence of this problem limits the use of wide-bodied implants in this region (see Fig 11-6c), as even the conventional diameter may protrude through the bony housing.

It may preclude implant placement and reestablish a conventional fixed prosthesis as the restoration of choice (Figs 11-11a to 11-11c). This decision may require the use of a questionable abutment with a marginal prognosis as a strategic tooth. In the absence of a reasonable choice, an autogenous block graft can be harvested from the chin or the iliac crest and connected to the recipient site[16] (see Chapter 15). It is very difficult to apply the concept of ridge splitting because there is little cancellous bone interspersed between the cortical buccal and lingual walls to lend plasticity to the procedure. The instrumentation with chisels is also difficult to apply to the area.

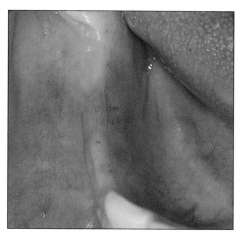

Fig 11-12a There is a significant difference in the width of the mandible in the proposed implant sites. The mesial implant site allows for choice of position, whereas the distal implant position is dictated by the size of the bone.

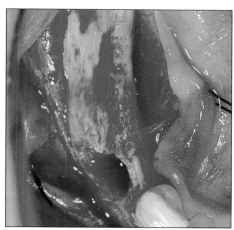

Fig 11-12b The thin, knifelike edentulous ridge is 6 to 7 mm high and, if reduced, would not permit implant placement.

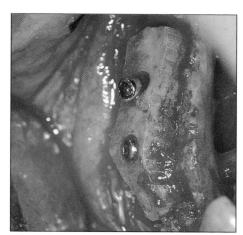

Fig 11-12c The thin ridge is augmented with a block of bone harvested from the chin.

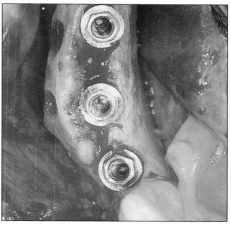

Fig 11-12d The bone-grafting procedure has resulted in a gain in width sufficient for the placement of dental implants.

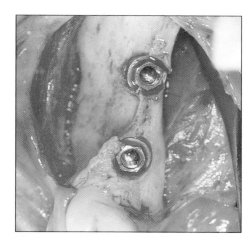

Fig 11-12e Note the knife-like mandibular edentulous ridge.

If the thin surface of the ridge widens quickly as it proceeds apically, implants can be inserted (Figs 11-12a to 11-12e). The angulation of the implants is determined by the bone morphology, but this may preclude implant placement.

The presence of a wide posterior mandible is a distinct advantage. It allows flexibility and the placement of wider implants when necessary. If one fixture is mobile at second-stage surgery, it can be removed and replaced with a fixture of wider diameter as a rescue procedure. It is necessary to remove all soft tissue from the site before a larger-diameter fixture is placed (Figs 11-13a to 11-13e).

There is much theater produced about the use of wide implants to replicate the emergence profile of mandibular molars, but this should be tempered for two reasons. The first is that thin and distorted ridges are far more common than wide ridges that could accommodate implants of a larger diameter. The second is that this is not an esthetic zone, and there is little reason to be overwhelmed by the emergence profile. There are more far-reaching difficulties encountered in achieving a finite treatment result with an implant prosthesis (Figs 11-14a and 11-14b).

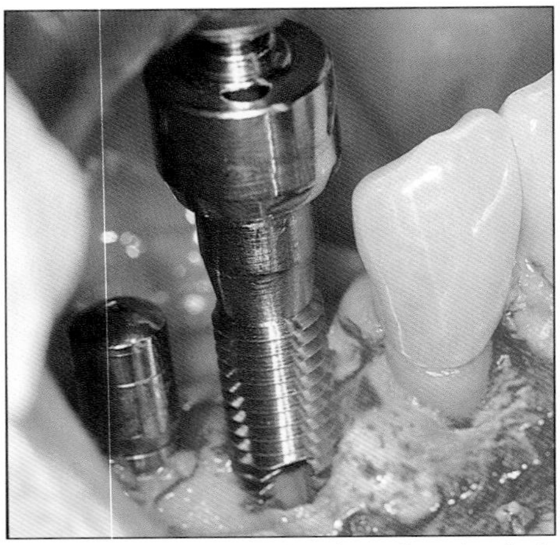

Fig 11-13a The fixture has been found to lack osseointegration and is removed at second-stage surgery.

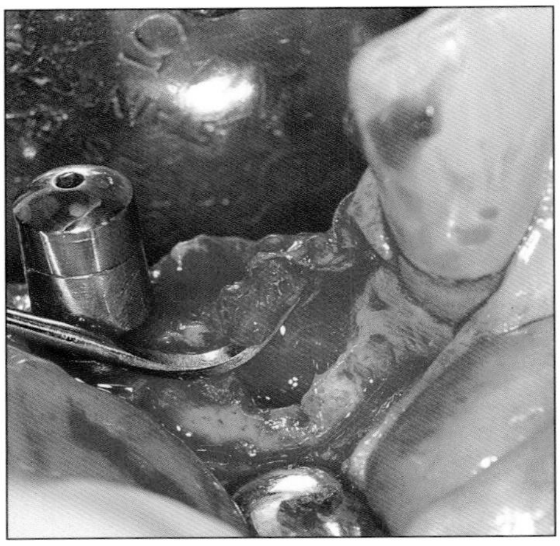

Fig 11-13b The explantation site is debrided of connective tissue.

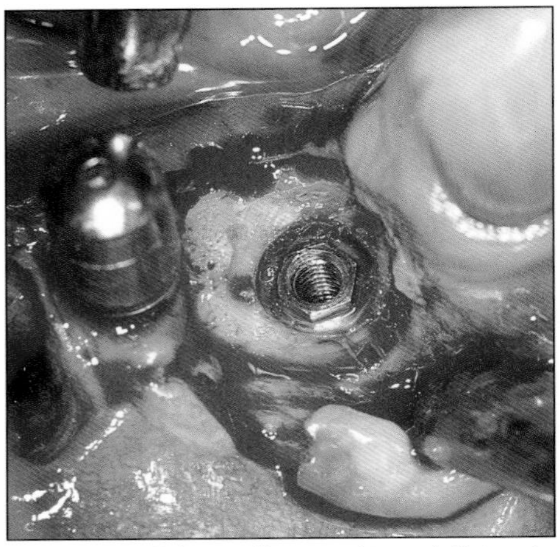

Fig 11-13c A larger-diameter (5-mm) fixture is inserted in a reprepared site.

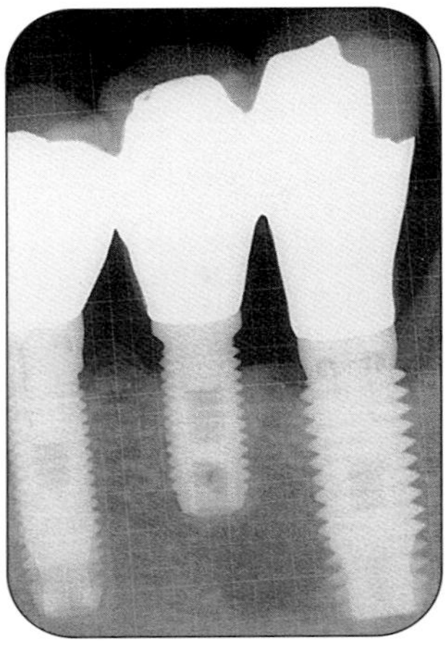

Fig 11-13d The larger-diameter fixture is shown following functional loading.

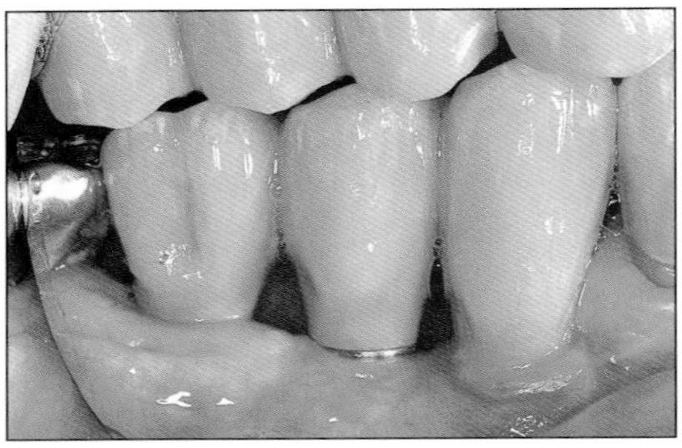

Fig 11-13e The final three-unit fixed partial denture restoration is in place.

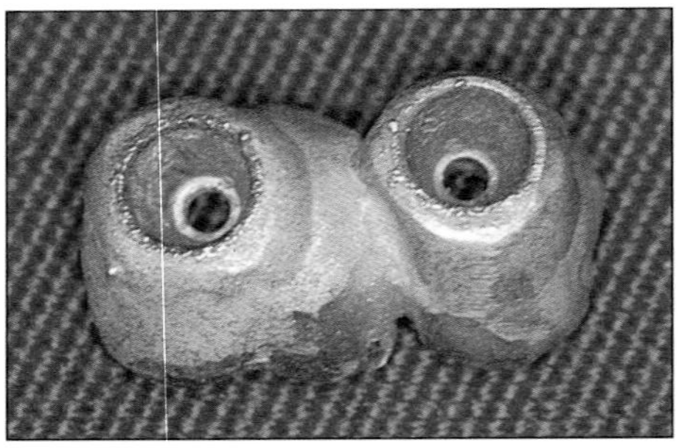

Fig 11-14a The improper finish of this final restoration will promote the accumulation of plaque and prevent the restoration from fitting properly. It cannot be polished to fit precisely.

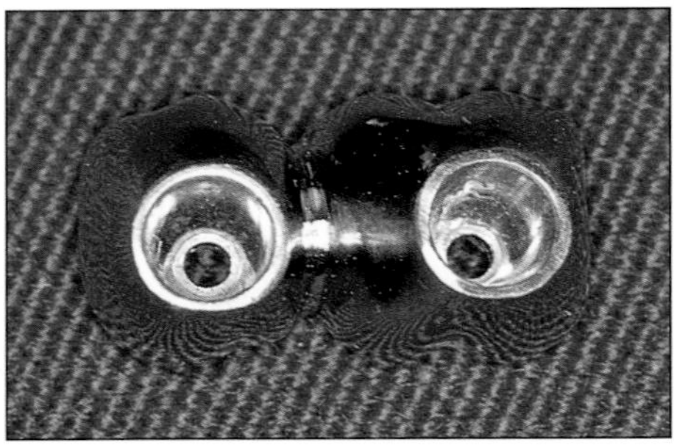

Fig 11-14b Smooth casting will facilitate the proper fit of the restoration and enhance soft tissue conditions.

Indications for Implant Therapy

A mandibular molar with compromised tooth structure should be evaluated for its possible restoration. Because a principal goal of treatment is to end the new restorative margin on sound tooth structure, a damaged tooth has to be considered within the limitation of lengthening the clinical crown. A tooth with fused roots or a long trunk is a better candidate than is the tooth with a normal-length trunk, because it is mandatory to reduce the periodontium to expose sound tooth structure without opening the furcation. This treatment is contraindicated if the removal of considerable quantities of bone to save a severely compromised tooth precludes the future placement of implants (see Chapter 1).

The periodontal prognosis of sectioned mandibular molars appears to be favorable, but the incidence of endodontic and restorative complications dictate caution.[17,18] A short edentulous span coupled with a large distal root will have a better prognosis than a long edentulous span or a mesial root that is more difficult to restore. Clinical evidence suggests that success increases as greater control is exercised over this multidisciplinary project. A resultant failure rate of 5.6% compares closely with the reported failure rate of mandibular posterior implants.[1–6] Because both therapies are reported to have a similar effectiveness, the burden of decision making becomes one of individual considerations when the tooth is stable and in a good state of repair, but is compromised periodontally.

The premature loss of mandibular first molars often results in the mesial tipping of the second molars, and the proximal discrepancies of the cementoenamel junctions are reflected by an angular mesial interproximal crest. This radiographic hemiseptum is correctable by orthodontic uprighting, if an inflammatory component has not been superimposed on it.[19]

When an inflammatory defect is superimposed upon a defect of tooth position, the additional loss of supporting structures is a compelling factor when deciding the prognosis of the tooth. The disease may be so advanced that extraction is the logical treatment, and guided bone regeneration is immediately implemented to prepare the area for future implants (see Chapters 5 and 6). If the teeth are stable and the pattern of bone loss is treatable, periodontal regenerative possibilities are considered. Tipped mandibular molars lose their contact points and exhibit the resultant diminishment of the embrasure space, reducing the possibilities for root resection and prosthetic restoration. Successful regenerative treatment may resolve the inflammatory defect, but it will be necessary to perform ostectomy to effectively create a flat edentulous ridge of bone.

A very treatable osseous lesion proximal to an edentulous region with implant treatment in the offing may offer the occasion for considerable debate. Is it necessary to save this tooth and thus commit the patient to a major surgical decision, or can it be added to the implant prosthesis by the use of a cantilever or another implant? (See Chapter 1.)

The easy decision occurs when the tooth structure and periodontium are severely compromised, and the pendulum of predictability swings completely to implant therapy. An intriguing situation occurs when a mandibular first molar is missing and the adjacent teeth are unrestored. Because the average mandibular first molar crown has a mesiodistal measurement of 10.5 mm, the edentulous area is generally too small to place two implants. Each implant is 3.75 mm, and two would measure 7.5 mm. Embrasure spaces of 2 mm proximal to adjacent teeth and between the two implants require an additional 6 mm, necessitating a total mesiodistal space of approximately 13.5 mm. Although a 5-mm implant is considered, the pattern of bone loss frequently presents a buccolingual bone width that is too narrow. An implant placed midway allows easy access for cleaning but traps food similarly to a sanitary pontic.

If the inferior alveolar nerve is near the surface, conventional fixed restorative dentistry should be performed. If there is enough dense bone to place a 13-mm implant, it should be placed in the space of the distal or mesial root, and the remaining space should be closed with a small cantilever. The restoration should only occlude in centric relation, and the patient can cleanse the interproximal and pontic areas with little difficulty (Figs 11-15a to 11-15d).

Overall, the posterior mandible is a common site for the consideration of implant placement because of the premature loss of the molars. The early loss of mandibular molars is often accompanied by the supraeruption of the maxillary molars, resulting in inadequate vertical space for the replacement of the missing teeth, even when the volume of bone is favorable. This circumstance exemplifies the need for a multidisciplinary approach to implant dentistry (Figs 11-16a to 11-16g). It is first important to consider the prevailing size of the embrasures of the maxillary molars and be sure that they can be restored. It is next critical to have teeth with long trunks, so that the furcations will not be exposed and worsen the prognosis of the teeth during crown-lengthening procedures. If these criteria are met and the reduction of tooth structure is perceived as involving endodontic treatment, the patency of the canals should be established. The supraerupted teeth can then be reduced to the anticipated occlusal plane and receive provisional crowns. This is accomplished before implant placement to accommodate the drilling procedures.

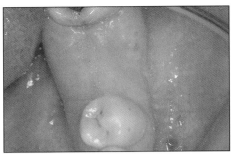

Fig 11-15a Treatment planning for implant placement in this edentulous space may be difficult. The mesiodistal dimension of the missing first molar does not permit the insertion of two implants with appropriate interproximal spaces.

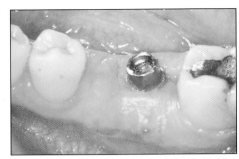

Fig 11-15b The implant has been placed in the position of the distal root.

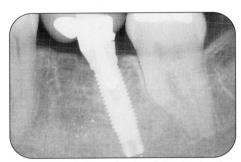

Fig 11-15c Radiograph taken following loading of the implant.

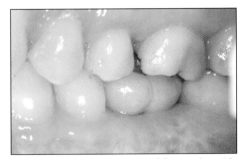

Fig 11-15d Final restoration of first molar with a cantilevered prosthesis. (Courtesy of Dr John Koslowska.)

The mesiodistal drilling site in the absence of the mandibular molars should be located so as to avoid the roots of the distalmost tooth, to allow sufficient embrasure space between the implants, and to avoid the need for an oversized crown on the mesial implant. The limited access for site preparation can be better managed by placing the first implant 6 mm distal to the last premolar and using a small mesial cantilever rather than an oversized crown that will probably precipitate gingival hyperplasia.

Conclusion

Mandibular posterior implants replace missing teeth with a similar predictability afforded by anterior implants. However, their use is complicated by the anatomic obstacle of the inferior alveolar nerve, a variety of malformations of the ridges, the presence of softer bone, and little or no possibility of reinforcement via bicortical stabilization.

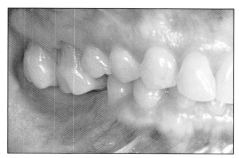

Fig 11-16a The maxillary molars are supraerupted and in contact with the mandibular soft tissues. There is no room for mandibular teeth.

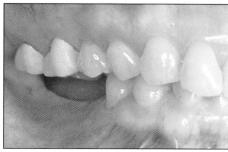

Fig 11-16b Endodontics was performed for both maxillary molars, and they were then shortened and provided with provisional crowns. This created space for the mandibular teeth and access for the drilling equipment needed to place implants.

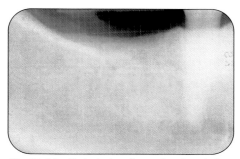

Fig 11-16c Periapical radiograph taken before implants were placed.

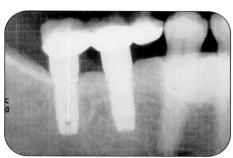

Fig 11-16d Periapical radiograph taken after implants were placed. Note the small mesial cantilever. This is preferable to an oversized awkward crown that is difficult to cleanse and may result in gingival hyperplasia. It also solves the problem of drilling without endangering the premolar root in an area with limited access.

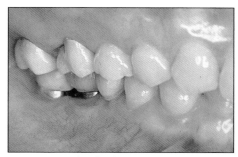

Fig 11-16e The final prosthesis is in place. (Courtesy of Dr Jeffrey Dornbush.)

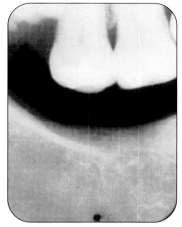 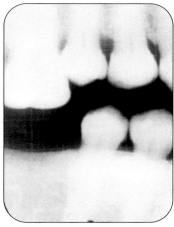

Fig 11-16f Pretreatment bitewing radiographs. Note the supraeruption and mesial drifting of the maxillary molars.

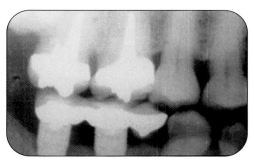 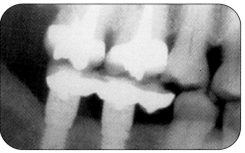

Fig 11-16g Posttreatment bitewing radiographs taken with the implant prosthesis in place.

References

1. Jemt T, Lekholm U, Adell R. Osseointegrated implants in the treatment of partially edentulous jaws: A preliminary study on 876 consecutively placed fixtures. Int J Oral Maxillofac Implants 1989; 4:211–217.

2. Buser D, Weber HP, Brägger U, Balsiger C. Tissue integration of one-stage ITI implants: Three-year results of a longitudinal study with hollow cylinder and hollow screw implants. Int J Oral Maxillofac Implants 1991;6:405–412.

3. Weber HP, Buser D, Fiorellini J, Williams R. Radiographic evaluation of crestal bone levels adjacent to nonsubmerged titanium implants. Clin Oral Implants Res 1992;2:181–188.

4. Jemt T, Lekholm U. Oral implant treatment in posterior partially edentulous jaws: A five-year follow-up report. Int J Oral Maxillofac Implants 1993;8:635–640.

5. Nevins M, Langer B. The successful application of osseointegrated implants to the posterior jaw: A long-term retrospective study. Int J Oral Maxillofac Implants 1993;8:428–432.

6. Lekholm U, et al. Osseointegrated implants in the treatment of partially edentulous jaws: A prospective 5-year multicenter study. Int J Oral Maxillofac Implants 1994;9:627–635.

7. Gher M, Richardson AC. The accuracy of dental radiographic techniques used for evaluation of implant fixture placement. Int J Periodont Rest Dent 1995;15:397–403.

8. Stella J, Tharanon W. A precise radiographic method to determine the location of the inferior alveolar canal in the posterior edentulous mandible: Implications for dental implants. Part 2. Clinical application. Int J Oral Maxillofac Implants 1990;5:23–29.

9. Quirynen M, Lamoral Y, Dekeyser C, et al. CT scan standard reconstruction technique for reliable jaw bone volume determination. Int J Oral Maxillofac Implants 1990;5:384–389.

10. Israelson H, Plemons J, Watkins P, Sory C. Barium coated surgical stents and computer assisted tomography in the preoperative assessment of dental implant patients. Int J Periodont Rest Dent 1992; 12:52–61.

11. Williams M, Mealey B, Hallmon W. The role of computerized tomography in dental implantology. Int J Oral Maxillofac Implants 1992;7:373–380.

12. Todd A, Gher M, Quitero G, Richardson A. Interpretation of linear and computer tomograms in the assessment of implant recipient sites. J Periodontol 1993;64:1243–1249.

13. Gher M, Richardson AC. The accuracy of dental radiographic techniques used for evaluation of implant fixture placement. Int J Periodont Rest Dent 1995;15:268–283.

14. Friberg B, Ivanoff CJ, Lekholm U. Inferior alveolar nerve transposition in combination with Brånemark implant treatment. Int J Periodont Rest Dent 1992;12:441–449.

15. Rugge G, Lekholm U, Nevins M. Osseointegration and nerve transposition after mandibular resection to treat an ameloblastoma: A case report. Int J Periodont Rest Dent 1995;15:397–403.

16. Buser D, Dula K, Belser U, Hirt HP, Berthold H. Localized ridge augmentation using guided bone regeneration. Part 2. Surgical procedure in the mandible. Int J Periodont Rest Dent 1995;15:11–29.

17. Langer B, Stein SD, Wagenberg B. An evaluation of root resections: A ten year study. J Periodontol 1981;52:719–722.

18. Carnevale G, DiFebo G, Tonelli MP, Marin C, Fuzzi MA. Retrospective analysis of the periodontal-prosthetic treatment of molars with interradicular lesions. Int J Periodont Rest Dent 1991; 11:189–205.

19. Wise RJ, Kramer GM. Predetermination of osseous changes associated with uprighting tipped molars by probing. Int J Periodont Rest Dent 1983;3:69–80.

CHAPTER 12

The Placement of Maxillary Posterior Implants

Myron Nevins, DDS
Joseph P. Fiorellini, DMD, DMSc

The maxillary posterior quadrant offers an intriguing area of decision making because of the complex root anatomy of the teeth, the anatomic obstacle of the maxillary sinus, and the limited quantity and quality of the alveolar process to support osseointegrated implants. There is a frequent finding of interproximal infrabony pocketing that may involve the invasion of interradicular areas on the multirooted teeth.

The issues that complicate the preservation of the natural teeth are:

1. The loss of supporting bone.
2. The length of the clinical roots.
3. The length of the root trunk (distance from the cementoenamel junction to the furcation).
4. The state of repair of the teeth.
5. Interproximal embrasures.
6. Malpositioning of teeth.
7. The success of endodontic procedures.

What do we know about the use of dental implants in the maxillary posterior region? Is the answer to efficacy found in the structure and surface finish of the implant or in the volume of bone and surgical strategy? Retrospective studies that have examined the performance of implants replacing maxillary posterior teeth include the learning curves when early treatment efforts lacked a specific protocol for the partially edentulous patient. An overall success rate of 95% has been reported with the screw-form of titanium-finish implant in three separate studies[1-3] (Figs 12-1a and 12-1b). The questions that require answers pertain to the volume and quality of bone that is necessary to support the occlusal load. It also is important to consider the vertical loss of the alveolar process and its effect on the crown-root ratio of the planned prostheses. The importance of these issues is magnified by the force that can be exerted because of the proximity of these implants to the temporomandibular joint.

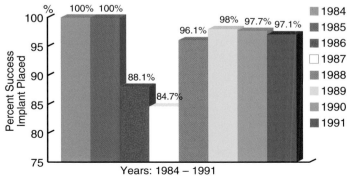

Fig 12-1a Success rate of implants placed in the maxillary posterior region. Very few were used in 1984 and 1985, but, in later years, the use was expanded and reflects the learning curve. (From Nevins and Langer.[2] Reprinted with permission.)

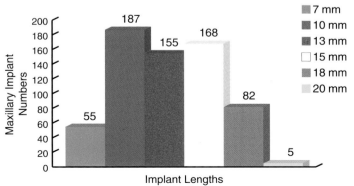

Fig 12-1b Many short implants have been successful, but there is an opportunity to use more long implants than in the mandibular posterior region. (From Nevins and Langer.[2] Reprinted with permission.)

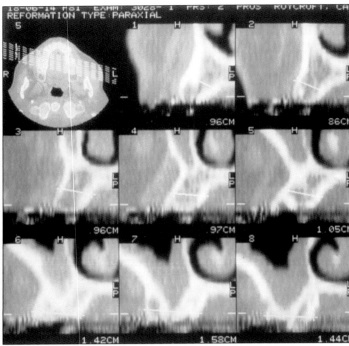

Fig 12-2a The CT scan is an important diagnostic tool for implant sites in the posterior maxilla. The information in the sagittal cross sections includes not only the bone height available below the sinus floor but also the shape and width of the ridge. These indicate adequate bone volume throughout the area and allow the angulation of the implant to be altered.

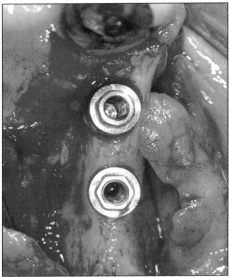

Fig 12-2b Note that there is minimal width of bone to contain the implants. It is not possible to alter the buccolingual position and keep the implant encased in bone.

Obstacles to Implant Placement

Bone Volume

The three-dimensional views provided by computerized tomography (CT) have both upgraded diagnostic capabilities and improved implant placement.[4-6] The placement of dental implants in the maxillary posterior region is challenging because of both the quantity and the quality of bone. Because the mandibular posterior teeth have a slightly lingual tilt, the maxillary teeth erupt and are positioned buccally, as evidenced by observation of the sagittal sections of the alveolar process in three-dimensional radiography. When the width of the alveolar process is 8 to 11 mm, the implant angulation is easily corrected to articulate with the opposing occlusal tables (Figs 12-2a and 12-2b). If the buccopalatal width is only 6 to 7 mm in the premolar region, the implant will be placed at an angle that will need to be corrected by an angulated abutment (Figs 12-3a and 12-3b), or the bone on the buccal surface will need to be supplemented before implant placement. Time, finance, and fear of morbidity are nontechnical factors that complicate this decision and may discourage the use of edentulous ridge augmentation.

A premolar occlusion offers a successful conclusion of treatment for many patients with or without dental implants (see Fig 12-3b and Figs 12-4a to 12-4d), although some individuals with a broad smile would suffer an esthetic compromise and may require a molar occlusion. Cantilevers offer a possible solution to this dilemma but must be supported by a reasonable number of teeth or implants and should be provided in a trial restoration before construction of a final prosthesis.[7]

The horizontal width of bone is frequently inadequate in the premolar region but is usually more than sufficient in the molar region, where the maxillary sinus results in an insufficient vertical height of bone. The drilling process for implant placement identifies less compact bone as one proceeds distally. Edentulous ridge augmentation procedures have evolved to provide the possibility of placing dental implants in a restorable position and of a size that can predictably support the load of occlusion.[8,9]

The first consideration of bone volume should be the preservation of the natural dentition and its periodontium. It is frivolous to allow untreated periodontal disease to slowly erode the alveolar process in this difficult area of the mouth and diminish or possibly preclude implants as an alternative. Although this is especially true in the molar region, the two-rooted first premolar is an interesting challenge in the premolar region (Figs 12-5a and 12-5b).

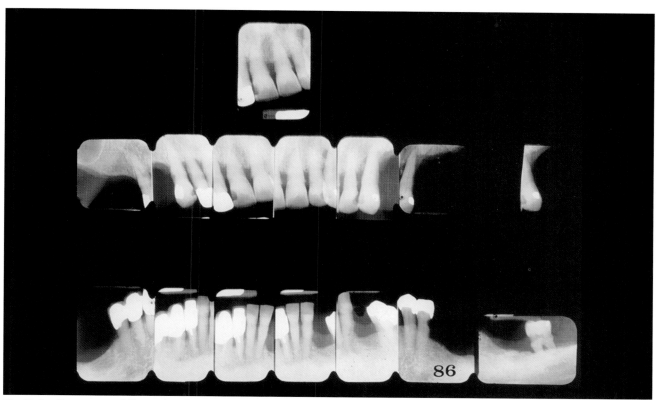

Fig 12-3a Pretreatment full-mouth radiographic survey (1986). This maxillary dentition is reduced to anterior teeth. The premolar bone measures horizontally between 6 and 7 mm. Implants were placed so as to be confined in bony housing, because treatment preceded many contemporary treatment regimens for edentulous ridges. The buccolingual angulation needed to be corrected with angulated abutments.

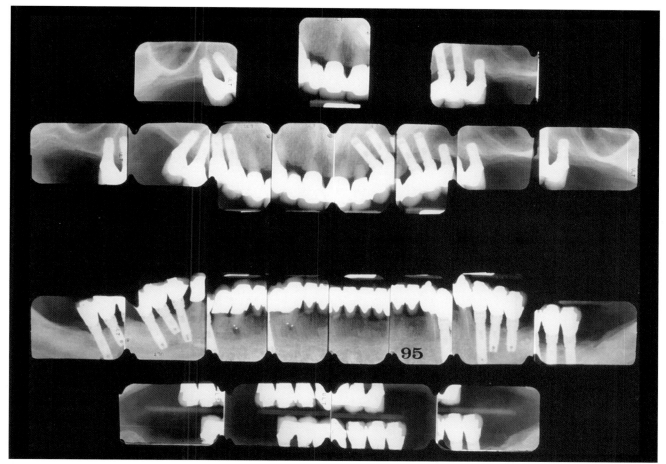

Fig 12-3b Full-mouth radiographic survey (1995). The implants have now been loaded for 8 years and present no problems. The angulation issues were resolved with cast abutments. (Prosthetics by Dr Howard M. Skurow.)

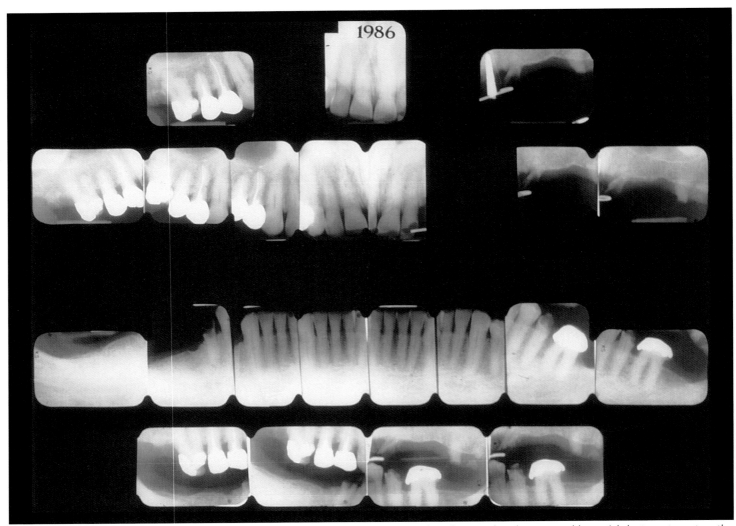

Fig 12-4a Full-mouth radiographic survey (1986). The patient selected osseointegrated implants, rather than removable partial dentures to restore the dentition.

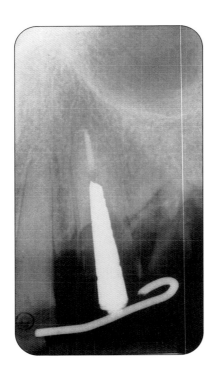
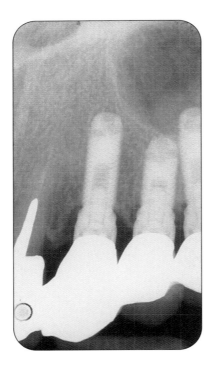

Fig 12-4b The maxillary left canine evidences caries around the post in the pulp chamber *(left)*. Crown-lengthening surgery would have jeopardized the lateral incisor and reduced the volume of bone available to place implants if the canine failed. Therefore, the canine has been replaced with an implant, and no periodontal surgery has been performed *(right)*.

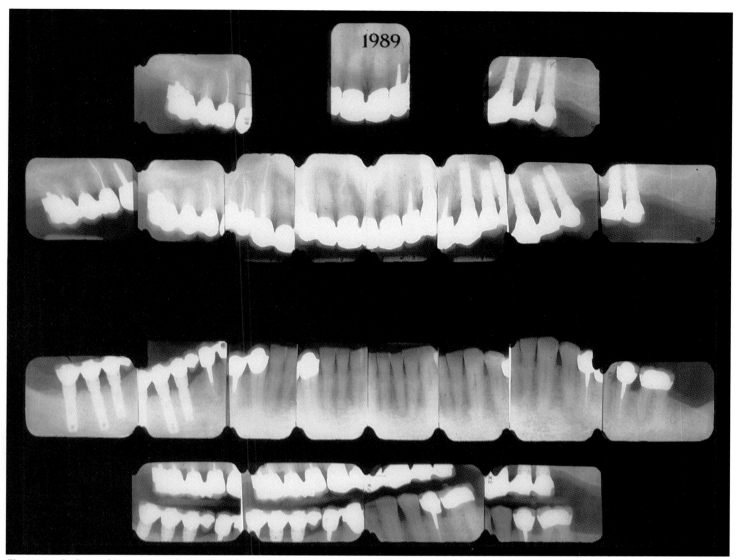

Fig 12-4c Radiographic survey made in 1989. The implants are 3 years old and have been loaded for 1½ years. The patient is comfortable with a premolar occlusion. (Prosthetic dentistry by Dr Janice Conrad.)

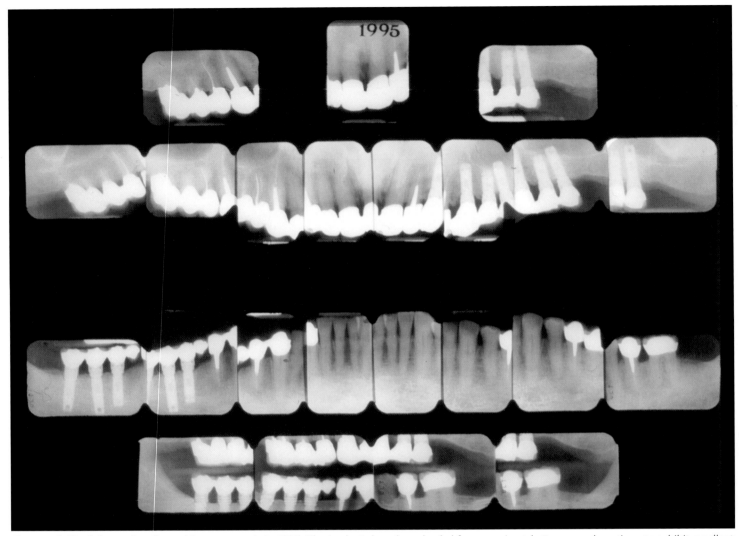

Fig 12-4d The full-mouth radiographic survey made in 1995. The implants have been loaded for approximately 8 years and continue to exhibit excellent bone height. There is no clinical symptomology. The implant prostheses are freestanding.

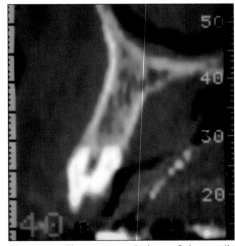

Fig 12-5a The root morphology of the maxillary first premolar can influence the treatment of the posterior maxilla. This CT scan reveals bone loss within the furcation. Fortunately, the bone available above the root apex is ample for implant placement.

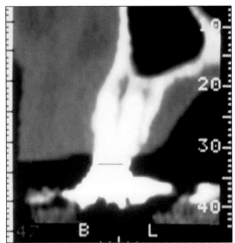

Fig 12-5b This maxillary first premolar has no furcation invasion, but, if it became periodontally compromised, quick extraction would be necessary to salvage sufficient bone to place an implant.

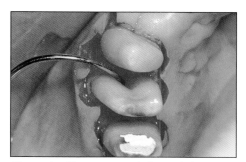

Fig 12-6a The root morphology of the maxillary first premolar reduces the prognosis of the tooth when the furcation is completely invaded. A more conservative and predictable therapy is extraction.

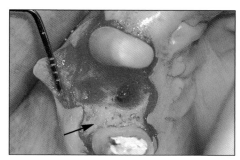

Fig 12-6b The extraction of the first premolar eliminates a most difficult cul-de-sac that is problematic to treat or maintain. Note the flat interproximal bone proximal to the canine and second premolar (arrow).

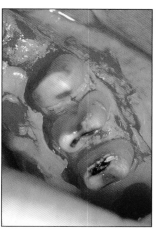

Fig 12-7 When the furcation invasion is minimal and there is a wide embrasure, osseous surgery can be performed. The furcation on the mesial surface can greatly influence several factors, including plaque retention. By ostectomy of the bone and odontoplasty, the architecture can be improved to provide access and enhance the prognosis.

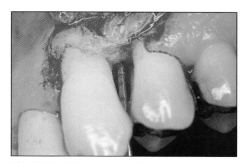

Fig 12-8a There is a shallow intrabony crater between the canine and first premolar. Both teeth are stable.

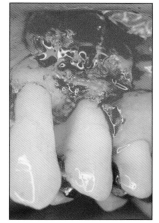

Fig 12-8b The crater is reduced by ostectomy to achieve a completely flat interdental crest of bone.

Premolar Region

The first premolar has buccal and palatal roots that separate in the apical third of their length. A mesial concavity begins approximately 1 mm apical to the cementoenamel junction and continues until the furcation begins, probably serving as a funnel for the inflammatory process and the continual loss of bone on this surface.[10]

Furcal invasion results in a defect that is impossible for the patient or the hygienist to clean. It is most unusual to be able to section a maxillary first premolar because the furcation occurs so far apically that very little clinical root remains. If the adjacent teeth are secure periodontally, a furcated first premolar should be extracted to establish a cleansable environment and preserve the interproximal bone (Figs 12-6a and 12-6b). If the furcation is only minimally involved, the principle of odontoplasty can be used to resolve the concavity in the presence of an embrasure

that can be cleansed (Fig 12-7). Angular osseous defects must be attended to, and a flat interproximal crest must be created by subtraction or addition[11] (Figs 12-8 and 12-9). Continued loss of bone lessens the prognosis for both the teeth and future implants.

A primary goal of periodontal regeneration is to convert an untreatable tooth into a functional, useful member of the dentition, but it may not be 100% successful. Because these individuals have already demonstrated their susceptibility to inflammatory periodontal disease, it is a poor decision to allow any osseous defect to remain after the regenerative procedure.[11] Any remaining angular crest is resolved in the future so as to provide a flat interdental septum. The introduction of guided tissue regeneration procedures has increased the possibilities of success when less contained osseous defects are encountered, although such areas have been successfully treated with both autografts and allografts in the past.[12–17]

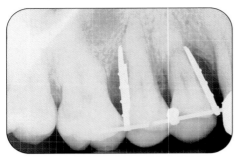

Fig 12-9a The pretreatment radiograph exhibits severe bone defects on the mesial surface of the maxillary first premolar and the distal surface of the second premolar (1970).

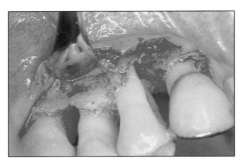

Fig 12-9b Clinical correlation of the radiograph.

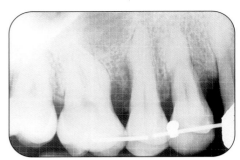

Fig 12-9c Posttreatment radiograph (1972). Note the interdental bone improvement. The areas were treated with frozen iliac grafts harvested with a trephine.

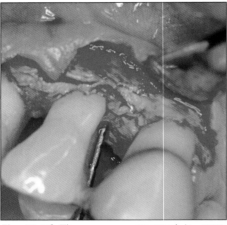

Fig 12-9d The area was reentered in 1988, when the patient agreed to replace the fixed prosthesis. There is obvious bone improvement 18 years later.

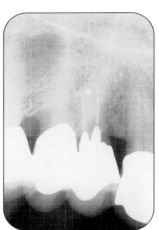

Fig 12-9e The 1997 radiograph, taken 25 years after treatment, clearly establishes the stability of the periodontal regeneration procedure.

An unrestored single-rooted first premolar demonstrating a deep vertical osseous defect is a candidate for periodontal regeneration (Figs 12-10a to 12-10e). The surgical procedure must extend to the far line angles of adjacent teeth, remove all infected granulation tissue, and provide a clean root surface. Periodontal regeneration must be accomplished without damaging the approximating bone surface of the canine and will follow the procedures suggested in Chapters 15 and 16.

There are rare occasions when first premolars are treated with root sectioning (Figs 12-11a to 12-11c). It may be reasonable to section a first premolar, and, when stability exists, the single root can be retained and used in a final prosthesis, although contemporary treatment will predictably offer extraction and replacement with an implant.

The thinness of the buccal plate of bone, together with endodontic and periodontal pathology, often results in fenestrations and encourages the palatal placement of maxillary

first premolar implants at the time of extraction (Figs 12-12a to 12-12d). This presents esthetic restorative complications and the need to cantilever ceramics buccally to satisfy the esthetic demands. However, the implant placed in the position of the palatal root is in excellent alignment for occlusion.

It has been proposed that an immediate implant can only succeed if it can be anchored apically in sufficient bone. However, the interradicular area of pronounced root concavities offers horizontal bone support to help stabilize the implant and allow an excellent buccolingual position (Figs 12-13a to 12-13d). It is an alternative to vertical bone stabilization of an immediate implant when the tooth apex approaches the sinus. The loss of the thin buccal plate following extraction contributes to the problem of an inadequate horizontal dimension of bone when implants are a future consideration and no effort is made to treat the extraction vault at the time of extraction (see Chapters 5 and 9).

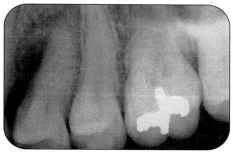

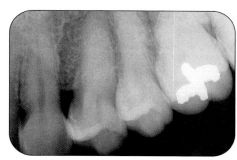

Fig 12-10a There is a deep mesial defect extending to the apex of the single-rooted maxillary first premolar (1988).

Fig 12-10b There appears to be remarkable evidence of periodontal regeneration in the 1996 radiograph (8 years posttreatment).

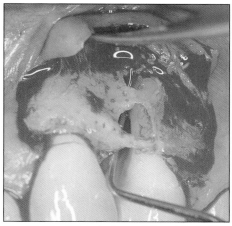

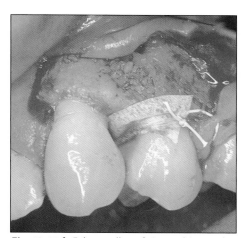

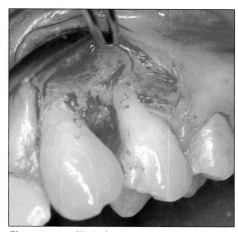

Fig 12-10c Clinical view of the defect. The small bridges of bone should be retained during debridement of the root surface and during removal of granulation tissue because they will help contain the graft material and create space for regeneration.

Fig 12-10d A bone allograft is used in combination with a membrane in this regeneration surgery. The shapes of the membrane were limited in 1988, so a large wraparound configuration was reduced to fit the narrow embrasure.

Fig 12-10e Clinical reopening procedure in 1989 (11 months later).

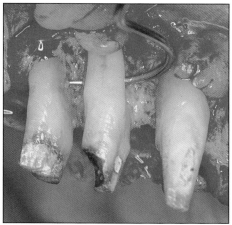

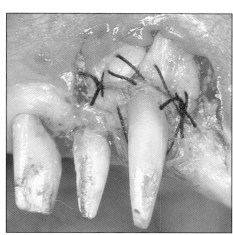

Fig 12-11a Complete furcation invasion of the maxillary first premolar.

Fig 12-11b The buccal root has been removed, and the palatal root is stable.

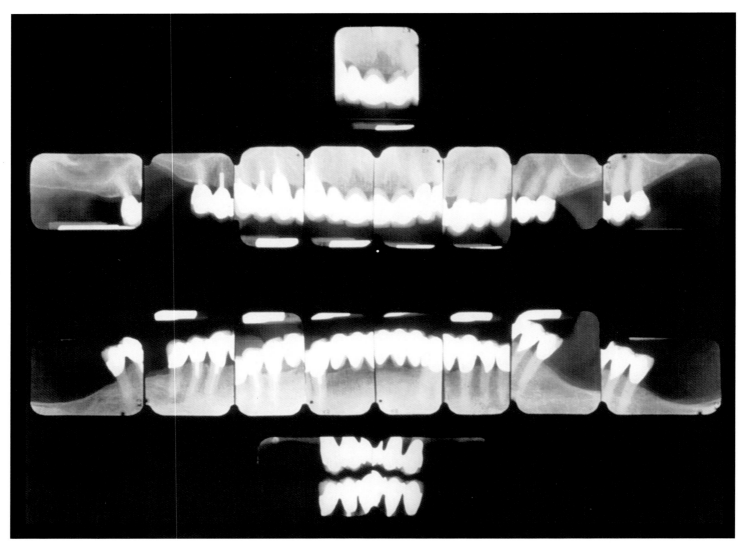

Fig 12-11c The prosthesis has been completed as a premolar occlusion. The palatal root of the first bicuspid offers the same stability as the other abutments.

The two-rooted maxillary first premolar is very difficult to restore with a post and core because it is narrow mesiodistally and somewhat resembles a biconcave disk. Crown-lengthening procedures are routinely successful, but it is necessary to decide how much bone should be removed, because this same bone will be needed for placement of an implant. The tooth's prognosis is further worsened by limited embrasures or previous apicoectomies (Figs 12-14a to 12-14d). It is prudent to reconsider the strategy of keeping a badly damaged maxillary premolar and to contemplate implant treatment, considering the successful record of osseointegration in this area. The maxillary premolar area has no impediment to achieving bicortical stabilization, offers good resistance to drilling, permits the use of maximum-length implants, and provides a strong resistance to occlusal loading.

An inadequate horizontal volume of bone can be enhanced by separating the cortical plates[18,19] or by using an onlay graft that is fixed in place.[20] The ideal candidate for ridge splitting is identified on a sagittal CT image as having the shape of an isosceles triangle with the base at the apical margin and an occlusal width of 3 mm (Figs 12-15a to 12-15e). It is difficult to split a thin rectangular ridge and maintain continuity. The initial gingival incision is made toward the palate to prevent membrane exposure and healing problems. The buccal flap dissection should be partial thickness to preserve the periosteal and connective tissue bone cover with its blood supply intact. The occlusal cortical bone is first cut with a non-crosscutting fissure bur to a depth of 2 mm to bypass the cortical cover. A thin chisel with a sharp, beveled cutting edge is then introduced to a depth of 6 mm, providing sufficient width to then engage larger

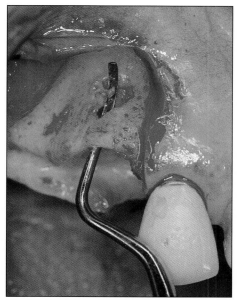

Fig 12-12a There is an obvious buccal fenestration of the buccal wall of bone after the extraction of the maxillary first premolar. Note the buccal cavity.

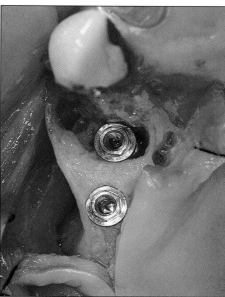

Fig 12-12b The implant is placed toward the position of the palatal root to avoid the buccal concavity and prevent exposure of implant threads. It makes the prosthesis more difficult to construct esthetically, although the implant is in excellent occlusal alignment.

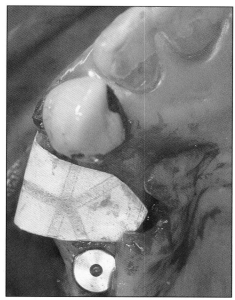

Fig 12-12c The implant and the defect are covered with a titanium-reinforced membrane (Gore-Tex, WL Gore, Flagstaff, AZ).

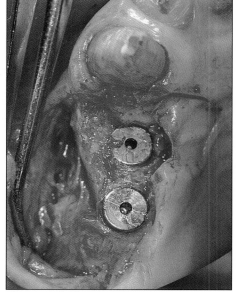

Fig 12-12d The second-stage surgery reveals complete fill of the bone defect, as expected, because it is within the envelope of bone.

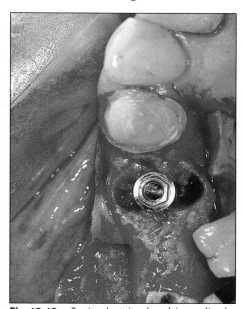

Fig 12-13a An implant is placed immediately into the extraction site of a maxillary first premolar where there is inadequate bone apical to the tooth to stabilize an implant. The implant is stabilized by wedging it into the bone convexities that fill the root concavities.

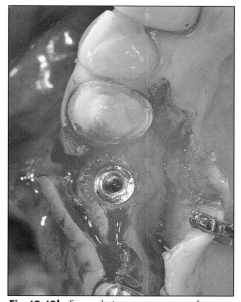

Fig 12-13b Second-stage surgery reveals complete bone fill and an implant in an excellent position to be restored.

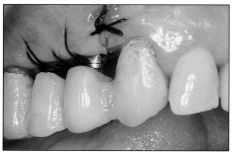

Fig 12-13c The provisional prosthesis is cemented over the implant abutment. Note the excellent alignment.

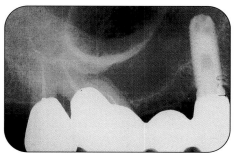

Fig 12-13d Posttreatment radiograph. (Prosthetic dentistry by Dr John Machel.)

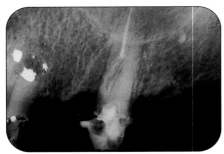

Fig 12-14a The maxillary first premolar is periodontally compromised, and its prognosis is further challenged by an apicoectomy.

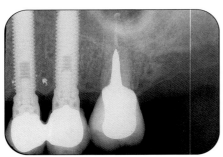

Fig 12-14d Posttreatment radiograph. The implants offer substantial improvement in the clinical root support and the prognosis of this quadrant. They are freestanding. (Prosthesis by Dr James Stein)

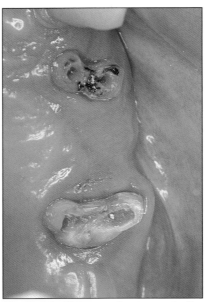

Fig 12-14b This premolar does not offer a strong prognosis as an abutment for a fixed bridge. There is very little clinical crown, and this tooth is not the best candidate for a post and core restoration. Using these two abutments for a fixed prosthesis would result in a high risk for problems.

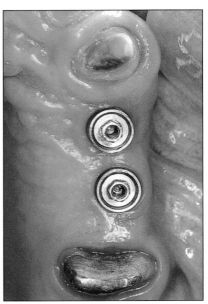

Fig 12-14c The premolar has been replaced by two implants that will support a freestanding implant prosthesis. The sectioned molar will have a single crown.

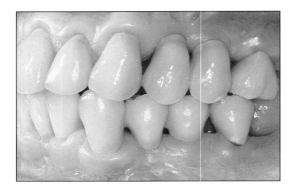

Fig 12-14e The final prosthesis is in place.

monobeveled chisels that are 10 mm long. The bevel faces the buccal plate, which is expanded buccally to result in a width of approximately 6 or 7 mm. The length of the longest beveled chisel is 10 mm, but it is important to maintain some portion of the most apical bone in one piece to fix the implant. This procedure can be done with simultaneous delivery of the implants or as a staged procedure with implants only inserted after the volume of bone increases (Figs 12-15f and 12-15g). The surgeon must not countersink the buccal plate or attempt to tap these sites because it is crucial to maintain complete attachment of the buccal plate and its blood supply. Self-tapping implants are used if possible, and smaller diameter implants are substituted when necessary. The trough is then filled with an autogenous or allograft bone graft and covered with a barrier membrane to ensure the growth of bone. Others report using only a membrane or nothing, but this is a complicated procedure and a comprehensive approach is suggested.[18,19] This procedure can be used

bilaterally in the edentulous patient but is not extended to the area of the incisive canal. Another approach would be to use a block of bone from an extraoral site[20] (see Chapter 15).

Guided bone regeneration can preserve a thin buccal plate or reconstruct a missing buccal plate if the patient is encountered before removal of the teeth or the failure of implants. Large defects are treated with block autografts, particulate autografts, or mineralized allografts and then covered with a barrier membrane that may or may not need to be fixed in place. Still larger defects may be better treated by adding a titanium mesh to help stabilize the bone graft when the palatal height of bone is compromised (Figs 12-16a to 12-16e) or a titanium-reinforced membrane to create space for regeneration.[21]

There is inconclusive evidence to support or contraindicate the use of implants of a smaller diameter to replace maxillary premolars. They do offer an alternative if the occlusal load is considered and not overextended with cantilevers.

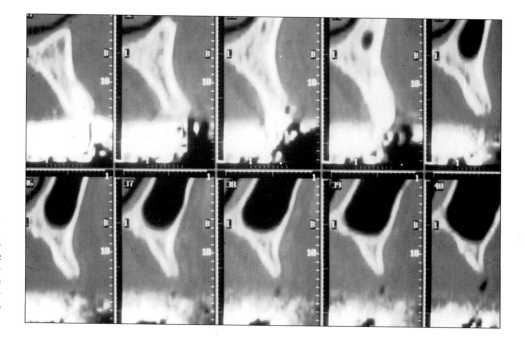

Fig 12-15a There are several techniques available to augment the severely resorbed ridge. One that is used when the base of bone has adequate width but the crestal area is thin is the ridge-splitting technique. The CT scan demonstrates the narrow buccal-to-palatal dimension of the crest, but bone that could support implants following separation of the cortical plates is present at the base.

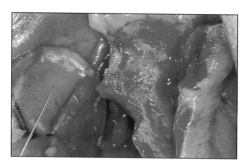

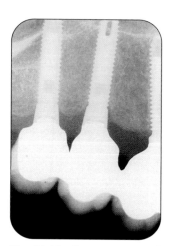

Fig 12-15b Following reflection of a mucoperiosteal flap, the ridge form is noted to be narrow and irregular. The cuspid had been extracted because of a vertical root fracture, and the area was regenerated.

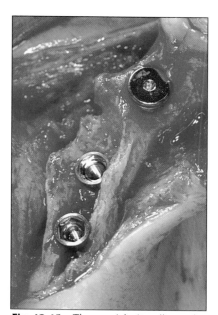

Fig 12-15c The mesial site allows the placement of a 3.75-diameter fixture; however, the distal ridge requires expansion first. The cortical plates are separated with a fissure bur; then they are wedged apart with chisels. The area is grafted and covered with a barrier membrane to regenerate bone within the expansion.

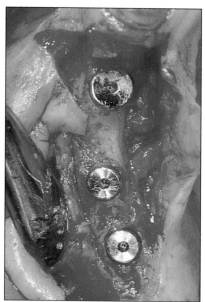

Fig 12-15d Second-stage surgery. The surgically created space between the cortical plates of bone has completely filled with bone. A bone allograft and a Gore-Tex Augmentation Membrane were used.

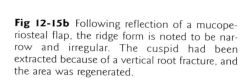

Fig 12-15e Posttreatment radiograph. Two 3-mm implants were used in the premolar region.

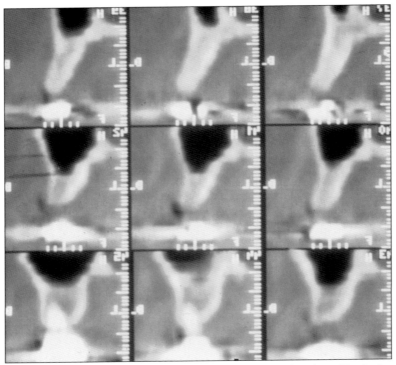

Fig 12-15f A presurgical CT scan demonstrates a narrow edentulous ridge in the maxillary bicuspid region.

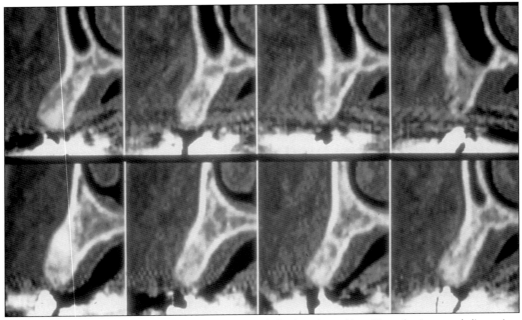

Fig 12-15g A postsurgical CT scan reveals an expanded edentulous ridge. Note the increased dimension coronally.

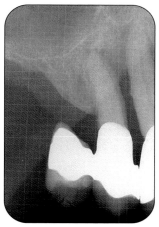

Fig 12-16a There is complete loss of interproximal bone between the maxillary canine and the first premolar. The maxillary sinus is an obstacle to placement of posterior implants unless it is enhanced with a regenerative procedure.

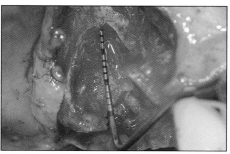

Fig 12-16b The extraction vault demonstrates complete loss of buccal plate (17 mm). Successful guided bone regeneration is necessary to avoid a removable partial denture without retention on the right side.

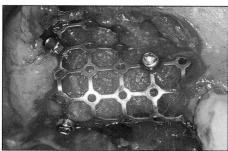

Fig 12-16c A mineralized bone allograft is covered with a titanium mesh that is held in place with Memfix screws. The mesh helps to stabilize the wound during healing.

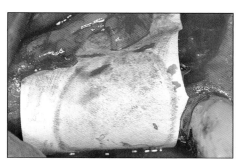

Fig 12-16d A Gore-Tex Augmentation Membrane is fitted over the assembly of graft and mesh as an exclusionary barrier that will limit the field to osteogenic precursor cells.

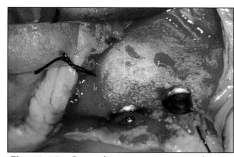

Fig 12-16e Second-stage surgery reveals significant bone formation. Implants have been placed at a vertical level that permits the prosthesis to be constructed.

Fig 12-16f Final radiographs of loaded implants.

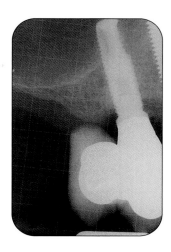
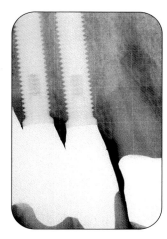

Molar Region

It is not the buccopalatal width, but the vertical height, of bone that is the limiting factor for implants in the maxillary molar region. The distance from the floor of the sinus to the hiatus of the furcation usually ranges from 4 to 8 mm; thus the premature removal of these teeth would do little to improve future implant placement. Therefore vertical osseous defects that do not encounter open proximal furcations should be committed to periodontal regeneration techniques in an effort to avoid the need for implants. The irony is that the same periodontal defects exhibited in the loss of interproximal and interradicular periodontium that reduce the prognosis of the natural teeth create a problematic encounter with dental implants. It is important to consider the future crown-root ratio and to make realistic decisions that avoid unmanageable clinical problems.

The early recognition of periodontal disease and its correction are immensely important in establishing a favorable prognosis for the maxillary molar region. A loss of attachment of 5 mm interproximally encounters the furcations, introduces deplaquing limitations, and portends continued bone loss. Periodontal regeneration procedures in this area are more likely to be successful in the Class II furcation on the buccal surface, but success is very limited interproximally.[22] The predictability of regenerative periodontics for maxillary molar Class III furcations is poor, and the procedures should be avoided.

167

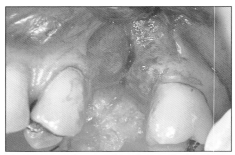

Fig 12-17a The maxillary first molar has been extracted after the failure of surgical endodontic treatment. There is a cleft in the edentulous ridge.

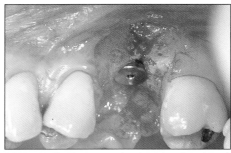

Fig 12-17b A 15-mm implant is placed and obscures most of the defect. Treatment consists of a bone graft and a Gore-Tex barrier membrane.

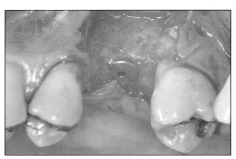

Fig 12-17c Six months later, at second-stage surgery, there is no evidence of the former bone defect.

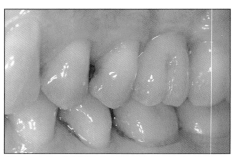

Fig 12-17d The final crown is in place. (Prosthetics by Dr Janice Conrad.)

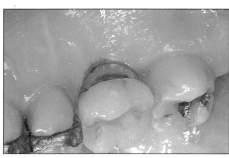

Fig 12-17e Palatal view of the final restora-

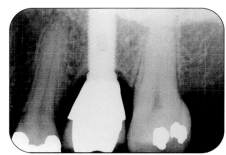

Fig 12-17f Posttreatment radiograph. There is sufficient bone to place a 15 mm implant and support the restoration.

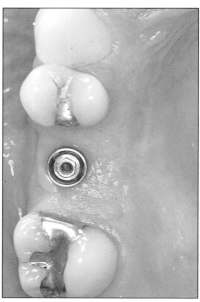

Fig 12-18a A single implant is used to replace a maxillary first molar. There is no clinical evidence of inflammation.

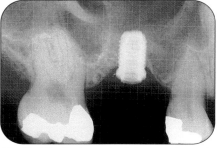

Fig 12-18b Radiograph of the area shown in Fig 12-18a. The selection of a short implant to replace a maxillary molar is a poor decision. Occlusal forces can dislodge the implant even in the absence of inflammation.

The ultimate goal is to attenuate the loss of bone because there is a precious small amount available in the nondiseased dentition of most patients in the maxillary molar region. It is realistic to supply one or more molar teeth with implants for the individual with a large alveolar process and a high sinus cavity (Figs 12-17a to 12-17e), but it is foolish to replace a missing first molar with a single short implant (Figs 12-18a to 12-18e). A traditional fixed partial denture should not be overlooked as an alternative for replacement of missing maxillary posterior teeth, as it has a favorable track record.

The quantity of bone can be altered by a sinus elevation procedure or by the use of an implant in the posterior maxilla where it fuses with the pterygoid and palatine bones (see Chapters 13 and 14). These procedures require considerable surgical experience and should be considered on a basis of need, because many patients will be agreeable to a premolar occlusion. Shorter implants with a larger diameter have been proposed and have evidenced some clinical success, but there is no long-term report to support their efficacious use in this region.[23]

Conclusion

There is a gap between the rapid development of guided bone regeneration procedures and patients' acceptance of them (see Chapters 5 to 8). This is a reflection of patients' concerns about the length of proposed treatment time, the financial expenditure involved, and fear of morbidity. Such concerns can result in the use of alternative-sized implants or alternative nonimplant treatment plans, because there is no dictum that every missing tooth will be replaced, let alone with an implant. Treatment of this area of the dentition frequently requires a maximum of ingenuity to reach a successful conclusion.

References

1. Bahat O. Treatment planning and placement of implants in the posterior maxillae: Report of 732 consecutive Nobelpharma implants. Int J Oral Maxillofac Implants 1993;8:151–161.

2. Nevins M, Langer B. The successful application of osseointegrated implants to the posterior jaw: A long-term retrospective study. Int J Oral Maxillofac Implants 1993;8:428–432.

3. Jemt T, Lekholm U. Oral implant treatment in posterior partially edentulous jaws: A 5-year follow-up report. Int J Oral Maxillofac Implants 1993;8:635–640.

4. Wisham MS, Bahat O, Kramer M. Computed tomography as an adjunct in dental implant surgery. Int J Periodont Rest Dent 1988; 8:31–47.

5. Mecall RA, Rosenfeld AL. Barium-coated surgical stents and computer assisted tomography in the preoperative assessment of dental implant patients. Int J Periodont Rest Dent 1991;12:53–62.

6. Borrow JW, Smith JP. Stent marker materials for computerized tomography–assisted implant planning. Int J Periodont Rest Dent 1996; 16:61–68.

7. Strub JR, Linter H, Marinello CP. Rehabilitation of partially edentulous patients using cantilever bridges: A retrospective study. Int J Periodont Rest Dent 1989;9:365–376.

8. Mellonig JT, Nevins M. Guided bone regeneration of bone defects associated with implants: An evidence-based outcome assessment. Int J Periodont Rest Dent 1995;15:168–185.

9. Nevins M, Mellonig JT, Clem DS, Reiser GM, Buser DA. Implants in regenerated bone: Long-term survival. Int J Periodont Rest Dent 1998;18:35–45.

10. Joseph I, Varna BRR, Bhat KM. Clinical significance of furcation anatomy of the maxillary first premolar: A biometric study on extracted teeth. J Periodontol 1996;67:386–389.

11. Papanou PN, Wennström JL. The angular bony defect as an indicator of further alveolar bone loss. J Clin Periodontol 1991;18:317–322.

12. Dragoo MR, Sullivan HC. A clinical and histological evaluation of autogenous iliac bone grafts in humans. Part I. Wound healing two to eight months. J Periodontol 1973;44:614.

13. Nyman S, Lindhe J, Karring T, Rylander H. New attachment following surgical treatment of human periodontal disease. J Clin Periodontol 1982;9:290–296.

14. Gottlöw J, Nyman S, Lindhe J, Karring T, Wennström J. New attachment formation in the human periodontium by guided tissue regeneration: Case reports. J Clin Periodontol 1986;13:604.

15. Schallhorn RG, McClain PK. Combined osseous composite grafting, root conditioning, and guided tissue regeneration. Int J Periodont Rest Dent 1988;8:9–31.

16. Bowers GM, Chadroff B, Cerveale R, Mellonig JT, Corio R, Emerson J, et al. Histologic evaluation of new attachment apparatus formation in humans. Part III. J Periodontol 1989;60:683–693.

17. McClain PK, Schallhorn RG. Long-term assessment of combined osseous composite grafting, root conditioning, and guided tissue regeneration. Int J Periodont Rest Dent 1993;13:9–27.

18. Simion M, Baldoni M, Zaffe D. Jawbone enlargement using immediate implant placement associated with a split-crest technique and guided tissue regeneration. Int J Periodont Rest Dent 1992; 12:463–473.

19. Scipioni A, Bruschi GB, Calesini G. The edentulous ridge expansion technique: A 5-year study. Int J Periodont Rest Dent 1994; 14:451–459.

20. Buser D, Dula K, Belser U, Hirt H-P, Berthold H. Localized ridge augmentation using guided bone regeneration. II. Surgical procedure in the mandible. Int J Periodont Rest Dent 1995;15:11–30.

21. Jovanovic SA, Nevins M. Bone formation utilizing titanium-reinforced barrier membranes. Int J Periodont Rest Dent 1995;15:57–70.

22. Pontoriero R, Lindhe J. Guided tissue regeneration in the treatment of degree II furcations in maxillary molars. J Clin Periodontol 1995; 22:756–763.

23. Langer B, Langer L, Herrman I, Jorneus L. The wide fixture: A solution for special bone situations and a rescue for the compromised implant. Part I. Int J Oral Maxillofac Implants 1993;8:400–408.

The Maxillary Sinus Floor Augmentation Procedure to Support Implant Prostheses

Myron Nevins, DDS
Joseph P. Fiorellini, DMD, DMSc

The maxillary posterior quadrant offers special challenges to the successful use of implant prostheses to restore dental function. The volume of alveolar process that is present in a healthy periodontium is limited, as observed in anterior-posterior, three-dimensional sagittal radiographs (Figs 13-1a to 13-1c). A periodontally compromised patient shows a continued deterioration, and the resultant edentulous quadrant presents with a paucity of alveolar bone and an increased maxillary sinus pneumatization (Figs 13-2a to 13-2c). The solution offered to counter this clinical problem and place dental implants is the raising and augmentation of the maxillary sinus floor, referred to as a *sinus floor augmentation*. This procedure was first described by Geiger and Pesh[1] and Tatum,[2] and the use of autogenous marrow from the iliac crest was introduced by Boyne and James.[3] Brånemark et al[4] reported a survival rate of 70% over a period of 10 years for implants in the grafted maxillary sinus. When successful, the procedure produces a meaningful quantity of bone to allow placement of implants and provide support for an implant prosthesis (Figs 13-3a to 13-3d).

The techniques utilized for this procedure are recent, and there is little offered as evidence to the long-term fate of the implants or the prostheses supported by them. On the other hand, the successful use of these procedures is gaining credibility based on the increasing numbers of respected clinicians observing and reporting results.[5–12]

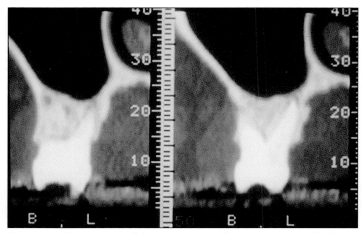

Fig 13-1a The anatomy of the posterior maxilla varies among individuals. In these cross-sectional CT scans of the first molar, the apices of the mesiobuccal and palatal roots are in contact with the inferior border of the sinus. The interradicular area is filled with bone; however, the buccal plates are thin. Anatomic cross sections also reveal the relationship of the sinus floor and roots. With the loss of posterior teeth in this situation, the bone available for implants below the sinus would be minimal.

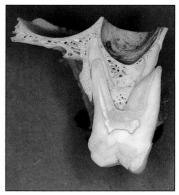

Fig 13-1b Sagittal section through the furcation of a cadaver molar. There is minimal bone available for implant placement before invasion by inflammatory periodontal disease.

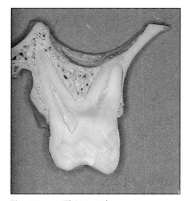

Fig 13-1c This tooth presents even less bone than the tooth in Fig 13-1b.

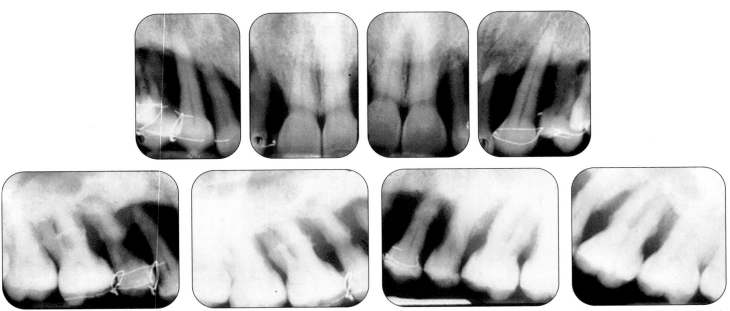

Fig 13-2a Maxillary radiographic survey. As periodontal disease resorbs bone in the posterior maxilla, the bone available for implant insertion is reduced. The loss of interradicular bone not only compromises the prognosis of the dentition but also complicates implant therapy because of the effect on the crown-root ratio.

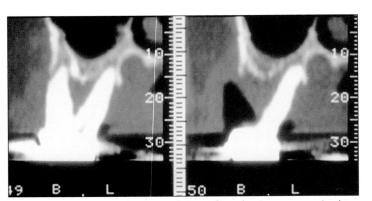

Fig 13-2b The periapical radiograph is confirmed using computerized to-mography.

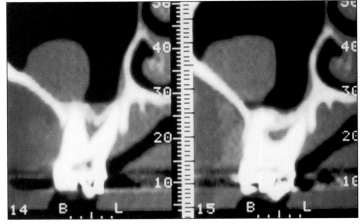

Fig 13-2c These sagittal CT scans reveal that there is insufficient bone for implants unless a sinus floor augmentation procedure is performed. Note the well-defined radiopacity that must be diagnosed before treatment.

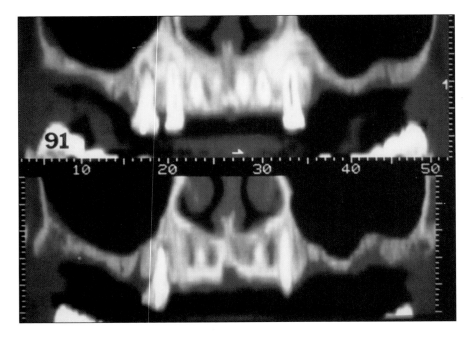

Fig 13-3a The panoramic CT view indicates an absence of bone height in the posterior maxilla (1991). The posterior teeth are missing, and a bilateral implant prosthesis depends on a successful sinus elevation procedure.

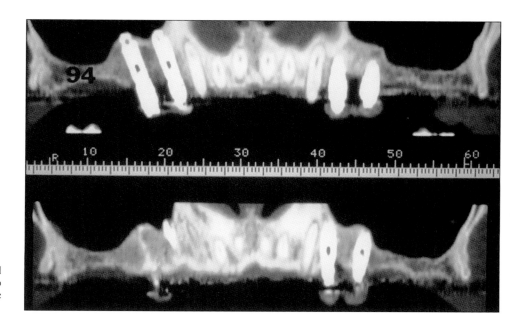

Fig 13-3b The implant prosthesis was removed to provide clarity in the CT scan (1994). Two implants were placed bilaterally 1 year after the sinus floor augmentation procedure.

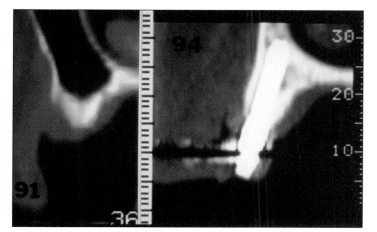

Fig 13-3c Maxillary left sagittal cut before *(left)* and after *(right)* bone regeneration and implant placement.

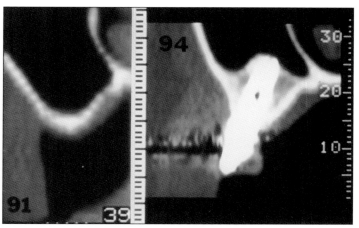

Fig 13-3d Maxillary left sagittal cut before *(left)* and after *(right)* bone regeneration and implant placement.

Contraindications

The sinus floor augmentation procedure is contraindicated:

1. For patients with excessive interarch distance (Figs 13-4a and 13-4b).
2. For patients with sinus pathoses.
3. In the presence of root tips in the sinus.
4. For patients with acute sinusitis.
5. For smokers.
6. For a variety of systemically compromised patients.

Careful radiographic analysis will indicate the proposed crown-root ratio of a prosthesis that will be supported by implants that have been placed in regenerated bone after the floor of the maxillary sinus has been elevated. The size of the proposed implant is easily calculated, and then the distance from the most occlusal bone to the occlusal plane is measured (Figs 13-4a and 13-4b). Although efforts are made to onlay meaningful vertical heights of bone, it is unlikely that there will be a remarkable change. The crown-root ratio may be overwhelming in some cases of advanced bone loss and is calculated at no better than a 2:1 ratio. This, in addition to the fact that the implants are placed almost totally in reconstructed bone, and in close proximity to the occlusal force of the temporomandibular joint, may preclude the procedure.

Because smoking has been implicated as a factor that worsens the prognosis of both periodontal and dental implant procedures,[13,14] there is every reason to request that the patient enroll in a smoking cessation program before proceeding.

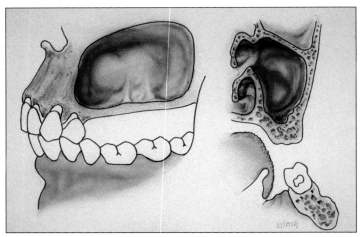

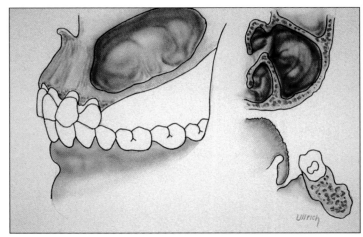

Fig 13-4a The anatomic considerations for sinus augmentation will contribute to the prognosis of the case. When the bone resorption in the posterior maxilla has been minimal and/or the sinus has expanded inferiorly, the implants placed in the grafted site will have an acceptable crown-root ratio.

Fig 13-4b Once there has been extensive bone resorption, the implant will be inserted more superiorly, resulting in an unfavorable crown-root ratio. It may negate the use of implant dentistry.

Anatomy of the Maxillary Sinus

The maxillary sinus is found within the maxilla, overlies the alveolar process and the roots of the maxillary teeth, particularly the molars, and is the largest paranasal sinus.[15] It is not unusual for its mesial extension to extend anteriorly to the canine or first premolar area, but there will usually be more alveolar process in this region. The delicate floor of the maxillary sinus covers the roots of the teeth and is itself covered by a periosteum that is inseparable from the respiratory epithelium on the sinus surface. The combined lining is commonly referred to as the schneiderian membrane.

The sinus extends about 3.0 cm anteriorly-posteriorly and is about 2.5 cm wide and 3.5 cm high in the molar region. The anatomic drainage of a healthy sinus is found high on the medial wall and is far removed from procedures aimed at extending the floor of the sinus to place dental implants. This may be more of a concern with a very flat sinus.

Treatment Options

There currently are two treatment options available for this procedure, and the selection is based on the volume of residual alveolar ridge. In the simultaneous procedure, the implants are placed and the sinus floor is elevated at the same visit. It is mandatory for an implant to be rigid at the time of placement, and this requires a minimum of 5 mm of bone.[10,16] The advantages of this approach are measured in a reduced number of surgical treatments, a reduced treatment time, and a reduced financial commitment. It is necessary to use radiographic interpretations because it is impossible to measure the degree of linear osseointegration on the implant surface.

The alternative is staged surgeries, the first to develop bone in the sinus and the second to place implants.[17,18] This offers the surgeon the clinical advantages of drilling and knowingly placing the implant into bone, and achieving a

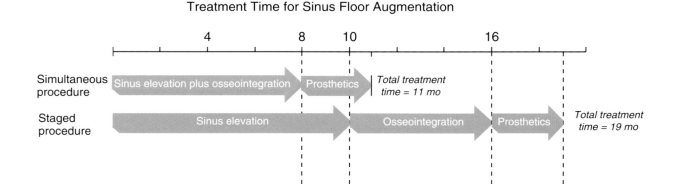

174

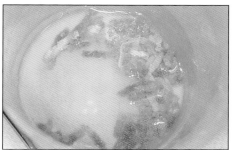

Fig 13-5a The grafting materials for sinus elevations vary; however, autogenous bone harvested from the iliac crest is preferred. Multiple cores from a trephine are defrosted at the time of surgery.

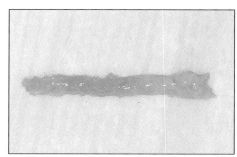

Fig 13-5b One core before it is crushed.

contact area of bone and titanium. If the quality or quantity of bone is insufficient, the procedure can be attenuated. The disadvantage is that the result of the bone-development surgery should not be tested for 9 to 12 months, and then another 6 months must be invested in the osseointegration process. Including prosthesis construction, the treatment time easily can approach 2 years, and this requires an understanding patient and treatment team.

Graft Materials

The reconstruction of the sinus floor occurs in an area that is not naturally bone forming. Graft materials proposed for this procedure include autogenous blocks of bone anchored in place by the implant fixture and particulate bone. The block procedure is described in Chapter 15.

At present, there are four categories of materials used to augment the bone that forms on the floor of the maxillary sinus. Case reports suggest success with intraoral and extraoral autografts, allografts, xenografts, and alloplasts, as well as combinations.[1–12,16–21] In this chapter, the use of freeze-dried human allograft, iliac crest autograft, and Bio-Oss (Osteohealth), a xenograft, will be discussed. Recent research success using recombinant human bone morphogenetic protein–2 in the animal model and humans will also be reported.

Each patient is first offered the possibility of using bone harvested from the posterior iliac crest with a trephine. This method obviates the need for an open reduction procedure and hospitalization, but most patients still prefer to avoid it for reasons of perceived morbidity and finance. It is most comfortably performed with a short-acting general anesthesia because the exit size with the captured bone core is wider than the entry size of the trephine. There is no need for hospitalization, and the patient is released after an obligatory stay related to anesthesia. The cores are immediately frozen in sterile saline or the patient's own blood, and not thawed until some days later, at the time of surgery.

It is reasonable to assume that multiple cores will be harvested from a single entry site and that enough bone will be available for the procedure (Figs 13-5a and 13-5b). They are easily reduced to small pieces. This appears to be the most osteogenic graft material available for collecting desired elements for bone induction (Figs 13-5c to 13-5i). It eliminates any discussion of disease transfer and must be more osteogenic than any allograft, alloplast, or xenograft. There is no concern of root resorption because there is no contact with natural teeth.[22]

For the sizable patient population that prefers to seek another approach, mineralized freeze-dried allogenic bone has proven to be efficacious[10] and appears to outperform demineralized bone for this particular procedure, although there are reports of success with both.[21] It is hydrolyzed with sterile saline, and a small amount of tetracycline is added empirically.

The particulate graft procedure requires the compartmentalized healing that is offered by an intact sinus membrane.[17] When the membrane is torn, the grafting material scatters in the sinus and the result is usually disappointing. Efforts to suture a torn membrane are unsuccessful, but small perforations can be blocked with strips of collagen.

Recent studies show less encouraging data with the use of Bio-Oss, a bone derived xenograft (Fig 13-6).

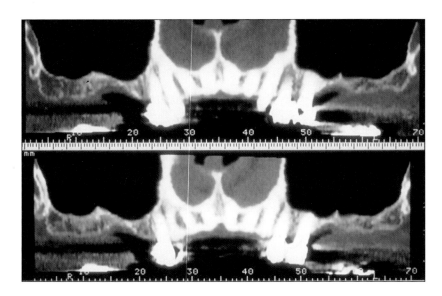

Fig 13-5c The panoramic CT view reveals the absence of sufficient bone to place maxillary posterior implants.

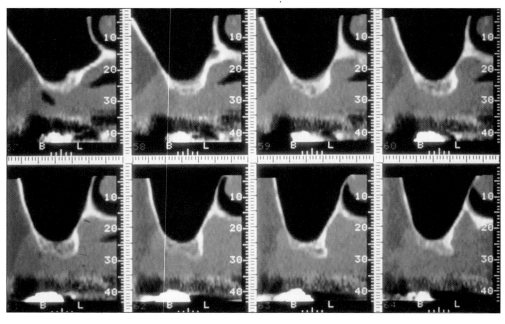

Fig 13-5d The maxillary sagittal CT sections substantiate the panoramic radiograph. There are no septae to interfere with the osteotomy.

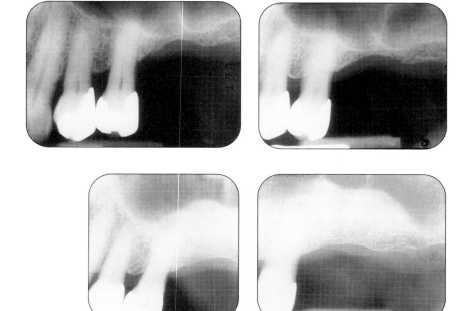

Fig 13-5e Periapical radiographs taken before the sinus elevation.

Fig 13-5f Periapical radiographs taken after the sinus elevation show that there is ample bone formation to place dental implants.

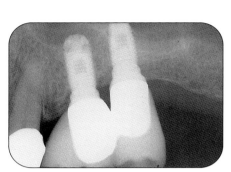
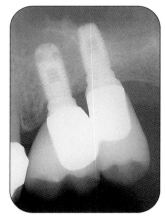

Fig 13-5g Implants have been placed and loaded.

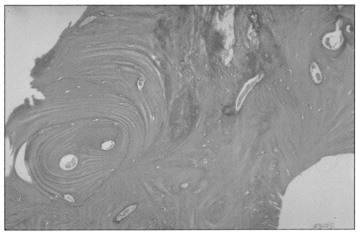

Fig 13-5h The histologic review of a core 1 year after a sinus floor elevation using a combination of iliac crest trephined cores and mineralized freeze-dried bone.

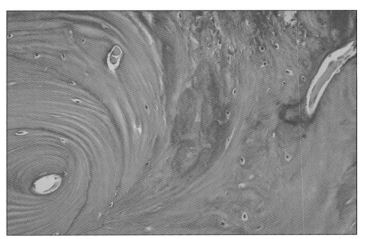

Fig 13-5i An enlarged view demonstrating dense vital bone surrounding a small particle of graft material.

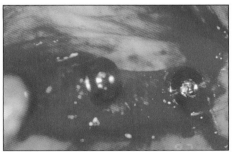

Fig 13-6b The osteotomy window is covered with Bio-Gide (Osteohealth), a slowly resorbing bilayer collagen membrane.

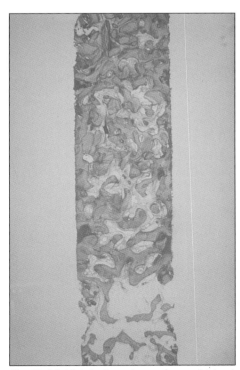

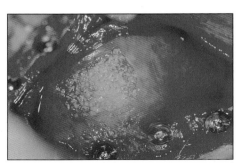

Fig 13-6a The medial and posterior aspects of the sinus are filled with Bio-Oss, and root form implants are placed. Additional Bio-Oss is then packed to fill the remainder of the sinus to a level even with the surrounding bone.

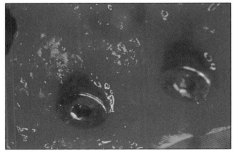

Fig 13-6c Nine-month re-entry of the original osteotomy site demonstrating complete closure of the original osteotomy window. Core biopsies were obtained for histologic analysis.

Fig 13-6d Histologic analyses of core obtained from the sinus floor graft using Bio-Oss demonstrated good bone formation on the surface of the graft particles. (Clinical case by Dr Vince Iacono; histology by Robert Schenk.)

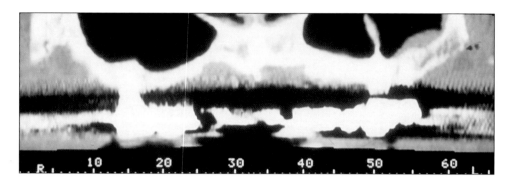

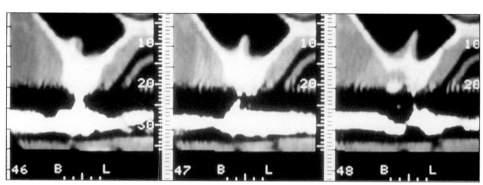

Fig 13-7a The maxillary sinus may contain bony septa that require presurgical diagnosis to plan the osteotomy. The panoramic view of the CT scan will indicate the position of the septa that are in the lateral-medial direction.

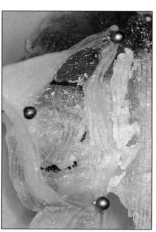

Fig 13-7b The cross sections will indicate the position and height of septa that are in the anterior-posterior direction. At times the septa may not traverse the sinus perpendicular to the buccal wall and may be several millimeters in thickness.

Fig 13-7c An acrylic resin model reformatted from the computerized tomography demonstrates the inferior surface of the sinus with two horizontal struts identified by black pencil .

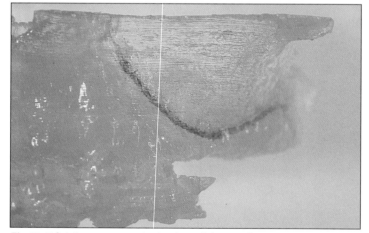

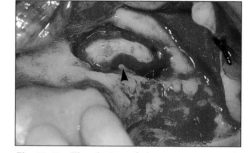

Fig 13-7d It is easy to see the borders of the maxillary sinus in this model constructed from the CT scan. This implements the presurgical treatment plan.

Fig 13-7e The design of the osteotomy is altered to account for a septum in the sinus *(arrow)*.

Sinus Elevation Procedure

Presurgical Planning

The presence of septa that totally or partially compartmentalize the sinus can be detected radiographically, but computerized tomography (CT) allows the surgeon to plan the osteotomy (Figs 13-7a to 13-7e). When possible, it helps to select one chamber to work in and to avoid the sharp angles of the spiny septa, because the elevation of the schneiderian membrane from these spines is precarious and likely to lead to perforations. This procedure is best performed with diagnostic procedures of the highest magnitude. The CT scan can be complemented with a three-dimensional replicate resin model constructed from a magneto-optical disk. Bone structures of interest are thresholded in each slice until the physical resin model is fabricated.[23]

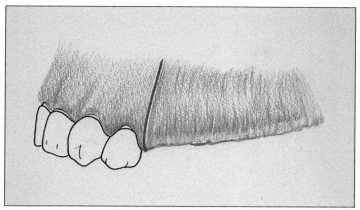

Fig 13-8a A deep vertical incision is connected to a horizontal incision palatal to the crest of the edentulous ridge.

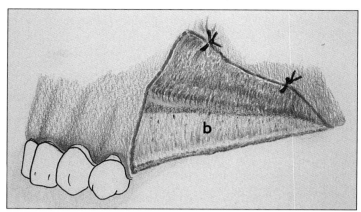

Fig 13-8b The full-thickness flap is reflected, exposing the buccal wall of bone (b).

Staged Approach

The technique of the two-stage procedure will be described and then amended to include the single-stage procedure (Figs 13-8a to 13-8q). Local anesthesia, lidocaine, is administered into the buccal vestibule and the palatal vault; no attempt is made to sedate the patient beyond oral medication unless there is an obvious anxiety problem.

A beveled incision is extended from the maxillary tuberosity to the distal surface of the most distal tooth or the canine area, so as to be anterior to the sinus (Fig 13-8a). This incision is slightly palatal to the crest of the soft tissue ridge and is connected to a vertical incision that extends deep into the buccal mucosa. When the premolars are present, the flap will be extended anteriorly to include these teeth, so as to provide a minimum of 8 mm between the soft tissue vertical incision and the anterior bone incision of the osteotomy. This provides soft tissue closure over a bed of bone with little or no chance of exposure of the underlying bone graft or the barrier membrane.

The flap is reflected with blunt dissection and tied back with two sutures to the buccal mucosa (Fig 13-8b). The outer wall of the remaining alveolar process and the maxillary sinus now are visible. Transillumination applied beneath the palatal soft tissues or directly to the bone surface of the ridge frequently will identify the demarcation of the residual alveolar process and the sinus and establish the location of the inferior bone incision 2 or 3 mm superior to it. This will allow horizontal access to the membrane on the sinus floor after the osteotomy is performed, and obviate the need to instrument it in a vertical direction (Figs 13-8c and 13-8d). Radiographic interpretation supplements this information and helps identify the anterior extent of the sinus and thus, the location of the anterior bone incision just distal to it (Figs 13-8e and 13-8f). The superior and distal bone incisions are placed and connected so as to offer the correct size of the proposed augmentation (Figs 13-8c and 13-8d). Both of these borders are limited by access and

must be made at levels where adequate retraction can provide easy visibility and access.

The ostectomy described above must not damage the lining membrane of the sinus. This can be recognized as a gray line that appears as the bone is gently removed with a diamond bur (Figs 13-8c and 13-8d). It is wise to stop periodically and test the membrane to identify those sites that are soft and require no further osteotomy. The window is also tested to see if it moves and is free.

The sinus membrane is then gently separated from the floor of the sinus and the surrounding walls, and the bone attached to it will form the roof of the compartment of bone development (Figs 13-8c and 13-8g). If there is a measurable tear in the membrane, the procedure is stopped and resumed in the future. After the membrane is disengaged from the osseous walls, it will pulsate with patient respiration (Figs 13-8g to 13-8i). This does not occur when there is a large hole in the membrane and is a good clinical test of membrane continuity. A small tear in the membrane can be managed by using a resorbable material such as a barrier membrane. If the membrane is intact, the compartment that has been created is filled with the bone graft to the bone surface to recreate the original wall of bone (Fig 13-8i), and then covered with a Gore-Tex Augmentation Membrane (WL Gore, Flagstaff, AZ) (Fig 13-8j). The flap is sutured in place with Gore-Tex suture material (Fig 13-8k).

The patient is prescribed an antibiotic regimen of 2 g per day for 10 days. Chlorhexidine rinses are used to cleanse the incision during healing, and decongestants are prescribed to minimize sneezing. The maxillary sinus is monitored periodically with radiographs for a minimum of at least 8 months before the placement of implants. The osteotomy site is routinely completely reconstructed when a barrier membrane is used and the membrane is removed at the time of implant placement (Figs 13-8l to 13-8m). Prosthetic loading is performed after second-stage abutment connection surgery (Figs 13-8n to 13-8p).

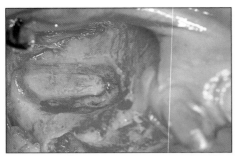

Fig 13-8c The osteotomy is prepared with a No. 6 round diamond. The inferior bone incision should allow horizontal deflection of the membrane, and the mesial bone incision should require minimal mesial instrumentation. A gray hollow develops as the membrane is approached.

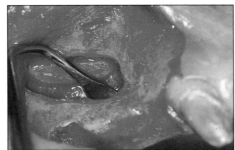

Fig 13-8d A spoon elevator is used to separate the intact membrane from the sinus floor; there is no need for vertical reflection. Note the distance between the soft and hard tissue vertical incisions. This provides insurance that neither the bone graft nor the barrier membrane will become exposed. The osseous window is reflected medially and superiorly. The bone of the window becomes the new floor of the sinus.

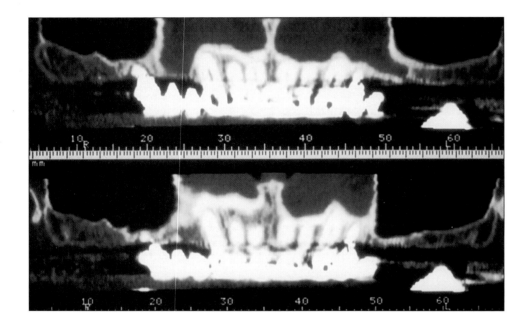

Fig 13-8e Panoramic CT view. Note the clear sinuses with no apparent septa.

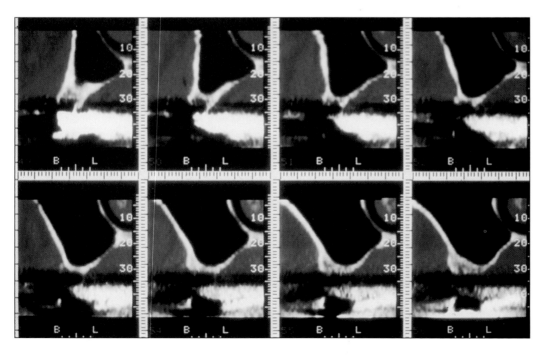

Fig 13-8f Sagittal CT cuts of the maxillary sinus.

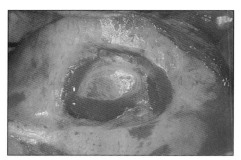

Fig 13-8g The osteotomy is complete and the membrane is intact.

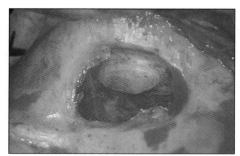

Fig 13-8h The membrane elevates and pulsates with respiration when it is intact.

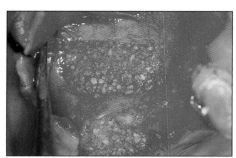

Fig 13-8i The bone graft is extended to the osteotomy borders.

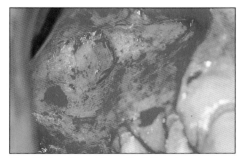

Fig 13-8j A Gore-Tex Augmentation Membrane is placed to cover the bone graft.

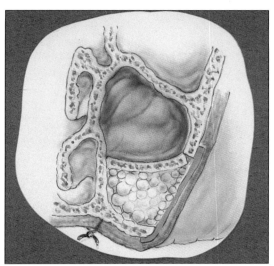

Fig 13-8k The palatal flap is sutured over the assembly of bone graft and membrane.

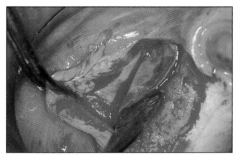

Fig 13-8l The surgical site is revisited for placement of implants after 10 months. The barrier membrane is removed.

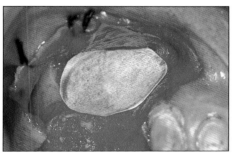

Fig 13-8m The side wall of the sinus is completely reconstructed.

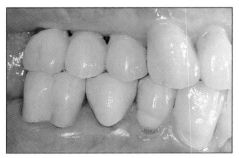

Fig 13-8n The final prosthesis is in place, and the implants shown in Fig 13-8p are now loaded.

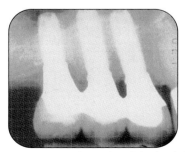
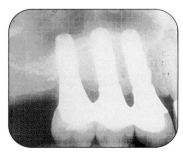
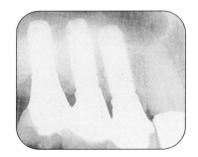

Fig 13-8o Radiographs of the loaded implants (right side).

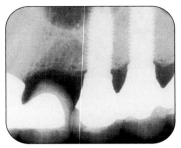
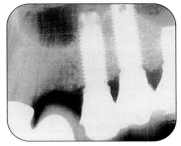
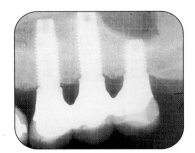

Fig 13-8p Radiographs of the loaded implants (left side).

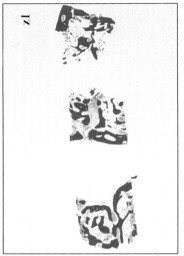
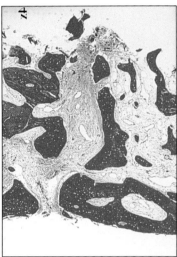
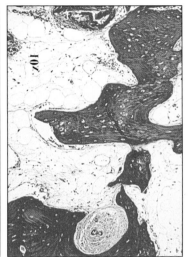
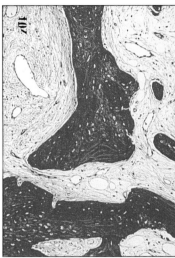

Fig 13-8q Bone core harvested from the maxillary sinus with a trephine at the time of implant delivery. Mineralized freeze-dried bone allograft was used for this sinus elevation. Note the presence of vital bone; there is little or no bone allograft remaining.

Simultaneous Approach

If there is more than 5 mm of residual alveolar process, implants can be placed at the time of the osteotomy and before or after the bone graft is applied[10] (Fig 13-9a). The soft tissue incision must be located considerably palatal and mesial to the osteotomy. The osteotomy is identical to that used for the staged procedure, and the sinus membrane's integrity must be preserved.

Some bone graft material is placed toward the medial and anterior walls of the compartment before the implant is inserted, to ensure that there will be no voids. An implant is selected that will extend to and support the remaining bone of the window that serves as the roof of the compartment (Fig 13-9b). The bone graft then is completed and covered with a Gore-Tex Augmentation Membrane (Fig 13-9c). Minimal countersinking is used for this procedure, because the remaining cortical bone is necessary to stabilize the fixture.[10]

At the abutment connection surgical procedure, there is routinely no sign of the original osteotomy when the barrier membrane is removed (Fig 13-9d). The results are evident with conventional periapical radiographs (Figs 13-9e, 13-10a, and 13-10b). This procedure is performed in the dental office under sterile conditions.

Planned Approach

A third treatment option is referred to as the *planned approach*. To increase the alveolar height, the floor of the maxillary sinus is grafted before the extraction of the hopeless teeth. This procedure was developed for a discerning patient who wanted to reduce the time spent without a fixed posterior prosthesis (Figs 13-11a and 13-11b). The surgical flap is elevated from the gingival sulcus with a mesial vertical incision extending deep into the buccal mucosa, because the procedure is only indicated if there is significant bone loss and a very limited prognosis for the natural teeth. The inferior bone incision of the osteotomy must be apical to the tooth apices, and considerable care needs to be exercised to avoid tearing the membrane as it is separated from the root convexities. The mesial extent of the osteotomy is extended either to the mesial wall of the sinus or to the site designated for bone growth. It is recommended that there be a waiting period of 1 year before the teeth are removed. Another 3 months should be allowed for healing before the implants are placed. The routine schedule of osseointegration is then followed.

This procedure requires careful judgment regarding the proposed crown-root ratio and the occlusal stress that will be placed on the prosthesis. It is intended for individuals

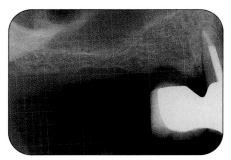

Fig 13-9a The single-stage, or simultaneous, sinus elevation procedure requires 5 mm of preexisting bone.

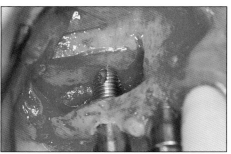

Fig 13-9b The size of the implant is established after the osteotomy is completed, the membrane is reflected, and the drill sites are prepared.

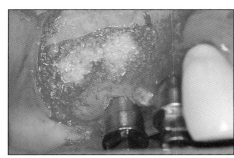

Fig 13-9c The bone graft is placed to fill the compartment. Bone is packed toward the anterior and medial walls before the implants are delivered.

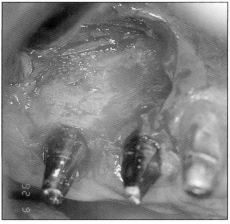

Fig 13-9d At second-stage surgery, there is no evidence of the window.

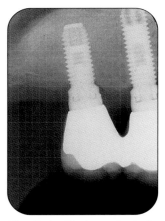

Fig 13-9e Final prosthesis in place.

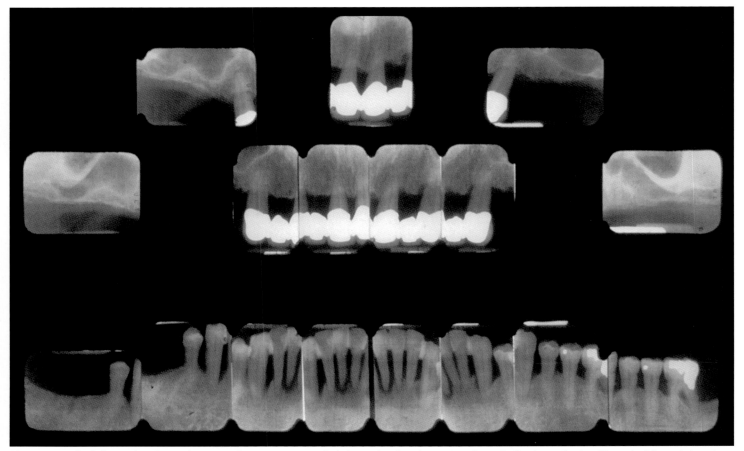

Fig 13-10a The full-mouth radiographic series demonstrates very little bone distal to the canine. A totally fixed prosthesis will require bilateral elevations of the sinus floor.

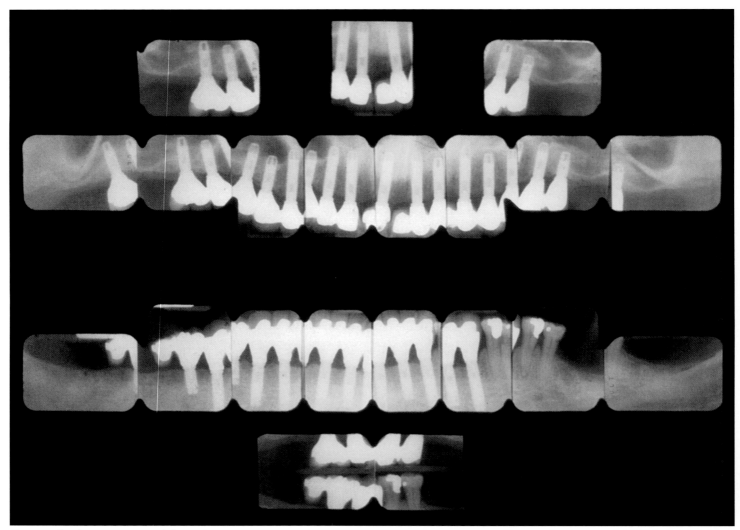

Fig 13-10b The posttreatment full-mouth radiographic series demonstrates the use of two additional implants in the premolar areas bilaterally. A total of eight implants easily support the prosthesis.

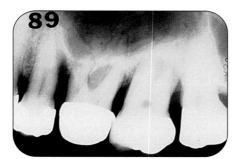

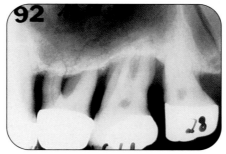

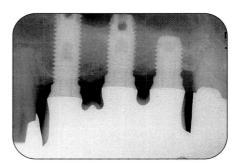

Fig 13-11a When the treatment plan of the posterior dentition takes into consideration that bone height below the sinus will be limited, a surgical procedure to augment the sinus can be done prior to extraction. This sequencing of the procedure will allow the patient to remain dentate during the sinus graft healing period of 1 year. As the teeth are extracted, the implants will then be placed in the remaining native bone and grafted bone.

Fig 13-11b Posttreatment radiograph of the three implants and the final prosthesis in place.

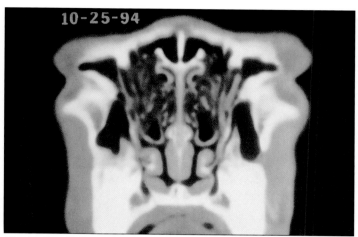

Fig 13-12a Eight-week CT scan showing increased radiopacity in the rhBMP-2/ACS–treated sinus *(right)* and an empty control sinus that collapsed to original size after resorption of the absorbable collagen sponge *(left)*.

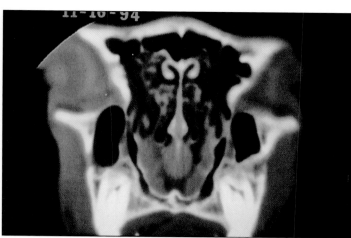

Fig 13-12b Twelve-week CT scan with rhBMP-2/ACS–treated sinus *(left)* and buffer/ACS–treated sinus *(right)*.

with an extreme loss of bone extending to the interradicular areas (furcations), where there is no possibility of recapturing the periodontium and it is necessary to consider future tooth replacement. The sinus floor augmentation procedure should result in bone formation, but it is necessary to compare the size of a proposed implant to the length of the crowns in the implant prosthesis. These implants, which are placed mostly in reconstructed bone, will be subjected to considerable force because they are close to the temporomandibular joint. It is similar to a nutcracker, where the greatest leverage is near the hinge. Extreme cases exceeding a crown-root ratio of 2:1 in dentitions of occlusal athletes (bruxers) should be reconsidered, and perhaps another treatment plan selected.

As mentioned previously, considerable periods of time should be allowed to pass for bone formation to occur before the implants are placed. There is some sentiment in favor of placing an interim prosthesis but little evidence that it is necessary. Every effort must be made to distribute the occlusal forces carefully and to avoid eccentric function completely.

Animal Studies

All autogenous and allograft bone graft materials that are thought to participate in osteoinduction contain some quantity of bone morphogenetic protein (BMP). More than 30 years ago, Urist[24] demonstrated that protein extracts from bone implanted into animals at nonbony sites are capable of inducing the local formation of new cartilage and bone. Since that time, at least nine BMPs have been cloned, and their osteogenic activities have been characterized.[25] The results of these experiments demonstrate that recombinant

human BMP-2 (rhBMP-2) has the ability to induce bone by targeting mesenchymal cells to differentiate into cartilage or bone-forming cells. It is found in minute quantities in human bone, and, before the recombinant form was available, it was necessary to purify 1 kg of bone to harvest 1 μg of crude BMP. The results of animal studies demonstrate that human rhBMP-2 has the ability to induce bone and repair bony defects at a variety of anatomic sites.[26–29]

The first maxillary sinus study assessed the efficacy, safety, and technical feasibility of inducing bone formation in an animal model of maxillary sinus floor augmentation using an absorbable collagen sponge (ACS) impregnated with rhBMP-2.[30] Bilateral antral maxillary sinus floor elevation procedures were performed in six adult female Alpine-Saanen goats. Bone formation in response to the implant was evaluated with sequential radiographs, computerized tomography, and gross pathologic and histologic analysis performed at necropsy. Sinuses implanted with rhBMP-2/ACS subsequently demonstrated increasing radiopacity local to the implant site, while the radiopacity of the negative control sinuses remained unchanged or decreased (Figs 13-12a and 13-12b). The results demonstrated the ability of an rhBMP-2/ACS implant to induce substantive new bone formation within the maxillary sinus of goats without adverse sequelae.

Histologic results observed at 4, 8, and 12 weeks substantiated the observations drawn from radiography and gross pathology (Fig 13-13). New trabecular bone covered by robust osteoblasts was observed at 4 to 8 weeks and demonstrated continuity (Figs 13-14a to 13-14e), whereas the control sinus was empty (Figs 13-14c and 13-14d). The 12-week results demonstrated the formation of concentric rings of a mature haversian system (Figs 13-15a and 13-15b). There were no significant immune responses or other adverse responses in these animals.

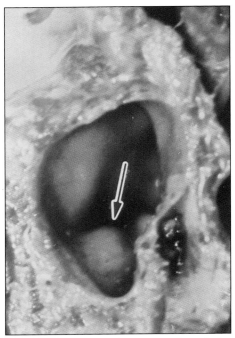

Fig 13-13 Twelve-week gross section of the right sinus treated with rhBMP-2/ACS *(arrow)*. (From Nevins et al.[29] Reprinted with permission.)

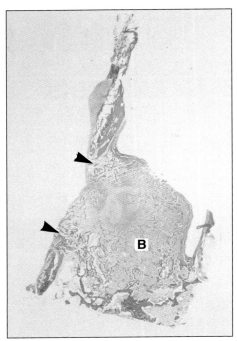

Fig 13-14a Section through the maxillary sinus treated with an rhBMP-2–impregnated implant and harvested at 4 weeks. Lateral edges of the osteotomy *(arrowheads)*; new trabecular bone (B). (Hematoxylin-eosin stain.) (From Nevins et al.[29] Reprinted with permission.)

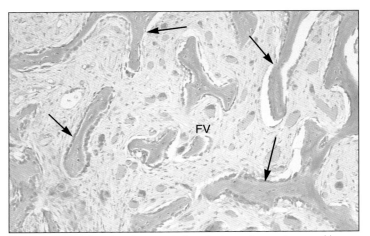

Fig 13-14b Section showing new trabecular bone *(arrows)* covered by active osteoblasts at 4 weeks. The new bone is embedded in fibrovascular tissue (FV). (Hematoxylin-eosin stain.) (From Nevins et al.[29] Reprinted with permission.)

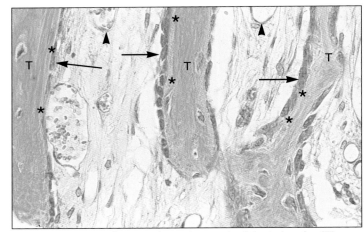

Fig 13-14c Increased power photomicrograph of the trabeculae (T) seen in Fig 13-13b. Cuboidal osteoblasts *(arrows)* rest on a layer of unmineralized osteoid (*). Blood vessels *(arrowheads)*. (Hematoxylin-eosin stain.) (From Nevins et al.[29] Reprinted with permission.)

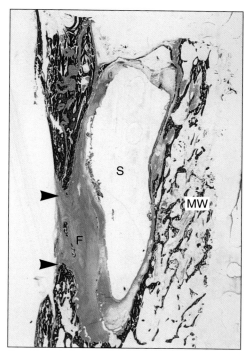

Fig 13-14d Section through the maxillary sinus treated with a buffer-impregnated implant and harvested at 8 weeks (control). Lateral edges of the osteotomy *(arrowheads)*. Fibrous tissue (F); sinus (S); medial wall of the sinus (MW). (Von Kossa stain.) (From Nevins et al.[29] Reprinted with permission.)

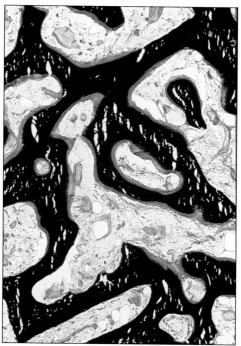

Fig 13-14e New trabecular bone at 8 weeks. (From Nevins et al.[29] Reprinted with permission.)

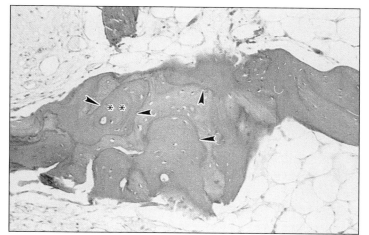

Fig 13-15a Section of a trabecula in fatty marrow at 12 weeks. Cement lines *(arrowheads)* separate bone deposited earlier (dark pink) from more recently deposited bone (light pink). Haversian system (*). (Hematoxylin-eosin stain.) (From Nevins et al.[29] Reprinted with permission.)

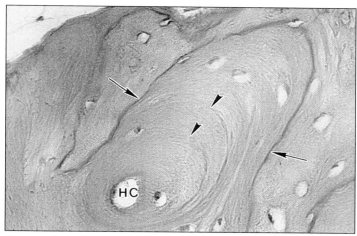

Fig 13-15b Higher-power magnification of the section shown in Fig 13-14a showing cement lines *(arrows)*, concentric rings of a haversian system *(arrowheads)*, and a haversian canal (HC). (Hematoxylin-eosin stain.) (From Nevins et al.[29] Reprinted with permission.)

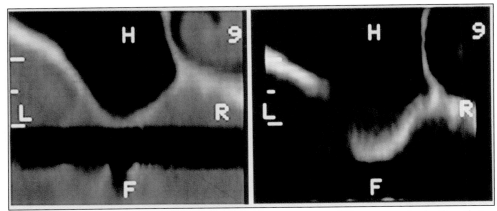

Fig 13-16a Comparison of the baseline and 16-week posttreatment CT scans reveals significantly increased radiopacity in the rhBMP-2/ACS–treated human sinus.

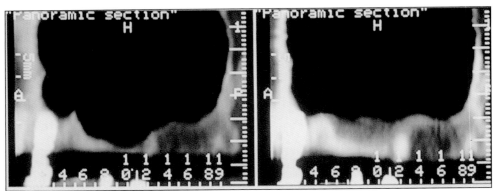

Fig 13-16b Comparison of the baseline and 16-week posttreatment panoramic CT views reveals significantly increased radiopacity in the rhBMP-2/ACS–treated human sinus.

Pilot Study in Humans

The next step was to treat patients with an edentulous posterior maxilla who presented with inadequate volume of bone to successfully support loaded dental implants. A four-center feasibility study was designed. In this study, rhBMP-2 was delivered on an absorbable collagen sponge to a total of 12 patients who required maxillary sinus floor augmentation.[29] CT scans were determined to be the best available method to obtain reproducible quantitative measurements. At 16 weeks, the CT scans for all 12 patients showed evidence of biologic activity, defined as an increase in radiodensity suggestive of mineralized tissue (Figs 13-16a to 13-16f).

Ten of the 12 patients formed enough bone to allow the placement of dental implants, and histologic specimens confirmed normal bone formation. The early trabeculation was continuous and covered by a cuboidal layer of osteoblasts on a surface of osteoid. Polarized light microscopy showed the woven bone converting to lamellar bone.

This pilot study resulted in plans to continue the investigation on a larger scale with an opportunity to vary the dosage (Fig 13-17). The availability of a product that can induce bone growth in a non–naturally occurring site portends exciting developments in the future. It would eliminate inconvenient, expensive secondary surgical sites for autogenous bone and provide a better product for bone induction that is readily available.

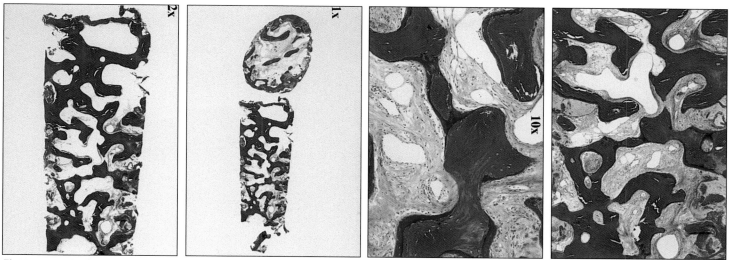

Fig 13-16c Histologic section of a bone core harvested from the maxillary sinus with a trephine at the time of implant placement. The new bone trabeculae (blue) are lined with a layer of osteoid (red). (Goldner's stain.)

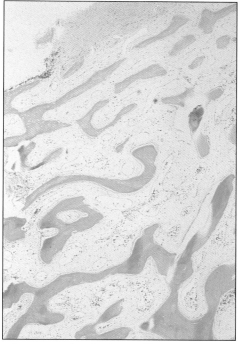

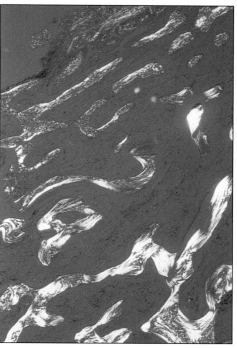

Fig 13-16d Section showing new trabecular bone. (Hematoxylin-eosin stain.)

Fig 13-16e Polarized light preparation to demonstrate maturation of the newly formed bone. The woven bone is being converted to lamellar bone.

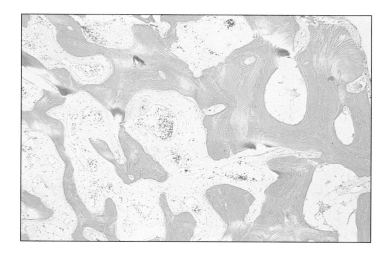

Fig 13-16f Increased power photomicrograph of the trabecular bone seen in Fig 13-16d. (Hematoxylin-eosin stain.)

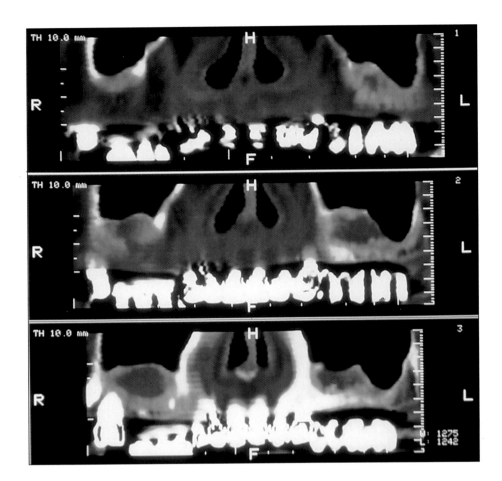

Fig 13-17a An 18-week postsurgical CT scan (panagraphic view, right side) demonstrates a marked increase in radiopacity in the maxillary sinus.

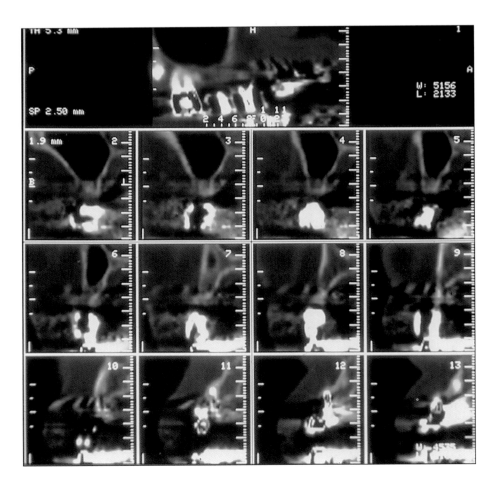

Fig 13-17b The presurgical CT scan. Note the paucity of bone to support dental implants.

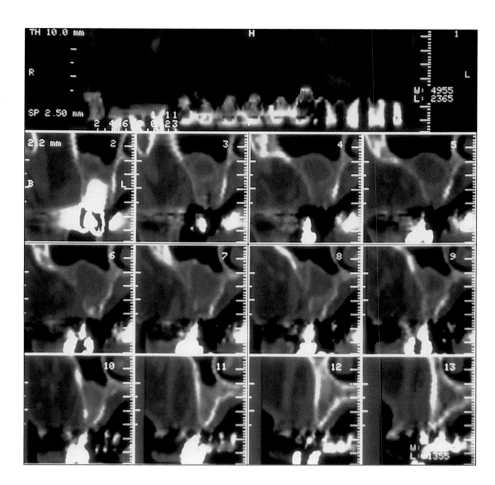

Fig 13-17c The 18-week postsurgical CT scan demonstrates a marked increase in radiopacity.

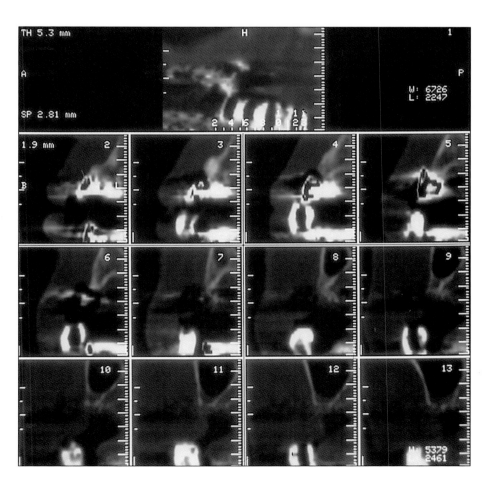

Fig 13-17d The presurgical CT scan reveals very little native bone to support dental implants.

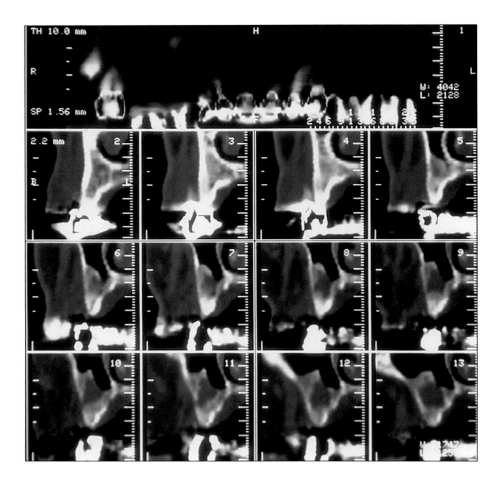

Fig 13-17e The postsurgical CT scan demonstrates a marked increase in radiopacity.

Alternative Treatments

Because many patients who present with edentulous maxillary posterior quadrants are not candidates for the maxillary sinus floor augmentation surgical procedure, but would prefer an implant prosthesis to a removable partial denture, it behooves the clinician to consider alternative treatments. Three-dimensional radiographs, tomography, or computerized tomography offer the opportunity to assay the existing volume of bone. One possibility is that the palatal plate of the maxilla extends further apically than it might appear on a conventional radiograph. This will allow a longer implant to be selected and offer greater resistance to occlusal loading (Fig 13-18). It is necessary to have the shoulder of the implant in a midcrestal position buccopalatally to ensure restorability.

Another alternative is to place a long implant distal to the sinus in the posterior maxilla or where the maxilla joins the sphenoid and the palatal bones. This approach can be united with a short, wide implant over the sinus to reduce the edentulous space and better distribute occlusal load. (Fig 13-19). This approach is particularly useful when the patient's physical history includes previous sinus surgery or a chronic unresolved sinusitis.

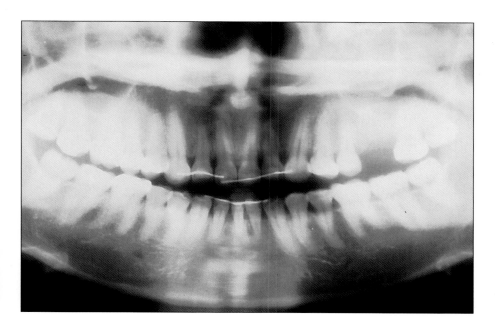

Fig 13-18a The maxillary left first molar is absent. The remaining bone appears insufficient to place an implant.

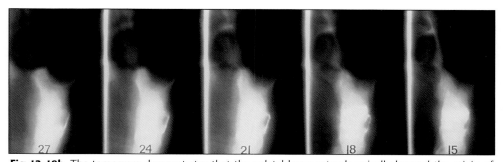

Fig 13-18b The tomogram demonstrates that the palatal bone extends apically beyond the origin of the sinus over the edentulous ridge.

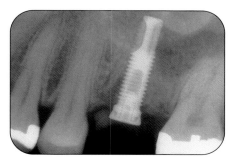

Fig 13-18c A 15-mm implant is placed using the palatal bone and bypassing the maxillary sinus.

Conclusion

The author has not encountered any serious sinus complications in patients who have undergone the sinus lift procedure, but there definitely has been a learning curve relative to success. Although the success rate is less than that reported for conventional implant procedures in the maxillary posterior region, a 90% fixture survival has been demonstrated, and no loaded implants have failed to date. This does not mean that sufficient bone formation always occurs as a result of the procedure; rather this figure should be interpreted as the success rate of implants that have been placed where significant bone formation did occur.

The use of an implant prosthesis supported by bone created on the floor of the sinus has proven to be an efficacious alternative for the replacement of missing maxillary posterior teeth in the partially edentulous patient. The sinus floor augmentation procedure should be performed by an individual with a well-developed surgical acumen. Short- and long-term reports are necessary for scientific analysis, but, for the moment, the procedure can be offered to patients with the appropriate caveats.

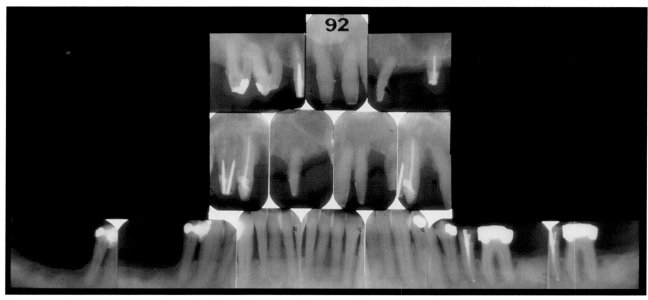

Fig 13-19a The pretreatment full-mouth radiographic survey. The maxilla has a paucity of bone bilaterally in the sinus area.

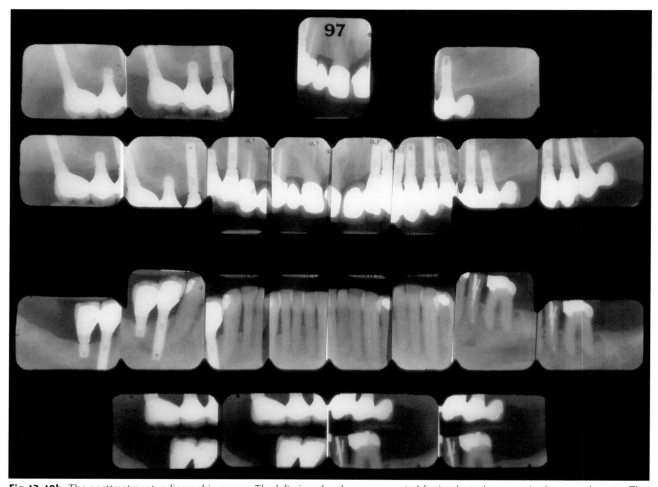

Fig 13-19b The posttreatment radiographic survey. The left sinus has been augmented for implant placement in the premolar area. The right sinus had been treated previously with a Caldwell-Luc procedure and continued to be an infectious problem. Therefore, one short implant was placed occlusal to the sinus, and a long implant was placed posterior to the sinus.

References

1. Geiger S, Pesh H. Animal and experimental studies of the healing around ceramic implants in bone lesions in the maxillary sinus region. Dtsch Zahnärtzl Z 1977;32:396.

2. Tatum H. Maxillary and sinus implant reconstruction. Dent Clin North Am 1986;30:207–229.

3. Boyne PJ, James R. Grafting of the maxillary floor with autogenous marrow and bone. J Oral Surg 1980;38:613–616.

4. Brånemark P-I, Adell R, Albrektsson T, et al. An experimental and clinical study of osseointegrated implants penetrating the nasal cavity and maxillary sinus. J Oral Maxillofac Surg 1984;42:497–505.

5. Small S, Zinner I, Panno F, Shapiro H, Stein J. Augmenting the maxillary sinus for implants: Report of 27 patients. J Oral Maxillofac Implants 1993;8:523–528.

6. Lozada J, Emanuelli S, James R, Boxkovic M, Linsted K. Root form implants placed in subantral grafted sited. J Calif Dent Assoc 1993;21:31–35.

7. Keller E, Eckert S, Tolman D. Maxillary antral and nasal one-stage inlay composite bone graft: Preliminary report on 30 recipient sites. J Oral Maxillofac Surg 1994;52:438–448.

8. Jensen J, Sindet-Pederson S, Oliver A. Varying treatment strategies for reconstruction of maxillary atrophy with implants: Results in 98 patients. J Oral Maxillofac Surg 1994;52:210–216.

9. Kent J, Block M. Simultaneous maxillary sinus floor bone grafting and placement of hydroxyapatite coated implants. J Oral Maxillofac Surg 1987;47:238–242.

10. Jensen OT, Greer R. Immediate placement of osseointegrated implants into the maxillary sinus augmented with mineralized cancellous allograft and Gore Tex: Second stage surgical and histologic findings. In: Laney WR, Tolman DE (eds). Tissue Integration in Oral, Orthopedic, and Maxillofacial Reconstruction. Chicago: Quintessence, 1992:320–333.

11. Daelemans P, Hermans M, Godet F, and Malevez D. Autologous bone graft to augment the maxillary sinus in conjunction with immediate endosseous implants: A retrospective study up to 5 years. Int J Periodont Rest Dent 1997;17:27–39.

12. Wallace SS, Froum SJ, Tarnow DP. Histologic evaluation of sinus elevation procedure: A clinical report. Int J Periodont Rest Dent 1996;16:47–51.

13. Bain C, Moy P. The association between the failure of dental implants in healthy and medically compromised patients. Int J Oral Maxillofac Implants 1993;8:609–615.

14. Gunsolley JC, Quinn SM, Tew J, Gooss CM, Brooks CM, and Schenkein HA. The effect of smoking on individuals with minimal periodontal destruction. J Periodontol 1998;69:165–170.

15. Snell R. Clinical Anatomy for Medical Students, ed 3. Boston: Little, Brown, 1986:853.

16. Kent JN, Block MS. Simultaneous maxillary sinus floor bone grafting and placement of hydroxyapatite-coated implants. J Oral Maxillofac Surg 1989;47:238–242.

17. Chanavez M. Maxillary sinus: Anatomy, physiology, surgery and bone grafting related to implantology: Eleven years of surgical experience (1979–1990). J Implantol 1990;16:199–209.

18. Tidwell JK, Blijdorp PA, Stoelinga PJW, Brouns JB, Hinderks F. Composite grafting of the maxillary sinus for placement of endosteal implants: A preliminary report of 48 patients. Int J Oral Maxillofac Surg 1992;21:204–209.

19. Smiler DG, Johnson PW, Lozada JL, Misch C, Rosenlicht JL, Tatum OH Jr, et al. Sinus lift grafts and endosseous implants: Treatment of the atrophic posterior maxilla. Dent Clin North Am 1992;36:151–188.

20. Raghoebar GM, Brouwer TJ, Reintsema H, Van Oort RP. Augmentation of the maxillary sinus floor with autogenous bone for the placement of endosseous implants: A preliminary report. J Oral Maxillofac Surg 1993;51:1198–1203.

21. Zinner ID, Small SA. Sinus lift graft using the maxillary sinuses to support implants. J Am Dent Assoc 1996;127:51–57.

22. Dragoo M, Sullivan H. A clinical and histological evaluation of autogenous iliac bone grafts in humans. Part I. Wound healing 2-8 months. J Periodontol 1973;44:599.

23. Bianci SD, Lojacono A, Nevins M, Ramieri G, Corrente G, Martuscelli G, Fiorellini J. The use of replicate resin models in the treatment of maxillary sinus augmentation patients. Int J Periodont Rest Dent 1997;17:349–357.

24. Urist MR. Bone: Formation by autoinduction. Science 1965;165:893–899.

25. Wozney JM. The bone morphogenetic protein family and osteogenesis. Mol Reprod Dev 1992;32:160–167.

26. Toriumi DM, Kotler HS, Luxenburg DP, Holtrop ME, Wang EA. Mandibular reconstruction with a recombinant bone-inducing factor. Arch Otolaryngol Head Neck Surg 1991;117:1101–1112.

27. Sigurdsson TJ, Lee MB, Kubota K, Turek TJ, Wozney JM, Wikesjö UME. Periodontal repair in dogs: Recombinant human bone morphogenic protein-2 significantly enhances periodontal regeneration. J Periodontol 1995;66:131–138.

28. Howell TH, Buser D, Fiorellini J, Stich H, Wozney J. Effect of bone morphogenetic protein on bone healing around endosseous implants: A pilot study in beagle dogs [abstract]. J Dent Res 1995;74:415.

29. Nevins M, Kirkerhead C, Nevins M, Wozney JA, Palmer R, Graham D. Bone formation in the goat maxillary sinus by absorbable collagen sponge implants impregnated with recombinant human bone morphogenic protein-2. Int J Periodont Rest Dent 1996;16:9–16.

30. Boyne PJ, Marx RE, Nevins M, Triplett RG, Lazaro E, Lilly LC, Alder M, Nummikoski P. A feasibility study evaluating rhBMP-2/absorbable collagen sponge for maxillary sinus floor augmentation. Int J Periodont Rest Dent 1997;17:11-25.

CHAPTER 14

Implant Use in the Tuberosity, Pterygoid, and Palatine Region: Anatomic and Surgical Considerations

Gary M. Reiser, DDS

The posterior maxilla frequently presents as a challenging site for implant placement. The poor bone quality characteristic of this region, coupled with limited vertical bone height related to damage caused by periodontitis and sinus pneumatization, creates difficulties in providing a significant number of implants of sufficient length to predictably support an implant prosthesis.

The placement of implants in the tuberosity region[1–5] and grafted sinus sites[6–11] and the availability of wide-diameter implants[12,13] have enhanced the prognosis of implants placed in the posterior maxilla. These procedures may be combined to allow distribution of a sufficient number of implants of adequate length and width to withstand posterior occlusal forces.

The purpose of this chapter is to evaluate more closely the use of implants placed in the tuberosity region. The anatomy is described, the surgical placement of implants in this region is discussed, and restored cases documenting site placement variations of the posterior implant are presented.

Anatomy of the Posterior Maxilla

Several articles have assigned various labels to the posteriorly placed maxillary implant. Implants in this region have been described as *tuberosity implants*,[1–3] *pterygoid plate implants*,[4] and *pterygomaxillary implants*.[5] The varied terminology arises as a result of the various anatomic structures that may be engaged in the placement of implants in this region. Anatomic investigations utilizing cadaver dissection have enabled the author to examine the articulation between the maxilla, the palatine bone, and the pterygoid process of the sphenoid bone. The precise structures offering potential support for implant placement are the tuberosity of the maxillary bone, the pyramidal process of the palatine bone, and the pterygoid process of the sphenoid bone[14] (Figs 14-1 and 14-2).

The tuberosity is the posterior convexity of the maxillary alveolar ridge. Its medial and posterior boundary is the pyramidal process. The pyramidal process of the palatine bone and the anterior surface of the pterygoid process of the sphenoid bone are located behind and slightly medial to the tuberosity.[15] This process binds to the anterior surface of the pterygoid plates of the sphenoid bone and is interposed between the inferior end of the pterygoid plates and the maxillary tuberosity. This junction of the palatine bone and pterygoid plates forms a narrow column of dense bone, referred to as the *pterygoid pillar*, into which the apical portion of an implant can be fixed.

If the tuberosity is of favorable dimension—height, width, and length—an implant may be successfully placed within this structure (Figs 14-3a and 14-3b) and a more distal placement of the implant apex avoided. However, if the dimension and/or quality of the tuberosity is insufficient, a more medially angled and posteriorly placed implant is determined by the angle of the posterior wall of the maxillary sinus.[4] The implant must be placed parallel to the posterior sinus wall to prevent penetration of the sinus (Figs 14-4, 14-5, and 14-6). Depending on the angle of placement and length of the posterior implant, four apical anatomic bone engagements are possible and can be classified as follows:

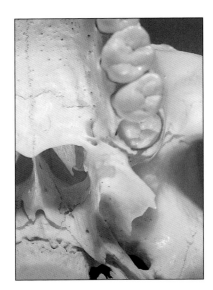

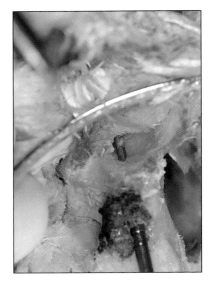

Fig 14-1a Region of a skull demonstrating the inferior relationship of the tuberosity, the pyramidal process of the palatine bone, and the pterygoid process of the sphenoid bone.

Fig 14-1b Cadaver dissection demonstrating the inferior view of the tuberosity (blue), the pyramidal process of the palatine bone (green), and the lateral and medial pterygoid plates (red). The path of a twist drill passing at an angle through the tuberosity and emerging into the pterygoid fossa is demonstrated. Actual surgical instrumentation would terminate in the pterygoid process or pyramidal process and not perforate the pterygoid fossa, thereby preventing damage to the medial pterygoid muscle.

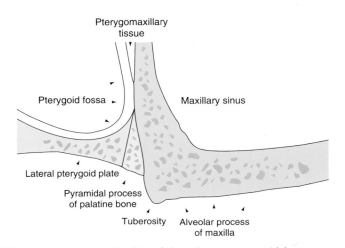

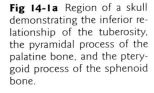

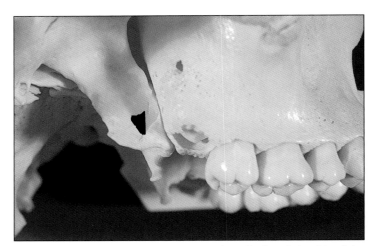

Fig 14-2a Lateral relationship of the tuberosity, pyramidal process, and lateral pterygoid plate. The alveolar process, maxillary sinus, pterygoid fossa, and pterygomaxillary fissure are also identified.

Fig 14-2b Region of a skull demonstrating laterally the relationship of the tuberosity, pyramidal process, and the pterygoid process. The hamulus extends inferiorly from the medial plate of the pterygoid process (*arrow*).

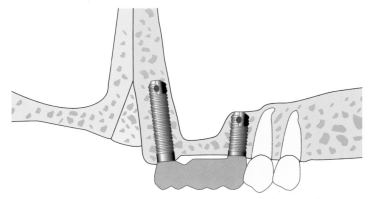

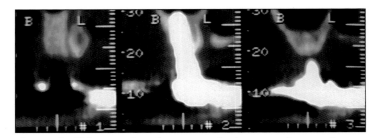

Fig 14-3a Three-unit implant-supported fixed partial denture. The posterior implant is located in the tuberosity and parallels the posterior wall of the maxillary sinus.

Fig 14-3b Oblique section of a computerized tomography scan demonstrating an implant placed within the maxillary tuberosity.

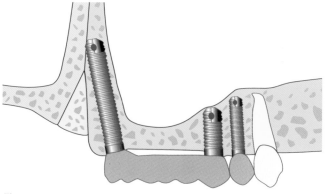

Fig 14-4 Posterior implant engaging the tuberosity and pterygoid process.

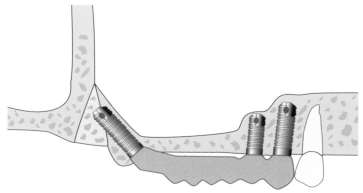

Fig 14-5 Posterior implant engaging the tuberosity and pyramidal process.

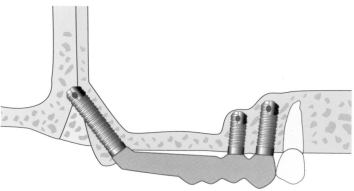

Fig 14-6a Posterior implant engaging the tuberosity, pterygoid process, and pyramidal process.

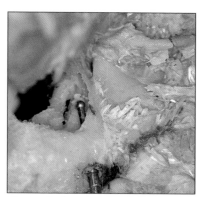

Fig 14-6b Incorrect path of a twist drill passing through the tuberosity and emerging into the maxillary sinus (cadaver).

Classification of the Posterior Maxillary Implant Based on Anatomic Location

1. Tuberosity (Figs 14-3a and 14-3b)
2. Tuberosity/pterygoid process (Fig 14-4)
3. Tuberosity/pyramidal process (Fig 14-5)
4. Tuberosity/pyramidal process/pterygoid process (Fig 14-6a)

The Tuberosity Implant

If the anatomy of the tuberosity is favorable, a long implant can be placed so that it is confined to this structure (Figs 14-3a and 14-3b). Care must be taken to avoid perforating the posterior wall of the maxillary sinus (Fig 14-6b), the location of which is determined radiographically. The bone within the tuberosity is typically of poor quality; therefore, if the dimensions of this structure are favorable, implants of wide diameter should be used. The wide-diameter implant fills a greater volume of the tuberosity and may provide an osteotome-like effect by condensing and compacting the internal bone of this structure between the implant and the cortical plates of bone (Figs 14-7 to 14-9).

Technique

A mucoperiosteal flap is elevated from the facial aspect and reflected palatally. The incision design is such that the entire tuberosity, including its posterior aspect, is uncovered for visualization and instrumentation. Sequential drilling procedures are followed in usual step-by-step fashion, as dictated by protocol for the placement of screw-type[16] implants. Radiographic information is used to determine the proper drilling angle necessary to avoid perforation of the posterior sinus wall. Because of the poor bone quality typically found in the tuberosity, tapping and countersinking of the bone should be avoided in order to gain optimal implant fixation and stabilization.

At the time of second-stage surgery to uncover the tuberosity implant, the surgeon should consider soft tissue reduction in order to reduce the submucosal extension of the abutment. The tuberosity implant may require an angulated abutment, depending on the angle of implant placement.

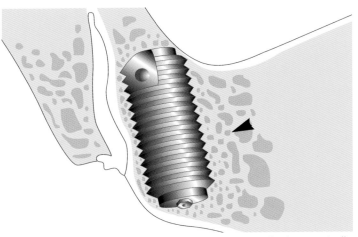

Fig 14-7 Wide-diameter implant placed in the poor-quality bone typically found to constitute the maxillary tuberosity. The fatty marrow is condensed because of the osteotome-like effect of the wide-diameter implant (*arrow*).

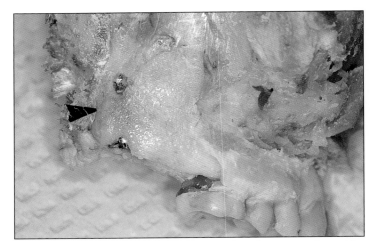

Fig 14-8 Cadaver maxilla demonstrating the placement of a wide-diameter implant within the tuberosity (*arrow*).

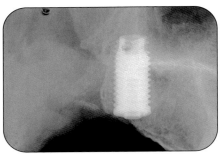

Fig 14-9 Periapical radiograph demonstrating the placement of a 6-mm-wide implant into the maxillary tuberosity (cadaver).

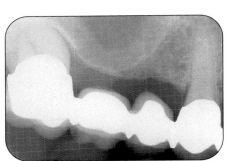

Fig 14-10a Periapical radiograph demonstrating severe periodontitis involving the maxillary right second molar.

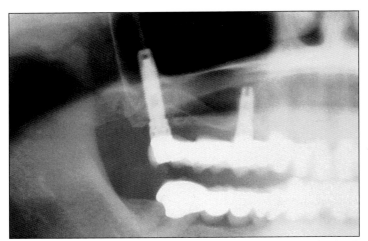

Fig 14-10b Three-unit implant-supported fixed partial denture. The distal implant is 18 × 4 mm and has been placed within the tuberosity.

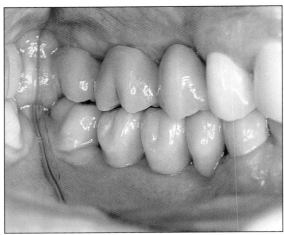

Fig 14-10c Completed three-unit implant-supported fixed partial denture.

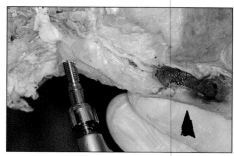

Fig 14-11 Angulation of implant placement of a tuberosity/pterygoid implant. The handpiece must be angled medially (cadaver). Exudate indicative of a chronic sinus infection is noted (*arrow*).

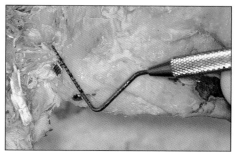

Fig 14-12 A tuberosity/pterygoid implant has been inserted, and bone has been removed from the apical region of the implant so that implant angulation may be visualized. A periodontal probe is in place, paralleling proper mesiodistal implant angulation. The shadow of the maxillary sinus is visualized through the thin maxillary process (cadaver).

Case

A second molar, serving as the distal abutment tooth for a fixed partial denture, was lost to advanced periodontitis. The tuberosity implant placed was 18 × 4 mm, and the second premolar implant placed was 10 × 4 mm (Figs 14-10a to 14-10c). A three-unit implant-supported fixed partial denture was provided.

The Pterygoid Process Implant

The dimensions of the tuberosity may not be sufficient for the placement of an implant. In such cases, the angle of the posterior wall of the sinus is determined radiographically. If the angle is not severe, and if the tuberosity provides ample dimension crestally, an implant of sufficient length can be placed so that it initiates in the tuberosity and terminates apically in the pterygoid process of the sphenoid bone.

Technique

The sequential steps followed are the same as for the placement of the maxillary tuberosity implant. To place the implant apex into the pterygoid plate, the surgeon must angle the handpiece medially (Fig 14-11). The thickest area of supporting bone is located in the middle part of the pterygoid process between the plates. This is 3 to 4 mm medial to the alveolar ridge. An implant must, therefore, be angled slightly medially to bisect this dense juncture of bone in the pterygoid region. The hamular process on the medial pterygoid plate is typically palpable in the oropharynx. The implant is placed just lateral to this key landmark.[4] There is a natural tendency for the surgeon to err by using the center of the maxillary ridge as a directional drilling guide for implant placement. Because the pterygoid process is located medial to the maxillary tuberosity, care must be taken to avoid perforation of the lateral pterygoid plate, otherwise the external pterygoid muscle may be traumatized and the opportunity to achieve osseointegration lost due to the implant apex being situated in soft tissue.

Again, care must be taken to avoid perforating the posterior wall of the maxillary sinus (see Figs 14-6b, 14-7, and 14-12 to 14-14). If the sinus is inadvertently penetrated, the surgeon can develop a second, more posterior, access. Angling the twist drill more distally enables the placement of a more angulated implant, thus avoiding re-entry into the sinus. The length of the pterygoid implant is determined during drilling by encountering the dense pterygoid plate (Figs 14-13 and 14-14).

Concern regarding the violation of the pterygoid vasculature may be somewhat overstated in that these structures are located superior to the planned apical placement of the pterygoid process implant. The internal maxillary artery courses superior and lateral to the pterygomaxillary suture and terminates in the sphenopalatine fossa. The internal maxillary artery crosses 1 cm superior to the pterygomaxillary suture as it enters the pterygopalatine fossa. The mean distance from the inferior pterygomaxillary suture to this artery is approximately 25 mm.[17]

Case

An existing fixed partial denture failed as a result of caries and periodontitis (Fig 14-15a). An 18 × 3.75-mm pterygoid process implant was placed in conjunction with first and second premolar implants (Fig 14-15b). The first premolar implant was 13 × 3.75 mm; the second premolar implant was 8 × 5 mm in diameter. The use of a standard and wide-diameter implant in conjunction with a long posterior implant contributed to the patient's ability to withstand significant posterior occlusal forces in a long-span fixed partial

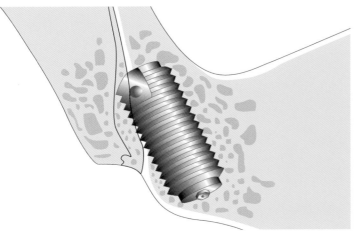

Fig 14-13 Placement of a tuberosity/pterygoid implant (distal/apical aspect). The implant is situated in the dense pterygoid plate.

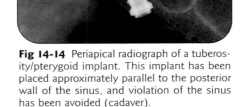

Fig 14-14 Periapical radiograph of a tuberosity/pterygoid implant. This implant has been placed approximately parallel to the posterior wall of the sinus, and violation of the sinus has been avoided (cadaver).

denture. To engage the pterygoid process, the vertical drill angle was significantly steeper than that used during tuberosity implantation.

A preangulated or cast custom abutment (Fig 14-15c) can be used in restoring the pterygoid process implant. In this case, a cast-gold framework was provided in order to engage the posterior implant, as well as the two premolar implants (Fig 14-15d). The framework was cemented to the two premolar custom implant abutments and was screw retained by the distal implant. The casting is a nonanatomic bar in the region extending distally beyond the mandibular dentition (Figs 14-15e to 14-15g).

The Pyramidal Process Implant

In patients demonstrating exaggerated angulation of the posterior sinus wall, an implant of sufficient length may be placed so that it initiates in the tuberosity and terminates apically in the pyramidal plate of the palatine bone (see Fig 14-5).

Technique

The surgeon must flatten the angle of the twist drill compared to the angle used for the placement of the pterygoid process implant, to avoid sinus perforation and to engage the pyramidal process of the palatine bone.

Case

An existing fixed partial denture failed as a result of severe periodontitis involving premolar abutment teeth. The posterior sinus wall was determined radiographically to be at a significantly greater angle than that shown in the previous patient, thus limiting the height and length of the tuberosity. As a result, a posterior implant of 18 × 3.75 mm was

placed at a greater angle, and the pyramidal process of the palatine bone was engaged (Figs 14-16a to 14-16c). Implants provided in the second premolar and first molar sites, both 15 × 3.75 mm, were placed simultaneously in conjunction with sinus graft procedures.

The Tuberosity/Pyramidal Process/Pterygoid Process Implant

In some cases the angle of the posterior wall of the sinus may permit a twist drill angulation that places the apex of the implant at the junction of the pyramidal process of the palatine bone and the pterygoid process of the sphenoid bone. The implant placed would then engage all three bone segments that constitute this region (see Fig 14-6a)

Technique

The sequential steps followed are the same as those used for the maxillary tuberosity implant. The drill angle approximately bisects the angles utilized in the placement of tuberosity and pyramidal process implants.

Case

A four-unit fixed partial denture failed because of periodontitis involving the maxillary right first premolar and second molar teeth. A 15 × 3.75-mm implant was placed in the region of the articulation of the tuberosity, pyramidal process, and pterygoid process in conjunction with two premolar implants. The first premolar implant was 13 × 3.75 mm, and the second premolar implant was 10 × 3.75 mm (Fig 14-17a). The restoration of the implant placed in this region was similar to that of the pterygoid process implant. (Figs 14-17a and 14-17b).

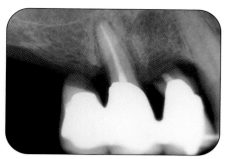

Fig 14-15a Failure of an existing three-unit fixed partial denture. The failure is due to a combination of periodontitis and caries.

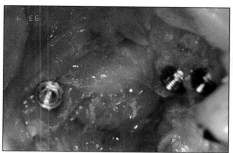

Fig 14-15b Placement of three implants in the maxillary right posterior segment from which the failed premolar teeth have been removed. The implant placed in the first premolar site is 13 × 3.75 mm. The implant placed in the second premolar site is 8 × 5 mm. The posterior implant placed in the pterygoid process is 18 × 3.75 mm.

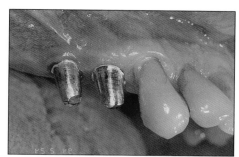

Fig 14-15c Custom cast-gold abutments retained by the two premolar implants.

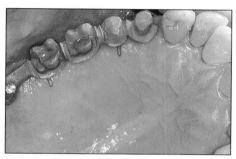

Fig 14-15d Cast-gold superstructure that is cemented onto the two premolar custom cast abutments and screw retained by the pterygoid process implant. The distal aspect of the superstructure is a bar design lacking dental anatomy. Dental anatomy in this posterior region is unnecessary because the bar is unopposed by mandibular teeth. The nonanatomic cast bar facilitates the patient's tongue adaptation and hygiene procedures.

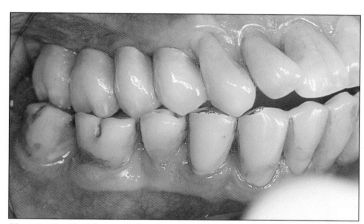

Fig 14-15e Final four-unit implant-supported fixed partial denture.

Fig 14-15f Periapical radiograph demonstrating the restoration of the two premolar implants. Note the 5-mm-wide implant replacing the second premolar tooth.

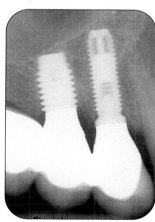

Fig 14-15g Panographic view showing the restoration of the implanted segment.

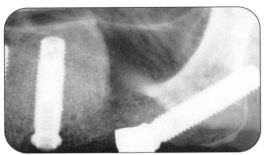

Fig 14-16a Periapical radiograph showing the placement of an 18 × 3.75-mm implant in the pyramidal process region. The angle of the drill is flatter for this implant placement than for placement in the pterygoid process. The distal of two implants placed in the premolar region is also visible. The two premolar implants were placed simultaneously in conjunction with sinus graft surgery, and each is 15 × 3.75 mm.

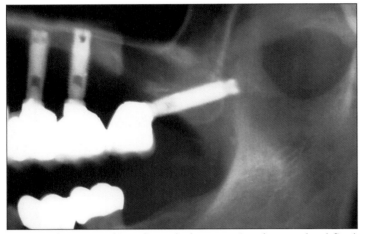

Fig 14-16b Panographic radiograph demonstrating the completed fixed restoration supported by two premolar implants and an implant located in the pyramidal process.

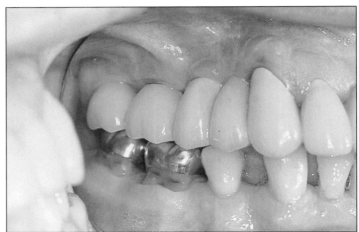

Fig 14-16c Buccal view of the completed implant-supported fixed restoration.

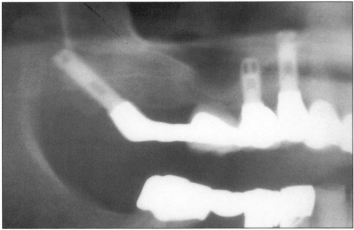

Fig 14-17a Panographic view of a maxillary right posterior segment showing the placement of two premolar implants and a tuberosity/pyramidal process/pterygoid process implant at the site of a failed four-unit fixed partial denture. The abutment teeth were lost to advanced periodontitis. The final implant-supported fixed partial denture has been placed.

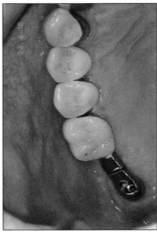

Fig 14-17b Occlusal aspect of the final implant-supported fixed partial denture.

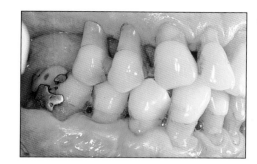

Fig 14-18a and 14-18b Patient suffering from advanced periodontitis and posterior tooth loss.

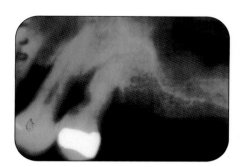

Fig 14-18c Periapical radiographs demonstrating the maxillary left and right posterior segments. The left second premolar has been lost, and the remaining premolars demonstrate severe periodontitis. The maxillary sinuses are pneumatized bilaterally.

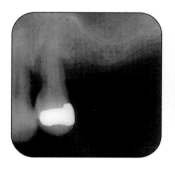

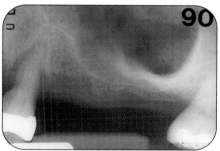

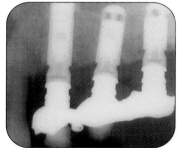

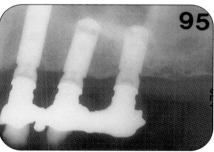

Fig 14-18d Comparison of the maxillary left posterior segment pretreatment (1990) and post–sinus grafting with the staged placement of three implants (1995), which have been occlusally loaded. The first premolar implant is 15 × 4 mm; the second premolar and first molar implants are 10 × 4 mm.

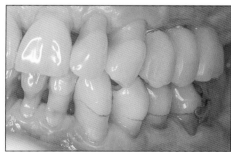

Fig 14-18e Left lateral view of implants loaded with a heat-processed, acrylic resin, gold-supported provisional fixed partial denture.

The Distal Implant Combined With Sinus Graft Implant Sites

A long posterior implant used with implants that are placed in conjunction with sinus elevation procedures offers yet another possible solution for managing the compromised maxillary posterior segment.

Case

An implant of the right pterygoid process was placed in conjunction with two premolar implants placed simultaneously with sinus graft surgery (Figs 14-18a to 14-18j). This treatment approach allowed longer implants in the premolar region, complemented by the long posterior implant. This approach was advantageous for the management of

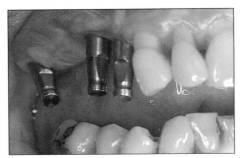

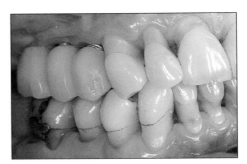

Fig 14-18f Right posterior maxilla with three implant impression copings seated. The first premolar implant was placed in mature bone and is 15 × 3.75 mm, the second premolar implant was placed simultaneously with a sinus graft procedure and is 15 × 3.75 mm, and a tuberosity/pterygoid process implant has been placed in the posterior site and is 18 × 3.75 mm.

Fig 14-18g Right side with implants occlusally loaded with a heat-processed, acrylic resin, gold-supported provisional fixed partial denture.

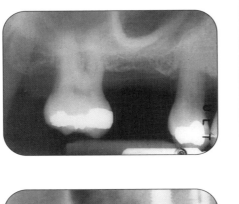

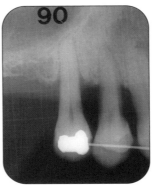

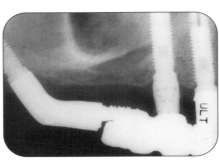

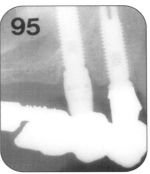

Fig 14-18h Comparison of the maxillary right posterior segment pretreatment (1990) and posttreatment (1995). Two long premolar implants and a tuberosity/pterygoid process implant are occlusally loaded.

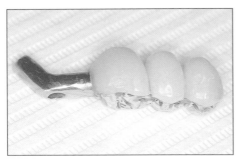

Fig 14-18i Occlusal and facial aspects of the provisional fixed partial denture. The posterior implant is screw retained and the occlusal aspect of the provisional restoration is cast gold. The cast-gold occlusal surface provides durability, rigidity, and the preservation of vertical dimension. The angle of the distal implant is indicated by the distal angulation of the casting.

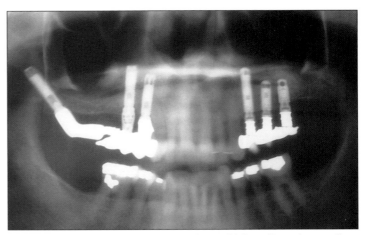

Fig 14-18j Occlusally loaded implants located bilaterally in the maxillary posterior segments. The right wall includes a tuberosity/pyramidal process/pterygoid process implant and a second premolar implant placed in a sinus grafted site. The left side includes two premolar implants and a first molar implant, all placed in sinus grafted sites.

posterior occlusal forces delivered to the implant-supported fixed partial denture. The posterior implant was 18 × 3.75 mm and the two premolar implants were each 15 × 3.75 mm. Three implants were placed in the left posterior segment in conjunction with sinus graft surgery.

Conclusion

Problems of bone quality and quantity create challenges for implant placement in affected maxillary posterior regions. Solutions for this region, when it is compromised, include the use of implants in the posterior site in sinus augmentation sites, in the placement of wide-diameter implants, and in implant placement in the posterior site. Anatomically, the posterior region is complex and comprises portions of three bones—the tuberosity of the maxillary bone, the pyramidal process of the palatine bone, and the pterygoid process of the sphenoid bone.

The location of the posterior implant is dictated by the dimensions and quality of the tuberosity. The mesiodistal angulation of the implant is dictated by the angle of the posterior wall of the sinus and its proximity to the posterior wall of the tuberosity. The buccopalatal angulation of the implant is dictated by the bone segments to be engaged. When indicated, and when sufficient bone structure is available, the surgeon may place the apical portion of the implant in the pterygoid process of the sphenoid bone and/or the pyramidal process of the palatine bone. A classification for the placement of implants in this region has been suggested. Cases using implants to demonstrate the classification have been presented.

Success of implant prostheses in the maxillary posterior region is dependent on the ability of implants to withstand occlusal forces. The use of the long posterior implant anchored in mature bone placed in conjunction with implants positioned in bone developed by sinus grafting, as well as the use of wide-diameter implants, can provide implant solutions for the compromised maxillary posterior segment.

Acknowledgments

The author wishes to thank Parker Mahan, DDS, PhD, and Lynn H. Larkin, PhD, for sharing their knowledge of the anatomy of the posterior maxillary region.

References

1. Bahat O. Osseointegrated implants in the maxillary tuberosity: Report on 45 consecutive cases. Int J Oral Maxillofac Implants 1992; 7:459–467.

2. Balshi TJ. Single tuberosity osseointegrated implant support for a tissue integrated prosthesis. Int J Periodont Rest Dent 1992;12:345–357.

3. Khayat P, Nader N. The use of osseointegrated implants in the maxillary tuberosity. Pract Periodontics Aesthet Dent 1994;6:53–61.

4. Graves SL. The pterygoid plate implant: A solution for restoring the posterior maxilla. Int J Periodont Rest Dent 1994;14:512–523.

5. Balshi TJ, Hy L, Hernandez RE. The use of pterygomaxillary implants in the partially edentulous patient. Int J Oral Maxillofac Implants 1995;10:89–99.

6. Boyne PJ, James RA. Grafting of the maxillary sinus floor with autogenous marrow and bone. J Oral Surg 1980;38:613–616.

7. Wood RM, Moore DI. Grafting of the maxillary sinus with intraorally harvested autogenous bone prior to implant placement. Int J Oral Maxillofac Implants 1988;3:209–214.

8. Tidwell JK, Blijdorp PA, Stoelinga PJ, Brouns JP, Hinderkes F. Composite grafting of the maxillary sinus for placement of endosteal implants. A preliminary report of 48 patients. Int J Oral Maxillofac Surg 1992;21:204–209.

9. Raghoeban GM, Brower JJ, Reintsema H, Van Oort RP. Augmentation of the maxillary sinus floor with autogenous bone for the placement of endosseous implants. A preliminary report. J Oral Maxillofac Surg 1993;51:198–203.

10. Small S, Zinner I, Panno F, Shapiro H, Stein J. Augmenting the maxillary sinus for implants; report of 27 patients. Int J Oral Maxillofac Implants 1993;8:523–528.

11. Moy PK, Londgen S, Holmes R. Maxillary sinus augmentation: Histomophonetic analysis of graft materials for maxillary sinus floor augmentation. J Oral Maxillofac Surg 1993;51:857–861.

12. Langer B, Langer L, Herrmann I, Jorneus L. The wide fixture: A solution for special bone situations and a rescue for the compromised implant. Int J Oral Maxillofac Implants 1993;8:400–408.

13. Graves SL, Jansen CE, Siddiqui AA, Beaty KD. Wide diameter implants: Indications, considerations and preliminary results over a two year period. Aust Prosthodont J 1994;8:31–37.

14. Grant JCB. An Atlas of Anatomy. Baltimore: Williams & Wilkins, 1956:541.

15. Tulasne JF. Implants pterygo-maxillaires experience sur 7 ans. Implant 1992;1(hors serie):39–48.

16. Brånemark PI, Zarb GA, Albrektsson T. Tissue-Integrated Prostheses. Chicago: Quintessence, 1985:211–227.

17. Turvey T, Fonseca R. The anatomy of the internal maxillary artery: its relationship in maxillary surgery. J Oral Surg 1980;38:92–95.

Osseous Regeneration With Bone Harvested From the Anterior Mandible

R. Gilbert Triplett, DDS, PhD
Sterling R. Schow, DMD

Augmentation of the deficient dental alveolar ridge has been the subject of clinical investigation for years. A number of surgical techniques have been devised to replace the deficient alveolar bone. These include the use of alloplastic materials such as hydroxyapatite, bone allografts such as freeze-dried demineralized bone, and autologous bone grafts. Although alloplastic and allogeneic materials have utility in the reconstruction of alveolar defects, autologous grafts provide the most rapid and predictable results in terms of resultant bone quality and quantity. All the above-mentioned materials, including autologous bone, have been used successfully with and without barrier membranes.

Endosseous dental implants must be surrounded by a sufficient quantity of viable bone to support and sustain osseointegration successfully. The purpose of this chapter is to discuss the use of autologous bone grafts obtained from the anterior mandible to create adequate alveolar ridge size and form for successful implant placement.

Various donor sites for autologous grafts are available to the surgeon, including the iliac crest, calvarium, tibia, ribs, and the maxillofacial skeleton (maxilla, mandible, and zygoma.[1,2] The donor site is chosen based on the type and quantity of bone required, the access to the donor site, the difficulty and time required in the bone harvest, the morbidity associated with the bone harvest, and the cost.[3–8] The anterior mandible is a favorable donor site because it has an excellent risk-benefit ratio. Access is excellent, the type and quantity of bone obtainable is suitable for augmentation of a one- to three-tooth alveolar segment, the operating time is short (24 to 40 minutes), and the morbidity is very low. Additionally, the cost is reasonable because few special instruments are required. Bone can be harvested from the symphysis on an outpatient basis using a local anesthetic with or without sedation. Autologous grafts are the most predictable and successful augmentation material.[1,5]

Surgical Technique

Preoperative Assessment

The patient's general oral health should be addressed prior to any grafting procedure. All chronic periodontal infection should be well controlled, and acute infection should be managed prior to surgery. Teeth with caries or that are not salvageable should be restored or removed prior to the surgery. Prophylactic antibiotics are chosen based on the area to be grafted. If the maxillary sinus is the graft recipient area, the antibiotic spectrum should be sufficient to control microorganisms known to inhabit the upper airway, eg, *Haemophilis influenza*.

Sound principles of prophylactic antibiotic administration require that the patient receive a bolus of antibiotic with 1 hour of the start of the procedure and a follow-up dose 6 to 8 hours later (depending on the antibiotic). This establishes circulating blood and indwelling tissue levels of the antibiotic of sufficient concentration for the duration of the surgery and early postoperative period. For example, a patient having alveolar ridge augmentation grafting could receive 2 to 3 g of amoxicillin orally 1 hour preoperatively or a similar dose of ampicillin intravenously if intravenous sedation is to be used for the procedure. This would be followed by an oral dose of either medication, equal to half the original dose, 6 hours later. For patients allergic to the penicillins, alternative antibiotics include the cephalosporins (oral Keflex or intravenous Kefzol are good choices) or clindamycin given either orally or intravenously.

The decision to carry antibiotic coverage beyond the perioperative period is based on the long-term needs of each individual patient clinically and *not* on operative prophylactic antibiotic principles. For most patients, antibiotics will not be required beyond the preoperative and early postoperative doses.

Having the patient rinse with 0.2% chlorhexadine for 1 minute before surgery is also helpful to reduce the total oral bacteria count before incisions are initiated.

Anesthesia

The use of local anesthesia for harvesting autologous bone from the anterior mandible is critical for both patient comfort and the quality of the operative site. Because the anterior mandible will be exposed from mental foramen to mental foramen, bilateral inferior alveolar and lingual nerve blocks are required. In addition, infiltration of the anesthetic in the labial vestibule from second premolar to second premolar to the inferior border of the mandible helps provide good hemostasis of the operative site and anesthetizes the sensory cutaneous cervical nerves, which also provide sensation to this region. Local anesthetic infiltration in the corresponding lingual soft tissues, to the inferior border of the mandible, also provides additional anesthesia and hemostasis.

Local anesthesia is usually obtained with a longer-acting bupivicaine and a vasoconstrictor for more prolonged patient comfort and analgesia. An epinephrine concentration of 1:200,000 provides maximum vasoconstriction. Concentrations greater than this have been shown to have no increased benefit for hemostasis, and concentrations of 1:50,000 have significant cardiovascular risk in the quantities needed for anesthesia for this harvest.

Incision

The incision is made to expose the anterior mandible sufficiently to assure gentle handling of the surgical flaps and protection of the mental nerves.

Vestibular Incision

For most harvests in a patient with anterior teeth, a vestibular incision allows good exposure and easy closure and is the incision of choice. The mouth should be closed or only slightly open to allow maximum relaxation of the obicularis musculature. The lower lip is retracted labially, tensing the vestibular mucosa. The incision is made obliquely through the mucosa in the depth of the vestibule

and at least 1 cm apical to the mucogingival junction in the symphysis region. The incision is carried to bone, incising the mentalis muscles. In its superior posterior extent, the incision moves slightly superiorly, while remaining in the alveolar mucosa, to pass above the mental foramen (Figs 15-1a to 15-1d). The mentalis muscle is identified and incised labial to its attachment to the mandible to allow sufficient tissue for a deep, layered closure at the completion of the procedure. This is important to prevent postsurgical ptosis of the chin.

A subperiosteal dissection is carried to the inferior border of the mandible and distal to the mental foramen. Depending on the graft size, either one or both mental foramina will require exposure to protect the mental nerve from stretch injury during the graft harvest. Management of the flap in this area is crucial because the mental nerve is easily injured by stretching, crushing, or excessive manipulation. The nerve should be carefully identified and protected by stable, gentle flap retraction.

Once the anterior mandible is exposed, the mouth should be closed and the exposure checked to ensure adequate access for harvesting the graft. It is better to spend a few additional minutes providing access and relaxation of the tissues than to deal with the intraoperative frustration of poor exposure. The best access is usually obtained if the subperiosteal dissection is carried to the midportion of the inferior border of the mandible.

— Alternative Incision —

In some circumstances, it may be desirable to use a crevicular incision around the necks of the teeth and to make vertical releasing incisions in the premolar region. When this incision is chosen, a one-layer subperiosteal dissection is used to expose the entire anterior mandible. It is crucial that the vertical releasing incision avoid the mental nerve branches as they course into the substance of the lower lip. When the releasing incisions are made distal to the second premolar teeth, there is usually an adequate margin of safety; if the incision is placed more anteriorly, the surgeon must accommodate for these branches to prevent nerve injury.

The crevicular truncated flap also requires detachment of the mentalis muscle from the anterior mandible. This muscle must be *reattached* at the end of the procedure to minimize postoperative chin ptosis. Reattachment can be accomplished by creating small bur holes in the mandible at the superior margin of the donor site to allow attachment of the mentalis muscle directly to bone at the position from which it was detached. This will depend on the site and size of the graft. Usually, a hole can be made at the edge of the superior cut of the donor site, and the suture can be passed through the muscle and mandible and secured.

A well-placed and maintained external pressure dressing is critical to ensure good tissue repositioning and hemostasis when this flap design is used.

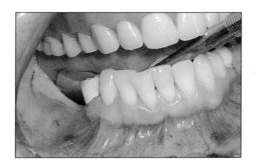
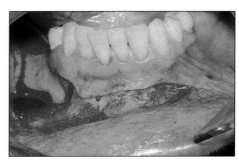

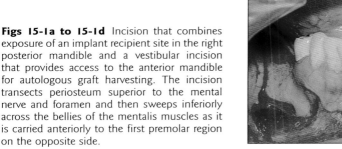
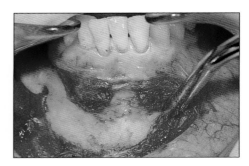

Figs 15-1a to 15-1d Incision that combines exposure of an implant recipient site in the right posterior mandible and a vestibular incision that provides access to the anterior mandible for autologous graft harvesting. The incision transects periosteum superior to the mental nerve and foramen and then sweeps inferiorly across the bellies of the mentalis muscles as it is carried anteriorly to the first premolar region on the opposite side.

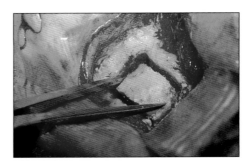

Fig 15-2 Measuring the graft with calipers.

Harvesting

The type of graft to be harvested depends on the defect to be restored and operator choice. Block grafts and particulate grafts, or combinations of both, can be obtained from the anterior mandible.

Block Grafts

- Partial-thickness cortical strips
- Corticocancellous blocks (labial cortex and cancellous marrow)
- Full-thickness block grafts (labial and lingual cortices)

Particulate Grafts

- Cores (trephine)
- Corticocancellous chips and particles
- Shavings

—— *Block Grafts* ——

The size and shape of the graft is outlined on the anterior surface of the mandible. The superior aspect of the graft must be 5 mm below the apices of the anterior teeth to minimize injury to these tooth roots, and the sides of the graft should be at least 6 mm anterior to the mental foramen to avoid injury to the nerve. A sterile marking pen is an ideal tool to outline the graft. The outline can be sketched on the bone (which must be dry and clean) and verified for size with calipers before the osseous cuts are begun (Fig 15-2). The surgeon should attempt to harvest a slightly larger block of bone than is required for the final graft to allow for shaping.

The osseous cuts are made with a bur or a thin saw blade to the desired depth and dimensions. If a bur is used, it should be used in a high-speed, high-torque handpiece. The bur should be a No. 699 or 700 crosscut fissure bur. The saw blade will be an oscillating angled or straight blade.

Frequently, the inferior border of the mandible will be included in the graft (Figs 15-3a and 15-3b). This is of no negative consequence to external facial esthetics, if a bone substitute is used to fill the defect. Including the inferior border may greatly facilitate bone harvest and improve the shape and contour of the graft.

If a block graft does not include the inferior border the margins of the host bone should be beveled to accommodate a small, sharp, curved chisel (Figs 15-4a to 15-4c). There must be adequate access for the blade of the chisel to reach

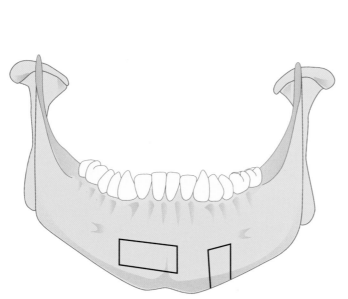

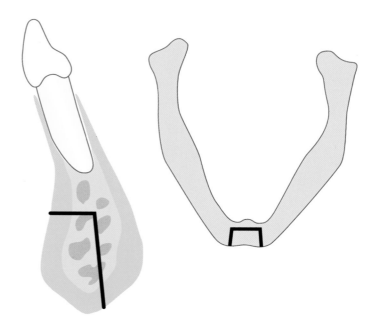

Fig 15-3a Two possible approaches to harvest of block grafts: On the right side, the rectangular graft preserves the inferior border of the mandible; on the left side, the graft includes the inferior border.

Fig 15-3b Cross-sectional view of a block graft that includes the inferior border of the mandible. *(right)* View from the inferior border of the mandible.

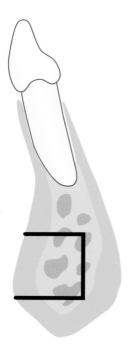

Fig 15-4a Cross-sectional view of a block graft that preserves the inferior border of the mandible. The labial margins of the cut should be beveled.

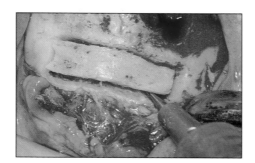

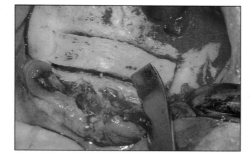

Figs 15-4b and 15-4c Beveling the cortical cuts to allow insertion of the osteotome.

the depth of the cut; otherwise the thickness of the graft may be irregular or inadequate. When the chisel is malleted, the occlusal surface of the teeth should be protected from those of the opposing arch. Mouthguard material is ideal for this task, and a piece can be cut and placed between the teeth to absorb the shock and protect the crowns from trauma.

The most inferior cut on the mandible will pose the greatest difficulty to access for the osteotome. For this approach, the patient's mouth should be closed to relieve the tension of

the lips and obicularis oris muscles. If self-retaining cheek retractors are used to maintain oral exposure during surgery, they should be removed to enhance exposure. If a thin strip of bone between the inferior cut of the block graft and the inferior border of the mandible is left when the graft is outlined, the leverage of the chisel should avoid the inferior edge of the mandible. This margin fractures easily when torqued and may result in a complete mandibular fracture. If the inferior border is included in the graft, placing the pa-

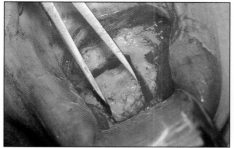

Fig 15-5a Corticocancellous block of bone outlined for an inlay graft.

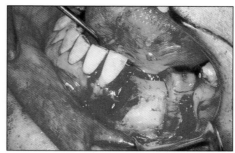

Fig 15-5b Bone wax used to form the pattern of the recipient site.

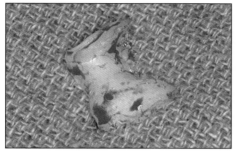

Fig 15-5c Wax pattern used to form the graft.

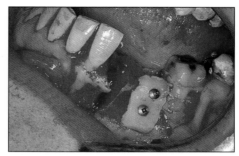

Fig 15-5d Inlay graft secured in place.

tient in a mouth-closed, chin-up position will allow maximum access for the bur to make the inferior cortical cut and to directly insert the osteotome for graft material.

Cutaneous sensory innervation to this area may require administration of additional local anesthesia along the muscle and periosteum of the inferior border. Once all of the cortical cuts are completed to the desired depth, the straight chisel is directed from the inferior cuts superiorly. This provides easy access for a clean osseous cut, and the graft can be delivered intact, usually with one or two taps on the chisel.

Once the graft is obtained, it can be stored in a moist, saline-soaked gauze while additional bone is harvested (if needed) and the mandibular wound is prepared for closure. Additional particles or chips can be harvested from the graft site as needed to fill voids and irregularities around the graft. Figures 15-5 to 15-7 show various block grafts being harvested and placed in a variety of recipient sites.

Full-Thickness Block Graft. Full-thickness grafts may occasionally be required in circumstances where increased depth of the graft is required. The approach is the same as for a partial-thickness harvest. The osseous cuts are made completely through the lingual cortical plates. An oscillating saw is ideal for this procedure. To maintain integrity to the mandible, the inferior border should not be violated. If a bur is used, the width of the cut should be wide enough to accommodate the bur shaft. Once the cuts are made, the lingual musculature is dissected free from the lingual plate.

Electrocautery is helpful for this harvest to control muscle bleeding, which can be a nuisance intraoperatively and can cause large sublingual hematomas if not controlled. The osseous defect can be filled with a bone substitute or a block

of hydroxyapatite on completion of the procedure. Complete bone repair of this defect may not occur, but it is usually of little consequence.

Particulate Grafts

Particulate grafts are ideal when the graft material can be confined to the recipient site without rigid fixation such as bone screws or plates. These grafts are appropriate in sinus grafting when the membrane is intact or in intraosseous alveolar defects that naturally limit movement of the graft if the material can be confined by a mesh or a barrier membrane. Particulate grafts include cores, corticocancellous particles, and shavings harvested from the anterior mandible or other regions.

Cores. Trephine burs can be used in the anterior mandible for bone harvest. A series of cores can be obtained within the limits previously described for the mandibular block grafts (a minimum of 5 mm below the apices of the mandibular teeth). Partial-thickness cores can be cut out while the lingual cortical plate is maintained. Trephine burs are commercially available in dimensions ranging from 3 to 5 mm in diameter. Approximately 3 to 5 cm^3 of bone can be obtained by harvesting multiple cores.

The particulate graft can be used alone, in combination with block grafts, or mixed with bone graft substitutes such as calcium phosphate, resorbable hydroxyapatite, or freeze-dried bone allografts. It is important with all of these graft materials to confine the materials to the area that is to be augmented. If the material becomes compacted or displaced, the results will be compromised.

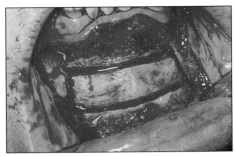

Fig 15-6a Corticocancellous block of bone outlined for a large veneer graft or to provide a block graft for a sinus lift.

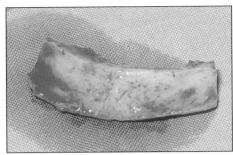

Fig 15-6b Large block graft.

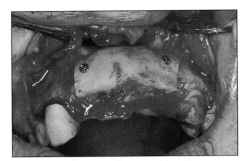

Fig 15-6c Veneer graft secured in place.

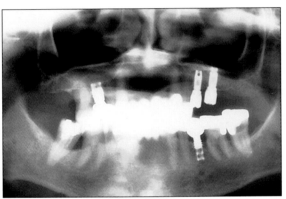

Fig 15-6d Totally reconstituted donor site, 18 months after harvesting.

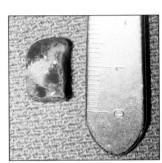

Fig 15-7a Corticocancellous block of bone for an onlay graft.

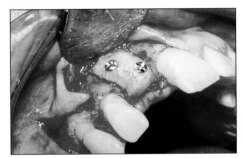

Fig 15-7b Onlay graft secured in place.

Corticocancellous particles. These grafts are harvested as small cortical and cancellous chips or small blocks that are then reduced with rongeurs or a bone mill. Although particles of this type are easy to obtain from the anterior mandible with drills and rongeurs, they are difficult to confine in the recipient area. These grafts must be confined with a nonresorbable barrier membrane, which itself should be fixed with miniscrews. If these chips and irregular particles are not confined and protected, they have a propensity to work themselves through the overlying mucosa, creating a nuisance for the patients, a potential infection or graft exposure, and a poor augmentation.

Shavings. Bone-collecting chambers that are commercially available make it possible to collect bone particles created with drills or burs (Fig 15-8). These collection devices are placed in the suction line only during the time that the shavings are being created. The bone collector consists of a fine mesh screen that "traps" the shavings. These shavings are similar in appearance and handling to a bone paste. The shavings are condensed with a compacting tool, which forms the particles into a defined mass that can be transplanted to the area needing augmentation. This graft material is easily adapted to dehiscences, sinus floors, and other confined spaces.

This harvesting method has promise as an addition to other techniques. It is simple to harvest moderate amounts of bone quickly and easily. A small window is drilled in the labial cortical plate on each side of the mandibular symphysis. The opening on either side of the symphysis should be at least 5 mm in diameter to accommodate a large round bur. The holes are connected by a slot cut in the cortex with a No. 703 fissure bur. This allows movement of a large round bur throughout the medullary areas of the anterior mandible. The collection apparatus is applied to the suction, and the suction tip is placed in one of the holes while the bur is moved through the medullary space, removing the bone shavings from the inner surface of the mandible.

Bleeding should be minimal while the bone shavings are collected because blood clots tend to occlude the collection screen. Excess blood is eliminated by copiously irrigating the area and only collecting while the shavings are being created with a bur. A large, round mastoid bur or a large round bur with deep flutes is ideal for creating the shavings. Once an adequate amount of bone has been obtained, the collector is removed from the suction line. The bone is compacted with a compacting device that comes with the set. The bone is then prepared for the graft procedure.

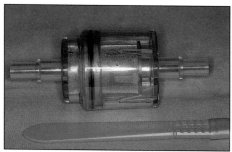

Fig 15-8 Bone-collecting chamber.

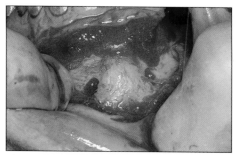

Fig 15-9a Exposed symphysis and drilled pilot holes.

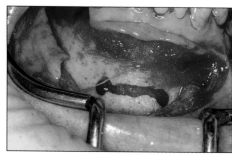

Fig 15-9b Joined pilot holes.

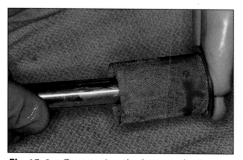

Fig 15-9c Compacting the harvest shavings.

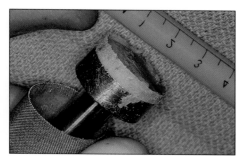

Fig 15-9d Compacted bone collected from the chamber.

Approximately 3 to 5 cm³ of bone shavings can be harvested in this manner. If this amount is not adequate to fill the defect at the recipient site, other areas of the mandible, such as the retromolar area and along the oblique ridge, can also be harvested in a like manner (Figs 15-9a to 15-9d).

Wound Closure

Prior to soft tissue closure of the mandibular donor site, the area is copiously irrigated and inspected. Sharp osseous edges and irregularities are reduced to minimize postoperative discomfort.

A filler material may be used to restore the contour of the donor site to minimize the possibility of a postoperative surface defect. With small donor sites that do not include the inferior border, this is rarely needed. For larger grafts, through-and-through defects, and grafts that include the inferior border of the mandible, use of a graft filler or bone substitute is desirable. A totally resorbable material is best because it will provide normal future architecture of the symphyseal bone should this area need to be imaged radiographically in the future. Additionally, it may also allow the site to be reused as a graft donor area in the future, should it be needed.

The filler material should have adequate resistance to displacement by the pressure dressing placed over the site. Resorbable calcium phosphate, resorbable hydroxyapatite, or a calcified bovine bone preparation all have suitable properties for this purpose. Placement of a resorbable membrane over the material is an option but is usually not necessary if the periosteum has been maintained intact.

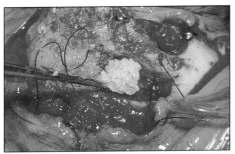
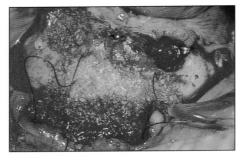

Figs 15-10a and 15-10b Resuspension of the mentalis muscle to holes drilled in the labial cortex of the superior osseous margin of the donor site.

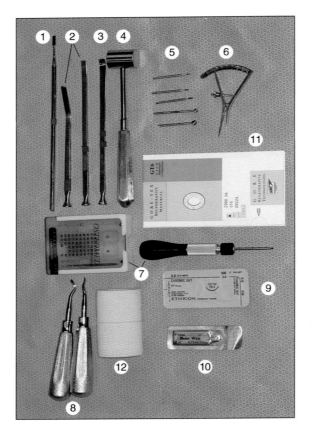

Fig 15-11 Special instruments needed to harvest autologous grafts from the anterior mandible.

1. Stout monobeveled osteotome
2. Straight 4- or 5-mm Lambote osteotome
3. Curved 4- or 5-mm Lambote osteotome
4. Surgical mallet
5. Burs: Nos. 699, 701, and 702 straight fissure burs; large, round mastoid bur
6. Surgical calipers
7. Microscrew set: 1.6-mm-diameter titanium screws of lengths 4 to 18 mm
8. Miller's dental elevators, right and left
9. Sutures: 2-0 chromic or polyglycolic acid for mentalis muscle suspension; 3-0 chromic; 3-0 polyglycolic acid; 4-0 chromic with tapered needle
10. Bone wax
11. Barrier membrane (eg, Gore-Tex, WL Gore)
12. Elastic or microfoam tape

A layered closure is important for the elimination of dead space and the minimization of postoperative donor site complications such as hematoma formation and wound dehiscence. The mentalis muscle should be reapproximated with a heavy-gauge resorbable suture, such as 2-0 chromic or 3-0 polyglactin 910. Proper approximation of the mentalis muscle is critical to prevent chin ptosis and labial mental fold irregularities (Figs 15-10a and 15-10b). The periosteal layer, lateral to the muscle, can be closed next, followed by the mucosal closure. Mucosal tissue is friable and will tear easily; therefore, use of a tapered (noncutting) needle with 3-0 or 4-0 resorbable material is recommended.

A pressure dressing should be applied to the chin and maintained for 5 days to minimize postoperative swelling and hematoma formation. Elastic tape is a good choice to provide pressure to the chin region.

Instruments

The instruments needed to harvest donor bone from the anterior mandible are already available in the surgical sets of most dentists who perform dentoalveolar and implant surgery. However, the special instruments shown in Figure 15-11 will be needed and should be readily available when this surgery is performed.

Acknowledgments

The authors acknowledge Dr Michael Zide for his generosity in providing photographs for the bone collection chamber, marketed by Ace Surgical, and Darlene Amos and Ellie Weigand for assistance in manuscript preparation.

References

1. Misch CM, Misch CE, Resnik RR, et al. Reconstruction of maxillary alveolar defects with mandibular symphysis grafts for dental implants: A preliminary procedural report. Int J Oral Maxillofac Implants 1992;7:360.

2. Buser D, Hirt HP, Dula K, et al. GBR-technique/implant dentistry. Simultaneous application of barrier membranes around implants with peri-implant bone defects. Schweiz Monatsschr Zahnmed 1992;102:1491.

3. Buser D, Brägger U, Lang NP, et al. Regeneration and enlargement of jaw bone using guided tissue regeneration. Clin Oral Implants Res 1990:1:22.

4. Buser D, Dula K, Belser UC, et al. Localized ridge augmentation using guided bone regeneration. II. Surgical procedure in the mandible. Int J Periodont Rest Dent 1995;15:11.

5. Borstlap WA, Heidbuchel KLWM, Freihofer HPM, et al. Early secondary bone grafting of alveolar clefts defects. A comparison between chin and rib grafts. J Craniomaxillofac Surg 1990;18:201.

6. Sindet-Pederson S, Enemark H. Reconstruction of alveolar clefts with mandibular or iliac crest bone grafts. A comparative study. J Oral Maxillofac Surg 1990;48:554.

7. Hirsch JM, Ericsson I. Maxillary sinus augmentation using mandibular bone grafts and simultaneous installation of implants. A surgical technique. Clin Oral Implants Res 1991;2:91.

8. El Deeb M. Reconstruction of alveolar clefts with mandibular or iliac bone grafts: A comparative study [discussion]. J Oral Maxillofac Surg 1990;48:559.

The Esthetic Management of Dental Implants

Burton Langer, DMD, MSD

Completely Edentulous Patients

While the development of osseointegration by Brånemark et al[1] has revolutionized the success and predictability of dental implants, the esthetic management has become the next hurdle to overcome. The completely edentulous patients who were the original group treated in Sweden were less of a problem because the objective was to offer an effective means to retain a loose-fitting denture. Inconsistencies in esthetics could be compensated for with artificial prosthetic means. This is still an effective approach in patients who have lost so much of their alveolus that the only method available to replace lost attachment apparatus is the fabrication of an acrylic resin or porcelain camouflage with overdentures or flanges that simulate lost anatomic structure (Figs 16-1a and 16-1b).

The completely edentulous condition is limited by previously lost structure; however, the prospectively completely edentulous individual may have avenues of hope to retain most of the dental anatomy; consequently, the final implant restoration will mimic a tooth-supported prosthesis. This will depend on the manner in which the teeth are extracted and the implants are inserted and will be addressed in the section on the partially edentulous condition (Fig 16-2). One approach that most certainly will produce the least desirable esthetic result will be the extraction of the teeth and collapse of the edentulous ridge.

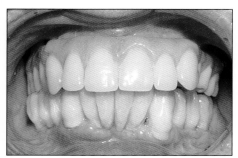

Fig 16-1a Severe alveolar atrophy necessitates the use of a labial flange attached to the fixed prosthesis. The flange avoids the need for excessively long teeth and offers lip support.

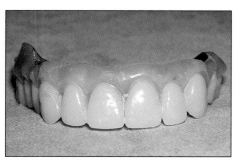

Fig 16-1b Fixed prosthesis with labial flange for a patient who requires lip support. This can also be used with a removable appliance.

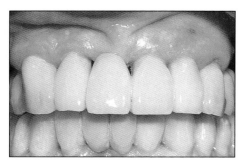

Fig 16-2 Implant-supported maxillary prosthesis that resembles a tooth-supported restoration. (Courtesy of Dr F. Kastenbaum.)

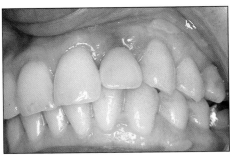

Fig 16-3a The maxillary right lateral incisor has a vertical fracture and is scheduled for extraction.

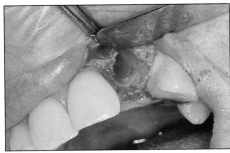

Fig 16-3b The tooth is extracted, and an implant fixture is inserted simultaneously. Note the buccal dehiscence, which usually causes a collapse of the edentulous ridge.

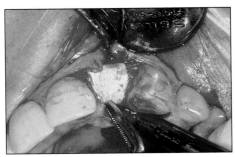

Fig 16-3c Gore-Tex membrane (WL Gore, Flagstaff, AZ) is placed over the implant site to prevent connective tissue from invading the space adjacent to the implant.

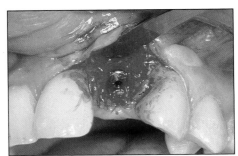

Fig 16-3d At the uncovering stage, new bone has grown around the implant, preserving the profile of the alveolus.

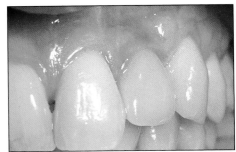

Fig 16-3e The final crown is in place. Tooth and tissue contour are normal. (Courtesy of Dr B. Croll.)

Partially Edentulous Patients

The introduction of osseointegration to the partially edentulous situation has changed the prosthetic alternatives. Consequently, the strategy of surgery to preserve tissue anatomy is crucial to optimizing cosmetics in the esthetic zone. The major objective of implant therapy is to place an anchoring unit that will support a fixed prosthesis and blend into the anatomic topography of the adjacent teeth. The clinician will be treating either a preexisting edentulous ridge or teeth scheduled for extraction and subsequent implant placement. Both categories allow a variety of different approaches.

When hopeless teeth are present, extraction and immediate implant placement with tissue augmentation must be weighed against extraction and socket retention procedures involving bone grafts and/or membrane placement and 6 months of healing prior to implant placement.[2–4] Although many find the latter approach more predictable, many sur-geons are comfortable with the technique of simultaneous extraction and implant placement.[5–9] They find it expedient for the patient and believe it may assist them surgically to retain the normal anatomy of the alveolus.

Extraction and Immediate Implant Placement

The surgical approach for the immediate extraction site requires both buccal and palatal or lingual flaps. The tooth to be extracted, if ankylosed, should be surgically dissected away from the alveolar bone with a thin diamond bur. This helps to prevent unnecessary loss of the labial plate during extraction and increases the predictability of bone regeneration around the implant. The buccal flap can be mobilized by making oblique cutback incisions. This will enable the operator to pull the flap coronally and facilitate closure over the implant site. Because the buccal tissue has such a rich vascular supply it is not necessary to keep the base of the flap wider than the coronal portion to avoid tissue necrosis (Figs 16-3a to 16-3e).

After extraction, debridement of the socket, and placement of the implant, the use of a barrier membrane, bone grafts, or both should be considered. Most clinicians would elect to have complete tissue coverage should a membrane be employed.[2,5,7] However, numerous reports have described complete bone regeneration over implants placed immediately after an extraction even though the membrane was exposed to the oral cavity during the healing stages.[6,8] Patients receiving this type of therapy should be examined frequently to monitor tissue health and prevent infection at the site. Antibacterial rinses have been advocated to reduce contamination of the area and subsequent damage to the underlying bone. The consensus is that the exposed membrane should be removed after approximately 8 weeks. It is to be hoped that underlying healing by secondary intention over the implant and below the membrane will cover the area and normal bone regeneration will ensue.

An advantage of this modality is its ease of manipulation. No attempt is made to mobilize the flap to the extent of creating primary tissue closure with the palatal flap. Therefore, the buccal flap is merely elevated with trapezoidal vertical incisions. Advocates of this approach also feel that there is better continuity of the mucogingival junction with the adjacent teeth. Vertical incisions should be made at least one tooth laterally to avoid unnecessary membrane exposure at the lateral borders, where the membrane is less occlusive and might admit more bacterial contaminants into the site.

Complete Coverage

The most predictable and biologically sound technique is aimed at covering all membranes and accompanying bone grafts. This objective can be accomplished by mobilizing the buccal flap and pulling it coronally to cover the implant site. Placement of interrupted horizontal mattress sutures tied to the palatal flap is often the most desirable method to close the crestal area because it capitalizes on greater vascular contact between the buccal and/or lingual connective tissue. Supplemental vertical interrupted sutures are also necessary to stabilize the buccal flap.

The major untoward result of this approach is the displacement of the mucogingival junction in a coronal direction. Often this displacement is self-correcting during the healing months between stage 1 and stage 2 surgery. Major tissue defects are not easily corrected with this technique unless additional ridge augmentation procedures are used. Beveled lateral incisions will help to prevent unsightly scarring and offer additional tissue to cover the implant area. Vertical interrupted sutures assist in stretching the elastic tissue laterally to the desired position to ensure complete tissue closure.

Connective Tissue Grafting

A third approach has been employed in the treatment of immediate extraction and fixture placement. This uses the same entry incisions on both the buccal and palatal or lingual; however, a subepithelial connective tissue graft[9–11] is harvested from the palate. The graft is obtained by making two parallel incisions, approximately 2 mm apart, starting at least 1 mm apical to the free gingival margin on the palate and meeting at a superior position between the midline of the palate and gingival margin. The epithelial band is removed from the connective tissue graft, and the graft is draped from buccal to lingual to cover the open socket (Figs 16-4a to 16-4g). The buccal and palatal flaps are sutured over the underlying connective tissue graft. If the clinician wishes to augment the buccal profile of the alveolus at stage 1 surgery, it would be advisable to add an extra piece of connective tissue underneath the buccal flap.

Because there may be a small area of connective tissue not covered at the crest of the ridge, especially when the implant area has been grafted with bone, a small island of tissue necrosis may develop during the first 10 days. The necrotic tissue can easily be removed without anesthesia, and well-vascularized connective tissue beneath the excised tissue will be covering the implant site. Bone grafts and/or barrier membranes may also be employed; however, it is advisable to avoid placement of extra pieces of connective tissue because the circulation could be impaired and some of the graft will slough.

Tissue Defects

Any major anatomic tissue defects should be addressed before the uncovering stage of osseointegration is reached. Exposure of the implant and placement of the cover screw impedes any further tissue grafting. Two-dimensional defects of buccopalatal width can be treated successfully at stage 2 with the connective tissue–grafting procedure. Some clinicians have also corrected small tissue defects by inverting palatal connective tissue at the uncovering site and tucking it inside the buccal flap. This approach, called the *roll technique*,[11,12] could be useful if the area in question is deficient in tissue in a buccolingual dimension only but would have some major dimensional limitations. It is generally advisable to build up tissue three dimensionally to avoid a curtain effect that is deficient of tissue on the palatal aspect of the implant, causing interproximal tissue cratering and eventual recession.

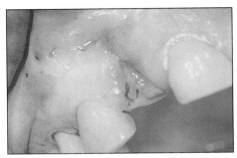

Fig 16-4a The maxillary right central incisor is fractured and has lost a significant amount of labial tissue.

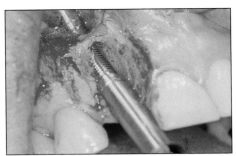

Fig 16-4b The tooth is extracted and an implant fixture is inserted at the time of extraction. A large deficiency of bone is present on the buccal surface of the implant.

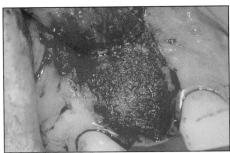

Fig 16-4c A bone graft is placed over the exposed threads.

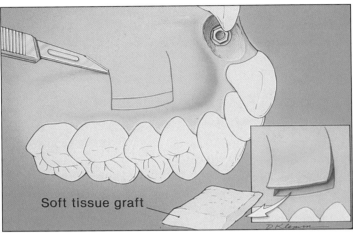

Fig 16-4d A connective tissue graft is harvested from the palate.

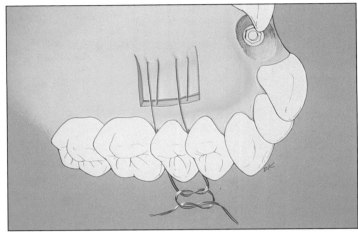

Fig 16-4e The donor site is closed with vertical mattress sling sutures.

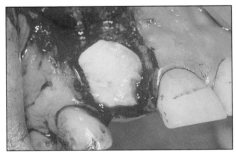

Fig 16-4f The connective tissue is placed over the grafted bone and below the overlying flap to supplement the deficiency in the original tissue.

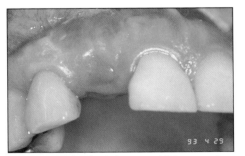

Fig 16-4g The healed area exhibits complete restoration of edentulous ridge architecture, which will be conducive to the placement of a single-tooth crown.

Delayed Implant Placement

If the area to be implanted is edentulous, tissue closure is not a surgical problem. Yet these areas are usually deficient in normal tissue dimensions as a result of previous extractions or trauma to the ridge and therefore may require augmentation. Because the intended site is scheduled for a two-stage surgery, it is suggested that tissue augmentation be anticipated at either of the surgical events to minimize a third surgical visit. A two-dimensional defect on the buccal aspect may be corrected at either stage 1 or stage 2 surgery

with a subepithelial connective tissue graft[13] placed on the buccal aspect of the ridge (Figs 16-5a to 16-5e).

If, however, the defect is also deficient occlusogingivally, then a connective tissue graft of thicker and longer dimensions is often necessary so that it may be draped over the alveolar ridge and lapped over from the buccal to the palatal aspects. This approach will help to provide adequate vascular nourishment to the coronal tissue covering the top of the implant, provide the necessary circulation to allow the crestal graft to survive, and thus offer additional coronal height (Figs 16-6a to 16-6c).

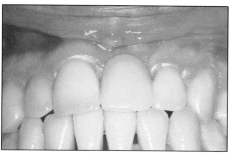

Fig 16-5a The edentulous ridge in the area of the maxillary left central incisor has a deficiency of tissue, creating the necessity for an elongated pontic.

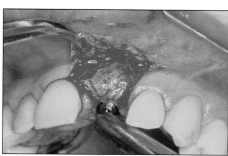

Fig 16-5b The underlying connective tissue over the implant is exposed.

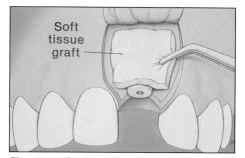

Fig 16-5c A connective tissue graft is placed over the central portion of the implant to create the illusion that there is a root prominence.

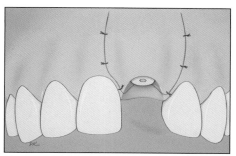

Fig 16-5d The overlying flap is coapted over the graft and sutured.

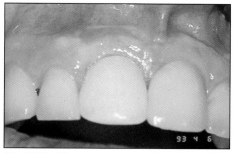

Fig 16-5e Two-year postoperative view of the final crown, which appears to be supported by a root prominence. (Courtesy of Dr L. Calagna.)

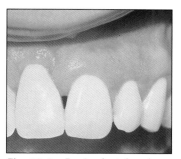

Fig 16-6a An implant has been placed; however, the gingival heights are uneven, creating an unsightly result.

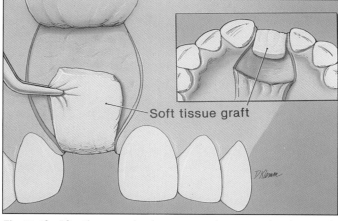

Fig 16-6b After the crown has been removed, a connective tissue graft is placed from the buccal to the palatal surface in an attempt to rebuild height of tissue.

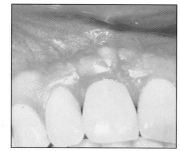

Fig 16-6c Gingival height has been restored, and a new crown has been placed on the implant in harmony with the adjacent tooth. (Courtesy of Dr D. Sullivan and Dr M. Stiglitz.)

If the first attempt does not fulfill the necessary esthetic requirements, an additional grafting procedure will be necessary before the uncovering stage. Exposure of the cover screw and/or placement of an abutment often will preclude additional grafting in tissue height. Should an abutment be in place, it is advisable to remove it and place either the cover screw or a space screw so that the titanium surface occupies the least area that would interfere with the vascular nourishment of the graft.

Spontaneous In Situ Gingival Augmentation

Recently a new approach has been developed that may stimulate the body to manufacture gingival tissue around a tooth scheduled for extraction.[14] This is intended to facilitate the surgical procedure for the clinician and the patient by reducing the need or the amount of extra tissue necessary to cover the newly placed implant in a fresh extraction site.

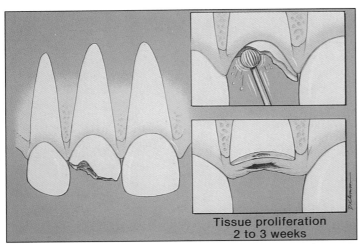

Fig 16-7 Tooth scheduled for extraction because of a fracture. The root is reduced to well below the free gingival margin.

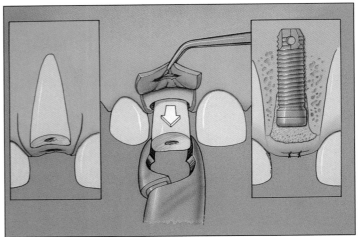

Fig 16-8 After approximately 2 to 3 weeks, the flap is elevated from the palatal line angle to the buccal, and the residual root is extracted. At that visit, the implant may be inserted with minimum tissue augmentation.

The tooth scheduled for extraction is reduced to the level of the free gingival margin. Then either a round bur or a safe-sided bur is used to reduce the remaining portion of the root below the free gingival margin of the gingiva to a level approximately 3 to 4 mm subcrestally. Care is taken to avoid unnecessary trauma to the surrounding tissue, which could ultimately cause permanent tissue damage. The perimeter of the tooth must be removed entirely so that the only tissue that is visible to the naked eye is gingival sulcus or bone and periodontal ligament (Fig 16-7).

A provisional prosthesis is fabricated in advance and inserted at this reduction visit. This might be a fixed or a removable partial prosthesis or even a complete denture. If the tooth in question is nonvital, nothing other than the reduction of the crown is necessary; however, if the tooth is vital, the residual root must receive either a pulp extirpation or simple pulp capping.

The patient is allowed to remain in this condition for a minimum of 3 to 4 weeks before the surgical visit. At this visit, the remaining root will be almost completely covered with a relatively thick layer of keratinized gingival tissue. There may be a residual opening in the tissue above the pulp chamber of the submerged tooth; however, this does not affect the ease of tissue manipulation.

The surgical flap is incised, starting from the palatal line angle, and this crestal tissue is incorporated into the buccal flap. The remaining buccal flap is elevated as in other stage 1 procedures. The remaining root is extracted and the implant is inserted (Fig 16-8). Membranes, bone grafts, and accessory tissue grafts can be added to the surgical site. The flap is coapted over the top of the implant and sutured to the palatal flap. The small opening at the crest of the tissue will be closed in most instances by simply suturing the flaps together. In some instances, small accessory sutures may be advisable to obtain complete closure.

In most cases, flap advancement or tissue grafts are not required to obtain complete closure. There will usually be an abundance of self-generated tissue to allow the surgeon to easily coapt the tissue. This will enhance the ability of complete tissue closure over membranes in the cases of immediate extraction and implant placement. The technique has also been extremely useful in patients who must wear complete dentures immediately after the implant procedure because the restorative dentist has the opportunity to fit the denture properly before the teeth are extracted and the implants are placed. The amount of relining is minimized because there is less tissue distortion between preoperative and postoperative visits. The reduction in tissue damage and proliferation of new tissue only enhances the gingival profile and the final esthetics (Figs 16-9a to 16-9e).

Peri-implant Tissue

Peri-implant tissue can be keratinized and firmly attached or movable mucosa. Most clinicians will agree that the patients have an easier task of cleaning the implant if they are brushing keratinized gingiva rather than movable mucosa. Yet it is not crucial that the tissue be keratinized for the health of the bone adjacent to the implant.

The simplest approach to maintaining keratinized tissue is to preserve it during either stage 1 or stage 2 surgery.[15,16] The placement procedure may help to retain or increase the amount of keratinized tissue. The uncovering visit may do

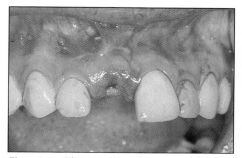

Fig 16-9a The maxillary right central incisor, scheduled for extraction, had been reduced approximately 3 mm subgingivally. Tissue has proliferated over the residual root.

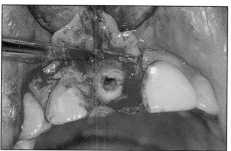

Fig 16-9b The flap is elevated from the palatal line angle, exposing the remaining root.

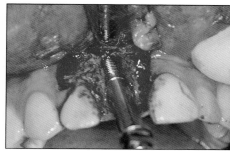

Fig 16-9c At the time of extraction, the implant is placed. A large defect present on the buccal surface was grafted with demineralized freeze-dried bone and a membrane.

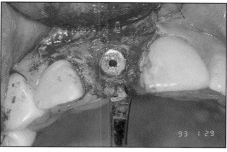

Fig 16-9d At the uncovering stage, the bone has filled the buccal dehiscence, which helps to restore the buccal profile.

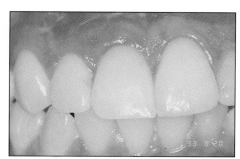

Fig 16-9e The final restoration blends into the profile of the adjacent teeth.

the same. It is customary to use a partial-thickness dissection flap on the buccal aspect rather than a punch procedure to locate the buried implant. This will allow the surgeon the flexibility to reposition the keratinized tissue to the desired position around the implant. Keratinized tissue may be borrowed from adjacent locations for areas that are deficient. Positioning tissue laterally or coronally by the use of pedicle or apically repositioned flaps at the uncovering stage avoids the need for additional surgery.

If, however, the area in question is totally devoid of keratinized tissue and it is desired for cosmetics or patient comfort, the most effective approach to create this tissue is the use of the autogenous tissue graft.[17] This is taken from the external surface of the palate. The donor site is prepared by taking a thin complex of epithelium and connective tissue of the same approximate dimensions as the recipient site. Rugae should be avoided because they will reappear at the recipient site and are unsightly. Interrupted suturing at the coronal and lateral borders is more than adequate to immobilize the graft for successful survival.

The most common error made in creating keratinized tissue with this technique is the failure to remove elastic and muscle fibers at the recipient site, resulting in an island of keratinized tissue that is not firmly attached to the underlying bone. This tissue is virtually useless and no better than alveolar mucosa. Another problem encountered is in patients with severe alveolar atrophy. There is virtually no vestibular fold because the residual alveolar ridge and floor of the mouth are at the same level.

Either vestibuloplasty or autogenous tissue grafting may achieve a desired result but is not always long lasting. Failure to achieve an optimum tissue border for the implant prior to the uncovering will certainly complicate a desirable result because the creation of attached keratinized tissue at this stage becomes more difficult and often impossible. The long-term survival of the bone around the implant may not be dramatically affected by the peri-implant tissue; however, the cosmetic acceptance and comfort to the patient for the life of the implant may relate to its soft tissue environment.

References

1. Brånemark P-I, Zarb GA, Albrektsson T (eds). Tissue-Integrated Prostheses: Osseointegration in Clinical Dentistry. Chicago: Quintessence, 1985:222.

2. Buser D, Dula K, Belser U, Dury HP, Bertold H. Localized ridge augmentation using guided bone regeneration. I. Surgical procedure in the maxilla. Int J Periodont Rest Dent 1993;13:29.

3. Bahat O, Koplin LM. Pantographic lip expansion and bone grafting for ridge expansion. Int J Periodont Rest Dent 1989;5:345.

4. Nevins M, Mellonig JT. Enhancement of the damaged edentulous ridge to receive dental implants: A combination of allograft and the Gore-Tex membrane. Int J Periodont Rest Dent 1992;12:97.

5. Dahlin C, Sennerby L, Lekholm U, et al. Generation of new bone around titanium implants using a membrane technique: An experimental study in rabbits. Int J Oral Maxillofac Implants 1989;4:19.

6. Lazzarra RJ. Immediate implant placement into extraction sites: Surgical and restorative advantages. Int J Periodont Rest Dent 1989;9:333–343.

7. Becker W, Becker B. Guided tissue regeneration for implants placed into extraction sockets and implant dehiscences: Surgical techniques and case reports. Int J Periodont Rest Dent 1990;10:377.

8. Gelb D. Immediate implant surgery: Three year retrospective evaluation of 50 consecutive cases. Int J Oral Maxillofac Implants 1993;8:388–399.

9. Langer B, Calagna L. Subepithelial connective tissue graft. J Prosthet Dent 1980;44:363.

10. Langer B, Calagna L. Subepithelial connective tissue graft: A new approach to the enhancement of anterior cosmetics. Int J Periodont Rest Dent 1982;2:23.

11. Abrams L. Augmentation of the deformed residual edentulous ridge for fixed prostheses. Compend Contin Educ Dent 1980;1:205.

12. Tarnow DP, Scharf DR. Modified roll technique for localized alveolar ridge augmentation. Int J Periodont Rest Dent 1992;12:415.

13. Langer B. Dental implants used for periodontal patients. J Am Dent Assoc 1990;121:505–508.

14. Langer B. Spontaneous in situ gingival augmentation. Int J Periodont Rest Dent 1995;14:525–535.

15. Langer B, Langer L. The overlapped flap: A surgical modification for implant fixture installation. Int J Periodont Rest Dent 1990;10:209.

16. Langer B, Sullivan D. Osseointegration. I. Its impact on the interrelationship of periodontics and restorative dentistry. Int J Periodont Rest Dent 1989;9:85.

17. Nabers JM. Free gingival grafts. Periodontics 1966;4:243.

CHAPTER 17

The Need for Keratinized Tissue for Implants

Yoshihiro Ono, DDS

Myron Nevins, DDS

Emil G. Cappetta, DMD

The early focus of implant research and treatment addressed the bone-implant interface, the quality and quantity of bone available for surgical procedures, and prosthetic design. This chapter will discuss the need for keratinized tissue for implants as it corresponds to the attached gingiva for natural teeth and its natural role in the long-term maintenance of implant health. No direct evidence is available to confirm an improved prognosis for implants with gingiva,[1] and there is every reason to believe that dental implants can exist and function in health in the absence of keratinized tissue.[2,3] Long-term retrospective evidence is indicative of exceptional survival of implants in the edentulous jaw, but does not address the esthetic and functional issues essential to the partially dentate patient.[2,4]

Osseointegrated dental implants were initially supplied as an alternative to complete edentulism and the problems inherent in ill-fitting dentures and atrophic jaws. The early generations of hybrid dentures were considerably elevated from the soft tissues and allowed for easy access for oral hygiene. The atrophic jaws usually had a paucity of keratinized tissue, and long-term observation seemed to indicate no need to enhance the gingival dimension. These early cases established the efficacy of osseointegration for implants, which continued to fulfill the patient's masticatory and psychological needs.

The partially dentate patient emerged as a candidate for osseointegration coincidentally with the training of North American dentists. These patients generally were not dental cripples, and their criteria for success encompassed more than implant survival. The restoration of function and psychological improvement continued to be important, but esthetics catapulted to the forefront. It became unacceptable to deliver the implant prosthesis on titanium "stilts." The evolution of abutment changes and designs that commenced allowed resolution of this obstacle but introduced new issues. The restorative margins approached or entered the soft tissues, and new inflammatory challenges emerged. The patient's appreciation of the dental correction diminished, and many partially dentate patients retreated to old habits and patterns of oral health care. Even the edentulous hybrid prostheses have been upgraded to fulfill esthetic and phonetic expectations and are much more difficult to cleanse.

Rationale for Mucogingival Augmentation Around Implants

The new paradigm of implant treatment has forced the issue of the need for attached gingiva to surround dental implants. Many factors must be considered in deciding whether the width of the keratinized tissue around the natural teeth is adequate. Traditional periodontal therapy is performed at sites at risk for mucogingival problems or sites at which problems have already occurred. In implant therapy, however, it is difficult to treat problems that occur after the implant is functioning.[4] It is not possible to achieve root coverage, as in the case of natural teeth, and the efficacy of regenerative therapy to restore lost supporting bone is limited. Therefore, in the case of implant therapy, it is reasonable to acquire an adequate width of keratinized gingiva *before* the placement of fixtures or at the time of second-stage surgery.

Factors To Consider When Determining If Attached Gingiva Around Natural Teeth Is Adequate

- Presence or absence of inflammation
- Degree and duration of gingival recession
- Patient's oral hygiene and compliance
- Relationship between gingiva and alveolar bone
- Tooth position
- Presence or absence of restorations
- Problems of esthetics or hypersensitivity

There has been much debate and some investigation of this question. Some studies demonstrate that implants will survive in the absence of keratinized gingiva,[2,3,5,6] while others say the presence of attached keratinized tissue is desirable and in fact necessary.[6–19]

Margins of keratinized attached gingiva have been advocated in the presence of tooth-supported restorations to reduce the possibility of radicular recession of soft tissue. The value of tissue augmentation to offset limitations in patient compliance has been noted even in the nonrestored dentition. There are few reports of recession of gingival tissue around implants, but the number of implants with cervical inflammation and early bone loss is of concern. Thus, it would seem reasonable to prepare the strongest possible environment to offset the likelihood of future problems. A complete lack of gingiva results in a mucosal margin that would be more likely to be retractable and to collect plaque, especially under the large hybrid dentures placed in atrophic patients.[18]

It seems rational to augment keratinized tissue to develop a tight adaptation to the implant and provide connective tissue that can form the circumferential fiber system needed to maintain a resistance to pull or deflection from the abutment surface and enhance a tight marginal seal.[16] Anterior implant restorations benefit esthetically from gingival augmentation, which helps to render the restoration inconspicuous.[17] Esthetic blending is possible and desirable in the partially edentulous patient, not only in the dimension of tissue available but also in the bulk of tissue. The presence of keratinized gingiva surrounding implants has several clinical advantages:

1. It facilitates impression making by the restorative dentist.
2. The tissues are less likely to collapse over the head of the implant.
3. The gingival height is maintained at a consistent level.
4. It provides a tight collar around the implant, which may be important in providing a fibrous "attachment" to the implant, as well as preventing trauma from plaque control procedures, especially if an implant thread becomes exposed.
5. It facilitates maintenance procedures by the hygienist.

A review of previous statements and conclusions provides support for interventive mucogingival surgery for dental implants. Restriction of gingival movement around implants seems important; hence it is recommended that dental implants emerge through keratinized mucosa because such implants are easier to maintain and more resistant to mechanical stress.[7–10,18–20] This is particularly important for implants in the posterior part of the mandible.[10] The clinical observation that inflamed peri-implant tissues tend to demonstrate a difference in probe penetration has been confirmed histologically.[21]

Poor oral hygiene and inadequate attached gingiva have been identified as the culprits in a substantial number of failures on long-term observation.[13,14] The presence of keratinized gingiva promotes resistance to mechanical trauma during oral hygiene exercises.[11,14,18] When movement of the buccal mucosa extends to the margin of the implant, it may lead to attachment loss, especially in those patients with severe mandibular atrophy in whom there is retraction of the lip and tongue.[18] The interdental brush is a very effective tool for the patient but is considerably less comfortable to use in the presence of alveolar mucosa and in the absence of a vestibule. The patient who is less than totally compliant will be less prone to follow instructions if oral hygiene procedures lead to discomfort and/or damage to the tissue. Although the rationale has been provided for the partially dentate patient, it may be the atrophic edentulous patient with a bulky prosthesis who presents the most difficult debridement problem. From the perspective of oral hygiene, which is indispensable to the long-term health of implants, adequate keratinized gingiva surrounding implants is desirable, because mucositis can often be intercepted by the early detection of soft tissue problems.[13,15,18] Schroeder et al[11] and Listgarten et al[19] state that it is preferable to locate implants within the masticatory mucosa because implants surrounded by movable mucosa may favor the disruption of the implant-epithelial junction and the development of inflammatory changes, especially for implant-supported dentures.

It has been reported that mobility of the marginal tissue and an inadequate width of masticatory mucosa have little significance for the health of the soft tissues of dental implants. A lack of masticatory mucosa does not impede oral hygiene, but it is noted that bleeding on probing, swelling, and redness occur in areas with less than 2 mm of masticatory mucosa. The quality of peri-implant mucosa may influence the apical spread of the inflammatory lesion, and peri-implant tissues may be more vulnerable than periodontal tissues to the spread of a plaque-induced lesion.[4]

The orientation of the supracrestal collagen fibers in the mucosa surrounding implants may be influenced by the mobility of the mucosa and the surface characteristics of the supracrestal portion of the implant.[19] Implants anchored in keratinized mucosa display horizontal connective tissue fibers that are perpendicularly arranged to the implant surface. The orientation of fibers around implants placed in nonkeratinized mucosa is predominantly parallel to the implant surface. It has been speculated that the maintenance and stability of function of the load-bearing implant are enhanced by a well-functioning barrier mechanism established at the transmucosal passage of the implant.[22]

It has been repeatedly postulated that the establishment of circumferential seal by a dense connective tissue collar at the site of implant penetration into the contaminated environment of the oral cavity is a prerequisite for long-term success of the implant.[6] This has not been substantiated in clinical or experimental studies.

Several efforts comparing the presence of bacterial pathogens in the sulcular area of dental implants placed in edentulous and partially edentulous patients have recorded a greater problem in the latter patients.[23–30] Colonies of periodontal pathogens were found in the sulci of implants in periodontally compromised patients. Crevicular fluid flow and the microbiota around implants were similar to the flow and the traditional periodontal pathogens found in the sulci of teeth.[30] The partially edentulous implant patient would seem to be at greater risk of peri-implant problems as a result of exposure to bacteria from sulci surrounding natural teeth. Some clinicians believe that, in the presence of adequate oral hygiene, the marginal tissues are commonly clinically healthy, even with nonkeratinized peri-implant mucosa, and that plaque and marginal inflammation do not appear to be related to the quality of the surrounding mucosa.[1]

One study has indicated a clear difference in the progression of plaque-induced peri-implant lesions at sites with nonkeratinized tissues and sites with keratinized tissues. Implants surrounded by mucosa demonstrate a higher susceptibility to tissue inflammation and destruction.[6] The amount of bone-implant contact is smaller in sites without keratinized tissue, indicating that keratinized mucosal tissue has a protective role as a tissue seal around implants.

In a 10-year study of 3,088 IMX implants, Kirsch and Ackerman[7] found that 61 implants were removed primarily because of soft tissue complications. Their conclusion was that "most notably insufficient mucogingival attachment or insufficient width of attached gingiva contributed to their failure."

Anatomy of the Oral Soft Tissues

The soft tissues through which transmucosal devices such as teeth and implants emerge function as an integument to seal the aseptic supporting structures from the oral sepsis. The barrier system is composed of a dense collagenous lamina propria, which is covered by stratified squamous keratinized oral epithelium that is continuous with the nonkeratinized sulcular epithelium that surrounds the implant as it emerges into the oral cavity. This sulcular epithe-lium is continuous with the junctional epithelium, which is attached to the teeth by hemidesmosomes and to implants in a similar fashion.[31–33]

The underlying connective tissue surrounding a tooth is composed of the gingival fiber complex, which attaches circumferentially via Sharpey's fibers, which engage the cemental surface. These supracrestal fibers are oriented perpendicular to the tooth surface and occupy approximately 1 mm of space between the crest of the alveolar process and the junctional epithelium.

The connective tissue surrounding dental implants does not demonstrate attachment to the implant surface and therefore only adheres to it. It has been suggested that the fiber orientation is influenced by the surface characteristics[11] and the mobility of the soft tissues.[9,19] Also, the attached gingiva and alveolar mucosa demonstrate a difference in fiber orientation; there is some tendency toward a perpendicular orientation in the gingiva.[6] Berglundh et al[22] confirmed that the fiber orientation is parallel to smooth implant surfaces, whereas Ruggieri et al[34,35] confirmed that alignment is more perpendicular with rougher surfaces. The size of the connective tissue adherence is a factor of the thickness of the soft tissues and the apical extension of the epithelium.

There is little evidence in the human to support a conclusion as to the value of the soft tissue attachment to the implant. The relationship between natural teeth and mucogingival tissues cannot be readily applied to implants. Tissues that have few blood vessels but are abundant in fibers are likely to be more resistant to inflammation because inflammation is a periovascular phenomenon. It would follow that a dense, relatively avascular tissue would offer greater resistance; therefore, it is advantageous and rational to have keratinized gingiva for long-term maintenance of this kind of weak adhesion.[36,37] The goal is a soft tissue resistant to abrasion, anchored to underlying bone, and dense enough to provide a cufflike seal or barrier via circular fibers to act as a protective barrier to inflammation.[16]

Clinical Significance of Attached Gingiva

- Prevents spread of inflammation to deep tissue (is less vascular)
- May prevent recession of marginal gingiva
- Prevents excessive movement of free gingiva
- Resists damage from brushing

If, in fact, implants require an adequate dimension of keratinized gingiva, how can the dimension be determined? Corrective therapy is reserved for areas considered to be at risk or for those teeth that have already demonstrated the need for correction. The criteria for teeth are more stringent when restorative margins approach the soft tissues, when orthodontics is required, or in the presence of frenum attachments. In implant therapy, however, it is difficult to

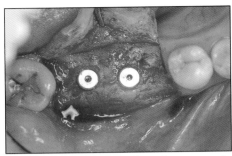

Fig 17-1a Two implants have been properly positioned in the mandibular molar region.

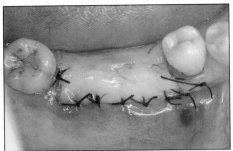

Fig 17-1b The incision was made in the mucobuccal fold and reflected lingually. There is an adequate dimension of attached keratinized tissue on the lingual, buccal, and occlusal surfaces of the ridge.

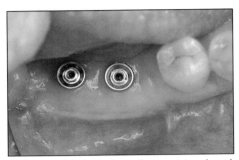

Fig 17-1c Implants have been retrieved and permanent abutments have been placed. Note the dimension of attached keratinized tissue on the buccal aspect.

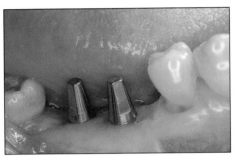

Fig 17-1d The permanent abutments are in place.

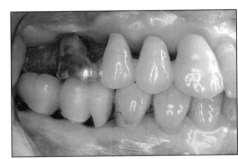

Fig 17-1e The final prosthesis has been placed.

treat problems that occur after the implant is functioning. It is not possible to achieve root coverage with connective tissue attachment, as it is in the case of natural teeth.[38,39] Therefore, it is apparent that early intervention is justified and it is appropriate to provide a significant zone of keratinized tissue before a prosthesis is completed. Such a policy is certainly unlikely to be detrimental.

In the case of natural teeth, emphasis is placed on the relationship between the thickness of the alveolar bone and the width of the attached gingiva. This diagnostic criterion is also useful in the case of implants. Mucogingival problems have a predilection for sites where the alveolar bone is thin on the buccal and lingual sides of the implant and there is little keratinized gingiva. When the margin of the restoration of natural teeth is to be placed below the gingival margin, Maynard and Ochsenbein prefer 5 mm of keratinized gingiva (2 mm of free gingiva and 3 mm of attached gingiva).[40]

This same criterion can be applied to implants. In natural teeth, gingival inflammation frequently occurs when the restoration is placed subgingivally. It is desirable to have at least 5 mm of keratinized gingiva for implants because the connective tissue attachment to the tooth is not well defined.

Classification of Attached Gingiva

The dimension of attached gingiva at the proposed implant site must be evaluated before fixture placement to determine whether it should be enhanced. Some clinical situations require no surgical intervention because an adequate zone of attached keratinized tissue is present (Figs 17-1a to 17-1e). The timing and method of mucogingival surgery will be a reflection of the quantity and location of existing keratinized gingiva. The following classification is suggested, based on the amount of keratinized gingiva at the proposed implant site. (Figs 17-2a to 17-2c).

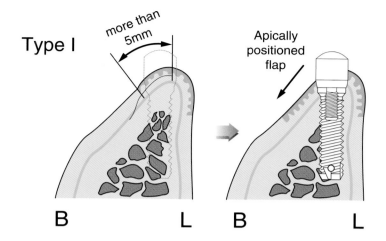

Fig 17-2a In a type I case, the flap can be apically repositioned to increase the zone of keratinized tissue on the facial aspect.

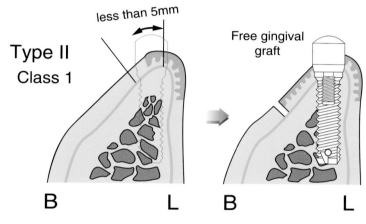

Fig 17-2b In a class I of type 2 case, there is minimal keratinized tissue on the ridge but little to none on the facial aspect. A gingival graft is recommended to increase the zone of keratinized tissue.

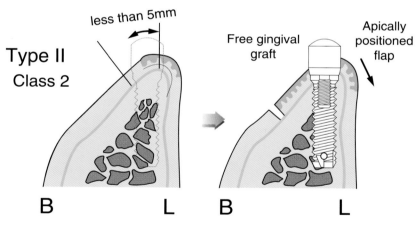

Fig 17-2c In a class II of type 2 case, most keratinized gingiva will be eliminated at the lingual site if the gingiva is festooned around the implants. A gingival graft is performed on the buccal site with an apically positioned flap on the lingual site to increase the zone of keratinized tissue on both aspects.

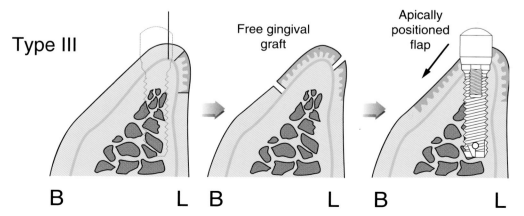

Fig 17-2d In a type 3 case, there is no attached keratinized tissue on the ridge or facial aspect. A gingival graft is used to increase the zone of keratinized tissue.

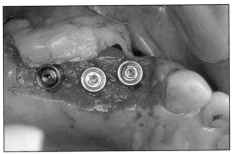

Fig 17-3a In a type I case, it is possible to apically position the tissue from the crest of the ridge along with the keratinized tissue that was present on the labial or buccal surface.

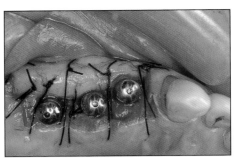

Fig 17-3b Healing abutments have been placed. The tissue is sutured into position, increasing the zone of attached keratinized tissue on the buccal aspect of all three implants.

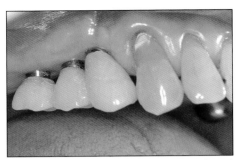

Fig 17-3c Implants have been retrieved and permanent abutments have been placed. Note the dimension of attached keratinized tissue on the buccal aspect.

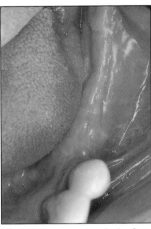

Fig 17-4a There is a lack of attached keratinized tissue on the buccal surface. Implants have already been placed, and this is the second stage of implant surgery.

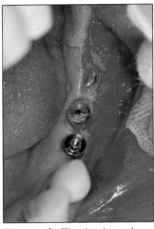

Fig 17-4b The implants have been uncovered, and abutments are being placed. The tissue bed is now prepared to accept the gingival graft.

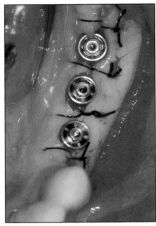

Fig 17-4c The gingival graft is sutured into position.

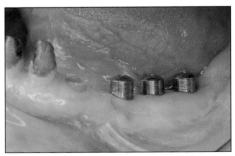

Fig 17-4d The area of the graft is shown 4 months postoperatively.

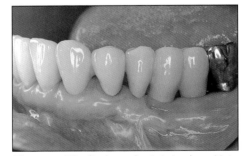

Fig 17-4e The final prosthesis is in place. Note the increase in vestibular depth and the increase in the zone of attached keratinized tissue along the facial aspect of the implant restoration.

Type 1. There is a minimum of 5 mm of keratinized gingiva covering the edentulous ridge from the lingual or palatal tangent to the buccal side of the proposed implant site (Figs 17-3a to 17-3c).

Type 2. There is keratinized gingiva on the top of the edentulous ridge and at the lingual or palatal tangent to the proposed implant site (Figs 17-4 to 17-6).

Class I. There is enough lingual keratinized gingiva at the site of the proposed implant.

Class II. Most keratinized gingiva will be eliminated at the lingual site if the gingiva is festooned around the implants.

Type 3. Keratinized gingiva of the alveolar ridge is present only on the lingual or palatal side of the proposed implant site (Figs 17-7 and 17-8).

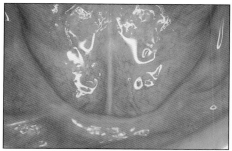

Fig 17-5a Type 2 class I mandibular anterior ridge prior to uncovering of the fixtures. Keratinized gingiva is present on the top and on the lingual surface of the alveolar ridge.

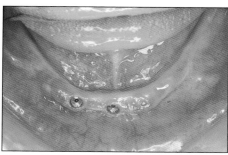

Fig 17-5b At second-stage surgery, the fixtures will be uncovered and a gingival graft will be placed on the facial surface.

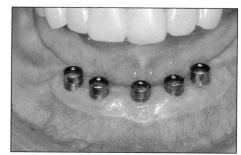

Fig 17-5c The implants have been uncovered. Final abutments have been placed. An adequate dimension of attached keratinized tissue is present on the ridge, as well as on the facial surface.

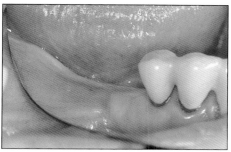

Fig 17-6a Type 2 (class II) case. There is little keratinized tissue remaining on the ridge or the buccal aspect. A gingival graft is needed to increase the zone of the keratinized tissue.

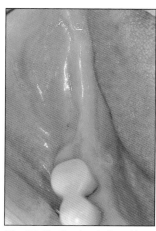

Fig 17-6b Occlusal view. Note the dimension of keratinized gingiva on the lingual surface.

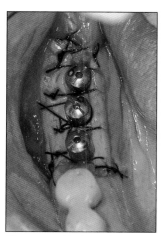

Fig 17-6c Healing abutments were placed at the second-stage surgery. A gingival graft was applied to the buccal surface. An apically positioned flap was performed on the lingual aspect at the same time.

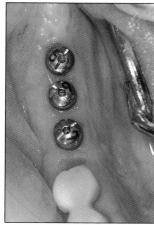

Fig 17-6d Three months after the secondary surgery, there is an increase in the zone of keratinized tissue along the buccal and lingual aspects.

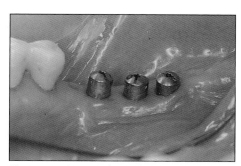

Fig 17-6e Increased vestibular depth and a zone of keratinized tissue are present on the lingual aspect, 4 months after the secondary surgery (lingual view).

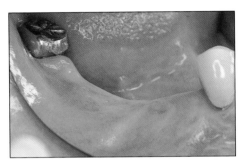

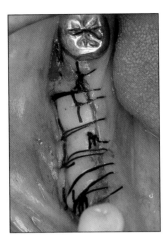

Fig 17-7a Two months after placement of the fixtures, there is no attached gingiva on the buccal or occlusal surface of the edentulous ridge (type 3).

Fig 17-7b A gingival graft has been placed on the top of the edentulous ridge and the facial surface.

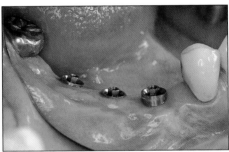

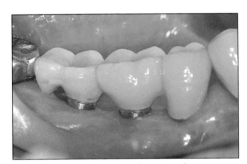

Fig 17-7c The implants have been uncovered 6 months after their placement and 4 months after the gingival graft.

Fig 17-7d The final prosthesis in place.

Procedure for Mucogingival Augmentation Around Implants

Gingival augmentation for implants can be accomplished with apically positioned flaps, free gingival grafts (strip or traditional design), de-epithelialized pedicle grafts, free connective grafts, or a variation of a "roll technique."[16,17] At second-stage surgery, the surgeon should consider the following factors:

1. The acquisition of adequate width of keratinized gingiva
2. The adjustment of gingival thickness
3. The selection and insertion of appropriately sized abutments
4. The shaping of alveolar bone and soft tissue to enhance cleansability and maintainability

An apically positioned flap is used to obtain keratinized gingiva at the second-stage surgery for type 1 ridges. An internal beveled incision is made in the gingiva toward the buccal from the lingual location of the implant, forming a partial-thickness flap. The 5 mm or more of keratinized gingiva is positioned apically to the buccal tangent of the implant. The buccal flap is elevated, and any tissue over the cover screws is removed. The appropriate abutment is connected, and the flap is sutured apically to the periosteum so that the coronal margin of the flap does not extend onto the abutment. This surgical technique makes it possible to augment keratinized gingiva around implants by utilizing existing keratinized gingiva.

For type 2 and type 3 ridges, a free gingival autograft is the procedure of choice because an inadequate amount of keratinized gingiva is available for an apically positioned flap. An internal beveled incision is made at the mucogingival junction, and the mucosa is removed from the buccal surface. The recipient site is prepared to receive a gingival graft. This can be accomplished at the time of second-stage surgery or between the first- and second-stage surgeries. The authors suggest the placement of the free gingival graft 2 to 3 months after implant placement in all type 2 and type 3 cases.

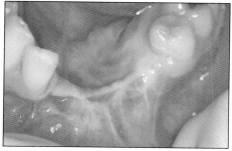

Fig 17-8a The teeth and a substantial portion of the alveolar process were lost in an automobile accident. There is minimal keratinized tissue on the ridge and no keratinized tissue along the facial aspect. The implants are in place, and the gingival augmentation procedure is performed before the second-stage surgery.

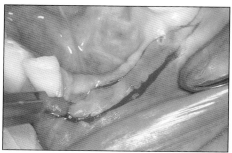

Fig 17-8b The recipient site is prepared to accept the gingival graft. The lingual portion of the alveolar process was lost to trauma, and the implants are positioned buccally.

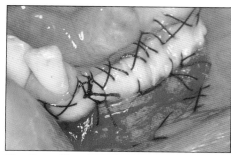

Fig 17-8c The gingival graft has been sutured into position.

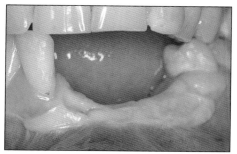

Fig 17-8d The area is shown 6 weeks postoperatively.

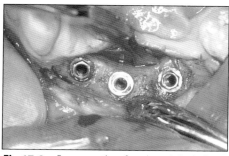

Fig 17-8e Four months after the original placement of the fixtures, the implants have been uncovered.

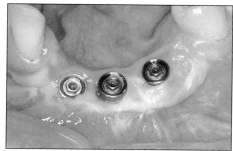

Fig 17-8f The tissues have healed with the permanent abutments in place. Compare the increased dimension of keratinized tissue to that shown in Fig 17-8a.

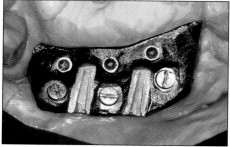

Fig 17-8g Try-in of the waxed base. Attachments are included to receive the superstructure.

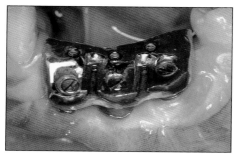

Fig 17-8h Try-in of the completed cast frame. Note the horizontal dovetail for lateral lock. The frame is screw retained to the implants, and there are screw holes to receive the superstructure. Note the space provided to clean the prosthesis.

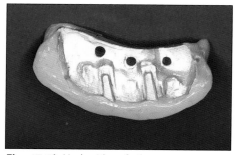

Fig 17-8i Underside of the superstructure. Note the internal anatomy of the casting, including the horizontal dovetails.

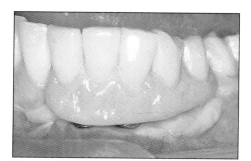

Fig 17-8j The final restoration is in place. (Prosthesis courtesy of Dr James Stein.)

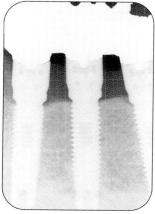

Fig 17-8k After the prosthesis has been in place for 7 years, there is no evidence of bone loss.

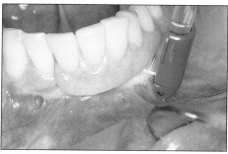

Fig 17-8l The patient is instructed in the use of the interdental brush, which fits beneath the prosthesis.

Conclusion

It must be reiterated that there is no direct evidence of the need for attached gingiva to establish long-term success of dental implants. However, there is room for clinical opinion expressed by an ever-growing population of experienced individuals. The possible benefits include esthetic blending for the partially edentulous patient, the ease of surgical management, the presence of less retractable tissues, and a reduction in plaque accumulation. The recognition of the presence of periodontal pathogens in the sulci of the partially edentulous patient underscores that these people are at risk. This, in combination with the poor compliance records of periodontal patients, suggests that the balance is favored toward implementation of mucogingival surgical enhancement for dental implants. The only negative factors are financial obstacles and the endurance of minor surgical procedures.

References

1. Schou S, Holmstrup P, Hjørting-Hansen E, Lang NP. Plaque-induced marginal tissue reactions of osseointegrated oral implants: A review of the literature. Clin Oral Implants Res 1992;3:149.

2. Adell R, Lekholm U, Rockler B, Brånemark P-I. A 15 year study of osseointegrated implants in the treatment of the edentulous jaw. Int J Oral Surg 1981;10:387–416.

3. Albrektsson T, Zarb G, Worthington P, Eriksson A. The long term efficacy of currently used dental implants: A review of proposed criteria of success. Int J Oral Maxillofac Implants 1986;1:11.

4. Wennström JL, Bengazi F, Lekholm U. The influence of the masticatory mucosa on the peri-implant soft tissue condition. Clin Oral Implants Res 1994;5:1.

5. Strub J, Gaberthuel T, Grunder U. The role of attached gingiva in the health of peri-implant tissue in dogs. Part 1. Clinical findings. Int J Periodont Rest Dent 1991;11:317–333.

6. Warrer K, Buser D, Lang NP, Karring T. Plaque-induced peri-implantitis in the presence or absence of keratinized mucosa: An experimental study in monkeys. Clin Oral Implants Res 1995;6:131.

7. Kirsch A, Ackerman KL. The IMZ osseointegrated implant system. Dent Clin North Am 1989;33:733–791.

8. Buser D, Weber HP, Brägger U. The treatment of partially edentulous patients with ITI hollow-screw implants: Presurgical evaluation and surgical procedures. Int J Oral Maxillofac Implants 1990;5:165–174.

9. Zarb GA, Schmitt A. The longitudinal clinical effectiveness of osseointegrated dental implants: The Toronto study. III. Problems and complications encountered. J Prosthet Dent 1990;64:185–194.

10. Block MS, Kent JN. Factors associated with soft and hard tissue compromise of endosseous implants. J Oral Maxillofac Surg 1990;48:1153–1160.

11. Schroeder A, van der Zypen E, Stich H, Sutter F. The reactions of bone, connective tissue, and epithelium to endosteal implants with titanium-sprayed surfaces. J Maxillofac Surg 1981;9:15–25.

12. McKenney RV, Steflick DE, Koth DL, Singh BB. The scientific basis for dental implant therapy. J Dent Educ 1988;52:696–705.

13. Simons A, Darany D, Giordano JR. The use of free gingival grafts in the treatment of peri-implant soft tissue complications—Clinical report. Implant Dent 1993;2:27.

14. Van Steenberghe D. Periodontal aspects of osseointegrated oral implants ad modem Brånemark. Dent Clin North Am 1988;32:355.

15. Worthington P, Bolender CD, Taylor TD. The Swedish system of osseointegrated implants: Problems and complications encountered during a 4 year trial period. Int J Oral Maxillofac Implants 1987;2:77–84.

16. Servor J. The use of free gingival grafts to improve the implant soft tissue interface: Rationale and technique. Pract Periodontics Aesthet Dent 1992;4:59.

17. Alpert A. Rationale for attached gingiva at the soft tissue/implant interface: Esthetic and functional dictates. Compend Contin Educ Dent 1994;20:356.

18. Rapley JW, Mills MP, Wylam Jr. Soft tissue management during implant maintenance. Int J Periodont Rest Dent 1992;12:373.

19. Listgarten MA, Lang HP, Schroeder HE, Schroeder A. Periodontal tissues and their counterparts around endosseous implants. Clin Oral Implants Res 1991;2.

20. Newman MG, Flemmig TF. Periodontal considerations of implants and implant-associated microbiota. J Dent Educ 1988;52:737–744.

21. Lang NP, Wetzel AC, Stich H, Caffesse RG. Histologic probe penetration in healthy and inflamed peri-implant tissues. Clin Oral Implants Res 1994;5:191–201.

22. Berglundth T, Lindhe J, Ericsson I, Marinello CP, Liljenberg B, Thomsen P. The soft tissue barrier at implants and teeth. Clin Oral Implants Res 1991;2:81.

23. Leonhardt A, Adolfsson B, Lekholm U, Wikstrom M, Dahlen G. A longitudinal microbiological study on osseointegrated titanium implants in partially edentulous patients. Clin Oral Implants Res 1993;4:113–120.

24. Leonhardt A, Berglundh T, Ericsson I, Dahlen G. Putative periodontal pathogens on titanium implants and teeth in experimental gingivitis and periodontitis in beagle dogs. Clin Oral Implants Res 1992;3:112–119.

25. Rosenberg ES, Torosian JP, Slots J. Microbial differences in two clinically distinct types of failure of osseointegrated implants. Clin Oral Implants Res 1991;2:135–144.

26. Rams TE, Roberts TW, Feik D, Molzan AK, Slots J. Clinical and microbiological findings on newly inserted hydroxyapatite-coated and pure titanium human dental implants. Clin Oral Implants Res 1991;2:121–127.

27. Mombelli A, Van Oosten MAC, Schurch E, Lang NP. The microbiota associated with successful or failing osseointegrated titanium implants. Oral Microbiol Immunol 1978;2:145–151.

28. Mombelli A, Merickse-Stern R. Microbiological features of stable osseointegrated implants used as abutments for overdentures. Clin Oral Implants Res 1990;1:1–7.

29. Quirynen M, Listgarten MA. The distribution of bacterial morphotypes around natural teeth and titanium implants ad modem Brånemark. Clin Oral Implants Res 1990;1:8–12.

30. Apse P, Ellen RP, Overall CM, Zarb GA. Microbiota and crevicular fluid collagenase activity in the osseointegrated dental implant sulcus: A comparison of sites in edentulous and partially edentulous patients. J Periodont Res 1989;24:96–105.

31. Gould TRL, Brunette DM, Westbury L. The attachment mechanism of epithelial cells to titanium in vitro. J Periodont Res 1981;16:611–616.

32. James RA, Schultz RL. Hemidesmosomes and the adhesion of junctional epithelial cells to metal implants: A preliminary report. J Oral Implantol 1973;4:294.

33. Listgarten M, Loll CH. Ultrastructure of the intact interface between and endosseous epoxy resin dental implant and the host tissues. J Biol Buccale 1975;4:13.

34. Ruggeri A, Franchi M, Marini N, Trisi P, Piatelli A. Supracrestal circular collagen fiber network around osseointegrated nonsubmerged titanium implants. Clin Oral Implants Res 1992;3:169–175.

35. Ruggeri A, Franchi M, Trisi P, Piatelli A. Histologic and ultrastructural findings of gingival circular ligament surrounding osseointegrated non-submerged loaded titanium implants. Int J Oral Maxillofac Implants 1994;9:636–643.

36. Kramer GM. In: Goldman HM, Cohen DW (eds). Periodontal Therapy, ed 6. St. Louis: Mosby, 1980.

37. Ruben MP. In: Goldman HM, Cohen DW (eds). Periodontal Therapy, ed 6. St. Louis: Mosby, 1980.

38. Han TJ, Klokkevold RP, Taher HH. Strip gingival autograft to correct mucogingival problems around implants. Int J Periodont Rest Dent 1995;15:405.

39. Pasquinelli K. The histology of new attachment utilizing a thick autogenous soft tissue graft in an area of deep recession: a case report. Int J Periodont Rest Dent 1995;15:249–257.

40. Maynard JG Jr, Wilson RDK. Physiologic dimensions of the periodontium significant to the restorative dentist. J Periodontol 1979; 50:170–174.

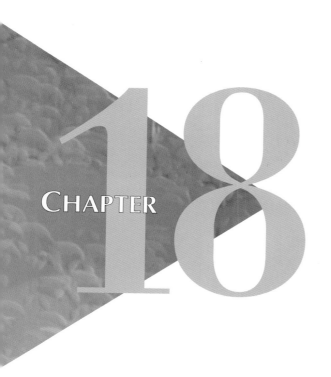
Implant Therapy for Patients With Refractory Periodontal Disease

James T. Mellonig, DDS, MS
Myron Nevins, DDS

Refractory periodontitis refers to disease in multiple sites in patients who continue to demonstrate attachment loss after apparently appropriate therapy (Figs 18-1a to 18-1d).[1] Patients with refractory periodontitis are also sometimes referred to as being *recalcitrant* or *downhill*.[2-6] These patients have a history of unsuccessful treatment, which usually consists of scaling and root planing, periodontal surgery, the use of tetracycline or other antibiotics, and regular periodontal maintenance recalls accompanied by progressive bone loss.[7-11]

The major reason for unsuccessful therapy in refractory periodontitis appears to be the inability of the clinician to eliminate a hidden reservoir of the causative organism in the soft tissues or on tooth surfaces inaccessible to mechanical instruments.[6,9,12-14] Other factors that may be responsible include poor oral hygiene, poor subgingival debridement, the patient's susceptibility, and a subgingival microflora resistant to therapy.[6] Some patients with refractory disease may exhibit a weakened periodontal defense that may allow even small numbers of pathogens to overwhelm the periodontium.[15] The most important factor appears to be that these are patients who are responsibly treated and observed but who have multiple sites that continue to demonstrate recurrent episodes of periodontal breakdown.[16,17]

Refractory periodontitis should not be confused with a recurring incidence of disease because of the lack of continued periodontal supportive care, or the presence of one or two "intractable" sites in an otherwise well-maintained patient.[17]

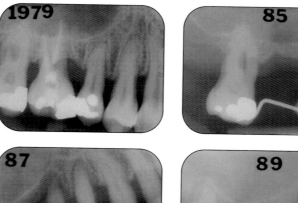

Fig 18-1a Posttreatment radiographic history of the continued loss of supporting structures that resulted in the loss of teeth (maxillary right posterior teeth).

be diagnosed longitudinally by careful monitoring of the   the gram-negative group

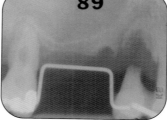

Fig 18-3d Final prosthesis in place together with the maxillary denture. (Prosthetics by Dr Howard M. Skurow.)

Chapter 18   Implant Therapy for Patients With Refractory Periodontal Disease

Chapter 18   Implant Therapy for Patients With Refractory Periodontal Disease

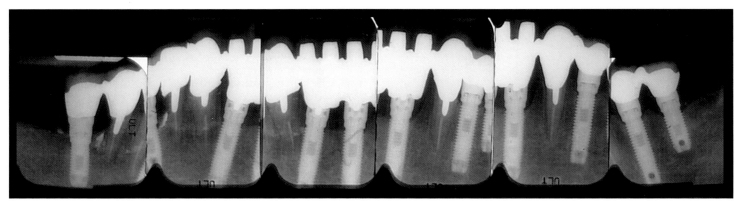

Fig 18-3e Updated mandibular radiographic survey (1995). There is very little change after 7 years.

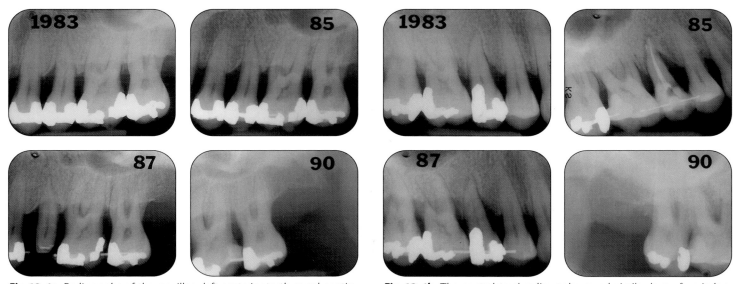

Fig 18-4a Radiographs of the maxillary left posterior teeth reveal continued loss of bone (1983 to 1990).

Fig 18-4b The contralateral radiographs reveal similar loss of periodontium.

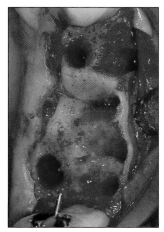
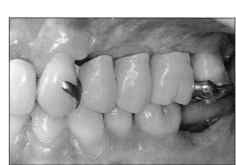
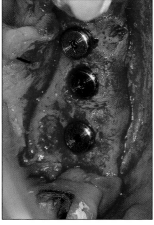
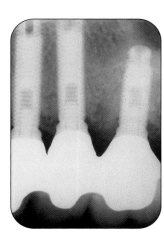

Fig 18-4c The two premolars and first molar have been extracted. The area was treated with mineralized bone allograft and a barrier membrane.

Fig 18-4d A resin-bonded fixed partial denture is used as the provisional prosthesis.

Fig 18-4e Three dental implants have been placed after a period of 8 months.

Fig 18-4f Five-year posttreatment radiograph.

A series of 196 subgingival microbial samples from refractory sites suggested that the most prevalent associated microbiota are, in descending order[19]:

1. *B forsythus* (84%)
2. spirochetes (83%)
3. motile rods (76%)
4. *Fusobacterium* spp (68%)
5. *P gingivalis* (63%)
6. *Campylobacter rectus* (47%)
7. *Capnocytophaga* spp (38%)
8. *P intermedia* (23%)
9. *Peptostreptococcus micros* (18%)
10. *A actinomycetemcomitans* (16%)
11. *Candida* (14%)
12. enteric rods (9%)
13. *Staphylococcus* spp, not including *S aureas* (5.6%)
14. *E corrodens* (3%)
15. *S aureas* (1.5%)
16. *Enterococcus* spp (less than 1%).

It is of interest that 19 of 21 subjects in one study[27] and 90% of subjects in another study[28] of refractory periodontitis had a history of smoking. Substantial data have identified tobacco smoking as a major risk factor for periodontitis.[38–41] Smoking may impair the outcome of periodontal therapy.[42] Smoking is also a significant risk factor for dental implants.[43] The success rate of 2,194 Brånemark implants placed in 540 patients over a 6-year period was 94%. It was found that a significantly greater percentage of failures occurred in smokers, and failure rates for each implant length were consistently higher in smokers than in nonsmokers.[43]

Bacterial Resistance

An antibiotic-resistant microbiota may also be an additional complicating factor in the patient with refractory periodontitis. Antimicrobial agents are often used in combination with subgingival debridement to eliminate the putative periodontal pathogens. The most frequently used antimicrobial agents are the tetracyclines.[44] As many as 75% of the bacteria in the subgingival flora may be resistant to tetracyclines after long-term, low-dose treatment,[44] and resistance is common in the patient with refractory sites.[17,45] In one study, 23% of the total cultivable subgingival flora was resistant to tetracycline.[46]

This resistance is not limited to tetracycline but also includes, to a lesser degree, penicillin, metronidazole, erythromycin, clindamycin, Keflex, dicloxacillin, and cephalosporin.[19,47] The results of a study of bacterial resistance in patients with refractory disease indicated that a substantial number of the microorganisms were resistant to commonly used antibiotics.[19] For this reason, it is advisable to perform antibiotic sensitivity tests when treating refractory disease.[6,33,34]

Treatment of the Patient With Refractory Disease

Treatment of refractory disease usually consists of additional scaling and root planing and further antibiotic therapy other than tetracycline. Clindamycin, Augmentin, and combination therapy with amoxicillin and metronidazole have been recommended. Other antibiotics, such as Temafloxin, a bone-seeking derivative of ciprofloxin, may also be effective in the treatment of resistant microbes.[47]

The findings of several studies[7,8,17,48,49] have indicated that clindamycin is useful in patients who do not respond to conventional treatment methods. Clindamycin is prescribed in a dose of 150 mg, four times a day, for 7 days. The adverse side effect of the most clinical significance is pseudomembranous enterocolitis, which is a serious gastrointestinal lesion that may result in diarrhea, abdominal cramps, fever, and leukocytosis. Therefore, clindamycin should be reserved for those patients for whom treatment modalities of lesser risk have been unsuccessful and in whom the subgingival flora is susceptible.

For selected patients, Augmentin may be the antibiotic of choice as an adjunct to scaling and root planing.[33] Augmentin consists of amoxicillin and potassium clavulanate, a potent β-lactamase inhibitor, and as such is effective against penicillin-resistant organisms. The antibiotic is administered systemically in a dose of 250 mg, three times daily, for 14 days. Collins et al[16] reported that the administration of Augmentin in conjunction with intrasulcular irrigation with povidone iodine, twice-daily chlorhexidine rinses, and repeated episodes of scaling and root planing is an effective treatment regimen for refractory periodontitis.

The combination of metronidazole, 250 mg, and amoxicillin, 250 mg, three times a day, for 7 days is also an effective treatment for refractory periodontitis, including cases that are resistant to tetracycline.[49,50] This combination is particularly effective in suppressing *A actinomycetemcomitans* in patients with refractory disease.[51]

Implants in the Patient With Refractory Disease

Unlike in the majority of general infections, in periodontal disease all the suspected pathogens are indigenous to the oral flora. Consequently, the long-term and total elimination of these microorganisms with antimicrobials will be very difficult to achieve because rapid repopulation with the indigenous bacteria will occur when therapy is concluded.[50] Therefore, it is not surprising that a significant number of patients with refractory disease require alternative modes of treatment.

It is not unusual for these patients to resist treatment with implants. They have already invested time, money, and emotion in an effort to maintain their teeth, and all efforts have proven unsuccessful. The routine, and expected, question is, "Why will implants be successful if my bone is not strong enough to support my teeth?"

There is a paucity of data regarding implants for the patient with refractory periodontal disease. Previous long-term studies have supported the efficacy of their use for tooth replacement in both the edentulous and partially edentulous patient (see Figs 18-1 to 18-4).[52–58] Jemt et al[53] reported on 876 consecutively placed implants in 244 patients over a 20-year period. Only four of 293 prostheses were lost, for a success rate of 98.7%. Similar results were documented by van Steenberghe.[55] Ericsson et al[59] demonstrated the success of osseointegrated fixtures in combination with natural teeth to support a fixed prosthesis (see Figs 18-3a to 18-3e). The success of using osseointegrated fixtures to replace missing posterior teeth has also been reported.[57,58]

However, Jaffin and Berman[60] reported on the efficacy of osseointegrated implants in a population that offers a specific factor that could offset routine success. They identified the quality of bone and reported a significant failure rate (35%) for jaws that were judged to contain poor trabeculation. Others disagree that the quality of bone limits success because short fixtures appear to support prostheses successfully when a rational functional load is applied.[57,58]

A study was undertaken to measure the efficacy of osseointegration for the treatment of the patient with refractory disease.[61] This study included 10 maxillary and 11 mandibular edentulous jaws and 33 maxillary and 27 mandibular partially edentulous jaws of 59 patients whose implants were placed over a 7-year period (Figs 18-5a and 18-5b). These individuals constituted less than 0.5% of the total treated periodontal patient population, and their overall periodontal regimens ranged from 2 to 27 years.

Efforts were made to develop treatment plans that would eliminate the need for interim removable prostheses for the partially edentulous patients. The edentulous patients were not allowed to use their dentures for 2 weeks after the first-stage surgery but were allowed to use them with soft liner adjustments anywhere from immediately to 1 week after second-stage surgery (see Figs 18-2a to 18-2f). Interim tooth replacement for the partially dentate patient included resin-bonded prostheses; acrylic resin provisional prostheses; the use of the old permanent prostheses, which were recemented; or removable partial dentures. Fixed restorations offered the advantage of preventing any possibility of premature loading (see Figs 18-3 and 18-4).

The maxillary prostheses represented 29 freestanding fixed prostheses, 10 hybrid fixed dentures, 11 fixed prostheses supported by a combination of natural teeth and osseointegrated implants, and no overdentures (Fig 18-6a). The mandibular prostheses included 27 freestanding prostheses, seven hybrid fixed dentures, four fixed prostheses supported by a combination of natural teeth and osseointegrated implants, and four overdentures (Fig 18-6b).

The maintenance recall period was 3 months but was sometimes stretched to 4 or even 5 months because of patients' excuses or appointment-scheduling problems. The success rate was predicated on the criteria presented by Albrektsson et al.[62]

Of 309 implants placed, three maxillary and four mandibular implants failed, for a success rate of 98% (Figs 18-7a and 18-7b). Three of the 177 original implants placed in the maxilla failed. Of the prostheses constructed on the 177 implants, none was lost. Two mandibular failures were removed prior to the second-stage surgery because of clinical symptoms including pain, swelling, and fistulation. The other two were removed at second-stage surgery. None of the 42 mandibular prostheses placed on the remaining 130 stable implants failed.

Several patients had one or more implants that lost bone surrounding the first or second thread, as witnessed radiographically. In addition, seven implants, four maxillary and three mandibular, lost bone to the fourth thread but demonstrated no further loss after the first year.

The results demonstrated 100% stability of the prostheses, suggesting the efficacy of the implementation of osseointegration as a treatment modality for the patient with refractory periodontitis.[61]

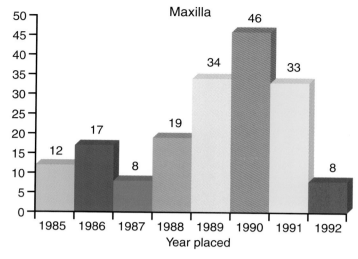

Fig 18-5a Number of maxillary implants placed each year during the course of the study.

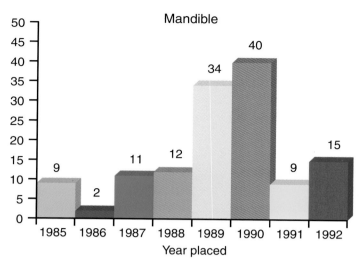

Fig 18-5b Number of mandibular implants placed each year during the course of the study.

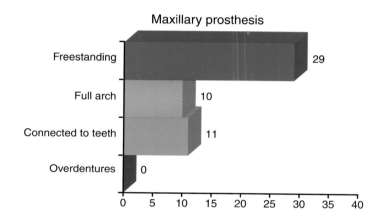

Fig 18-6a Distribution of maxillary prosthesis types in this study of implants in patients with refractory disease.

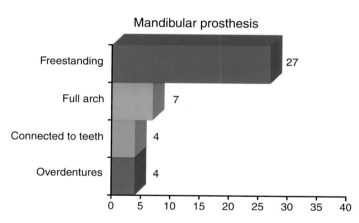

Fig 18-6b Distribution of mandibular prosthesis types in this study of implants in patients with refractory disease.

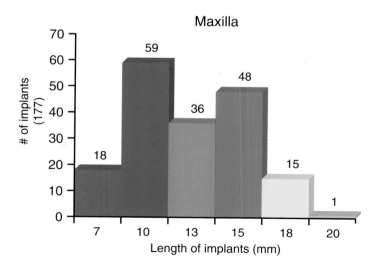

Fig 18-7a Length of implants used in the maxilla. Lengths ranged from 7 to 20 mm. Most were 10 to 15 mm, but the shorter implants were also successful.

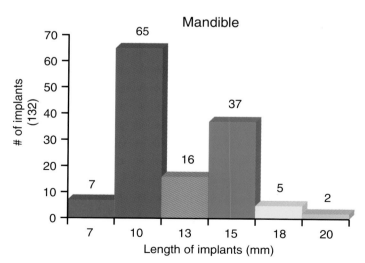

Fig 18-7b Length of implants used in the mandible. Lengths ranged from 7 to 20 mm. Most were 10 to 15 mm, but the short implants were also successful.

Figs 18-5 to 18-7 From Nevins and Langer.[61] Reprinted with permission.

References

1. Caton J. Periodontal diagnosis and diagnostic aids. In: Nevins M, Becker W, Kornman K (eds). Proceedings of the World Workshop in Clinical Periodontics. Chicago: American Academy of Periodontology, 1989:I-1–I-32.

2. Nevins M, Langer B. The successful use of osseointegrated implants for the treatment of the recalcitrant periodontal patient. J Periodontol 1995;66:150–157.

3. Hirschfeld L, Wasserman D. A long-term survey of tooth loss in 600 treated periodontal patients. J Periodontol 1978;49:225–237.

4. McFall WT. Tooth loss in 100 treated patients with periodontal disease. A long-term study. J Periodontol 1982;53:539–549.

5. Rosenberg E, Torosian J, Hammond B, Cutler S. Routine anaerobic bacterial culture and systemic antibiotic usage in the treatment of adult periodontitis: A 6-year longitudinal study. Int J Periodont Rest Dent 1993;13:213–243.

6. Van Winkelhoff AJ, de Graaff J. Microbiology in the management of destructive periodontal disease. J Clin Periodontol 1991;18:406–410.

7. Gordon J, Walker C, Socransky S. Efficacy of clindamycin hydrochloride in refractory periodontitis: 24-month results. J Periodontol 1990;61:686–691.

8. Walker C, Gordon J. The effect of clindamycin on the microbiota associated with refractory periodontitis. J Periodontol 1990;61:692–698.

9. Van Dyke TE, Offenbacher S, Place D, Dowell VR, Jones J. Refractory periodontitis: Mixed infection with *Bacteroides gingivalis* and other unusual *Bacteroides* species. A case report. J Periodontol 1988; 39:184–189.

10. Magnusson I, Marks RG, Clark WB, Walker CB, McArthur WP. Clinical, microbiological and immunological characteristics of subjects with "refractory" periodontal disease. J Clin Periodontol 1991; 18:291–299.

11. Hernichel E, Kornman KS, Holt SC, Nichols F, Meador H, Klung JT, Thomas C. Host responses in patients with generalized refractory periodontitis. J Periodontol 1994;65:8–16.

12. Pertuiset JH, Saglie FR, Lofthus J, Rezende M, Sanz M. Recurrent periodontal disease and bacterial presence in the gingiva. J Periodontol 1987;58:553–558.

13. Leon LE, Vogel RI. A comparison of the effectiveness of hand scaling and ultrasonic debridement in furcations as evaluated by darkfield microscopy. J Periodontol 1987;58:86–94.

14. Adriaens PA, DeBoever JA, Loesche WJ. Bacterial invasion in root cementum and radicular dentin of periodontally diseased teeth in humans. A reservoir of periodontopathic bacteria. J Periodontol 1988;59:222–230.

15. Oshrain HI, Telsey B, Mandel ID. Neutrophil chemotaxis in refractory cases of periodontitis. J Clin Periodontol 1986;14;52–55.

16. Collins JG, Offenbacher S, Arnold RR. Effects of a combination therapy to eliminate *Porphyromonas gingivalis* in refractory periodontitis. J Periodontol 1993;64:998–1007.

17. Walker CB, Gordon JM, Magnusson I, Clark WB. A role for antibiotics in the treatment of refractory periodontitis. J Periodontol 1993;64:772–781.

18. Goldman MJ, Ross IF, Goteiner D. Effect of periodontal therapy on patients maintained for 15 years or longer. A retrospective study. J Periodontol 1986;57:347–353.

19. Listgarten MA, Chen-Hsiung L, Young V. Microbial composition and pattern of antibiotic resistance in subgingival microbial samples from patients with refractory periodontitis. J Periodontol 1993;64:155–161.

20. Löe H, Anerud A, Boysen H, Morrison E. Natural history of periodontal disease in man. Rapid, moderate and no loss of attachment in Sri Lankan laborers 14 to 46 years of age. J Clin Periodontol 1986; 13:431–440.

21. Manji F, Baelum V, Fejerskov O. Tooth mortality in an adult rural population in Kenya. J Dent Res 1988;67:496–500.

22. Slots J, Rams TE. New views on periodontal microbiota in special patient categories. J Clin Periodontol 1991;18:411–420.

23. Jin LJ, Soder PO, Asman B, Soder B, Puriene A, Bergstrom K. Variations in crevicular fluid elastase levels in periodontitis patients on long-term maintenance. Eur J Oral Sci 1995;103:84–89.

24. Reinhardt RA, Masada MP, Kaldahl WB, Dubis LM, Kornman KS, Choi JI, et al. Gingival fluid IL-1 and IL-6 levels in refractory periodontitis. J Clin Periodontol 1993;20:225–231.

25. Lee HJ, Kang IK, Chung CP, Choi SM. The subgingival microflora and gingival crevicular fluid cytokines in refractory periodontitis. J Clin Periodontol 1995;22:885–890.

26. Haffajee AD, Socransky SS, Dzink JL, Taubman MA, Ebersole JL. Clinical, microbiological and immunological features of subjects with refractory periodontal diseases. J Clin Periodontol 1988;15:390–398.

27. Magnusson I, Low SB, McArthur WP, Marks RG, Walker CB, Maruniak J, et al. Treatment of subjects with refractory periodontal disease. J Clin Periodontol 1994;21:628–637.

28. MacFarlane GD, Herzberg MC, Wolff LF, Hardie NA. Refractory periodontitis associated with abnormal polymorphonuclear leukocyte phagocytosis and cigarette smoking. J Periodontol 1992;63:908–913.

29. Noble RC, Penny BB. Comparison of leukocyte count and function in smoking and non-smoking young men. Infect Immun 1975; 12:550–555.

30. Kraal JH, Kenney EB. The response of polymorphonuclear leukocytes to chemotactic stimulatory for smokers and non-smokers. J Periodontal Res 1979;14:383–389.

31. Kenney EB, Kraal JH, Saxe SR, Jones J. The effect of cigarette smoke on human oral polymorphonuclear leukocytes. J Periodontal Res 1977;12:227–234.

32. Seow WK, MacFarlane GD, Thong YH, Herzberg MC. Nicotine effects on PMN chemotaxis and phagocytosis [abstract 577]. J Dent Res 1992;71:178.

33. Magnusson I, Clark WB, Low SB, Maruniak J, Marks RG, Walker CB. Effect of non-surgical periodontal therapy combined with adjunctive antibiotics in subjects with refractory periodontal disease. J Clin Periodontol 1989;16:647–653.

34. Telsey B, Oshrain HI, Elison SA. A simplified laboratory procedure to select an appropriate antibiotic for treatment of refractory periodontitis. J Periodontol 1986;57:325–327.

35. Claffey N, Egelberg J. Clinical indicators of probing attachment loss following initial periodontal treatment in advanced periodontitis patients. J Clin Periodontol 1995;22:690–696.

36. Mejia GI, Botero A, Rojas W, Robledo JA. Refractory periodontitis in a Columbian population. Predominant anaerobic bacterial flora and antibiotic susceptibility. Clin Infect Dis 1995;20(suppl 2):S311–S313.

37. Rodenburg JP, van Winkelhoff AJ, Winkel EG, Goene RJ, Abbas F, de Graaff J. Occurrence of *Bacteroides gingivalis*, *Bacteroides intermedius* and *Actinobacillus actinomycetemcomitans* in severe periodontitis in relation to age and treatment history. J Clin Periodontol 1990; 17:392–399.

38. Preber H, Bergstrom J. Cigarette smoking in patients referred for periodontal treatment. Scand J Dent Res 1986;94:102–108.

39. Bergstrom J, Eliasson S. Cigarette smoking and alveolar bone height in subjects with a high standard of oral hygiene. J Clin Periodontol 1987;14:466–469.

40. Bergstrom J. Cigarette smoking as a risk factor in chronic periodontal disease. Community Dent Oral Epidemiol 1989;17:245–247.

41. Haber J, Kent R. Cigarette smoking in a periodontal practice. J Periodontol 1992;63:100–106.

42. Preber H, Bergstrom J. Effect of cigarette smoking on healing following surgical therapy. J Clin Periodontol 1990;17:324–328.

43. Bain CA, May PK. The association between failure of dental implants and cigarette smoking. Int J Oral Maxillofac Implants 1993; 8:609–615.

44. Olsvik B, Tenover FC. Tetracycline resistance in periodontal pathogens. Clin Infect Dis 1993;16(suppl 4):S310–S313.

45. Olsvik B, Olsen I, Tenover FC. The tet(Q) gene in bacteria isolated from patients with refractory disease. Oral Microbiol Immunol 1994; 9:251–255.

46. Olsvik B, Hansen BF, Tenover FC, Olsen I. Tetracycline resistant microorganisms recovered from patients with refractory periodontal disease. J Clin Periodontol 1995;22:391–396.

47. Fine DH. Microbial identification and antibiotic sensitivity testing, an aid for patients refractory to periodontal therapy. J Clin Periodontol 1994;21:98–106.

48. Gordon J, Walker C, Lamster I, West T, Socransky S, Seiger M, Fasciano R. Efficacy of clindamycin hydrochloride in refractory periodontitis. 12 months results. J Periodontol 1985;56(suppl):75–80.

49. Gordon JM, Walker CB. Current status of systemic antibiotic usage in destructive periodontal disease. J Periodontol 1993;64:760–771.

50. Seymour SA, Haesman PA. Pharmacological control of periodontal disease. II. Antimicrobial agents. J Dent 1995;23:5–14.

51. van Winkelhoff AJ, Tijhof CJ, de Graaff J. Microbiological and clinical results of metronidazole plus amoxicillin therapy in *Actinobacillus actinomycetemcomitans* associated periodontitis. J Periodontol 1992; 63:52–57.

52. Adell R, Lekholm U, Brånemark PI. A 15 year study of osseointegrated implants in the treatment of the edentulous jaw. Int J Oral Surg 1981;6:387–416.

53. Jemt T, Lekholm U, Adel R. Osseointegrated implants in the treatment of partially edentulous patients: A preliminary study of 876 consecutively placed fixtures. Int J Oral Maxillofac Implants 1989;4:211–217.

54. Zarb GA, Schmitt A, Baker G. Tissue-integrated prostheses: Osseointegration research in Toronto. Int J Periodont Rest Dent 1987; 7:9–35.

55. van Steenberghe D. A retrospective multicenter evaluation of the survival rate of osseointegrated fixtures supporting fixed partial prostheses in the treatment of the partial edentulism. J Prosthet Dent 1989; 61:217–222.

56. Jemt T, Lekholm U, Grondahl K. A 3-year follow-up study of early single implant restorations ad modem Brånemark. Int J Periodont Rest Dent 1990;10:341–349.

57. Nevins M, Langer B. The successful application of osseointegrated implants to the posterior jaw: A long-term retrospective study. Int J Oral Maxillofac Implants 1993;8:428–432.

58. Jemt T, Lekholm U. Oral implant treatment in posterior partially edentulous jaws. A 5-year follow-up report. Int J Oral Maxillofac Implants 1993;8:635–640.

59. Ericsson I, Lekholm U, Brånemark PI, Lindhe H, Glantz PO, Nyman SA. A clinical evaluation of fixed bridge restorations supported by the combination of teeth and osseointegrated titanium implants. J Clin Periodontol 1986;13:307–312.

60. Jaffin RA, Berman CL. The excessive loss of Brånemark fixtures in Type IV bone. A 5-year analysis. J Periodontol 1992;62:2–4.

61. Nevins M, Langer B. The successful use of osseointegrated implants for the treatment of the recalcitrant periodontal patient. J Periodontol 1995;66:150–157.

62. Albrektsson T, Zarb GA, Worthington P, Eriksson AR. The long-term efficacy of currently used dental implants. A review and proposed criteria of success. Int J Oral Maxillofac Implants 1986;1:11–25.

INDEX

Page numbers followed by "f" indicate figures; numbers followed by "t" indicate tables.

A

Abutments
 teeth, 2f–3f, 3
 titanium, for guided gingival growth, 121
Allografts, for guided bone regeneration
 bone morphogenetic proteins. *See* Bone morphogenetic proteins.
 decalcification of, 75
 description of, 72, 74, 87
 disease transmission
  bacterial infections, 76
  Creutzfeldt-Jakob disease, 76–77
  hepatitis, 76
  human immunodeficiency virus, 74–76
  syphilis, 76
 freeze-dried. *See* Freeze-dried bone allograft.
 in mandibular anterior implants, 134f
 processing of, 74–75
 procurement of, 74–75
 safety of, 74–77
Alveolar process
 anatomic center of, 40
 anatomy of, 32–33, 33f
 bone loss of
  bone graft and physical barrier technique treatment for, 62, 65f
  effect on implant position
   horizontal, 40
   vertical, 39–40
 computerized tomographic evaluations of
  accuracy rates, 34
  axial composite image, 35–36
  cross-sectional views, 36–37
  guidelines, 35
  images produced, 35, 35f
  overview, 34
  panoramic views, 36, 36f
  procedure, 35
 defects
  dehiscence
   barrier membranes
    bioresorbable, 72, 73f
    titanium-reinforced. *See* Titanium-reinforced barrier membrane.
   description of, 59–60
  fenestration
   demineralized freeze-dried bone allograft, 59, 87, 88f
   description of, 59–60

 illustration of, 163f
 implant stability, 85, 86f
 nonspacemaking, 55
 spacemaking, 55
 pathologic changes of, effect on implant placement, 34
 ridge. *See* Alveolar ridge.
 tooth and, relationship between, 33
Alveolar ridge
 augmentation of
  for maxillary posterior implants, 154
  using guided bone regeneration
   advantages of, 60, 61f
   and autogenous bone grafting, 65
   barrier membranes. *See* Barrier membranes.
   buccal plate, 64
   disadvantages caused by delaying implant placement, 62
   graft material, 65, 67f
   overview, 69
   resorption, 62, 63f
   split-ridge technique, 68, 68f
   success rates, 64, 66f
   timing of, 60
  vertical
   autogenous bone chip grafts, 108–109
   clinical studies of, 69
   discussion, 107, 108f
   methods and materials, 105–107, 106f
   results, 106f, 107–109, 109f
   titanium-reinforced barrier membranes. *See* Titanium-reinforced barrier membranes.
 computed tomographic evaluations of
  accuracy rates, 34
  axial composite image, 35–36
  cross-sectional views, 36–37
  guidelines, 35
  images produced, 35, 35f
  overview, 34
  panoramic views, 36, 36f
  procedure, 35
 narrow
  augmentation methods, 136
  dehiscence defects associated with. *See* Dehiscence defects.
  fenestration defects associated with. *See* Fenestration defects.
  illustration of, 166f
  preimplant considerations for, 122–125, 123f–125f
 pathologic changes of, effect on implant placement, 34
 reconstruction of, 65, 67f
 resorption, 34

 shape of, 34
Anodontia, 135, 135f
Anterior implants
 buccolingual placement considerations, 11
 mandibular
  description of, 129
  guided bone regeneration, 134f, 135
  placement obstacles
   buccolingual discrepancies, 135–136, 136f–138f
   mesiodistal discrepancies, 129–131, 130f–131f
   occlusal discrepancies, 139
   vertical discrepancies, 132–135, 133f–134f
  treatment considerations, 129
 maxillary
  in adolescents, 114
  bone regeneration after extraction, 118, 119f–120f
  clinical examination, 111, 112f
  factors that affect
   guided bone regeneration failure, 122, 122f
   high smile line, 125, 126f
   narrow buccolingual ridge, 122–125, 123f–125f
  versus fixed partial denture, 114, 118f
  guided gingival growth, 120f, 121
  illustration of, 16f
  pretreatment considerations, 111, 112f
  provisional restoration, 121
  for refractory periodontitis, 247f
  submergence profile
   bone loss considerations, 113f–114f, 113–114
   bone volume maximization, 114, 115f–116f
   canine impaction, considerations for, 114, 118f
   cementoenamel junction, 112, 112f–113f
   definition of, 111
Augmentation procedures
 for alveolar ridge
  for maxillary posterior implants, 154
  using guided bone regeneration
   advantages of, 60, 61f
   barrier membranes
    expanded polytetrafluoroethylene. *See* Expanded polytetrafluoroethylene.
    exposure problems, 62
    support devices, 68
    titanium-reinforced. *See* Titanium-reinforced barrier membranes.
   buccal plate, 64
   disadvantages caused by delaying implant placement, 62

graft material, 65, 67f
overview, 69
resorption, 62, 63f
split-ridge technique, 68, 68f
success rates, 64, 66f
timing of, 60
vertical
autogenous bone chip grafts, 108–109
clinical studies of, 69
discussion, 107, 108f
methods and materials, 105–107, 106f
results, 106f, 107–109, 109f
titanium-reinforced barrier membranes. See
Titanium-reinforced barrier membranes.
for maxillary sinus floor
anatomic considerations, 174f
animal studies of, 185, 186f–188f
autogenous bone graft, 171, 173f
contraindications, 173, 174f
description of, 171
edentulous patients
alternative treatments, 192, 193f–194f
bone regeneration, pilot studies in humans, 188–192
elevation procedure
identification of septa, 178
planned approach, 182, 184f–185f, 184–185
presurgical planning, 178, 178f
simultaneous approach, 182, 183f–184f
staged approach, 179–182
graft materials
harvest sites, 175
histologic results, 185, 186f
mineralized freeze-dried allogeneic bone, 175
types of, 175
illustration of, 176f–177f
success rate, 193
treatment options
description of, 174
factors that affect, 174
simultaneous approach, 174
staged approach, 174–175
treatment time, 174f
Autogenous bone grafts
from anterior mandible
anesthesia, 210
harvesting
of block grafts, 211–213, 212f–214f
full-thickness block graft, 213
particulate grafts, 213–215, 215f
incisions
crevicular, 210
vestibular, 210, 211f
instruments, 216, 216f
preoperative assessment, 209–210
wound closure, 215–216, 216f
augmentation uses
alveolar ridge, 65, 67f, 136, 138f
maxillary sinus floor, 171, 173f
bone formation
advantages, 99
factors that affect, 104
illustration of, 101f
bone morphogenetic proteins. See Bone morphogenetic proteins.

disadvantages of, 99
donor sites, 29
harvesting of, 87
osteoinductive activity of, 104
Autologous bone grafts. See Autogenous bone grafts.
Avulsed teeth, reimplantation of, 10, 117f

B

Barrier membranes, in guided bone regeneration
for alveolar ridge
augmentation of, 68
bone loss, 62, 65f
bioresorbable, 72, 73f
bone regeneration, 85
for clot protection and stabilization, 86
for dehiscence defects, 59
effect of exposure on bone fill, 58
exposure, 70f–71f, 70–71
failure, 99
for fenestration defects, 59
hydroxyapatite, 58
reinforced
bone grafts and, concomitant use, 95
healing duration, 93
indications, 95–97
placement of, 93, 94f
removal of, 93, 95f
with titanium, 91, 92f
support devices, 60f–65f, 64, 68
wound closure, 71
BMP. See Bone morphogenetic protein.
Bolton index deficiency, 120f, 121
Bone formation
protected space development for, 91
using autogenous bone grafts
advantages, 99
factors that affect, 104
illustration of, 101f
osteoinductive activity, 104
using barrier membranes. See Titanium-reinforced barrier membranes.
using guided bone regeneration. See Guided bone regeneration.
Bone grafts
allografts. See Allografts.
autogenous. See Autogenous bone grafts.
for extraction site defects, 55–56, 56f
and titanium-reinforced barrier membranes, concomitant use, 95
Bone loss. See also Resorption.
illustration of, 2f, 14f
in maxillary molar region, 11, 15f
of residual ridge, 42, 43f
vertical
evaluation of, 42
illustration of, 132f
in mandibular anterior implants, 132–135, 133f–134f
Bone morphogenetic proteins, 74, 185
Bone regeneration. See Guided bone regeneration.
Brånemark implant
for edentulous patients
anatomic conditions, 23–24

biomechanical considerations, 24
microbiologic state, 24
oral hygiene state, 24
history of, 29–30
for partially edentulous jaw, 24–26
Buccinator, 31, 31f
Buccolingual ridge, effect on anterior implants
mandibular, 135–136, 136f–138f
maxillary, 122–125, 123f–125f
Buccopalatal ridge, effect on maxillary posterior
implants, 154, 155f

C

Canine impaction, effect on lateral incisors, 114, 118f
Cementoenamel junction (CEJ), in maxillary
anterior implants, 112, 112f–113f, 115f
Ceramometal prostheses
cantilevered, 42, 43f
conventional, 42
Clot, for bone regeneration
barrier membrane positioning for, 86
formation of, 86
protection of, 86, 87f
space requirements, 87
stabilization of, 86, 87f
Computerized tomography
alveolar process evaluations using
accuracy rates, 34
axial composite image, 35–36
cross-sectional views, 36–37
guidelines, 35
images produced, 35, 35f
overview, 34
panoramic views, 36, 36f
procedure, 35
of inferior alveolar nerve, 142f
prosthetic-guided development using, 30
Computer profile image
barium-coated template for forming, 39
function of, 38
implant site analysis, steps involved in, 39–42, 41f
panoramic view of, 36
prosthetic designs
cantilevered ceramometal, 42, 43f
clip-retained overdenture/spark-erosion, 42, 44, 44t
conventional ceramometal, 42
fixed hybrid, 42
predictor modifiers, 44
Connective tissue
anatomy of, 229
grafting of, for immediate extraction implant in
partially edentulous patients, 221, 222f
Contained bone lesions, 55
CPI. See Computer profile image.
Creutzfeldt-Jakob disease, transmission via bone
allografts, 76–77
Crown-lengthening surgery
description of, 10
illustration of, 10f
CT. See Computerized tomography.

D

Dehiscence defects in implants, guided bone regeneration for
  barrier membranes
    bioresorbable, 72, 73f
    titanium-reinforced. *See* Titanium-reinforced barrier membrane.
  description of, 59–60
Demineralized freeze-dried bone allograft, in guided bone regeneration
  for alveolar ridge augmentation, 65, 67f
  autogenous bone grafts and, comparisons, 74
  bone formation
    description of, 100, 102f–103f
    factors that affect, 104
  for dehiscence defects, 59
  description of, 87
  expanded polytetrafluoroethylene barrier membrane and, concomitant use, 104
  for fenestration defects, 59, 87, 88f
  healing process of, 74
  for nonspacemaking defects in extraction sites, 55–56, 56, 57f
  studies of, 74
Dental implants. *See* Implants.
Dentition, maintenance strategies for, 1–3, 2f
Depressor anguli oris, 31f
Depressor labii inferioris, 31f
DFDBA. *See* Demineralized freeze-dried bone allograft.
Diagnostic waxup, for determining fixture compatibility equation, 37, 38f

E

Edentulous patients
  implants for
    anatomic conditions, 23–24
    biomechanical considerations, 24
    description of, 219
    esthetic management, 219, 219f
    microbiologic state, 24
    oral hygiene state, 24
  maxillary sinus floor augmentation in
    alternative treatments, 192, 193f–194f
    bone regeneration, pilot studies in humans, 188–192
  versus partially edentulous patients, treatment plan differences, 23–24
e-PTFE. *See* Expanded polytetrafluoroethylene membrane.
Ethylene oxide, effect on bone induction, 75
Expanded polytetrafluoroethylene membrane
  animal studies of, 53–54
  bacterial contamination, 71
  clinical uses
    dehiscence defects, 59
    fenestration defects, 59
    implants placed in extraction sites, 55–56
  exposure, 70–71
  factors that affect, 55
  function of, 55
  for large alveolar ridge deformities, 64
  predictability of, 84–85
  procedure, 54–55

titanium-reinforced, 91, 92f
  description of, 91
  healing duration, 93
  illustration of, 92f
  indications, 95–97
  limitations, 96
  placement of, 93, 94f
  removal of, 93, 95f
Extraction sites
  bone graft and physical barrier technique, concomitant treatment using, 62, 65f
  guided bone regeneration
    for implant placement, 55–58, 56f–58f
    in wounds, 118, 119f–120f

F

FDBA. *See* Mineralized freeze-dried bone allograft.
Fenestration defects in implants, guided bone regeneration for
  demineralized freeze-dried bone allograft, 59, 87, 88f
  description of, 59–60
  illustration of, 163f
  implant stability, 85, 86f
Fistulae, 115f–116f
Fixed hybrid prosthesis, 42
Fixture compatibility equation
  description of, 37
  determinants of
    clinical, 38
    diagnostic waxup, 37, 38f
    reformatted computerized tomography, 38
Flaps, periodontal
  full-thickness, 88, 89f
  for maxilla, 93, 94f
  partial-thickness, 88, 89f
  for soft tissue coverage in guided bone regeneration, 88f, 88–89
Freeze-dried bone allograft
  demineralized
    for alveolar ridge augmentation, 65, 67f
    autogenous bone grafts and, comparisons, 74
    bone formation
      description of, 100, 102f–103f
      factors that affect, 104
    for dehiscence defects, 59
    description of, 87
    expanded polytetrafluoroethylene barrier membrane and, concomitant use, 104
    for fenestration defects, 59, 87, 88f
    healing process of, 74
    for nonspacemaking defects in extraction sites, 55–56, 57f
    studies of, 74
  mineralized
    description of, 59, 87
    for large alveolar ridge deformities, 64
    for maxillary sinus floor augmentation, 175

G

GBR. *See* Guided bone regeneration.
GGG. *See* Guided gingival growth.

Gingiva
  attached, for implants
    advantages of, 228
    amount of, 230
    anatomy of, 229–230
    classification of, 230–235
    clinical importance of, 229
    esthetic blending, 228
    oral hygiene and, 228
    success rates and, 228
  guided growth of, for maxillary anterior implants, 120f, 121
  minimum amount of, for teeth, 121
  spontaneous in situ augmentation, 223–224, 225f
Grafts. *See* Allografts; Autogenous bone grafts.
Guided bone regeneration
  alveolar ridge, localized augmentation
    advantages of, 60, 61f
    barrier exposure problems, 62
    barrier support methods, 68
    buccal plate, 64
    disadvantages caused by delaying implant placement, 62
    graft material, 65, 67f
    overview, 69
    resorption, 62, 63f
    split-ridge technique, 68, 68f
    success rates, 64, 66f
    timing of, 60
  animal studies of, 53–54, 99
  barrier membranes. *See* Barrier membranes.
  bone graft materials
    allografts. *See* Allografts.
    autogenous. *See* Autogenous bone grafts.
  for bone loss associated with mandibular anterior implants, 134f, 135
  definition of, 53
  dehiscence defects, 59–60
  description of, 99
  failure of, 122, 122f
  fenestration defects, 59–60
  guided tissue regeneration and, comparisons, 53
  for implants
    in extraction sites, 55–58, 56f–58f
    failure, 69–70
    ideal placement
      expanded polytetrafluoroethylene membranes, 84–85
      factors that affect success
        clot protection and stabilization, 86, 87f
        implant stability, 85, 86f
        infection prevention, 88
        soft tissue coverage, 88f, 88–89
        space, 86, 87f
        surgical site preparation, 86
        unimpeded healing, 85–86
        wound healing, 89
    indications, 83–84
    overview, 83
    predictability, 83–84
  infection-related bone loss, 69
  for mandibular molars, 17, 17f
  periradicular defects, 69
  procedure, 54–55
  rationale for, 54–55
  using harvest cover screws

bone formation, 100–104, 101f–104f
  factors that affect, 104
  methods and materials, 99–100, 100f
  results, 100–104, 101f–104f
Guided gingival growth, 120f, 121
Guided tissue regeneration, 53

H

Harvest cover screws, bone formation using
  bone formation, 100–104, 101f–104f
  factors that affect, 104
  methods and materials, 99–100, 100f
  results, 100–104, 101f–104f
Hepatitis, transmission via bone allografts, 76
Human immunodeficiency virus (HIV), transmission via bone allografts, 74–76
Hydroxyapatite, for nonspacemaking defects in extraction sites, 58

I

Implants. See also Prostheses.
  anterior. See Anterior implants.
  attached gingiva around. See Gingiva, attached.
  bone loss and, 11, 15f–16f
  Brånemark. See Brånemark implant.
  buccolingual placement of, 11
  computerized tomography for determining need for, 11, 12f, 15f–16f
  description of, 4, 5f
  for edentulous patients
    anatomic conditions, 23–24
    biomechanical considerations, 24
    microbiologic state, 24
    oral hygiene state, 24
  for extraction site defects, 55–58, 56f–58f
  failure of
    bacterial etiology, 69
    occlusal trauma, 69
  guided bone regeneration. See Guided bone regeneration.
  intraosseous blade-vent, 4, 8f
  loading effects, 4
  mandibular anterior. See Mandible, anterior, implants.
  mandibular posterior. See Mandible, posterior implants.
  maxillary anterior. See Maxilla, anterior, implants.
  maxillary posterior. See Maxilla, posterior implants.
  maxillary sinus floor augmentation to support. See Maxillary sinus floor augmentation.
  for partially edentulous patients
    anatomic conditions, 23–24
    biomechanical considerations, 24
    microbiologic state, 24
    oral hygiene state, 24
  patient characteristics, 1
  placement
    anatomic elements that influence, 33–34
    effect of alveolar process pathology, 34
    ideal

expanded polytetrafluoroethylene membranes, 84–85
factors that affect success
  clot protection and stabilization, 86, 87f
  implant stability, 85, 86f
  infection prevention, 88
  soft tissue coverage, 88f, 88–89
  space, 86, 87f
  surgical site preparation, 86
  unimpeded healing, 85–86
  wound healing, 89
indications, 83–84
overview, 83
predictability, 83–84
posterior. See Posterior implants.
radiographs to determine need for, 11, 12f
root-form, 4, 6f–8f
single-tooth, 6f, 26
surface, detoxification of, 69
team approach to, historical development of
  hardware, 29–30
  prosthetic component development, 30
  prosthetic-guided development, 30
teeth and, connections between
  biomechanical aspects, 49
  connectors, 49
  considerations, 48, 49f
  description of, 47–48
  joint strength, 49
  multiple implants, 50, 50f–51f
  occlusion, 48
  principles, 49–51
  rigid attachment, 50, 50f
Incisors, implant replacement of, 6f, 129, 131f
Inferior alveolar nerve
  anatomic course of, 33, 143, 144f
  bone height above, pretreatment considerations for augmenting, 145, 145f
  in mandibular posterior implants
    illustration of, 141, 141f–142f, 145, 145f
    treatment indications, 149
Intraosseous blade-vent implants, 4, 8f

K

Keratinized tissue
  adequacy determinations, 228
  for attached gingiva
    advantages of, 228
    amount of, 230
    anatomy of, 229–230
    classification of, 230–235
    clinical importance of, 229
    esthetic blending, 228
    oral hygiene and, 228
    success rates and, 228
  augmentation of, 228
  autogenous tissue grafting for creating, 225
  maintenance of, 224–225

L

Lateral pterygoid plate, 197, 198f

M

Mandible
  anatomy of, 33, 33f
  anterior
    autogenous bone grafts from
      anesthesia, 210
      harvesting
        of block grafts, 211–213, 212f–214f
        full-thickness block graft, 213
        particulate grafts, 213–215, 215f
      incisions
        crevicular, 210
        vestibular, 210, 211f
      instruments, 216, 216f
      preoperative assessment, 209–210
      wound closure, 215–216, 216f
    implants in
      description of, 129
      guided bone regeneration, 134f, 135
      placement obstacles
        buccolingual discrepancies, 135–136, 136f–138f
        mesiodistal discrepancies, 129–131, 130f–131f
        occlusal discrepancies, 139
        vertical discrepancies, 132–135, 133f–134f
      for refractory periodontitis, 247f
      treatment considerations, 129
  bone quality of, 33
  edentulous. See Edentulous patient.
  partially edentulous. See Partially edentulous patient.
  posterior implants
    bone quality considerations, 143
    criteria for, 149
    description of, 141
    difficulties associated with, 11
    indications, 149–150, 150f
    inferior alveolar nerve considerations, 141, 141f–142f, 145, 145f
    for inflammatory defects associated with tooth position defects, 149
    mesiodistal drilling site, 150
    placement obstacles
      emergence profile replication, 147
      inferior alveolar nerve, 141, 141f–142f, 145, 145f
      mandible shape, 145–147, 146f–148f
      mental foramen, 142–143, 144f
    shape of, effect on posterior implant placement, 145–147, 146f–148f
Mandibular canal, 33
Mandibular molars
  compromises in, 16f
  guided bone regeneration for, 17, 17f
  prerestoration evaluation of, 11, 16f–17f, 149
  sectioned, periodontal evaluations for restorative procedures, 11, 149
  tipped, 17, 149
Masseter, 31f
Maxilla
  anatomy of, 32–33, 33f, 197, 198f–199f
  anterior teeth
    implants
      in adolescents, 114

bone regeneration after extraction, 118, 119f–120f
clinical examination, 111, 112f
factors that affect
  guided bone regeneration failure, 122, 122f
  high smile line, 125, 126f
  narrow buccolingual ridge, 122–125, 123f–125f
  versus fixed partial denture, 114, 118f
guided gingival growth, 120f, 121
illustration of, 16f
pretreatment considerations, 111, 112f
provisional restoration, 121
for refractory periodontitis, 247f
submergence profile
  bone loss considerations, 113f–114f, 113–114
  bone volume maximization, 114, 115f–116f
  canine impaction, considerations for, 114, 118f
  cementoenamel junction, 112, 112f–113f
  definition of, 111
resorption of, 62
bone resorption, 172f
bone type, 33
flap design, 93, 94f
posterior implants
  buccopalatal width, 154, 155f
  illustration of, 156f–158f
  overview, 153
  placement obstacles
    bone volume, 154, 155f–158f, 171
    molar region, 167–169, 168f
    premolar region. *See* Maxillary premolars.
  in pterygoid process of sphenoid bone
    case, 201–202, 203f
    description of, 201
    distal, 205–207, 206f
    technique, 201, 201f–202f
    and tuberosity and pyramidal process implant, 202, 204f
  ridge augmentation considerations, 154
  success rates, 153f
  in tuberosity
    case, 200f, 201
    description of, 199, 200f
    illustration of, 197, 198f
    and pyramidal process and pterygoid process implant, 202, 204f
    technique, 199
Maxillary molars
  bone loss associated with, 11, 15f–16f
  description of, 11
  in maxillary posterior implants
    bone quantity considerations, 168f, 169
    description of, 167–169
    periodontal regenerative procedures, 167, 168f
Maxillary premolars, in posterior implants
  compromised, considerations for, 162, 164f
  extraction site, 163f
  fenestration defects, 160, 163f
  furcal invasion, 159, 159f
  guided bone regeneration, 164, 167f

horizontal bone augmentation, 160, 162, 163f, 165f
periodontal regeneration, 159–160, 161f
ridge splitting, 162, 164, 165f
roots, 159
sectioning of, 160, 161f–162f
two-rooted, 162
Maxillary sinus
  anatomy of, 174
  sinus floor augmentation. *See* Maxillary sinus floor augmentation.
Maxillary sinus floor augmentation
  anatomic considerations, 174f
  animal studies of, 185, 186f–188f
  autogenous bone graft, 171, 173f
  contraindications, 173, 174f
  description of, 171
  edentulous patients
    alternative treatments, 192, 193f–194f
    bone regeneration, pilot studies in humans, 188–192
  elevation procedure
    identification of septa, 178
    planned approach, 182, 184f–185f, 184–185
    presurgical planning, 178, 178f
    simultaneous approach, 182, 183f–184f
    staged approach, 179–182
  graft materials
    harvest sites, 175
    histologic results, 185, 186f
    mineralized freeze-dried allogeneic bone, 175
    types of, 175
  illustration of, 176f–177f
  success rate, 193
  treatment options
    description of, 174
    factors that affect, 174
    simultaneous approach, 174
    staged approach, 174–175
  treatment time, 174f
Membrane. *See* Barrier membranes.
Mental foramen, effect on placement of mandibular posterior implant, 142–143, 144f
Mentalis, 31f, 210
Mineralized freeze-dried bone allograft
  description of, 59, 87
  for large alveolar ridge deformities, 64
  for maxillary sinus floor augmentation, 175
Molars
  mandibular
    guided bone regeneration for, 17, 17f
    prerestoration evaluation of, 11, 16f–17f, 149
    sectioned, periodontal evaluations for restorative procedures, 11, 149
    tipped, 17, 149
  maxillary
    bone loss associated with, 11, 15f–16f
    description of, 11
    in maxillary posterior implants
      bone quantity considerations, 168f, 169
      description of, 167–169
      periodontal regenerative procedures, 167, 168f
Mucogingival augmentation, for implants
  drawbacks of, 236
  procedure, 234, 235f

rationale for, 227–229
using keratinized tissue. *See* Keratinized tissue.

N

Neutral zone, 31
Noncontained bone lesions, 55
Nonspacemaking defects, definition of, 55

O

Occlusion
  effect on maxillary posterior implants, 207
  for implant–teeth connections, 48
  in mandibular anterior implants, 139
  trauma, implant failure and, 69
Orbicularis oris, 31f
Orofacial musculature
  augmentation procedures and, 32
  illustration of, 31f
Osseointegration
  Brånemark
    history of, 29–30
    for partially edentulous patients, 24–26
  definition of, 9
  illustration of, 8f, 9f
  loading considerations, 9
  for partially edentulous patients, 4, 5f, 227
Osseous defects
  dehiscence
    barrier membranes
      bioresorbable, 72, 73f
      titanium-reinforced. *See* Titanium-reinforced barrier membrane.
    description of, 59–60
  fenestration
    demineralized freeze-dried bone allograft, 59, 87, 88f
    description of, 59–60
    illustration of, 163f
    implant stability, 85, 86f
  nonspacemaking, 55
  spacemaking, 55

P

Partially edentulous patients
  versus edentulous patients, treatment plan differences, 23–24
  implants for
    anatomic conditions, 23–24
    biomechanical considerations, 24
    Brånemark
      complications, 26
      results, 24–26
    placement
      delayed, 222–223, 223f
      description of, 220
      immediate extraction
        buccal flap, 220, 220f
        complete coverage, 221
        connective tissue grafting, 221, 222f
        tissue coverage, 221

tissue defect considerations, 221
spontaneous in situ gingival augmentation, 223–224, 225f
teeth and, connections between
biomechanical aspects, 49
connectors, 49
considerations, 48, 49f
description of, 47–48
joint strength, 49
multiple implants, 50, 50f–51f
occlusion, 48
principles, 49–51
rigid attachment, 50, 50f
microbiologic state, 24
oral hygiene state, 24
single-tooth, 26
Particulate grafts
cores, 213
corticocancellous particles, 214
indications, 213
shavings, 214, 215f
Peri-implantitis
bone defects from, guided bone regeneration for, 69
definition of, 69
Periodontitis. See Refractory periodontitis.
Platysma, 31f
Posterior implants
mandibular
bone quality considerations, 143
criteria for, 149
description of, 141
indications, 149–150, 150f
inferior alveolar nerve considerations, 141, 141f–142f, 145, 145f
for inflammatory defects associated with tooth position defects, 149
mesiodistal drilling site, 150
placement obstacles
emergence profile replication, 147
inferior alveolar nerve, 141, 141f–142f, 145, 145f
mandible shape, 145–147, 146f–148f
mental foramen, 142–143, 144f
maxillary
buccopalatal width, 154, 155f
distal, combined with sinus graft implant sites, 205–207, 206f
illustration of, 156f–158f
occlusal forces, 207
overview, 153
placement obstacles
bone volume, 154, 155f–158f, 171
molar region, 167–169, 168f
premolar region. See Maxillary premolars.
in pterygoid process of sphenoid bone
case, 201–202, 203f
description of, 201
distal, 205–207, 206f
technique, 201, 201f–202f
and tuberosity and pyramidal process implant, 202, 204f
ridge augmentation considerations, 154
success rates, 153f
in tuberosity, implant placement
case, 200f, 201
description of, 199, 200f

illustration of, 197, 198f
and pyramidal process and pterygoid process implant, 202, 204f
technique, 199
Premolars. See Maxillary premolars.
Prostheses. See also Implants.
criteria for, 3
designs
cantilevered ceramometal, 42, 43f
clip-retained overdenture/spark-erosion, 42, 44, 44t
conventional ceramometal, 42
fixed hybrid, 42
predictor modifiers, 44
failure of, 3
historical development, 30
treatment plan, 1, 2f–4f
Protected space, for bone formation
description of, 91
using reinforced barrier membranes. See Barrier membranes, reinforced.
Pterygoid pillar, 197
Pterygoid process implant
case, 201–202, 203f
description of, 201
distal, 205–207, 206f
technique, 201, 201f–202f
and tuberosity and pyramidal process implant, 202, 204f
Pyramidal process
anatomy of, 197, 198f
implant
case, 202, 204f
technique, 202
and tuberosity and pterygoid process implant, 202, 204f

R

Radiographs, for determining treatment plan, 11, 12f
Rami, 33
Refractory periodontitis
bacterial resistance, 245
characteristics of, 239, 241, 242f–244f
definition of, 239
etiology of, 241, 245
factors that affect treatment success, 239
illustration of, 14f, 240f
immunologic features, 241
implants for, 246, 247f
incidence of, 241
polymorphonuclear neutrophil defect and, 241
recurring disease and, differential diagnosis, 239
treatment approaches, 245
Remaining ridge angle, 40
Residual ridge, of alveolar process
augmentation of
for maxillary posterior implants, 154
using guided bone regeneration
advantages of, 60, 61f
barrier membranes
expanded polytetrafluoroethylene. See Expanded polytetrafluoroethylene.
exposure problems, 62
support devices, 68

titanium-reinforced. See Titanium-reinforced barrier membranes.
buccal plate, 64
disadvantages caused by delaying implant placement, 62
graft material, 65, 67f
overview, 69
resorption, 62, 63f
split-ridge technique, 68, 68f
success rates, 64, 66f
timing of, 60
vertical
autogenous bone chip grafts, 108–109
clinical studies of, 69
discussion, 107, 108f
methods and materials, 105–107, 106f
results, 106f, 107–109, 109f
titanium-reinforced barrier membranes. See Titanium-reinforced barrier membranes.
computed tomographic evaluations of
accuracy rates, 34
axial composite image, 35–36
cross-sectional views, 36–37
guidelines, 35
images produced, 35, 35f
overview, 34
panoramic views, 36, 36f
procedure, 35
pathologic changes of, effect on implant placement, 34
resorption, 34
shape of, 34
Resorption, of bone. See also Bone loss.
horizontal, 44t
vertical, 44t
Root-form implants
osseointegration of. See Osseointegration.
results of, 6f–8f

S

SIM/Plant, 36, 37f
Sinus floor augmentation, for maxillary sinus
anatomic considerations, 174f
animal studies of, 185, 186f–188f
autogenous bone graft, 171, 173f
contraindications, 173, 174f
description of, 171
edentulous patients
alternative treatments, 192, 193f–194f
bone regeneration, pilot studies in humans, 188–192
elevation procedure
identification of septa, 178
planned approach, 182, 184f–185f, 184–185
presurgical planning, 178, 178f
simultaneous approach, 182, 183f–184f
staged approach, 179–182
graft materials
harvest sites, 175
histologic results, 185, 186f
mineralized freeze-dried allogeneic bone, 175
types of, 175
illustration of, 176f–177f
success rate, 193
treatment options

description of, 174
 factors that affect, 174
 simultaneous approach, 174
 staged approach, 174–175
treatment time, 174f
Smile
 cosmetic individuality of, 32
 creation of, 32
 line, effect on implant, 125, 126f
Smile zone
 definition of, 31
 muscles associated with, 31f, 31–32
Smoking, 89, 245
Spacemaking defects
 definition of, 55
 illustration of, 87f
 titanium-reinforced barrier membranes for vertical ridge augmentation, 96
Split-ridge technique, for alveolar ridge augmentation, 68, 68f, 135, 146, 164, 165f
Staphylococcus epidermis, transmission via bone
 allografts, 76
Submergence profile, of maxillary anterior
 implants
 bone loss considerations, 113f–114f, 113–114
 bone volume maximization, 114, 115f–116f
 canine impaction, considerations for, 114, 118f
 cementoenamel junction, 112, 112f–113f
 definition of, 111
Syphilis, transmission via bone allografts, 76

T

Team concept, historical development in
 implant dentistry
 hardware, 29–30
 prosthetic component development, 30
 prosthetic-guided development, 30
Teeth
 alveolar process and, relationship between, 33
 gingiva necessary for, 121
 implants and, connections between
  biomechanical aspects, 49
  connectors, 49
  considerations, 48, 49f
  description of, 47–48
  joint strength, 49
  multiple implants, 50, 50f–51f
  occlusion, 48
  principles, 49–51
  rigid attachment, 50, 50f
 replacement, indications for, 18, 19f–20f
Tissue. *See* Connective tissue; Keratinized tissue.
Titanium-reinforced barrier membranes, in
 guided bone regeneration
 description of, 91
 healing duration, 93
 illustration of, 92f
 indications, 95–97
 for maxillary premolars, 164, 167f
 placement of, 93, 94f

removal of, 93, 95f
 vertical ridge augmentation
  discussion, 107, 108f
  illustration of, 167f
  methods and materials, 105–107, 106f
  results, 106f, 107–109, 109f
Trabecular bone, 186f–187f
Treatment plan
 implants. *See* Implants.
 optimal type of, methods for selecting, 10–17
 for periodontal prostheses, 1, 2f–4f
 stages of
  implant placement, 1, 3
  removal of hopeless teeth, 1
  resolution of inflammatory disease, 1, 4f
Tuberosity, maxillary
 anatomy of, 197, 198f
 implant placement
  case, 200f, 201
  description of, 199, 200f
  illustration of, 197, 198f
  and pyramidal process and pterygoid process
   implant, 202, 204f
  technique, 199

Z

Zygomaticus major, 31f
Zygomaticus minor, 31f

THE
NEW COMPLETE
BOOK OF THE
DOG

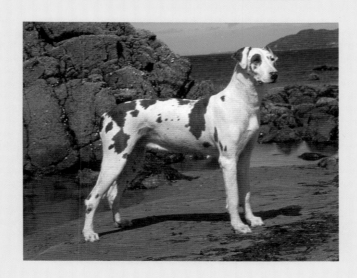

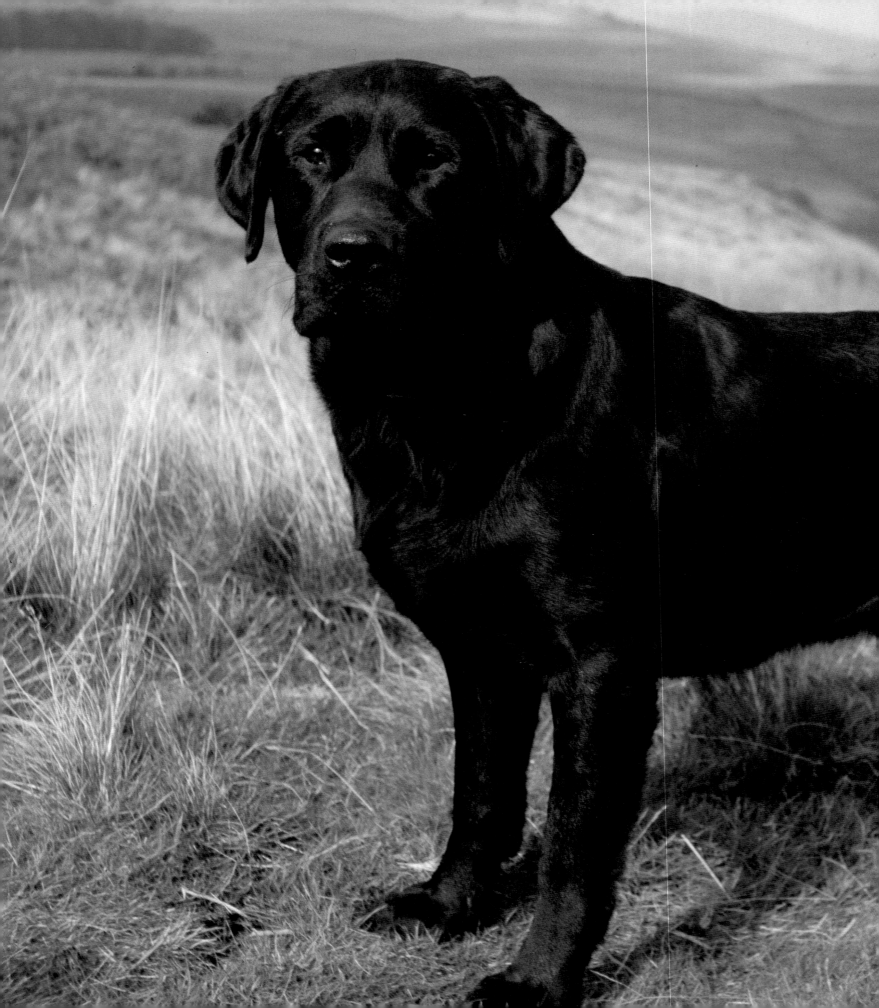

THE
NEW COMPLETE
BOOK OF THE
DOG

Foreword by Anne Rogers Clark

General Editor
Joyce Robins

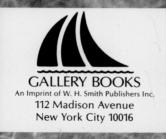

GALLERY BOOKS
An Imprint of W. H. Smith Publishers Inc.
112 Madison Avenue
New York City 10016

ACKNOWLEDGEMENTS

The publishers wish to thank the following photographers and agencies for their kind permission to reproduce their photographs in this publication:

Alton Anderson; AFIP, A M Berenger; Animal Graphics; Animal Photography; Animals Unlimited; Ardea; K Barkleigh-Shute; S C Bisserot; M Buzzini; Hanson Carroll; Bruce Coleman; Ann Cumbers; A Hamilton-Rowan; Michael Holford; Jacana; Octopus Group Picture Library; Dick Polak; Diane Pearce; Pictor; Anne Roslin-Williams; Michael Serlick; Spectrum; Tony Stone Worldwide; Guy Trouillet; US Customs; Mireille Vautier; Zefa Picture Library.

Published in Great Britain in 1991 by
The Octopus Publishing Group
as *The Complete Book of the Dog*

This edition published in 1990 by Gallery Books
an imprint of W.H. Smith Publishers Inc.
112 Madison Avenue
New York City 10016

ISBN 0 8317 6350 7

Produced by Mandarin Offset

Printed and bound in Hong Kong

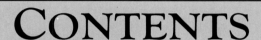

CONTENTS

FOREWORD 6

1 INTRODUCING THE DOG 8

Evolution . Domestication . Development of breeding . Senses . Communication .
The skeleton . Muscles and nerves . Respiration . Teeth and digestion .
Reproduction . Instincts and behavior .

2 CHOOSING A DOG 20

Dog or bitch . Two dogs or one . Puppy or adult dog . Pedigree or mongrel .
Which breed . Long or shorthaired . Family dogs . Guard dogs . Amount of
exercise . Breed drawbacks . Where to find your dog . Choosing from the litter

3 BREEDS OF THE WORLD 32

An A–Z of more than 150 breeds from all over the world

4 THE NEW PUPPY 110

Dogproofing your home . Equipment . Collecting your puppy . Children and
puppies . Introduction to other pets . Diet . Puppy health . Learning its name .
Early lessons . Play . Collars and leads . Grooming . Housetraining . Car travel .
Dogs and the law . Responsible dog ownership .

5 TRAINING AND OBEDIENCE 126

Joining a class . Choke collars . Training sessions . 'Come!' . The release word .
'Heel!' and 'Sit' . 'Sit and Stay' . 'Wait!' and 'Come' . 'Down and stay' . 'Leave!' .
The retrieve . Tricks . Curing bad habits . Aggression . Climbing on furniture .
Pulling . Wandering . Mounting . Phobias . Destructive dogs . Barking . Jumping
up . Stealing food . Chasing cats . Chasing vehicles . Digging holes . Resentment of
handling . Urinating indoors . Coprophagia . Car travel . Fights .

6 CARE OF THE DOG 146

Food . Special grooming . Nails . Anal sacs and glands . Baths . Health and sickness .
Signs of a healthy dog . Giving medication . First aid . Consulting a veterinarian .
A–Z of ailments . The older dog . Traveling . Boarding .

7 BREEDING 166

Preparations . Mating . Gestation . Whelping . The litter . Weaning . Hand-rearing
puppies .

8 SHOWING 178

Show organization . Show judging . Preparing for showing . Handling . The show
day . Obedience competitions . Field trials .

INDEX 188

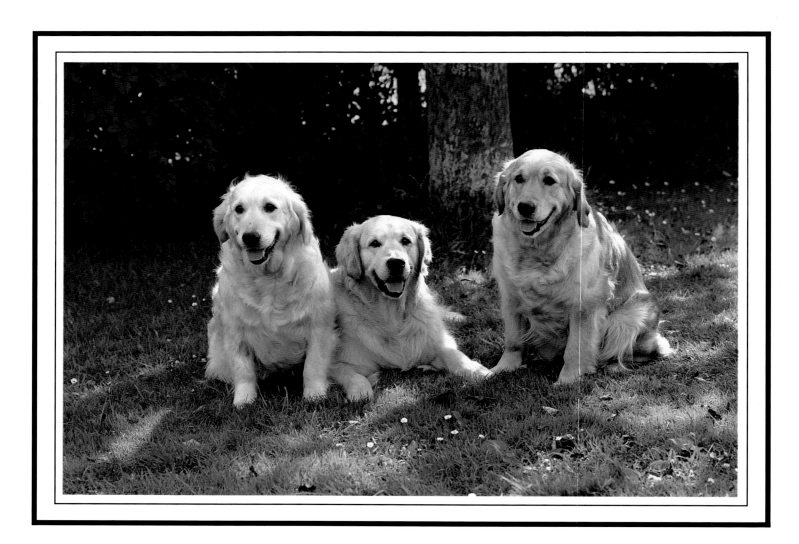

FOREWORD

My husband and I have traveled extensively, visiting every state in our vast country, as well as other countries all over the world: our purpose – to judge dog shows and to lecture on the many aspects of the sport of dogs.

Whether we find ourselves in Alaska, Hong Kong, Japan, Singapore, Canada, Australia, New Zealand, South America, the United Kingdom or the Scandinavian countries, we are ever amazed and pleased at the worldwide interest in and dependence on man's best friend – the dog.

Purebreds as well as regular dogs are a part of man's life and existence. The sport of breeding good dogs, raising them correctly and having them become useful members of society is universal in its appeal.

Dogs as companions for young and old, dogs as guards and sentries, dogs that assist in the hunt, dogs that rescue people from drowning, dogs that lead the blind and hear for the deaf; these must all be carefully chosen, reared and trained.

The New Complete Book of the Dog will be of immeasurable assistance in all of these pursuits. Comprehensive, informative, well-planned, it is a must on any dog lover's bookshelf – whether specialist dog fancier or just regular dog owner who wishes to be well read on the subject. Every aspect of dog ownership from choosing the correct breed of dog for one's purposes and raising and training it, to an introduction to the sport of showing dogs and a well-researched section on illnesses – is found here.
This is not a 'how to' book, but rather a complete and well-rounded work, on our friend, the dog.

ANNE ROGERS CLARK

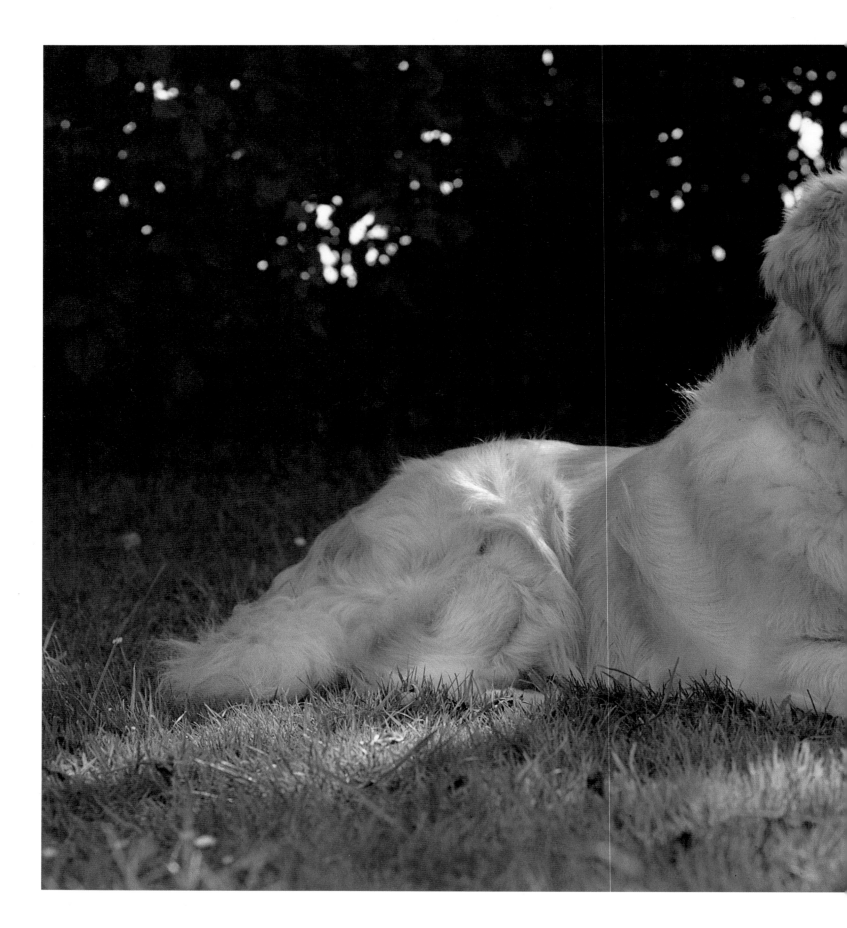

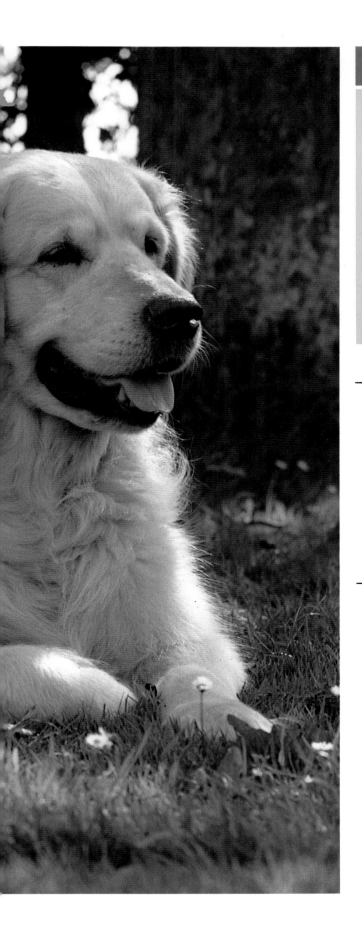

INTRODUCING THE DOG

The dog has always had a special place in man's affections and the relationship between the two goes back for thousands of years, with dogs being bred first for their usefulness as hunters, drovers and guards and later, by careful selection, for their distinctive looks and value in the show ring. You will get more out of your relationship with your pet if you understand the basic design of the dog, how its body works, the benefits of its highly developed sense of smell and hearing, and how its instincts and patterns of behavior are related.

The dog was the first wild animal domesticated by man and it has been his constant companion for thousands of years. Its basic nature makes it uniquely adaptable to the needs of man; it is essentially a pack animal, happily living under the dominance of a pack leader and ready to accept its human family as a substitute pack and its owner as the leader. The dog is an enthusiast, always keen to join in family activities, unquestioning in its loyalty and totally reliable in giving companionship and returning affection. Its ready submission to its owner means that it is easier to train than other animals; in fact, it eagerly welcomes training and man has been able to breed dogs for guarding, hunting, fighting, haulage, and as eyes for the blind and ears for the deaf. Since man's early days as a nomad hunter, the dog has earned its place as his best friend.

Dogs readily accept man as the substitute pack leader and so are easily trainable to fulfill a variety of roles.

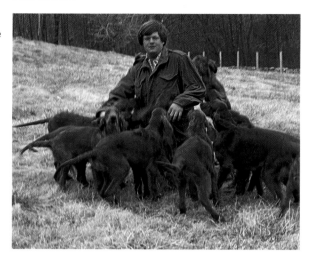

The origins of the dog have been the subject of much argument among the experts but it is now generally accepted that it is descended from the wolf.

EVOLUTION

Despite their huge range of shapes and sizes, all dogs belong to the same species, *canis familiaris*. The many breeds we know today are the result of selective breeding by man. The earliest ancestor of the *canidae* family, to which the dog belongs, along with other carnivores such as wolves, jackals and foxes, was the small carnivorous mammal called *Miacis*. This was a long-bodied, short-legged, tree-climbing animal rather like today's polecat, which flourished about 40 million years ago, during the late Eocene and early Oligocene periods. Various transitional forms evolved from *Miacis* until, some 10–20 million years ago, the forerunners of present-day *canidae* existed: first *Cynodictus*, with five toes, partly webbed, then *Tomarctus*, a primitive form of dog with longer jaws. About one million years ago, the forms we know as wolves, jackals and coyotes were already developing.

Scientists have never produced certain proof of the dog's immediate ancestor. In the nineteenth century Charles Darwin held that two species, the wolf and the golden jackal, might have given rise to the domestic dog, with some degree of cross-breeding. Certain breeds, it was argued, displayed a high degree of wolf ancestry, while others displayed mainly jackal ancestry. However, this theory has since been discredited and it is now generally accepted that the wolf alone is the dog's direct ancestor and that domestication of certain breeds of wolf probably happened in various geographical sites – North America, China and Africa as well as the Middle East – at around the same time, and this could help to explain some of the variations seen between today's breeds of dogs.

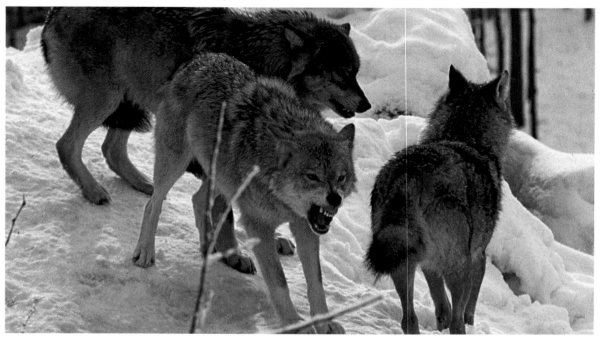

DOMESTICATION

The earliest fossil finds of domestic dogs date from about 12,000 years ago and include finds from Iraq and northern Israel. There are several other dog fossils dating from about 8,000 to over 10,000 years ago, from such widespread sites as Idaho in the United States, Turkey, Czechoslovakia and Yorkshire, England. However, the exact process of domestication is still a subject for debate among scientists.

It is possible that the relationship between dog and man first developed on a basis of mutual advantage. They were both hunting the same prey and though man was no match for the wolves as a hunter, he would have been able to drive them from their kill and enjoy the benefit of their stalking and killing skills. In turn, the wolves may have learned to exploit food discarded by man, as well as hunting the rats and other species that might have lived on grain stored by man. Tamer individuals, or cubs that grew up around humans, might have been tolerated for their use in keeping down vermin and were then befriended by man. Dogs and men might then have become hunting companions, cooperating in the gathering of food.

Another possibility is that dogs were pets or companions rather than working animals right from the start. Cubs orphaned when their mothers were killed by predators, or by man, might have been brought home as playthings for children, who brought them up much as today's youngsters might bring up an orphaned fox or badger. The working uses of the dog may have grown out of the understanding that developed between the children and their pets.

An alternative theory is that the early domestic dogs were kept as guards rather than hunters. Their superior senses of smell and hearing could have alerted man to the presence of wild animals or other

Wall paintings in the tomb of Rameses VI in the Valley of the Kings in Egypt show hunting dogs similar to modern greyhounds.

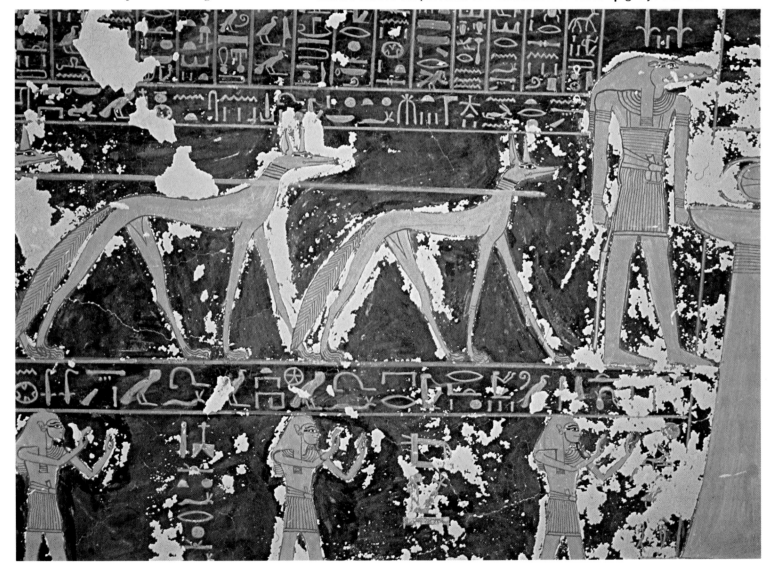

humans that might threaten his campsite. This may explain why barking is common behavior for the domestic dog but not for the wolf. Once man began keeping cattle and sheep, the dog's guarding skills would have been extended to protecting the flocks.

Whatever the details of domestication, it seems obvious that in time, the offspring of the wolf came to live in close association with man, learning to respond to his moods, fit in with his ways and obey his commands, eventually turning into the reliable worker and companion of modern times.

DEVELOPMENT OF BREEDING

Once the process of domestication had begun, man was able to breed dogs for a variety of uses. As long ago as 4000 BC the civilizations of the Middle East were breeding dogs with some care and selectivity. Egyptian murals of this period show several types of greyhounds: one has upright bat ears like the modern Ibizan Hound, while another has the small drop ear and the feathering of the modern Saluki. There is a theory that some type of greyhound, one of the ancestors of the Afghan Hound, reached Afghanistan along the trade routes of the ancient world between the Middle East and China. It was discovered there by British military men in the late nineteenth century and introduced to the western world.

The greyhound family were at their most successful in desert countries where the hot, still air makes for bad scenting conditions but visibility is excellent. This suits all types of greyhounds, since they hunt by sight rather than scent and use speed to overtake their prey. For this reason, they are also known as gazehounds.

Early Assyrian wall paintings portray a much larger, heavier Mastiff-like dog with a wrinkled head and curled tail. These were apparently used for hunting lions and were taken into battle by their Assyrian masters in 625 BC. The Greeks knew of the heavy, robust Molussus dog, also a Mastiff-type, that became famous for its courage and ferocity in tackling wild boar in the sixth century BC. Dogs of this type may have reached Britain with the Phoenician traders who came to buy tin. By the time the Romans invaded Britain, the British Mastiff was sufficiently impressive for several to be sent back to Rome to fight in gladiatorial contests.

The Middle Eastern peoples had no use for hounds that hunt by scent and the scent hounds evolved in cooler, milder climates, where the thickness of vegetation would prevent a sight hound from seeing the game. From the time of the peak of Greek civilization through to the Middle Ages in Europe, hunting with packs of scent hounds was a passion with the nobility.

Spaniels are the oldest of the gundog breeds and were widely used in medieval times to find and spring birds for the falconers' hawks, or flushing

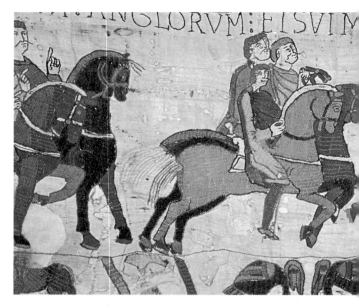

birds into a net for huntsmen.

Not all dogs were bred for their usefulness; many of the toy breeds have histories as long and well-documented as the more utilitarian varieties. Small dogs, though scorned by sportsmen, have been coveted and cosseted throughout the civilized world. The mummified remains of very small dogs have been found in Egyptian tombs. A tiny, long-coated dog was known in Malta in the time of the Phoenicians, and the Maltese seems to have existed in much its present form at the time of the Apostle Paul. In AD 100 the Chinese were breeding 'pai' dogs, described as short-legged, short-mouthed dogs which belonged under the table. The earliest of the flat-faced Chinese dogs to reach Europe was the Pug, brought home by Dutch and Portuguese traders in the sixteenth century; the first Pekingese seen in the western world came as part of the booty when the French and English troops sacked the Imperial Palace in Peking in 1860.

Many of the working breeds of the past, as opposed to the hunting dogs, have an undocumented history, for they did not attract the attention of artists and writers. We know that the vermin-hunting terriers, the cattle-droving dogs and the sheepdogs have been in existence for centuries, but we know little about their appearance before the nineteenth century.

Although some dogs have been bred over so many centuries, it was not until the advent of dog shows and the formation of the Kennel Club in Britain in 1873 and in other countries shortly afterwards that pedigrees as records of ancestry became the universal practice. The Kennel Club's first positive action was to organize a stud book and to rule that only registered dogs were allowed to enter its shows. The purpose of this was to eliminate some of the unscrupulous practices and confusion that reigned at the early shows.

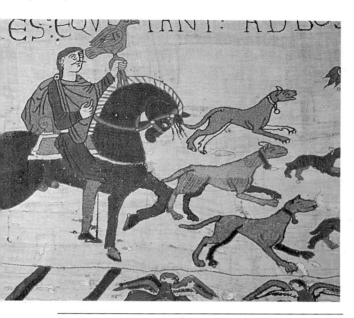

The Bayeux Tapestry, depicting the Norman Conquest, is one of the many pieces of artistic evidence showing that man has been breeding dogs for selected purposes for hundreds of years.

move their heads more frequently. They have better peripheral vision than ours, giving a larger visual field. It is movement that attracts a dog's attention to a distant object but it is remarkably difficult to point out a stationary object to a dog. The way a dog's eye lights up in the glare of car headlights is an indication of the animal's ability to make the best use of available light and see well in dim conditions. Light is reflected from a layer at the back of the animal's eye and passes twice through the light-sensitive retina, thus doubling sensitivity.

SENSES

To the dog, the most important sense is that of smell; it is estimated that its sense of smell is at least 100 times better than ours. Man has always put the dog's superior sense of smell to his own use and dogs have been trained to locate a wide variety of objects, from edible fungi such as truffles, to explosives or hidden drugs in a cargo. A dog concentrating on a track may become so absorbed in following its nose that it falls over the object of its search before its eyes register the find. As so much of its knowledge of the world is gained through its nose, the dog adapts very well to the handicap of blindness and its owner may not realize that a pet is losing its sight. A blind dog can still retrieve a ball, apparently locating it by smell and sound.

The dog's hearing is also better than ours and it is more sensitive to some sounds, especially those at high frequencies; hence the use of 'silent' dog whistles, audible to the dog but not to humans. Dogs seem to detect nuances of voice that humans are unaware of, so that a nervous person saying 'Good boy' may be conveying more about his fear than his good intentions to the dog. Most dogs can distinguish the sound of their owner's car from a medley of other traffic noises and this ability of the animal to hear an approach long before the sound is perceptible to human ears makes them valuable as sentries, watch dogs and border patrol guards. This acute hearing means that some dogs are 'sound shy', meaning that they are nervous or afraid of some noises and need a good deal of training before they become indifferent to the feared noise.

There is some controversy over whether dogs are colorblind or not; it seems likely that they see only in black and white. They cannot move their eyeballs in the sockets as freely as humans but compensate for this by the longer, more mobile neck and they

COMMUNICATION

Dogs use body signals, sounds and chemical smells in communicating with one another. The position of ears and tails indicates a great deal about a dog's mood. Two strange male dogs will approach one another with a jaunty step, heads and tails held high. Nervous dogs will make themselves appear smaller by crouching slightly and laying back their ears; they hold their tails tightly between their legs and will not allow another dog to sniff their rear. The aggressive dog, on the other hand, makes itself seem larger by raising the hair on the back of its neck and along its spine. The dog will be tense and stiff and it will fix its opponent with an intimidating glare. A stare is usually a threat signal and if an owner stares at a dog it will usually look away and become submissive, perhaps rolling on its back.

The use of smell is very important. When two dogs first meet they usually smell each others' faces

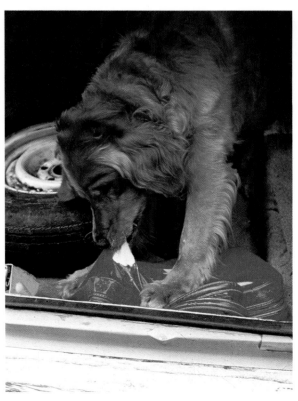

The dog's sense of smell is far superior to that of humans. It is so highly developed that a dog can be trained to detect hidden drugs or explosives.

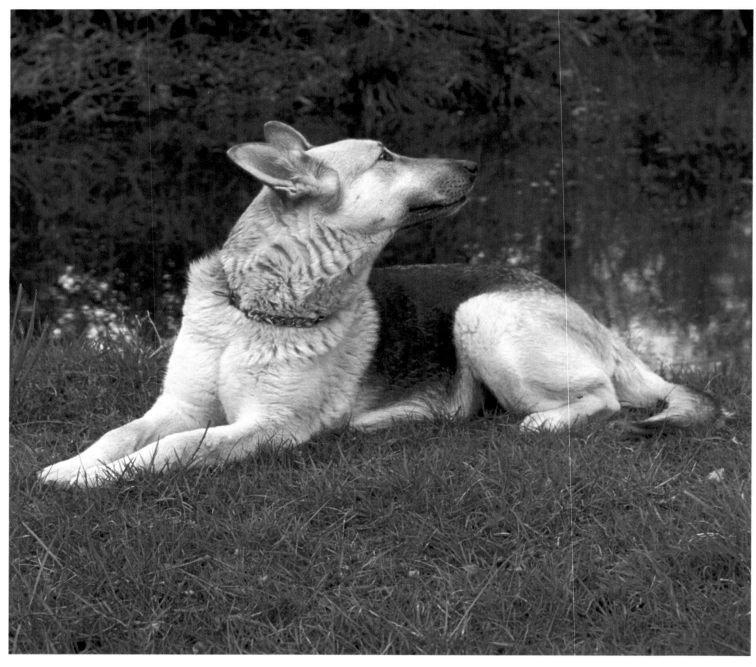

and then their hindquarters. A male dog cocks its leg to mark prominent objects while out walking in order to mask the smell of dogs that have passed recently and claim the territory as its own. Scratching with the back feet, seen mainly in male dogs after defecation, leaves a chemical signal, known as a pheromone, from special glands between the toes. Feces may be used as scent markers and a dog has anal glands that secrete a mixture of chemicals.

Sounds used include barking, whining and howling. Barking is usually to gain attention, perhaps as an excited greeting or a request for a game. Whining, often heard when a dog is left alone, is a distress call aimed at the owner and is hardly ever used towards another dog. Howling is probably a warning sound used to protect a territory.

THE SKELETON

The dog's basic skeletal structure remains the same in a tiny Chihuahua or a huge St Bernard though the size and thickness of individual bones varies from breed to breed.

Many dogs have skulls that differ little from their wild ancestors. However, in the short-faced breeds, the jaws are considerably shortened and the curva-

This German Shepherd shows that it has sensed a friendly presence; its ears are pricked and moving round in the direction of a sound and its nose has picked up a scent.

ture of the cheekbones increased, giving the appearance of a greater width of skull: this shape is known as brachycephalic. In some of the breeds, such as the Bulldog, the lower jaw is slightly longer than the upper, causing the lower teeth to meet outside the upper set, a condition known as 'undershot'.

The neck has seven vertebrae, known as the cervical vertebrae. The first (the atlas) allows the head to nod up and down and the second (the axis) allows the head to rotate. The remainder of the neck vertebrae permit the dog to bend its neck to look behind much more efficiently than a human being. Behind the neck are 13 thoracic vertebrae which protect the spinal cord and support the ribs. The seven lumbar vertebrae support the abdomen and lead to the sacrum, which usually consists of three vertebrae fused together. The sacrum supports the pelvic girdle and the hind limbs. The number of tail bones varies greatly according to breed.

The thoracic vertebrae, the ribs and sternum form what is commonly known as the ribcage, which encloses the heart and two lungs. It is particularly deep and roomy in the racing breeds, such as the Greyhounds. The heart of a racing Greyhound is measurably larger than that of a dog of similar size not subjected to so much exertion.

The structure of the shoulder, particularly the relationship between the shoulder blade (scapula) and upper arm (humerus), determines what kind of movement the dog has. Many breeds require the forelegs to move straight forward parallel to each other, covering the maximum of ground with the most efficiency. In this case the ideal is a shoulder blade at an angle of 45 degrees to the perpendicular, with the upper arm at right angles to it. The 'straight' front required by some terrier breeds is

The skeleton is made up of two parts: the axial skeleton comprises the skull and spinal column and the appendicular skeleton comprises the shoulders, pelvic girdle and the limbs.

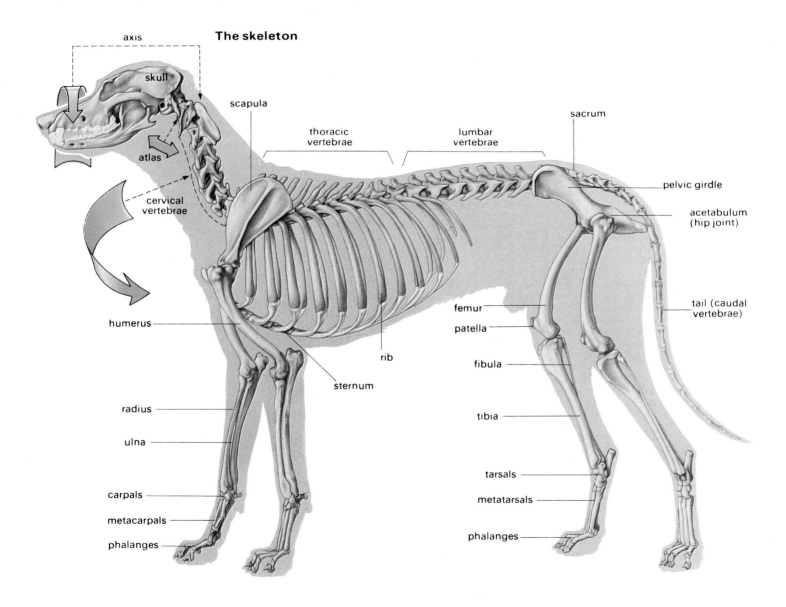

The skeleton

axis

skull

scapula

sacrum

thoracic vertebrae

lumbar vertebrae

pelvic girdle

atlas

cervical vertebrae

acetabulum (hip joint)

tail (caudal vertebrae)

humerus

femur

patella

rib

fibula

sternum

radius

tibia

ulna

tarsals

carpals

metatarsals

metacarpals

phalanges

phalanges

The action of the muscles in extending and contracting can be seen in the action of the racing Greyhound, a dog designed for great speed.

achieved by a short upper arm which brings the elbow of the dog up above the line of the brisket. Conversely, many of the racing breeds have a very long upper arm.

In the very short-legged dog, the leg bones have been shortened by selective breeding, rather than reducing the size of the animal, so that the result is quite a large dog set very low to the ground, for example Dachshunds and Basset Hounds. The long back comes from the length of rib cage and loin.

MUSCLES AND NERVES

The dog's skeleton is covered by layers of muscles and these provide the complex system necessary for the precise control of movement. Muscles always act in pairs or groups in which some contract to bend a joint while others contract to straighten a joint. Muscles are richly supplied wth blood vessels and nerves. The nerves carry messages to and from the brain, which contains the majority of nerve cells within the body. Messages from the brain control functions: for instance, instructing a muscle to contract or a gland to discharge its contents. Messages to the brain inform it of what is happening all over the body. If, for example, the dog's skin is inflamed, a message indicating pain will be transmitted to the animal's brain, which may then 'instruct' a leg to scratch the area concerned. If a nerve is seriously damaged the message will not get through and the result will be loss of feeling and motor paralysis.

RESPIRATION

Air is drawn in through the dog's nose and down the trachea, or windpipe. From the trachea the air

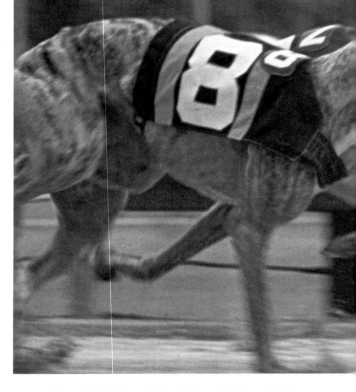

passes through the bronchi and bronchioles, which are extensions of the trachea and which gradually reduce in diameter, and finally into the air sacs in the lungs. These sacs have a rich supply of tiny blood vessels called capillaries which absorb the oxygen from the air and release waste carbon dioxide from the blood into the air sacs. This waste gas is then expelled when the dog breathes out.

The technique of panting, by which the dog regulates its body temperature, is connected with the respiratory system. Cold air is drawn in over the tongue and passed out again, taking with it moisture. It thus reduces the dog's body heat by evaporation.

TEETH AND DIGESTION

The dog has two sets of teeth in its lifetime. There are 28 milk teeth which appear at 3–5 weeks of age; then these are pushed out by the adult teeth which begin appearing at about four months, though the time varies between breeds with large dogs teething rather earlier than the toy breeds. There are 42 permanent teeth: the lower jaw has six incisors, two canines, eight premolars and six molars and the upper jaw has two less molars. The last premolar of the upper jaw and the first molar of the lower jaw are modified into 'carnassial' teeth, a type found only in carnivores. The sharp edges of these teeth slide over one another like scissor blades. These teeth can best be seen in action when a dog gnaws meat from a bone, using the side of its mouth.

This Deerhound is cooling itself by panting, which causes evaporation and therefore loss of excess heat.

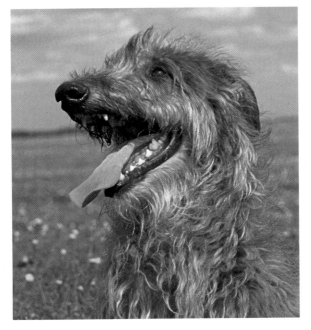

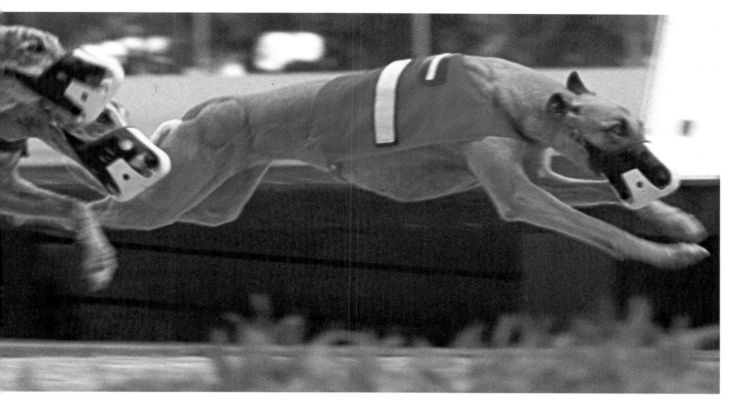

Food is roughly chopped by the teeth and softened with the help of saliva secreted by the three pairs of salivary glands that empty into the mouth. It then passes down the esophagus, or food pipe, into the stomach. There, acids and enzymes work on the food, preparing it for passage through the pylorus, a ring-shaped muscle around the hind end of the stomach and into the small intestine where useful parts of the diet are absorbed into the bloodstream. After all the nutrients have been extracted the remainder of the food moves into the large intestine, where excess fluid is removed and feces are formed before elimination through the rectum.

The main task of the liver, the largest single organ in the body, is to aid the digestion of food taken

The dog's adult teeth replace the milk teeth of the puppy when it is about four months old.

Dentition

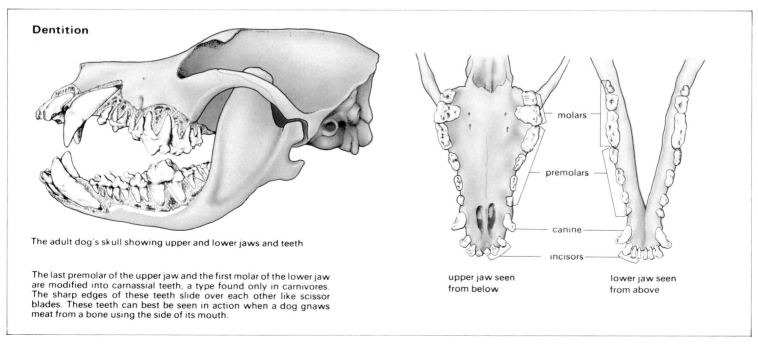

The adult dog's skull showing upper and lower jaws and teeth

The last premolar of the upper jaw and the first molar of the lower jaw are modified into carnassial teeth, a type found only in carnivores. The sharp edges of these teeth slide over each other like scissor blades. These teeth can best be seen in action when a dog gnaws meat from a bone using the side of its mouth.

molars

premolars

canine

incisors

upper jaw seen from below

lower jaw seen from above

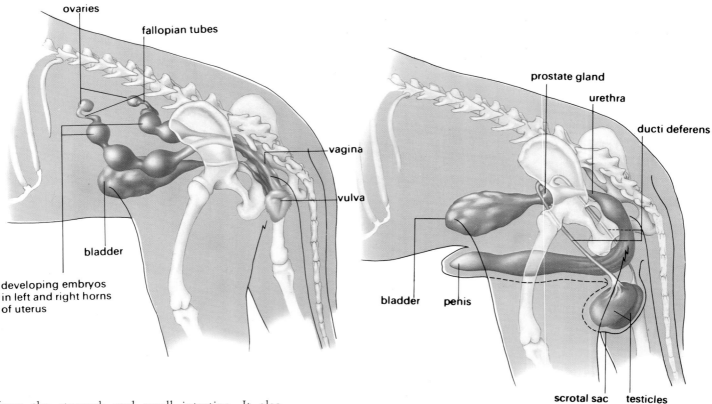

from the stomach and small intestine. It also produces bile, which assists in the digestive process and is stored in the gallbladder. The kidneys act as a sophisticated filter, ridding the blood of waste products and toxic substances, passed through the ureters to the bladder in the form of urine.

The illustrations above show the male and female reproductive organs which enable puppies to be conceived, carried and born after a dog and bitch have mated successfully. The horns of the uterus in the female show bulges of the developing embryos.

REPRODUCTION

The male dog is easily distinguished from the female by its external genitals: the penis and the two testicles, where the sperm is stored, ready to be ejaculated at mating. Of the bitch's reproductive organs, only the slit of the vulva, the end of the genital canal, is visible. The other organs of the reproductive system are the vagina (into which the penis is inserted), the cervix (a valve-like construction between the vagina and the uterus) and the uterus itself, which has two 'arms' or horns, each leading to a fallopian tube and an ovary. Each ovary produces female hormones and eggs.

Most bitches come into season or heat twice a year. A season lasts about 21 days, beginning with the discharge of a fluid opaque at first, then stained with blood. This happens when the walls of the uterus prepare to receive fertilized eggs. After 10 to 14 days the discharge loses its color; this is when the eggs produced by the ovaries are liberated and flow into the fallopian tubes ready for fertilization and eventual implantation.

At mating, seminal fluid is released via the dog's penis and the sperms in the fluid travel towards the cervix, which opens to allow them to pass into the uterus and from there to the fallopian tubes where the eggs are stored. Mating will only succeed if male sperms fertilize the eggs; then the fertilized eggs travel to the uterus and attach themselves to its walls. The embryos that form will develop into puppies which will be expelled through the vagina after about 63 days.

INSTINCTS AND BEHAVIOR

Some of the dog's most basic instincts result in behavior that is useful in its relationship with man. Chief among these is the pack instinct. The dog is a highly sociable animal and in the wild, dogs would live as a group, remaining close together, doing the same sort of thing at the same time and observing a set hierarchy. Therefore the dog is content with its position in a human family, where the owner dominates. However, there is one aspect of pack behavior that is often overlooked. It is easy for man to take over as pack leader for his dogs – but only if he is capable of leading. Nearly anyone can train a submissive dog but a dominant dog needs a dominant trainer. Within a household, a dog will often obey some members of the family and not others.

Fear is instinctive in the wild dog and is necessary to its survival but in a domestic dog, nervousness makes it less predictable, more difficult to train and control. Nerves and fear probably account for many of the dog bites suffered by children. Some dogs, for example, are easily frightened by a child rushing up with outstretched arms and misinterpret this friendly gesture as an attack. On the occasions where a dog bites its owner, it is often because the dog fears that it will be hurt and decides to attack first.

The dog's predatory instincts have been turned to good account in the hunting dogs. In pets it means that dogs will enjoy chasing balls and sticks but they also love to chase cats or rabbits. The herding instinct is only a slight deviation from the hunting instinct and in some dogs, like the Border Collie, it is strong enough to make it attempt to herd anything that moves, such as the ducks on the local pond.

Instinctive protective behavior can be useful to the human owner and is seen at its most extreme in trained guard dogs. Even a peaceful family pet will often defend its territory strenuously. Tradesmen who wear a distinctive uniform are often on the receiving end of this behavior: if they retreat when a dog barks or rushes towards the gate, the dog will regard this as a victory and will be encouraged to threaten even more fiercely when it next sees the uniform.

The dog's natural instincts can be put to use by man. Aggression can be useful in a guard dog and only a brave, or foolhardy, trespasser would ignore the menacing stance of the dog pictured below. The Golden Retriever (below left) makes a valuable companion on a pheasant shoot.

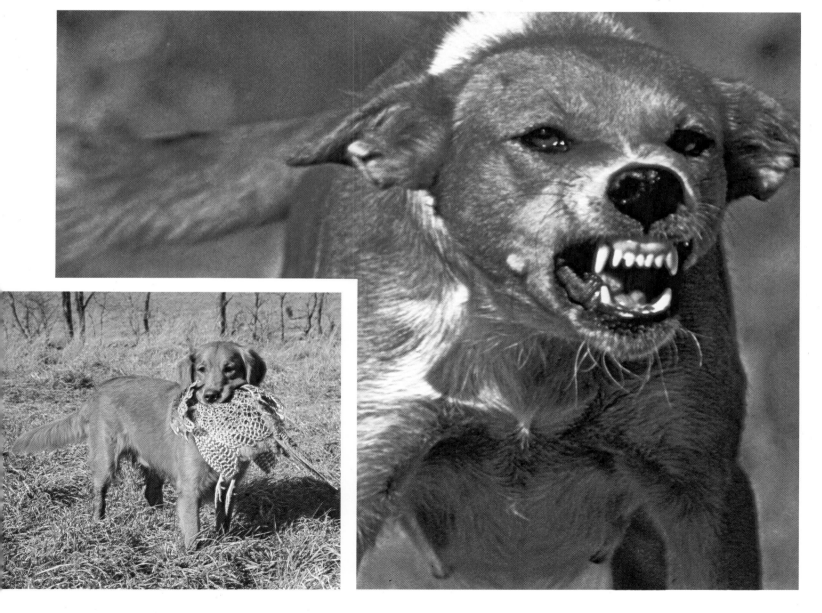

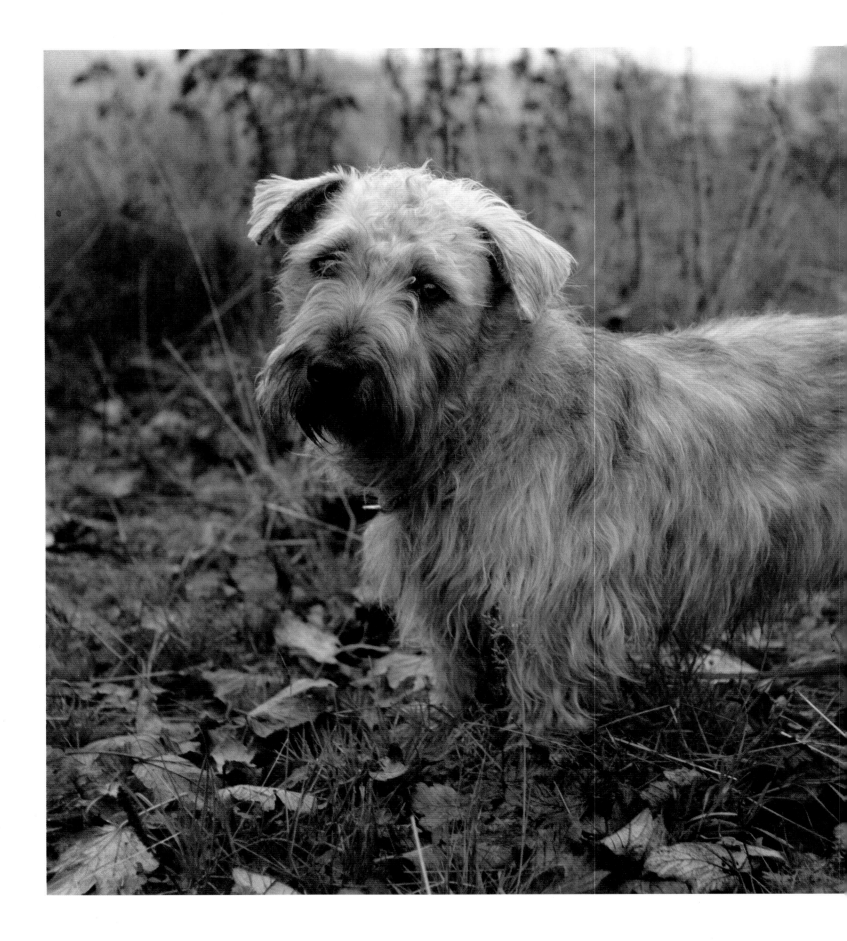

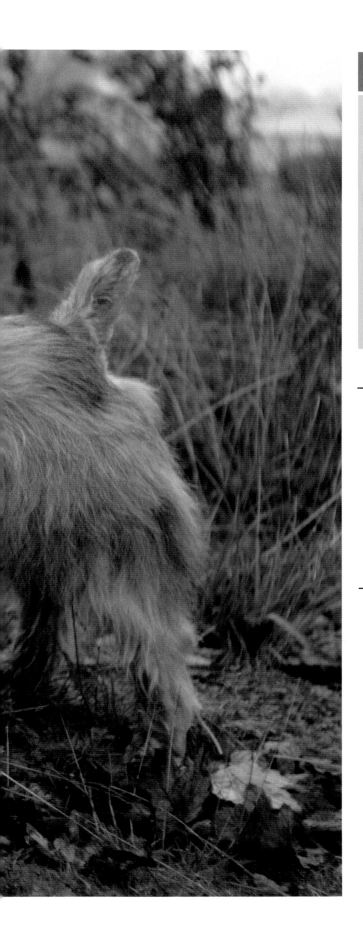

CHOOSING
A DOG

There are so many types of dog that you will be spoiled for choice but taking a dog into your home should never be a spur of the moment decision. You will need to be sure that its size, temperament and energy level suits your family's way of life, so that you can enjoy many happy years together. You will have to consider whether you want a pet or a show dog, whether your home needs a watchdog or your children a protector. Once you find a litter of suitable puppies, you will want to be sure of picking a healthy specimen.

Taking a dog into your home brings many pleasures and benefits; it also brings responsibilities. It will be dependent on you for years to come and you will be in charge of its well-being for the span of its life. No dog should have to change an established home for a new one unless unforeseen circumstances make it unavoidable. You will be responsible for its behavior at all times, as no pet should be allowed to roam unsupervised. You should only consider taking on a dog if everyone in the family wants one and you are sure that you can care for it over a long period. It should never be simply a child's plaything, to be overindulged as a puppy then, when it is no longer a furry little bundle, neglected in favor of a new toy.

Your choice of dog will depend on your lifestyle and on what you expect to get from your pet. It is no use thinking about a Great Dane or St Bernard if you live in an apartment or a mobile home; these dogs need plenty of room and once they spread themselves out, you may end up with nowhere to put your feet. You may want a dog primarily as a watchdog, or as a playmate for your children, or a cuddly armful to share your evenings in front of the television. There is little point in choosing a Pekingese if you want a companion on long country walks or a Golden Retriever if you want a guard dog to strike fear into the hearts of would-be burglars.

Before looking for a particular dog you must be sure that you can house and care for it properly. Companionship is high on the list of the dog's own needs and the happiest of dogs are those that spend most of their time with their owners, especially if they can participate in their activities in some way. If everyone in the household is at work for eight hours a day, or you spend most of your evenings and weekends out with friends, you would be wise to choose a more independent pet, a cat for instance.

A dog means extra expense, so calculate the amount you will need to spend on food, vaccinations, grooming equipment, collars and leads, baskets and bowls. There will also be veterinary fees over the years and perhaps boarding and training fees. On the whole, large dogs cost more and produce more waste, which may be a real problem for town dwellers; on the other hand, you may feel much safer walking a large dog at night through city streets.

Apart from size, you will need to decide whether to have a dog or a bitch, puppy or adult, pedigree or mongrel and how much time you are willing and able to spend on exercise and grooming.

DOG OR BITCH

Dogs and bitches do differ in temperament and a bitch may be more suitable as a family pet as the relationship between the male dog and its owner can become very intense. Male dogs are often bolder and more independent by nature, and may also be more aggressive and eager to roam. The male dog kept as a pet should be kept away from sexual temptation; it is a great mistake to allow him to mate a bitch as he may become disorientated and begin to wander. He may start marking out a territory in the home and become aggressive with other male dogs. Dogs used for stud work are specially trained from a young age and lead a completely different style of life from a pet. Though it is possible to castrate a male dog by a simple operation, this is not usually advised as it changes the animal's personality. A castrated dog will be less active and is liable to become overweight unless its diet is carefully monitored. It will probably be less protective and may lose its instinct to guard the home.

Bitches are often more affectionate and home-loving, needing less discipline, but they have the disadvantage of coming into season twice a year. Each time there is a three-week period when the bitch is 'in heat'; this begins with a blood-stained discharge from the vagina which changes to straw color at about the tenth day. During this time, she is very attractive to males who will track her down by her scent and may haunt your house and annoy you and your neighbors. The bitch will be eager to find a mate so she will escape if given the slightest opportunity and this may happen even before you realize she's in heat. If you do not want your bitch to have puppies, you will need to take great care, securing doors, gates and windows so that it is impossible for her to get out.

The alternative is to have her spayed, a major operation involving removal of the ovaries and the uterus. The spayed bitch will not have any further heats and cannot produce an unwanted litter. She will keep her female character and continue to be a home-loving pet but you may have to watch her diet if she shows signs of putting on too much weight. Your veterinarian will advise on the best age for spaying; some favor around five months, well before the first 'season'; others prefer to wait until the first heat has passed, believing that this cuts the risk of side effects, such as obesity.

TWO DOGS OR ONE

Though the human family takes the place of the pack for the dog, it is beneficial to have more than one dog wherever possible. They will keep one another company if you are often out and they will be less dependent on you for games. Dogs needing lots of exercise can run off their excess energy together without exhausting their owners.

Two bitches will usually get along well together with only an occasional squabble. If you plan to keep two male dogs in the household, choose one of the more placid-natured breeds as some males, particularly those of the terrier groups, are inclined

The right dog can be a protector, a playmate and a faithful companion from puppyhood to old age.

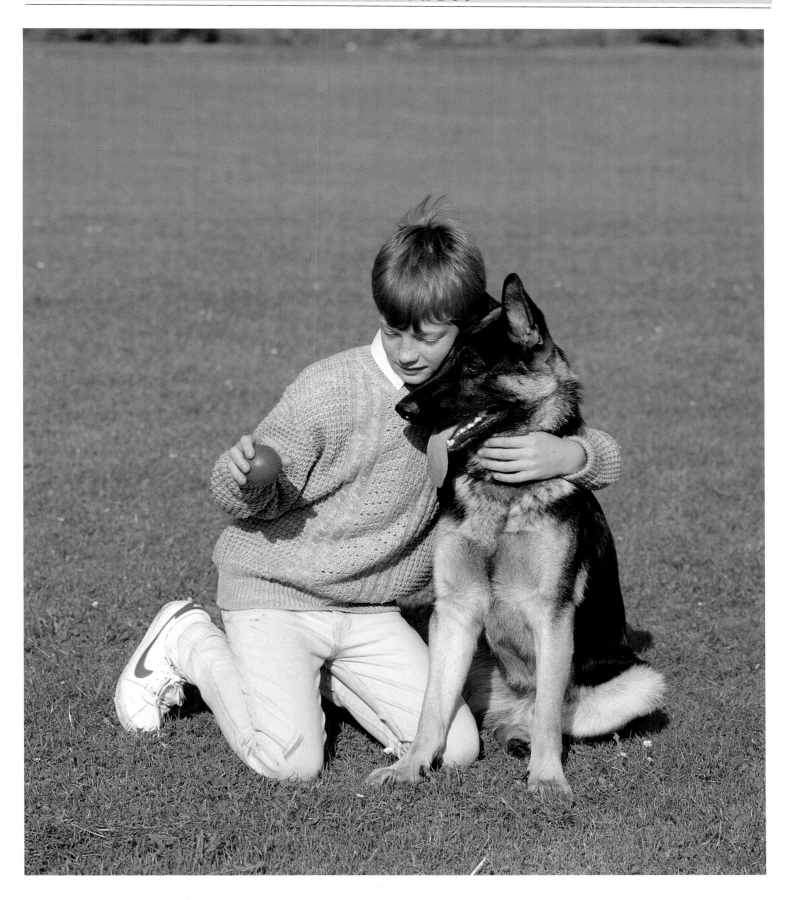

Two puppies brought into the family at the same time will play and exercise together and form a firm and lasting friendship.

A dog can provide valuable companionship for an elderly person but it should be carefully chosen for a quiet nature and the need for a minimum of exercise.

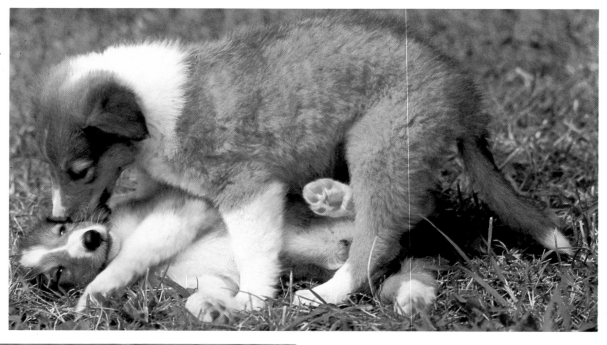

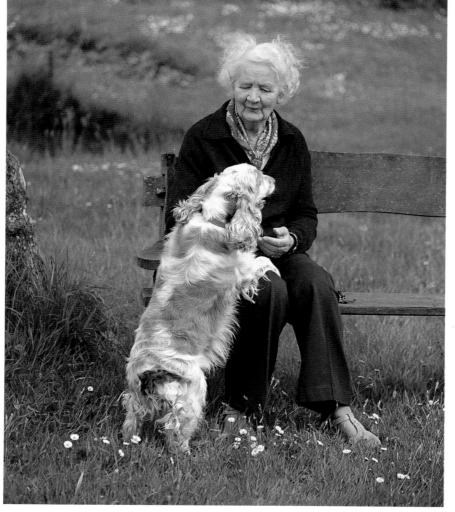

to fight. Keeping a dog and a bitch will mean problems when the bitch is in season, unless she has been spayed.

PUPPY OR ADULT DOG

It is normally more satisfactory to buy a puppy rather than a full-grown dog as a family pet. Of course, you will have to tackle housetraining and basic training as well as vaccinations but as the puppy grows up it will fit readily into your home life.

Taking an older dog can present difficulties; its habits and patterns of behavior are already formed. However, some dogs really need new homes, through no fault of their own. Sometimes owners die or emigrate or someone in the house becomes allergic and a healthy, well-behaved dog may find itself in need of a new owner. Occasionally a breeder has a young dog, kept because of its showing potential, which has been well trained and cared for but has to find a new owner because it has not lived up to its early promise. For an elderly person, who might find a lively puppy too much of a handful, or a busy household with children of various ages and a great deal of coming and going, an adult dog may be a more suitable pet.

If you take a dog from a pound or shelter, beware of sentimentality. A pair of brown eyes gazing out from a pen may be appealing but, sadly, some dogs have been passed from hand to hand, perhaps because of serious behavior problems, and may be difficult to rehabilitate. It is unwise to take such a dog unless you are sure that you can devote a great deal of time and patience to training and care. Some people have a knack of rescuing 'incorrigible' dogs but it is a special skill and not everyone can be successful. Remember that you will be doing an abandoned dog no favors if you take it in, only to find that you are unable to cope and have to return it several weeks later, adding another upheaval to its already unsatisfactory life.

PEDIGREE OR MONGREL

When you buy a pedigree puppy, you can be sure of its eventual adult size, shape, coat length and texture, as well as having a fair idea of its temperament, suitability for your lifestyle and the amount of time you will have to spend on grooming and exercise. With a mongrel, all these things are a gamble. Mongrel puppies may be very cheap to buy but may cost just as much to keep as a pedigree dog of the same size. Many mongrels prove to be intelligent and make good family dogs. As they are cross-bred they rarely show any hereditary defects and it is sometimes possible to buy first-cross puppies, either from a mismating or from a mating that was intended to combine the characteristics of both breeds. Such puppies may combine the best traits of both parents, in which case the results can be delightful but you need to be aware that they could combine the less desirable characteristics.

WHICH BREED

Try to look at some adults of any breed that attracts you and talk to the owners about possible problems before buying a puppy. Generalizations about breed characteristics can be very misleading as there are always exceptions but knowledge of the breed's original use may be a guide to the usual temperament you can expect. For instance, the gundogs' original role was to find game for the sportsman but to refrain from chasing it, so they had to be extremely obedient. Most gundogs, therefore, are amenable to discipline but they also have plenty of energy and stamina that needs an outlet. Few gundogs make good guard dogs but most of them are superb with children.

The greyhound family make gentle and dignified house dogs but the instinct to chase and kill can be triggered off by the sight of a small, moving object in the distance, and once in pursuit of anything they are virtually unstoppable. The scent hounds, like the Basset or Beagle, originally bred to live and work in packs, are surprisingly sociable, friendly and nonaggressive types. However, they can be obstinate and conveniently deaf when following their own interests. Sight hounds like the Afghan can be very aloof and retain a strong hunting instinct.

The Bulldog may look ferocious but it makes a lovable, intelligent and trainable family pet and is very good with children.

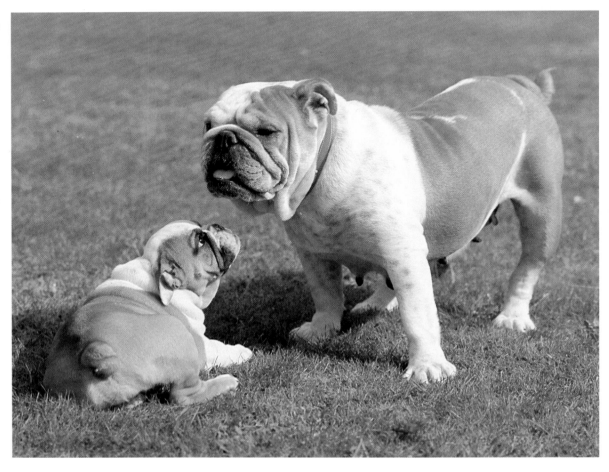

Long haired dogs, like this Rough Collie, need frequent and careful grooming, so prospective owners should take this into account.

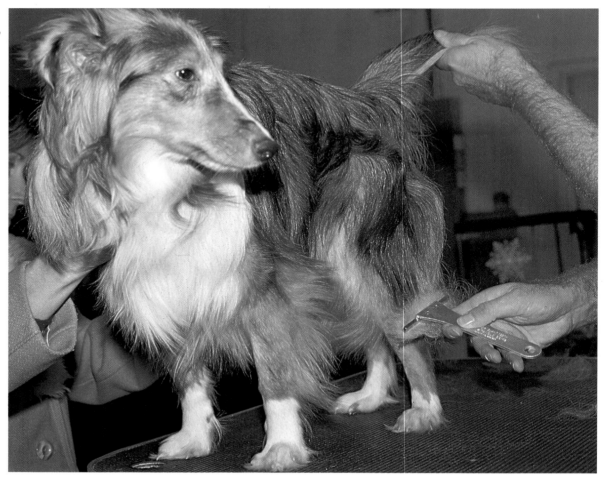

Dogs can be important in a child's life and Border Terriers (above right) make affectionate family pets.

Even in the White House the English Springer Spaniel Millie (below right) belonging to President Bush and his wife Barbara, claims pride of place after producing six puppies.

The terriers are very varied in appearance; many are named after the regions in which they were originally developed to hunt and kill vermin. They are all basically similar in temperament – very quick, agile and alert with fast reactions that cause them to snap first and ask questions later. They can also be noisy and excitable.

The giant breeds are expensive to keep and need a great deal of space. Though they do not need as much exercise as many of the smaller, lighter breeds, their bulk makes them unsuitable for many modern homes. Toy dogs, on the other hand, can fit into the most compact home and are often very good watch dogs. They make lively and amusing companions, so long as they are not spoiled by their owners.

The Spitz breeds are usually bold, hardy, adaptable dogs with strong wills. One or two of the Spitz breeds tend to be rather noisy.

Some breeds enjoy more robust health than others. This is because the basic dog shape is that of a medium-sized dingo type of animal and the further the breeds deviate from the norm, the more likely it becomes that the exaggeration of proportion represents a health risk to the dog. Giant breeds or those with large heads and very flattened muzzles tend to

have a shorter life span than other breeds. Miniature sizes or very long backs, heavily wrinkled faces, protruding or very small eyes – all these can be weaknesses from a health point of view. Serious dog breeders are always well aware of the strengths and defects of their chosen breeds and take both health and temperament into account when planning their breeding program.

LONG OR SHORTHAIRED

Too many owners have fallen in love with a shaggy Old English Sheepdog or a silky Afghan on the TV screen, only to find that the splendid appearance is the result of long and painstaking grooming, which does not fit into their busy lives. Many of the longhaired breeds need daily grooming but with others, a short session once a week is sufficient. Among the breeds needing minimum grooming are: Basenji, Basset Hound, Beagle, Bloodhound, Boston Terrier, Boxer, Bulldog, Bull Terrier, Corgi, Smoothhaired Dachshund, Dalmatian, Doberman Pinscher, Labrador Retriever, Miniature Pinscher, Norfolk Terrier, Papillon, Pug, Staffordshire Bull Terrier, Weimaraner, Whippet.

Whether you choose a long or a shorthaired

animal, remember that almost all dogs will molt in spring and autumn. Long hairs look more obvious on your upholstery but short hairs can be even more difficult to remove sometimes. The only way around this is to choose a breed that does not molt: these include Poodles, Bedlington Terriers and Kerry Blue Terriers.

FAMILY DOGS

Most dogs that grow up with a family will get on well with the children of the household, though it is important that children are taught never to tease an animal. However, a placid breed is a better choice than an excitable one that can get too carried away with rough and noisy games. Taking on a puppy when there is a toddler in the house is not really fair to either of them. The child will be too young to appreciate what will hurt or frighten the dog and the puppy may get carried away in a rough and tumble and hurt the child unintentionally.

Breeds with the reputation of being affectionate family dogs, good with children, include: Pointer, Golden Retriever, Labrador Retriever, English Setter, Cocker Spaniel, Basset Hound, Beagle, Finnish Spitz, Border Terrier, West Highland White Terrier, Cavalier King Charles Spaniel, Border Collie, Schipperke, Shih Tzu.

Some breeds, including Pekingese, Chihuahua and Scottish Terrier are less likely to make good pets for children, and Afghans react badly to teasing. Most Poodles prefer older children.

GUARD DOGS

You may like the idea of a dog that will warn of intruders and scare away burglars but do not forget that a domestic watchdog is very different from a guard dog, which will attack if necessary.

The breeds famous for their guarding potential need a high standard of training – and so do their handlers. Untrained or undertrained guard dogs can be rather like carrying around a loaded gun – it can go off with disastrous results. A well-trained Doberman Pinscher can make an excellent guard and companion but needs careful handling and firm discipline. They are powerful, muscular dogs with a strong sense of loyalty. The German Shepherd has a reputation as a 'one-man' dog though it has sometimes earned a bad reputation because in the wrong hands it can become dangerous; it is essentially a working dog and becomes very frustrated if given nothing to do. The Rottweiler first became known to the world as a German police and army dog and the power and strength of the breed is evident. It is a fearless and highly intelligent dog but, again, it needs expert training and skilled handling.

Other, less potentially ferocious, breeds may be more suitable for a suburban neighborhood. Though not usually thought of as guard dogs,

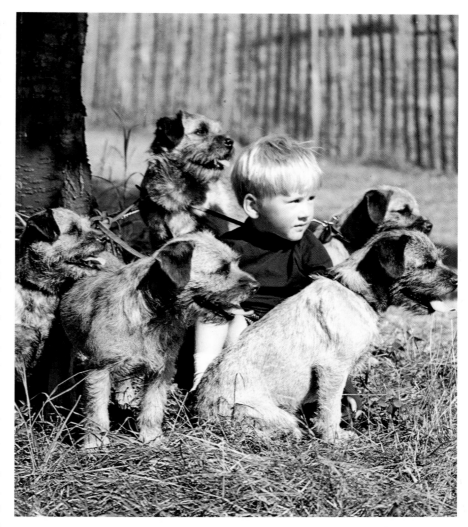

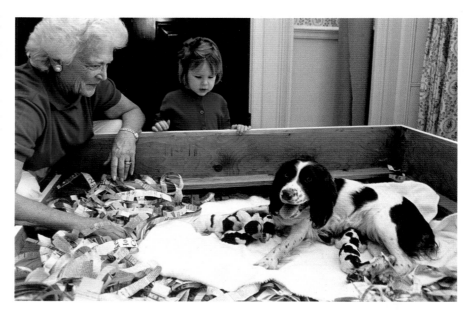

Dalmatians have a long tradition in this field; at one time they were used as war dogs and in the nineteenth century their normal duty was as carriage guards. The Great Dane looks the part and its awe-inspiring appearance and deep-throated bark would scare away all but the very bold or foolhardy.

Many small breeds do a good job as watchdogs, such as the small, tailless Schipperke, once used on Flemish canal barges to repel boarders. They are active, bustling, vigilant little dogs and their shrill piercing bark gives obvious warning of strangers. The happy little Lhasa Apso makes a courageous little guard and is quick to give a warning.

AMOUNT OF EXERCISE

Unless you are a keen walker and you live in an area where your dog has the opportunity to run free as part of its regular exercise, do not choose the muscular, active dogs that need a great deal of exercise. The Labrador Retriever, Border Collie or Dalmatian, for instance, need at least an hour's exercise a day and fare best if half of it is at the gallop!

All dogs appreciate a change of scene and fresh air but among the breeds that can manage with just a daily game with their owners are: Chihuahua, Chinese Crested Dog, Griffon, King Charles Spaniel, Lhasa Apso, Maltese, Miniature Pinscher, Papillon, Pekingese, Pomeranian, Pug, Shih Tzu, Yorkshire Terrier.

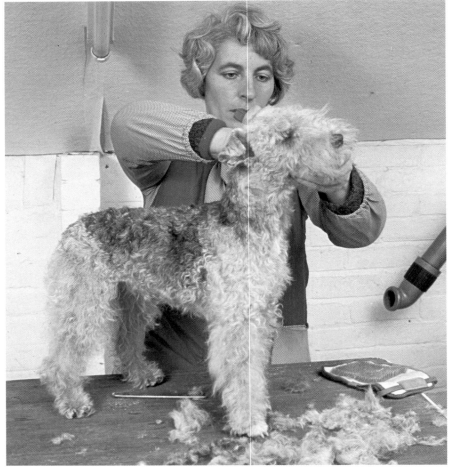

The rough haired Lakeland Terrier needs careful brushing and trimming.

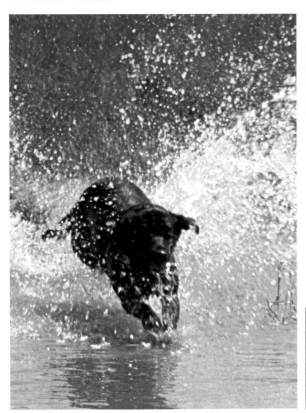

Some dogs need a great deal of vigorous exercise to keep in the peak of condition and a sedate walk around the block will not be sufficient.

BREED DRAWBACKS

Some popular dogs have particular problems from the point of view of ownership and it is important to consider whether or not these will cause you trouble:

Weimaraner: easily bored, can become destructive
Basset Hound: tends to roam
Irish Wolfhound: may be overprotective
Airedale Terrier: may be overprotective

Fox Terrier
Kerry Blue Terrier
Irish Terrier
Sealyham Terrier
Boxer
Doberman Pinscher } like to fight

Basenji
Scottish Terrier
Rough Collie
Doberman Pinscher
Shetland Sheepdog
Welsh Corgi
Lhasa Apso
Schnauzer } dislike or are suspicious of strangers

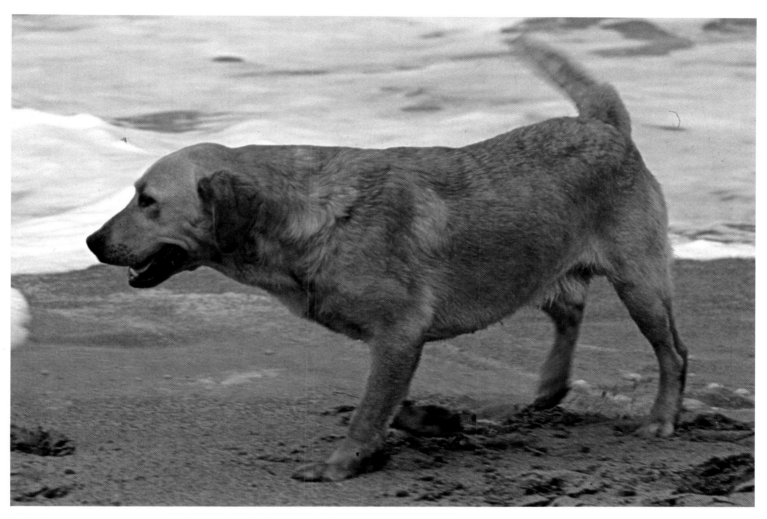

The Labrador Retriever is one of the most popular dogs in the USA: it is bright, alert, friendly and easily trained to obedience standards.

WHERE TO FIND YOUR DOG

Puppies, both pedigree and mongrel, are often offered for sale through the classified advertisements in local newspapers, or 'For Sale' cards in shops or stores. Veterinarians in your locality may know of available litters and specialist magazines covering the dog world will usually carry particulars of breeders who are likely to have puppies for sale. If you have decided on a particular breed, you can obtain the addresses of local breeders from the breed society. Your local library should be able to find the address for you; otherwise contact the head office of your Kennel Club. The secretaries of breed societies usually work on a voluntary basis, so send your request in writing, enclosing a large, stamped addressed envelope.

It is always best to obtain your puppy direct from the breeder, if possible. You will then be able to see the conditions in which the dogs are kept and get advice from the breeder on diet, exercise and so on. You will also get a much better idea of the likely temperament of your puppy if you see the mother and watch the puppies playing together. Most breeders are concerned about the future welfare of their puppies and will want to make sure that they are going to the right sort of home. Normally, they will be pleased to advise on any problems that arise after you have taken the puppy home.

Pet shops or dealers, who buy in many different breeds and offer them for sale, are not the best places to buy your pet. When puppies come from several different places and are kept in close proximity the chances of infection are much higher. The puppies may be stressed by long journeys and may be handled by several strangers in the course of a day. None of this contributes to their well-being. If you do buy from a pet shop or from a dealer, make sure that the establishment is scrupulously clean, that it is staffed by knowledgeable, caring people and that all the puppies look healthy. If you see any signs of diarrhea, discharge from the eyes or noses – on any puppies, not just the one you are thinking of buying – do not consider buying. If a puppy becomes ill after you have taken it home and made it part of the family, you will go through a great deal of worry and unhappiness, and no refund or replacement can make up for the sadness of losing a pet.

CHOOSING FROM THE LITTER

Choosing a puppy from the litter is not as simple as it sounds and you should take care not to allow sentimentality to cloud your judgment. Virtually all puppies are irresistibly attractive and it is easy to buy on impulse, so before you go shopping for your dog you should make contingency plans and stick to them rigidly. Do *not* take any family, friends, or children with you: it is easy to be swayed into buying a puppy for the wrong reasons.

The smallest and weakest pup may look the most appealing, but it might require a great deal of attention and veterinary help during rearing. It is quite a good idea to choose the puppy that first comes to you (if it is of the right sex). You should be able to handle it without the puppy showing fear or aggression. The puppies in the litter should look healthy and clean and not smell too 'doggy.' There should be no signs of discharge from the eyes or nostrils (some breeders may try to excuse these symptoms by saying they are due to sawdust or bedding). The ears should be spotless inside and the teeth should be sharp and white. The breath should smell sweet. Healthy puppies are plump, but without the extreme pot-bellied effect that could indicate a heavy worm burden. The skin should be very mobile and seemingly too large for the puppy's frame. The skin should be clean without any sign of soreness or redness anywhere, particularly under

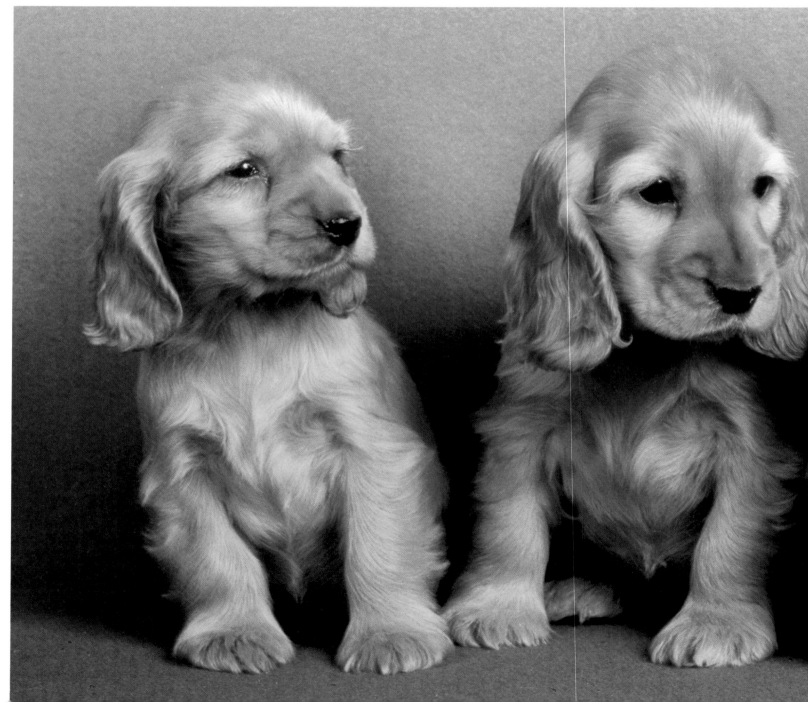

the belly or between the thighs, and there should be no black specks indicating the presence of fleas. Look under the tail for any staining – a sign of diarrhea – and examine the umbilicus area for any sign of a hernia. Make sure that you see your chosen puppy running around and that it moves correctly. If you arrive during the litter's sleep period, be prepared to wait until the pups have had a chance to wake up properly – after a long sleep it takes some minutes before their natural bounce returns.

Buying a pup with a pedigree does not necessarily mean that you acquire a show dog. If you do eventually hope to show or breed, you must make this quite clear to the breeder from the outset. High-quality puppies with show potential may cost several times more than a pedigree pup of only pet potential. It is in the breeder's interests to sell you the puppy most suitable for your needs. If you just want a healthy, happy pet, do not pay the extra money for one that excels in all physical features; it is equally pointless to buy a standard puppy if you hope to win top prizes.

If you do decide to go in for a show dog, you may have to wait longer for your puppy. The reason is that the breeder may decide that he needs to 'run on' several of the puppies for a few months before he will be able to be certain that they are of show standard. Naturally, this will increase the purchase price, but it is worth it if you want to win in competition.

It would be hard to choose from this litter of irresistible English Cocker Spaniel puppies but you should check each animal carefully before making your final selection.

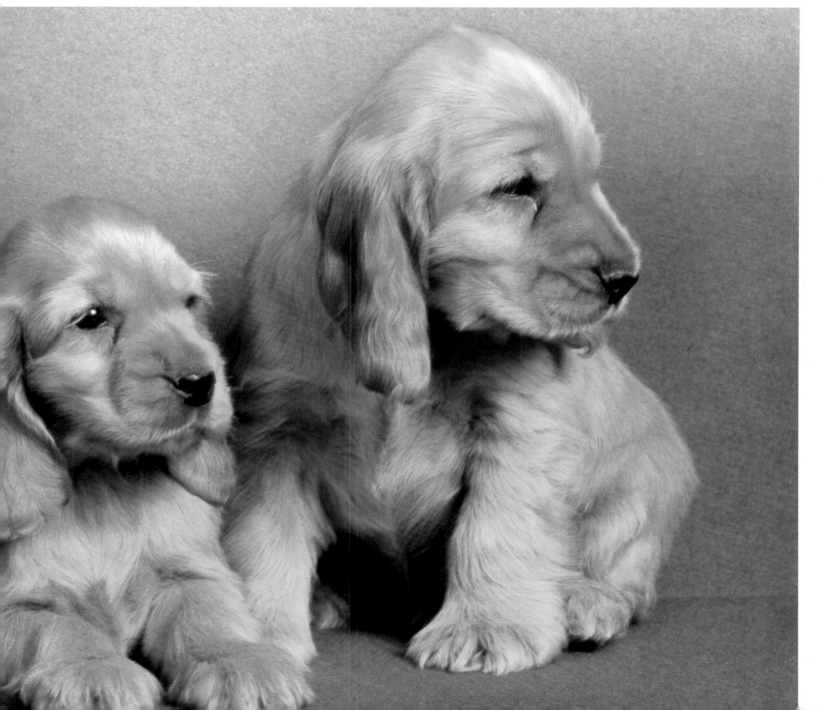

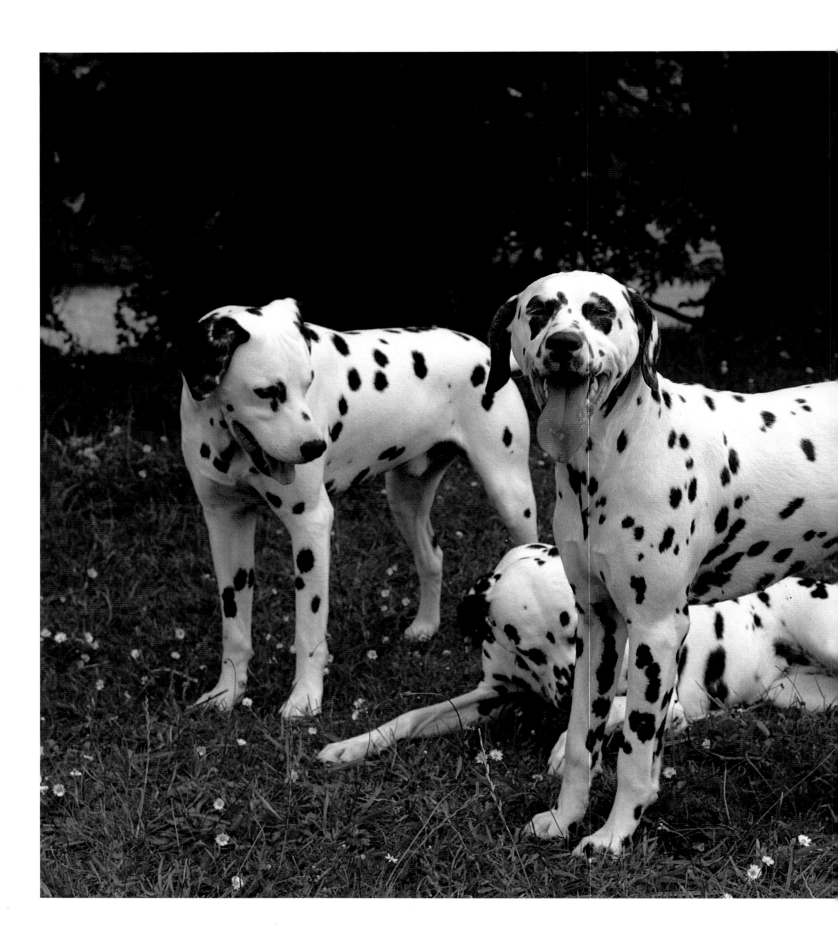

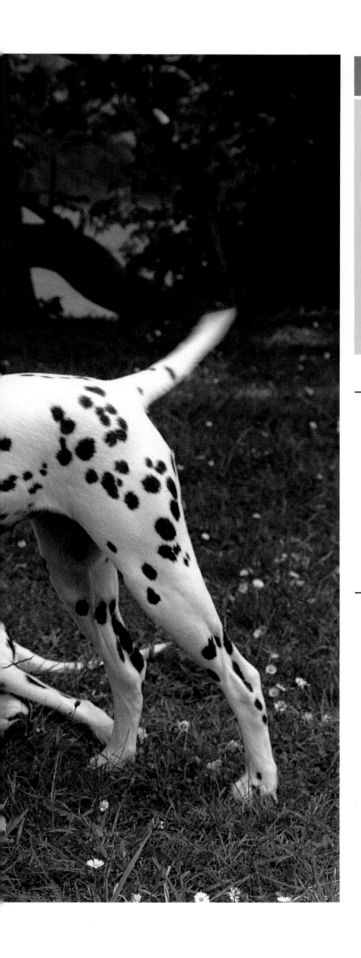

BREEDS OF THE WORLD

Dogs come in all shapes and sizes and colors, from the glamorous little pets like the Shih Tzu to hardy working animals like the Samoyed. They may be as tiny as the Chihuahua or as large as the Great Dane; they may have the extraordinary corded coats of the Komondor and the Puli or no coats at all, like the Chinese Crested Dog. Each country has its own traditional dogs and its own domestic favorites. This section describes a wide range of breeds from all corners of the world, with details of their origins, their original uses, their appearance and temperament.

BREEDS OF THE WORLD

Each breed has a detailed standard, covering every facet of its appearance, but these vary from one country to another so the descriptions in this section are designed to give an overall picture of the look of each dog, as well as its origins and temperament. If you wish to show your dog, you will need to contact your kennel club for full details.

Ideal sizes and weights are prescribed for the breeds by each kennel club and these also vary, so in the following pages, dogs are graded according to average heights – small (up to 38 cm, 15 in), large (over 56 cm, 22 in) and medium – as a general guide for prospective owners. Specific figures are only given if the breed is especially large, small or heavy.

For showing purposes, breeds are divided into groups, as follows: American Kennel Club (AKC): Sporting; Hounds; Working; Terriers; Toys; Non-Sporting; Herding; Miscellaneous. Kennel Club in Britain (KC): Hound; Terrier; Gundog; Toy; Utility; Working. Australian National Kennel Club (ANKC): Terrier; Toy; Gundog; Hound; Working; Non-Sporting. The Fédération Cynologique Internationale, which governs dog shows in Europe and some Latin American countries, has its own groupings; these are mentioned here only when the dogs concerned are not registered in Britain or the USA.

GLOSSARY

Brindle: fine even mixture of black hairs with hairs of a lighter color.
Cropped ears: ears cut at the top so that they stand erect. In some countries, including Britain, this operation is illegal.
Docked tail: tail shortened by surgery.

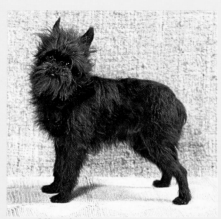

▲ **Affenpinscher**

Hound color: white, tan or black.
Grizzle: bluish-gray.
Pied: large patches of two or more colors.
Points: the ears, face, legs and tail of a contrasting color.
Undershot: where lower incisors lie in front of the upper ones when the jaw is closed.
Spitz: hardy dogs originating in the far north where they were bred for working under rigorous conditions.
Wheaten: pale yellow or fawn color.

▼ **Afghan Hound**

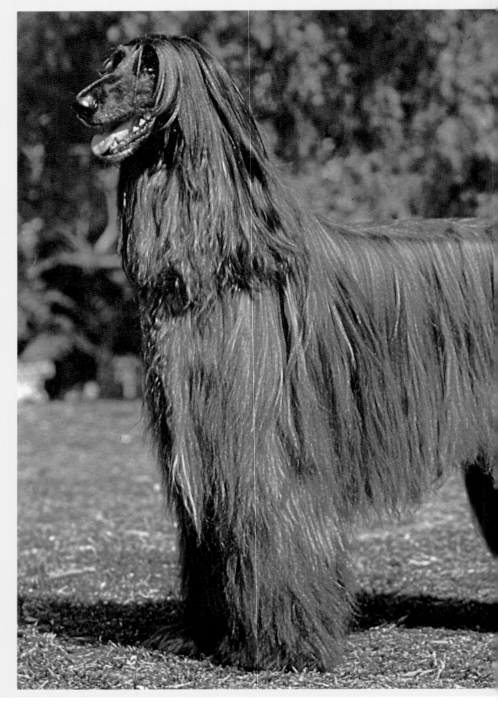

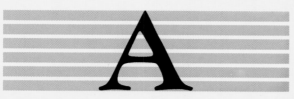

AFFENPINSCHER

Origins. Dogs which look very like the modern breed are to be seen in many paintings dating from the fourteenth century, but it was not until the turn of this century that the breed attracted enough attention in Germany, its country of origin, to be scheduled at shows.

Characteristics. Facially the Affenpinscher resembles a monkey and has some of that animal's mischievousness and humor. The face is flat with round dark eyes. The teeth fit closely together and many dogs are slightly undershot. The ears are small and pointed, in the USA they may be cropped. The body is short, compact and square with a docked tail.

Group. Toys.
Size. Small.

Coat. *Color:* Usually black. *Texture:* Short and dense, hard and wiry.
The head should carry a good crop of whiskers.

AFGHAN HOUND

Origins. This is a coursing hound from two distinct types, now almost entirely intermingled, from the mountains and plains of Afghanistan, its country of origin. Afghans were first imported into Britain in 1894 and into North America in 1926.

Characteristics. A dignified hound, but capable of playing the willful fool. The movement of the Afghan should be smooth and springy with considerable style. The dog gives the impression of strength and dignity. The head is long and lean, the body strong and deep.

Group. Hounds.
Size. Large: average 71 cm (28 in).
Coat. *Color:* Various. *Texture:* Long and fine.

AIREDALE TERRIER

Origins. The Airedale is by far the largest of the terriers and for that reason is sometimes referred to

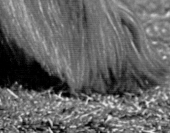

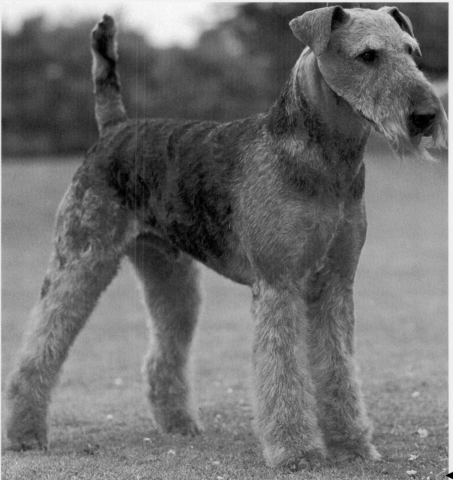

◀ **Airedale Terrier**

as the King of Terriers. In fact, the breed's size makes it something of an oddity and probably, both in origin and function, it owes as much to the hound group as it does to the terriers. The breed was developed to combine some of the capabilities of both terrier and hound, terrier characteristics being inherited from the Old English Rough-Coated Black and Tan Terrier, and hound characteristics, including size, from the Otter Hound. The breed's size, courage and intelligence make it an excellent guard and police dog.

Characteristics. The Airedale's character is shown by the expression of the eyes and by the carriage of the ears and tail. The head is long and flat, the jaws deep, powerful, strong and muscular. The eyes are dark, small, with a look of keenness and intelligence, the neck muscular, set into long, well-laid-back shoulders. The back is short, strong and level, the chest is deep but not broad. The tail is carried gaily.

Group. Terriers.

Size. Large.

Coat. *Color:* Black or dark grizzle with tan head and legs. *Texture:* Hard, dense and wiry.

ALASKAN MALAMUTE

Origins. First used as a sledge dog by the Mahlemut people in Alaska, its country of origin, the Malamute is one of the northern Spitz breeds and the largest of the sledge dogs. These dogs are very tough, capable of great feats of endurance and will survive in conditions to which other dogs would quickly succumb.

Characteristics. A powerful and substantially built dog with deep chest and strong, compact body. The head is strong and like a wolf's with a distinctive white cap or mask. The ears are pricked, the eyes alert and wolflike. The tail, as in all Spitz

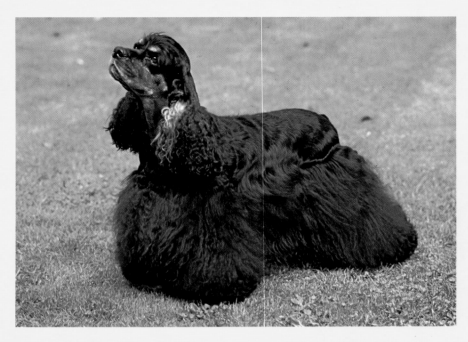

breeds, is carried over the back and is thickly plumed. The dog is affectionate, friendly, loyal, an excellent guard and formidable fighter when roused.

Group. Working.

Size. Large.

Coat. *Color:* Usually various shades of gray with white underbodies, legs, feet and part of the face. *Texture:* Thick and dense guard coat, not long nor soft. Coat is shorter when the winter coat is shed.

▲ American Cocker Spaniel

AMERICAN COCKER SPANIEL

Origins. A distinctive and glamorous gundog, developed in America from Cocker Spaniels imported from England. It has now achieved a

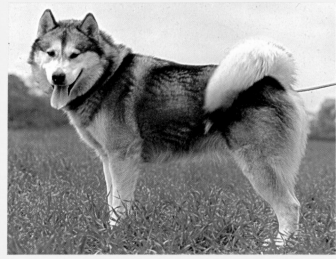

▲ Alaskan Malamute

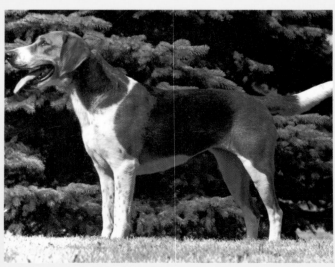

▲ American Foxhound

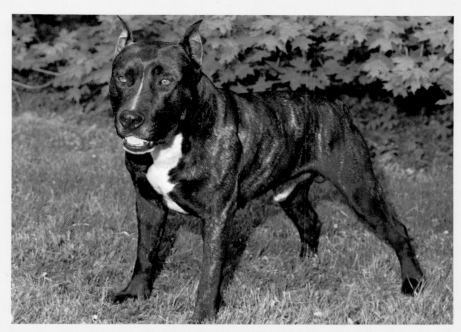

Group. Hounds.
Size. Large.
Coat. *Color:* Any color. *Texture:* Close, hard, medium length.

AMERICAN STAFFORDSHIRE TERRIER

Origins. The American Staffordshire Terrier is one of a handful of breeds which has developed in the USA into a breed with very different characteristics from the British version. The Stafford was registered in the USA in 1935, but it was only in 1972 that the changes which had taken place were officially recognized by a change of name to American Staffordshire Terrier. However, since the nineteenth century, a distinctive breed has been developing under the various names of Pit Dog, Pit Bull Terrier, Yankee Terrier or American Bull Terrier. The first two names give a clue to the breed's use: they were and are used for organized fights against each other in the 'pit.' The breed, though a terror with other dogs, is gentle with people, impressive in appearance and, in the right hands, tractable.
Characteristics. The breed gives an impression of great strength, muscularity, agility and considerable courage. The shoulders are wide and slope into a fairly short back. The chest is broad, the front legs are straight, the hindquarters well-muscled.
Group. Terriers.
Size. Medium.
Coat. *Color:* Various. *Texture:* Short, glossy, close and stiff to the touch.

ANATOLIAN KARABASH DOG (ANATOLIAN SHEPHERD DOG)

Origins. The Karabash is a herding and guard dog much valued by Anatolian shepherds who developed the breed over very many centuries from the

considerable degree of popularity on both sides of the Atlantic, both as a companion and as a show dog.
Characteristics. The breed is the smallest member of the sporting group. It is sturdy and compact with a refined head. The eyes are round, full and look directly forward, the ears long and well feathered. The body is short and compact, the back strong, the chest deep and the quarters wide and well muscled. The tail is docked short. The dog makes a loyal and affectionate pet.
Group. Sporting. Gundog (KC).
Size. Small.
Coat. *Color:* Various. *Texture:* Silky, flat or slightly wavy and profuse.

▲ **American Staffordshire Terrier**

AMERICAN FOXHOUND

Origins. Foxhunting in America is very different from foxhunting in Britain and it follows that the hounds used will also be very different. The American breed, however, is to a large extent the product of a pack of hounds imported into the country in 1650 by Robert Brooke and of later imports, such as those in 1742 made by Thomas Walker in the USA. Foxhounds are run in field trials, used for hunting a fox with a gun or raced along a predetermined trail.
Characteristics. The skull is fairly long and domed, the ears set moderately low, fine in texture, broad, long and pendulous. The eyes are large with a soft expression, the muzzle is fairly long. The chest is deep and narrower than in the English Foxhound, the hindquarters strong and well muscled. The tail is carried gaily with a slight brush. The American Foxhound is quite popular as a show dog in the USA but does not make a suitable pet.

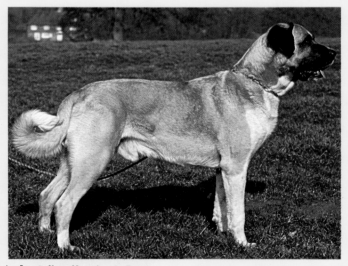

▲ **Anatolian Karabash Dog**

mastiff dogs which existed in the Babylonian Empire over 3000 years ago. The breed retains a considerable likeness to these ancient mastiffs.

Characteristics. The head is large and broad, the ears V-shaped and pendant. The back is long, and the powerful loins slightly arched. The tail is long and carried low.

Group. Working (KC).

Size. Large.

Coat. *Color:* Cream, fawn or brindle with black points. *Texture:* Short and dense.

AUSTRALIAN CATTLE DOG

Origins. From imported stock Australia has produced two distinctive and impressive working breeds, the Australian Kelpie and the Cattle Dog. The Cattle Dog has been known as the Australian, Blue or Queensland Heeler, Heeler being an old British word applied to cattle dogs. In its veins runs the blood of several working breeds which have combined to produce this superlative cattle dog.

Characteristics. The head is broad and wedge-shaped, the ears pricked, and the eyes dark. The chest is broad, the hindquarters are powerful. The tail is long, carried and furnished like a fox's.

Group. Herding. Working (KC).

Size. Medium.

Coat. *Color:* Usually blue, blue mottled with or without black markings, with some tan on legs and feet. It may also be red speckled. *Texture:* Short.

AUSTRALIAN KELPIE

Origins. The Australian Kelpie appears to have emerged, from crosses between imported herding dogs, as a distinct breed in the 1870s. Nowadays the Australian Kelpie works side by side with the ubiquitous Border Collie on the huge sheep farms of Australia where its keen sight, scenting powers and hearing make it highly valued.

Characteristics. The Australian Kelpie is a tough and muscular dog, rather foxlike in appearance with a strong, arched neck, moderately long back, and bushy tail carried low.

Group. Miscellaneous. Working (KC).

Size. Medium.

Coat. *Color:* Black, black and tan, red, red and tan, fawn, chocolate or smoke-blue. *Texture:* Short, straight, thick and harsh.

▼ **Australian Cattle Dog**

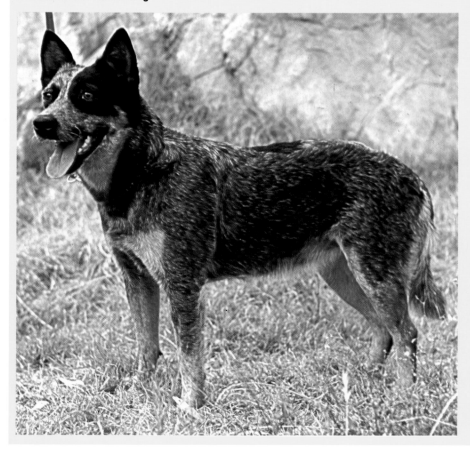

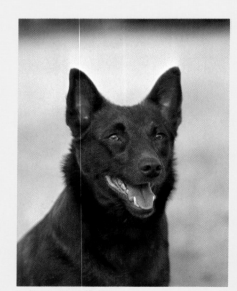

▲ **Australian Kelpie**

AUSTRALIAN TERRIER

Origins. One of very few terrier breeds which originated outside the British Isles, though undoubtedly bred from old British breeds. The Australian's slightly old-fashioned appearance is probably closer to some of these old breeds than are their modern counterparts. Recognition of the breed came in 1892 and they were first registered by the AKC in 1960.

Characteristics. The Australian Terrier is a rather low-set dog, compact and active with a long head, a soft topknot and a low powerful jaw. The eyes are small, keen and dark in color; the ears are small, set high on the skull, pricked or dropped towards the front and fringed with long hair. The neck is inclined to be long in proportion to the body, with a frill of hair. The forelegs are perfectly straight; the body is long in proportion to its height and the tail is docked. This little dog is spirited and affectionate.

Group. Terriers.

Size. Small.

Coat. *Color:* Blue or silver-gray body with tan color on legs and face, and the topknot blue or silver. Alternatively clear sandy or red. *Texture:* Straight hair 5–6 cm (2–2½ in) long, of hard texture.

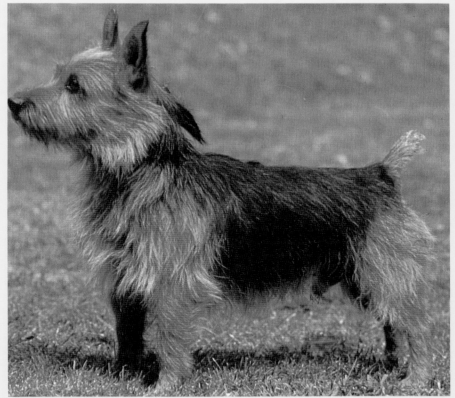

▲ **Australian Terrier**

AUSTRALIAN SILKY TERRIER (SILKY TERRIER)

Origins. The Silky Terrier may be regarded as a second generation Australian since it is said to have originated from a cross between the Australian Terrier and imported Yorkshire Terriers. It is just as likely to be a smaller, silkier-coated variation of the Australian, retained and bred for its attractive appearance. In its homeland it has been recognized as a distinct breed since the early years of the century. It was first exhibited in 1907, had its original standard drawn up in 1909 and was recognized in the USA in 1959.

Characteristics. The Silky is a lightly built, moderately low-set toy dog of pronounced terrier character and spirited action. The head is strong, wedge-shaped and moderately long. The ears, V-shaped and pricked, are set high and carried erect; the eyes are small and dark, with a piercingly keen expression. The body is low set and fairly long, and the tail is set high and carried erect. This happy little dog makes an affectionate pet.

Group. Toys.

Size. Small.

Coat. *Color:* Blue and tan, the topknot silver or fawn. *Texture:* Flat, fine in texture, glossy and silky.

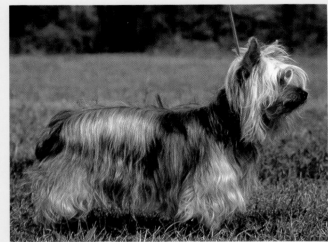

▲ **Australian Silky Terrier**

B

BASENJI

Origins. This breed originated in Zaire. It is unique as a nonbarking dog though it is an accomplished yodeler, and as a Spitz breed from Africa, still very close to its wild ancestors. Known as a guard, hunter and companion in Western Africa for centuries, it was not known in the Western world until two were brought to Britain in 1895; unfortunately both died shortly afterwards. It was not until 1937 in Britain and 1941 in America that imports became more successful and breeding stock became established.

Characteristics. The breed is remarkable for its great cleanliness, produced not only by its short coat but by its personal habits. Basenjis are lightly built, finely-boned aristocratic animals, tall, poised, alert and intelligent. The wrinkled head, with pricked ears, is carried proudly on a well-arched neck.

Group. Hounds.
Size. Medium.
Coat. *Color:* Pure bright red, or pure black, black and tan, all with white feet, chest and tail tip. *Texture:* Short, sleek and close, very fine.

BASSET GRIFFON VENDÉEN

Origins. A descendant of the white variety of the ancient St Hubert hound. As a hunting hound the breed is said to lack stamina.

Characteristics. The Basset Griffon Vendéen is an intelligent dog, sure of itself, distinguished in physique and gait. The head is well-rounded, not too broad. The eyes are large, dark and vivacious and the pendulous ears soft and narrow. The overall build is that of a Basset; its temperament is cheery, friendly and inquisitive.

Group. Hound (KC).
Size. Small/Medium.

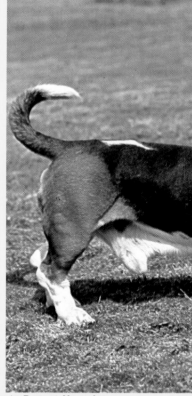

▲ **Basset Hound**

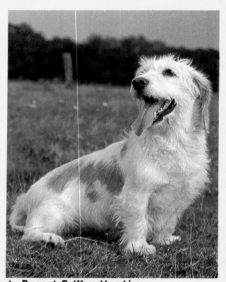

▲ **Basset Griffon Vendéen**

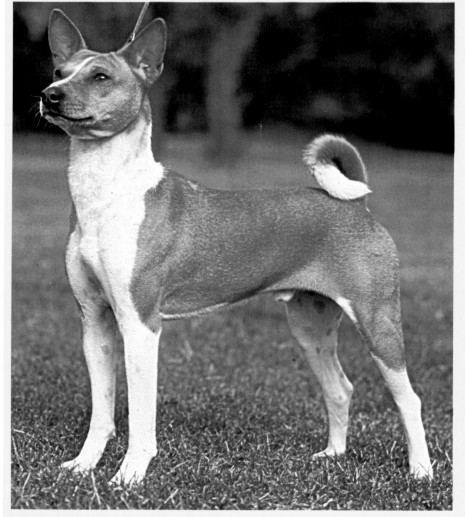

◄ **Basenji**

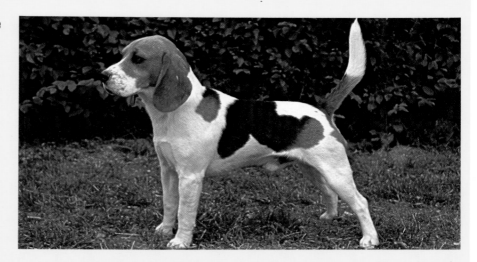

▶ Beagle

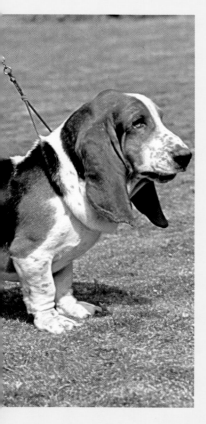

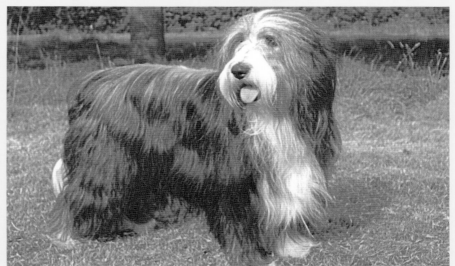

▲ Bearded Collie

Coat. *Color:* Fawn, white and orange, white and gray, tricolor. *Texture:* Long, bushy and heavy.

BASSET HOUND

Origins. This breed originated with the old French hounds, which were crossed with Bloodhounds to produce the dog which Shakespeare compared with Thessalian bulls. The breed was developed in Britain from a litter imported in 1872. Bassets are slow-moving, ponderous, deep-voiced pack hounds used for hunting the hare. Hounds bred for work and those bred for the show ring may nowadays be very different animals.

Characteristics. A somewhat hefty dog with very short legs, capable of moving smoothly. The head is big, domed and heavy, owing a lot in appearance to the Bloodhound; the ears are long and pendulous. It is a gentle, affectionate, good-mannered dog.

Group. Hounds.

Size. Medium: a heavy body set on short legs.

Coat. *Color:* Generally black and white and tan or lemon and white. *Texture:* Smooth, short and close without being too fine.

BEAGLE

Origins. This English breed is the smallest of the pack hounds and is used for hunting the hare with followers on foot. By the time Thomas Bewick was writing his *History of Quadrupeds* in 1790, he was able to speak of these small hounds which had already been known for over 300 years.

Characteristics. Certainly one of the most popular hounds and one that makes a cheerful companion. The Beagle is compactly built giving the impression of great stamina and activity. It has a short body and very muscular hindquarters.

Group. Hounds.

Size. Small/Medium.

Coat. *Color:* Any recognized hound colors. *Texture:* Close, hard and of medium length.

BEARDED COLLIE

Origins. This Collie is one of the oldest of Scottish herding dogs though it is probably of central European origin. The breed was recognized in Britain in 1944 and admitted to the AKC stud book in 1976.

Characteristics. Should be alert, lively and self-confident, the body strong without giving a heavy appearance. The Beardie's face has a quizzical expression. The dog has a good temperament as well as plenty of energy and high spirits.

Group. Herding. Working (KC).

Size. Medium.

Coat. *Color:* Slate gray or reddish fawn, black, all shades of gray, brown and sandy, with or without white markings. *Texture:* The undercoat is soft, furry and close, the outercoat hair strong and flat. A long beard is a characteristic of the breed.

BEDLINGTON TERRIER

Origins. This is one of the sporting terriers which have their origins among the valleys of northeast England. As a breed it owes much to the old rough-coated breeds kept as vermin killers by the sporting farmers and shepherds of Northumbria. The first Bedlington club was formed in 1877, since which time the breed's original hardness and fighting qualities have been overlaid with a quiet gentle disposition.

Characteristics. A graceful, lithe, muscular dog. The head is pear or wedge-shaped and the expression in repose mild and gentle, though not shy or nervous. When roused, the eyes sparkle and the dog looks full of temper and courage. Bedlingtons are capable of galloping at great speed. Movement is distinctive: rather mincing, light and springy in the slower paces, and may have a slight roll when in full stride.

Group. Terriers.

Size. Small/Medium.

Coat. *Color:* Blue, blue and tan, liver or sandy. *Texture:* Very distinctive, thick and soft, standing out well from the body.

BELGIAN SHEEPDOG (GROENENDAEL)

Origins. The herding dogs of mainland Europe are all closely related and share several strong family characteristics. However it was not until Professor Reul at the end of the nineteenth century embarked on a study of these dogs, then generally simply referred to as Chien de Berger, that the various local breeds were accorded separate recognition. Among the three basic types recognized by Professor Reul was one with rather long black hair. The principal breeder of this type was Monsieur Rose of Groenendael.

Characteristics. The breed is intelligent, courageous, alert and faithful, protective of the person and property of its owners. It responds well to training and has been widely used as a working dog by the Belgian police force. The Belgian Sheepdog is a well balanced, square dog, elegant in appearance with a pronounced proud carriage of the head and neck. The head is strong, the ears stiffly erect, the chest deep. Forelegs are straight and strong, hindquarters are broad and heavily muscled. The tail is long and undocked.

Group. Herding. Working (KC).

Size. Large.

Coat. *Color:* Black. *Texture:* The outer coat is long, straight and abundant, of medium harshness. The undercoat is very dense.

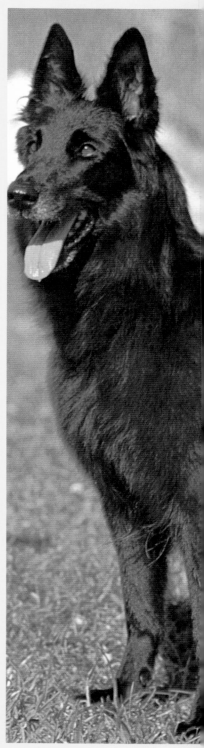

▶ **Belgian Malinois**

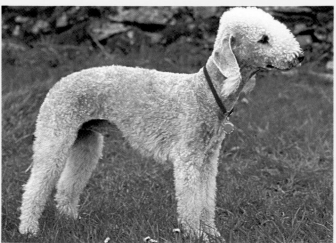

▲ **Bedlington Terrier**

▶ **Belgian Sheepdog (Groenendael)**

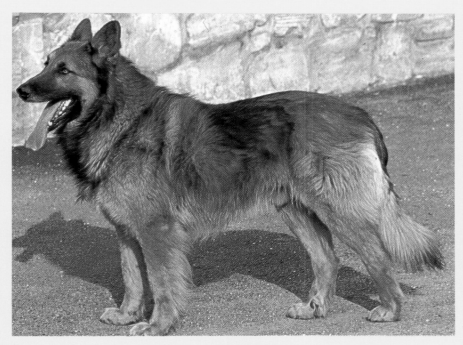

BELGIAN MALINOIS

Origins. One of the three breeds of Belgian herding dogs now growing in popularity throughout the world.

Characteristics. As for the Belgian Sheepdog (Groenendael).

Group. Herding. Working (KC).

Size. Large.

Coat. *Color:* Rich fawn to mahogany with black overlay, black face and ears. *Texture:* Comparatively short, straight with dense undercoat.

BELGIAN TERVUEREN

Origins. One of the Belgian Sheepdog breeds.

Characteristics. This breed differs from the Groenendael in little other than color.

Group. Herding. Working (KC).

Size. Large.

Coat. *Color:* Fawn with black tips to the hairs. *Texture:* Long and fairly harsh.

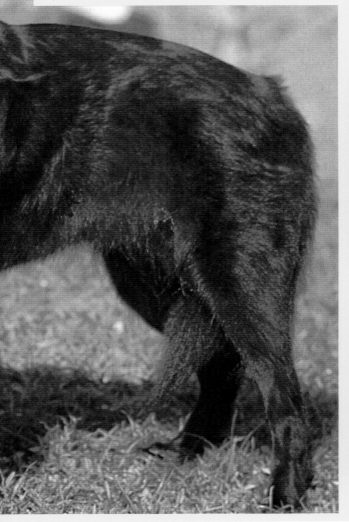

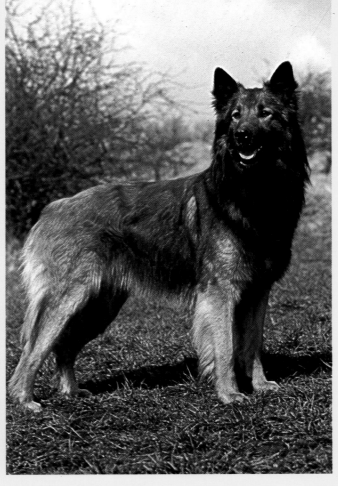

▲ **Belgian Tervueren**

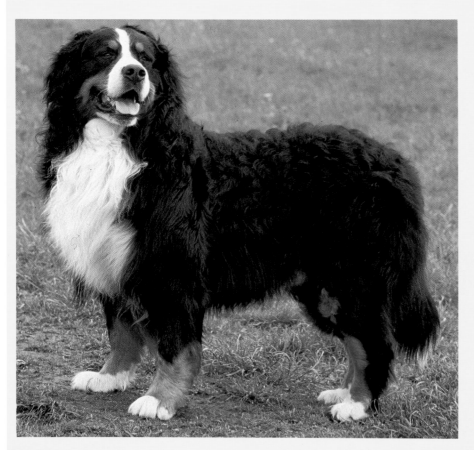

◀ **Bernese Mountain Dog**

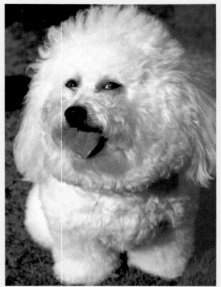

▲ **Bichon Frise**

BERNESE MOUNTAIN DOG

Origins. This is one of the European herding dogs developed from dogs left behind by Roman legions. Switzerland is home to four varieties of mountain dogs but it is the breed developed in the canton of Berne which, because of its rich black and tan silky coat, is the most distinctive.

Characteristics. The Bernese Mountain Dog is well balanced, active and alert. The eyes are dark, hazel-brown and full of fire, and the ears are V-shaped, set on high and in repose hang close to the head. The body is rather short, compact and strong.
Group. Working.
Size. Large.
Coat. *Color:* Jet black with tan and white markings. *Texture:* Soft and silky with bright, natural sheen, long and wavy.

BICHON FRISE

Origins. Italian traders returning from the Canary Islands in the fourteenth century brought with them some of the attractive little dogs which they had found in the islands. The dogs probably were descended from the Old Barbet or Water Spaniels from which the original name of Barbichon was derived. Later the name was contracted to 'Bichon' or changed to 'Teneriffe' and the breed began to gain favor in the Royal Courts of Europe.

Characteristics. The breed is sturdy and lively with a stable temper, has a stylish gait and an air of dignity and intelligence. The skull is broad and somewhat round with a dense topknot. The ears hang down and are covered with long flowing hair; the large, round eyes are dark and expressive. The neck is long and the head carriage is high. The tail is covered with long flowing hair, carried gaily and curved to lie on the back.
Group. Non-Sporting. Toy (KC).
Size. Small.
Coat. *Color:* Solid white, or white with cream, apricot or gray on the ears and body. *Texture:* Profuse, silky and loosely curled.

BLACK AND TAN COONHOUND

Origins. This is the only recognized breed of half a dozen Coonhounds which include the very impressive Redbone Coonhound and the surprisingly named English Coonhound. These hounds hunt by night as the raccoon is a nocturnal animal. The Black and Tan Coonhound is only recognized in the USA and was admitted to registry by the AKC in 1945.

Characteristics. Slightly resembles a lightly built Bloodhound, essentially a working dog, powerful, agile and alert. Its expression is friendly, eager and aggressive and its movement is easy, powerful and rhythmic.

Group. Hounds.

Size. Large.

Coat. *Color:* Coal black, rich tan markings. *Texture:* Short and dense.

BLOODHOUND

Origins. In 1553, the physician and dog expert Dr Caius was able to describe the Bloodhound very much in terms which are applicable today and was perhaps one of the first to mistakenly attribute the source of the breed's name to their ability to follow a blood trail. In fact the word is used in the same sense as in 'blood stock' as a reference to aristocratic breeding. Even so the breed's reputation as a formidable tracking dog had obviously already been established and has survived up to the present day. The breed is yet another of the English hound breeds originally derived from French stock.

▼ **Bloodhound**   ▶ **Black and Tan Coonhound**

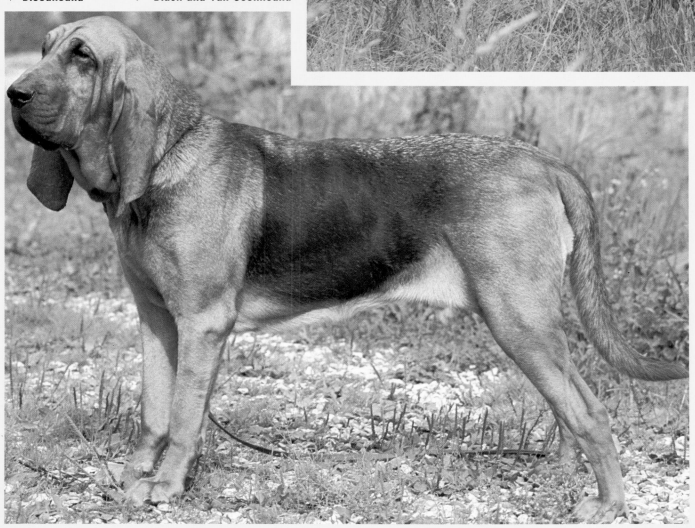

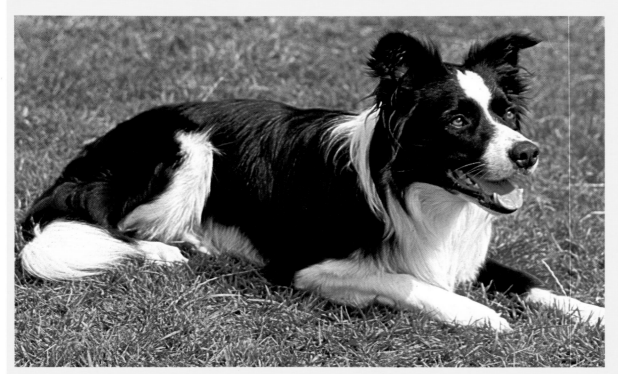

◀ **Border Collie**

▼ **Border Terrier**

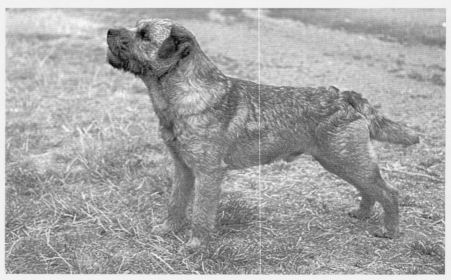

Characteristics. The Bloodhound is a powerful animal, larger than most hound breeds. It is characterized by a thin loose skin which hangs in deep folds, especially about the head, and gives the well-known lugubrious expression. The Bloodhound is a reserved dog, good-tempered and gentle with children.

Group. Hounds.

Size. Large.

Coat. *Color*: Black and tan, red and tan, red, called fawny in the USA. *Texture*: Smooth, short and glossy.

BORDER COLLIE

Origins. Arguably the world's finest sheepdog and now found wherever sheep are kept in appreciable numbers, often in environments very different from those in which the breed originated, in the hills of Scotland. By the mid-nineteenth century the breed was already well established but it was only recognized by the British Kennel Club in 1976.

Characteristics. A well-proportioned dog with a smooth outline which shows quality, grace and balance while giving the impression that the dog is capable of enduring long periods of active duty. The breed is very intelligent and loyal to its master but can become neurotic if not given enough to do.

Group. Miscellaneous. Working (KC).

Size. Medium/Large.

Coat. *Color*: Black and white, black, white and tan. *Texture*: Double, dense, moderately long, with a medium textured topcoat and short dense undercoat.

BORDER TERRIER

Origins. The Border Terrier was developed to run with hounds, and to be able to eject a fox from its earth, and so was an essential part of the system of fox control in the hilly sheep country of Northumbria in northern Britain.

Characteristics. The Border Terrier is essentially a working terrier able to follow a horse and must combine activity with gameness. The head is a distinctive feature of the breed, resembling that of an otter, moderately broad in skull, with a short strong muzzle. The eyes are dark with a keen expression, the ears V-shaped and dropping for-

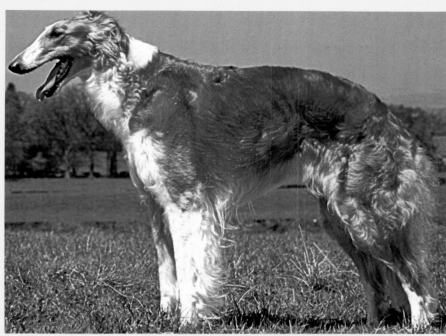

▲ **Borzoi**

ward close to the cheek. The body is deep, narrow and fairly long, the hindquarters strong. The tail is undocked, moderately short, and thick at the base. It is a good-natured, affectionate little dog.

Group. Terriers.

Size. Small.

Coat. *Color:* Red, wheaten, grizzle and tan or blue and tan. *Texture:* Harsh and dense and not overlong with a close undercoat.

BORZOI

Origins. Until comparatively recently, when the Borzoi's name was changed from Russian Wolfhound, its origins were obvious. Before the Revolution every Russian nobleman maintained a pack of these hounds which were used in pairs for coursing wolves.

Characteristics. A very graceful, aristocratic and elegant dog possessing courage, muscular power and great speed. The head is long and lean, the neck is slightly arched and powerful, the back rising in a graceful curve, more marked in dogs than bitches.

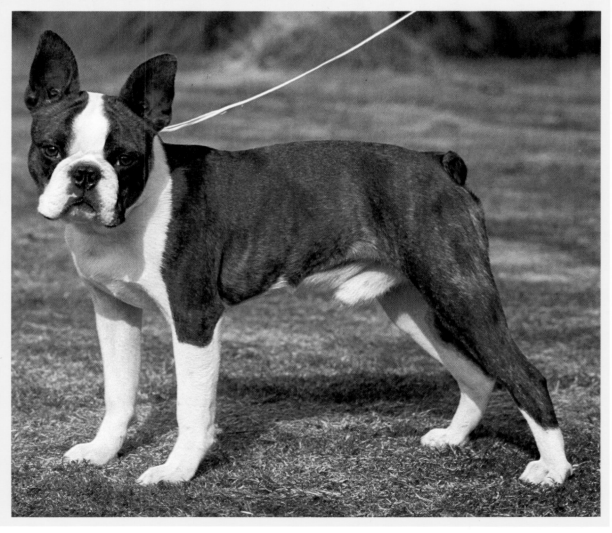

▶ **Boston Terrier**

The legs are long, the feet harelike and the tail long and well-feathered.

Group. Hounds.

Size. Large: 73 cm (29 in) upwards.

Coat. *Color:* Various. *Texture:* Long and silky, flat, wavy or rather curly.

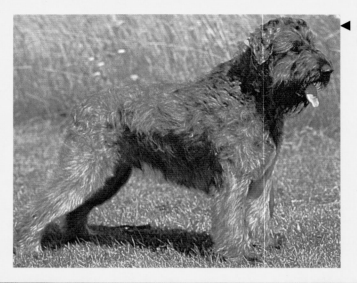

◀ **Bouvier des Flandres**

BOSTON TERRIER

Origins. An American breed, the Boston Terrier was the result of crosses between imported English Bulldogs and terriers bred in Boston in the 1870s. They were first exhibited as Round Heads or Bull Terriers, but as a distinct and stable type developed the name was changed to Boston Terrier. In 1891 the first breed club was formed in the USA and in 1893 the breed was recognized by the AKC.

Characteristics. The breed has a characteristi-

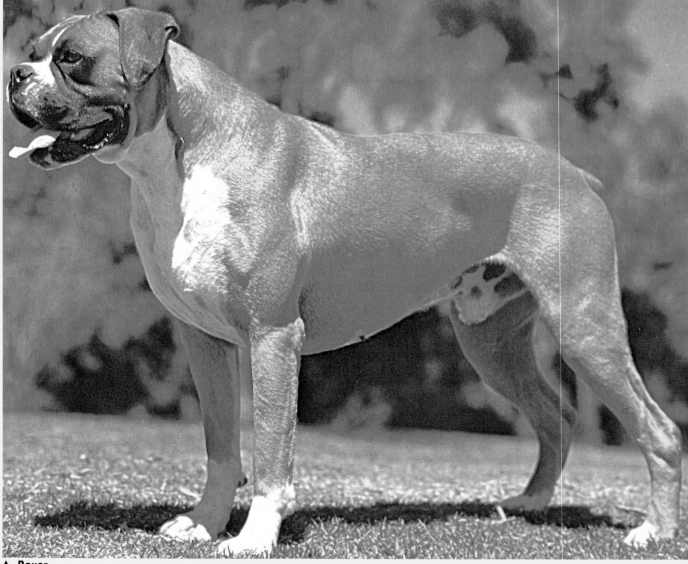

▲ **Boxer**

cally gentle disposition and is eminently suitable as a companion and as a house pet as it is both affectionate and protective. The Boston is smooth-coated, short-headed, compactly built and well balanced. The head is square, the muzzle short and the eyes large and round. The ears are carried erect and may be cropped. The shoulders are sloping, the back is short, the loins short and muscular. The tail is short, fine or tapering and may be straight or screw.

Group. Non-Sporting. Utility (KC).
Size. Small.
Coat. *Color:* Brindle with white markings. *Texture:* Short, smooth, bright and fine.

BOUVIER DES FLANDRES

Origins. This dog is one of a small group of Flemish drovers' dogs used partly for herding cattle and partly as guards. Bouviers are now used as police and army dogs.

Characteristics. A compactly bodied, powerfully built dog of upstanding carriage and alert, intelligent expression.

Group. Herding. Working (KC).
Size. Large.
Coat. *Color:* Fawn to black. Pepper and salt, gray and brindle. *Texture:* Rough, tousled and unkempt in appearance. Topcoat harsh, rough and wiry, undercoat fine and soft.

BOXER

Origins. A German breed, this is one of several European breeds which have their origins in the mastiffs of Southern Europe, and which in the Middle Ages were developed as hunting dogs. Nowadays working Boxers are mainly used as police dogs and guard dogs.

Characteristics. A medium-sized sturdy dog of square build with a short back, strong limbs and short, tight-fitting coat. It is clean and hard in appearance and has a firm, springy stride. The head is square and short, with skin forming deep wrinkles. In the USA the ears may be cropped, but in Britain the ears lie flat and close to the cheeks. The mouth is normally undershot.

Group. Working. Non-Sporting (ANKC).
Size. Large.
Coat. *Color:* Fawn, brindle and fawn in various shades from light yellow to dark deer red. *Texture:* Short, shiny, lying smooth and tight to the body.

BRIARD

Origins. The Briard comes from one of several ancient sheepdog breeds which probably came to Europe with the Mongol invaders and developed into different and localized breeds. This one is from France. A club was formed in France in 1900 to protect the breed and by 1930 an agreed standard had finally been adopted. The breed came to Britain after the First World War and to the USA in 1922.

Characteristics. A strong and substantially built dog, fitted for field work, lithe, muscular, well proportioned, alert and active. It is an intelligent dog, good-natured and tractable.

Group. Herding. Working (KC).
Size. Large.
Coat. *Color:* Various. *Texture:* Long, slightly wavy, stiff and strong.

BRITTANY

Origins. Oppian in AD 150 wrote of the uncivilized people of Britain and of their dogs. He, like other contemporary writers, used Bretagne to refer to Britain, whereas in a later period the word was used

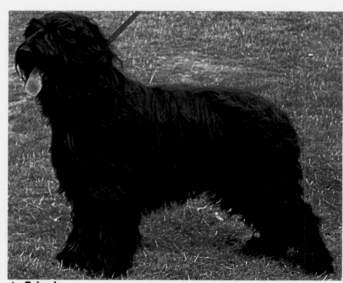
▲ **Briard**

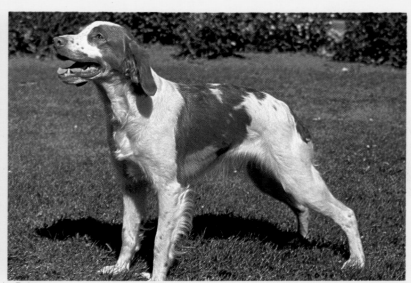
▲ **Brittany**

to refer to Brittany in France. The breed shares many characteristics with the Setter.

Characteristics. In appearance the breed has some resemblance to a very lightly built Springer: a compact, closely knit dog of medium size, with the agility and stamina to cover a lot of ground. The ears are dark, lying flat and close to the head. The body is square in outline, the shoulders sloping and muscular, the back short and straight, the chest deep. Hindquarters are broad, strong and muscular with powerful thighs. Some puppies are born without tails, others are docked short.

Group. Sporting. Gundog (KC).

Size. Medium.

Coat. *Color:* Dark orange and white or liver and white. *Texture:* Dense, flat or wavy.

BULLDOG

Origins. The Bulldog was originally used for bull-baiting, a sport which began in the early 13th century and continued until it was made illegal in 1835. The Bulldog as a distinct breed had evolved by the mid-17th century from crosses between mastiffs and more active terriers, and was then more like a Boxer or an old-type Staffordshire Bull Terrier. After bull-baiting became illegal the breed evolved to its present exaggerated form.

Characteristics. The general appearance is of a thickset dog, rather low in stature but broad, powerful and compact. The head is strikingly massive and large in proportion to the dog's size. The face is extremely short, flattened and wrinkled, which can lead to health problems. The tail is short and screwed, the forelegs are bowed. The formidable looks of the Bulldog hide a kindly and rather 'soft' nature.

Group. Non-Sporting. Utility (KC).

Size. Medium; weighing about 25 kg (55 lb).

Coat. *Color:* Various, either whole or with a black mask around eyes and muzzle. *Texture:* Fine in texture, short, close and smooth.

BULLMASTIFF

Origins. Shakespeare commended the British mastiffs as being very valiant creatures of unmatchable courage. The Bullmastiff is a nineteenth-century development of these ancient mastiff breeds, the product of a cross with terriers to produce a smaller, more active dog.

Characteristics. The dog's temperament combines high spirits, reliability, activity, endurance and alertness. It is powerfully built, showing great strength but not cumbersome. The head is large and square, and the skin wrinkles when the dog becomes interested in something. The neck is well arched and very muscular, the chest broad and deep, the back short and straight. It is loyal and patient with children, but needs firm handling.

Group. Working. Non-Sporting (ANKC).

Size. Large and heavy: average 54.3 kg (120 lb).

Coat. *Color:* Any shade of brindle, fawn or red with a dark muzzle. *Texture:* Short and hard, lying flat to the body.

BULL TERRIER

Origins. The USA differentiates between white and colored Bull Terriers, but in Britain no such

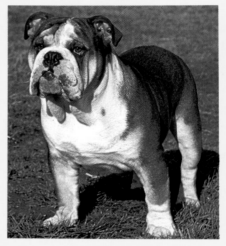

▲ **Bulldog**

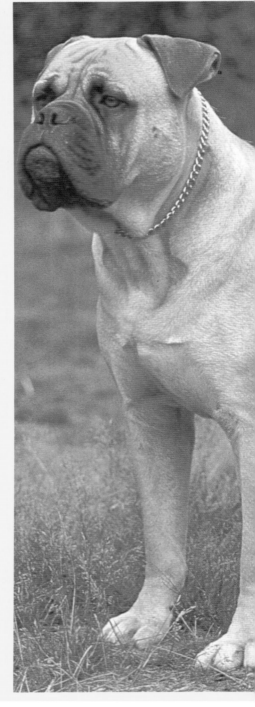

▶ **Bullmastiff**

difference exists and they remain, white or colored, the same breed. The breed is not of ancient origin, but was produced by crosses of the now extinct English White Terrier with the type of Bulldog which existed in the early nineteenth century to produce a 'gladiator' for dog fighting.

Characteristics. The Bull Terrier is strongly built, muscular, symmetrical and active, with a keen, determined and intelligent expression. It should be full of fire and courage, but amenable to discipline. The head is a characteristic of the breed being long, egg-shaped and free from hollows or indentations. The eyes are narrow, triangular and black or dark brown; the ears are small, thin and erect. The neck is long, arched and very muscular, fitting into strong and muscular shoulders. The body is well-rounded, the back short and strong, the hindquarters powerfully muscled. It is good with children but may be less friendly towards other pets.

Group. Terriers.

Size. Medium, but varies considerably. There is a miniature version, with a height of 35.5 cm (14 in) or less.

Coat. *Color:* White or colored. *Texture:* Short, flat, even and harsh to the touch with a fine gloss. The skin should fit the dog tightly.

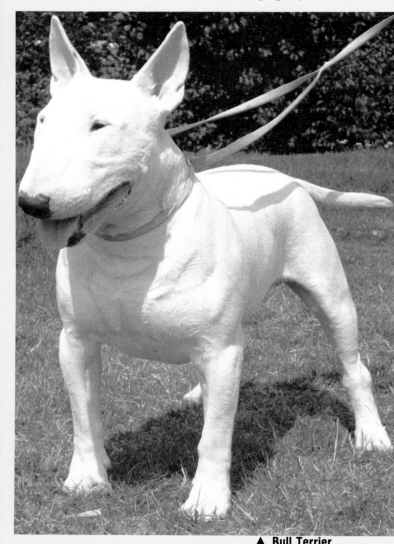

▲ **Bull Terrier**

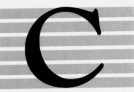

CAIRN TERRIER

Origins. A descendant of the working terriers used in Scotland and the Isle of Skye and, though no longer in demand as a working terrier, the breed retains much of the appearance and some of the characteristics of the older breeds. Authorities in the past often saw the Cairn as a short-haired Skye Terrier, but after a protest by Skye Terrier breeders the name was changed to Cairn Terrier at the beginning of this century.

Characteristics. This terrier is an active, game and shaggy little dog, strong though compactly built, very free in movement. The hindquarters are very strong, the tail short with plenty of hair. It is a cheeky, courageous little dog; good company as a pet.

Group. Terriers.
Size. Small.
Coat. *Color:* Red, sandy, gray, brindled or nearly black with dark points. *Texture:* Profuse, hard but not coarse outer coat, and a short, soft, close undercoat.

CAVALIER KING CHARLES SPANIEL

Origins. The Cavalier King Charles Spaniel is a re-creation of the toy dog favored by King Charles II and which bears his name, but which over the years had departed from its original form. Impetus to re-create this attractive toy Spaniel in its original form was given by a Mr Eldridge, an American, who, in 1920, offered prizes of £25 for Blenheim Spaniels possessing 'long faces, flat skulls, no inclination to be domes, no stop and a beauty spot in the center of the forehead'. By 1928, a club had formed and the breed was established.

Characteristics. The breed is active and graceful.

The head is flat, the muzzle tapered. The eyes are large, dark and set well apart, the ears are long and set high. It is a good-natured, docile and very clean little dog.

Group. Miscellaneous. Toy (KC).
Size. Small.
Coat. *Color:* Black and tan, rich red, chestnut and white, tricolor. *Texture:* Long, silky and free from curl, with ample featherings.

CHESAPEAKE BAY RETRIEVER

Origins. In the early part of the nineteenth century the nondescript indigenous Retrievers used in Maryland, USA, received an unexpected influx of new blood as a result of two dogs having been rescued from a wrecked English brig. The new blood so improved the native stock that other crosses were used and by the end of the century a distinct breed of Retriever had emerged. This dog was expected to work in the icy waters of Chesapeake Bay retrieving fallen duck.

Characteristics. The head and body, to some degree, resemble the Labrador Retriever. The skull is broad and round, the muzzle short, the ears small and pendulous and the eyes fairly large, clear and yellow or amber in color. The chest is barrel round and deep, the body of medium length. Hindquarters are especially powerful to supply driving power for swimming. The Chesapeake Bay is a rugged individualist, full of courage, and needs firm handling.

Group. Sporting.
Size. Large.
Coat. *Color:* Any color varying from dark brown to a faded tan. *Texture.* The coat is thick and short with a dense fine woolly undercoat. The outer coat is harsh and oily and resists water.

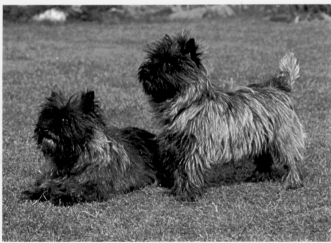

▲ **Cairn Terrier**

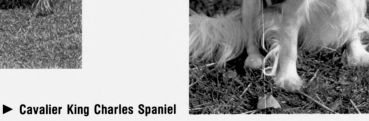

▶ **Cavalier King Charles Spaniel**

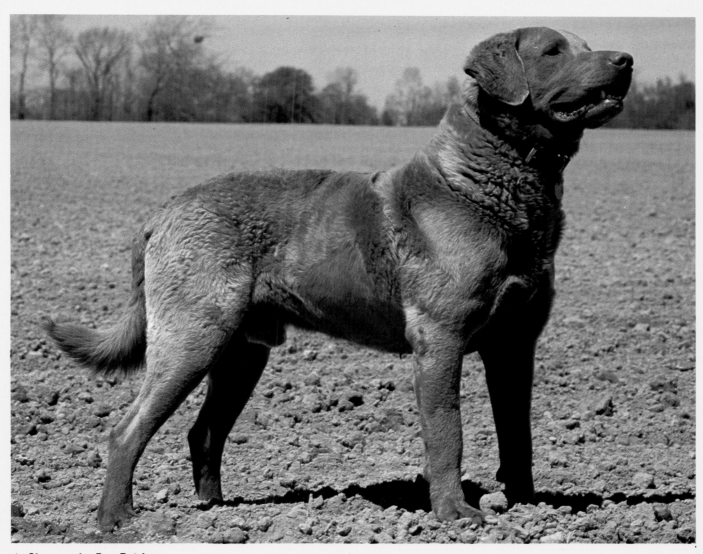

▲ **Chesapeake Bay Retriever**

CHIEN FRANÇAIS

Origins. The French hound derives from the Billy and the Poitevin and in 1957 was divided into three varieties, by size and color. The Blanc et Noir is the largest of the three and, apart from having a more domed skull, longer and narrower head, and thinner stern, is similar in appearance to the Foxhound. The Blanc et Orange and the Tricolore are similar in appearance, smaller than the Blanc et Noir; the Tricolore may have light colored eyes.

Group. Hounds for big game. (FCI).

Size. Large.

Coat. *Color:* White and black, tricolor or white and orange depending on the variety. *Texture:* Short, dense and rugged.

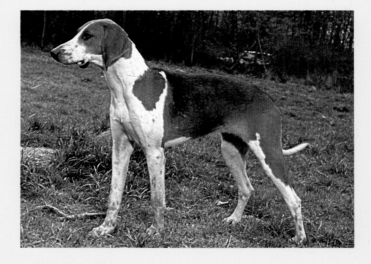

▲ **Chien Français**

▶ **Long Coat
Chihuahua**

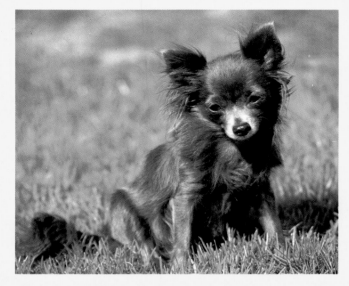

▶ **Smooth Coat
Chihuahua**

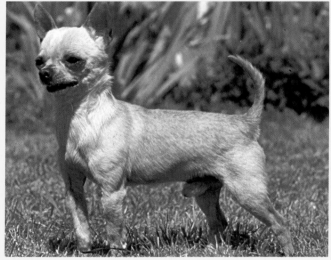

▼ **Chinese Crested Dog**

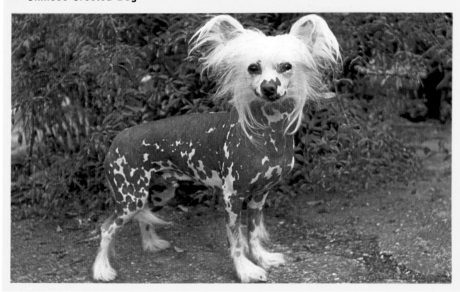

CHIHUAHUA

Origins. The immediate origin of the world's smallest breed of dog was the Mexican state after which the breed is now named, but whether it arrived there via trade routes to China or Japan or whether the breed was developed by the native Aztecs or Toltecs it is not possible to say. The first Chihuahua to be registered by the AKC was Midget registered in 1904.

Characteristics. The most obvious characteristic is its extremely small size. The head, too, is very distinctive, being round with an 'apple dome' skull, a characteristic also sometimes found in toy Japanese breeds. The eyes are full and round, though not protruding, and the ears large, set at an angle of about 45°. The dog is alert and swift with a saucy expression, it is small with a dainty compact appearance which is coupled with a brisk and forceful personality. There are two types, the Long Coat and the Smooth Coat; the Smooth Coat is still the more popular in the USA.

Group. Toys.

Size. Small; weight of 0.9–2.7 kg (2–6 lb).

Coat. *Color:* Various. *Texture:* In the Long Coat, the coat is soft, and either flat or slightly waved. Feathering on feet, legs, pants and ruff. The tail should be long and full as a plume. The Smooth Coat has a soft, close and glossy coat.

CHINESE CRESTED DOG

Origins. This is a breed from China. Hairless dogs exist in many parts of the world, such as Africa, Turkey, China and Mexico. Whether each shares a common origin or whether each is a mutant produced from a local breed it is not possible to say.

Characteristics. A small, active and graceful dog, medium to fine boned with a smooth hairless body, with hair on feet, head and tail only. The skull is slightly rounded with a fairly long muzzle, the eyes round and set wide apart, the ears large and upstanding. The tail is carried over the back or looped. The dog is very affectionate and becomes devoted to its owner.

Group. Miscellaneous. Toy (KC).

Size. Small.

Coat. *Color:* The skin can be any color, plain or spotted. *Texture:* The crest on the head is flat, either high or long-flowing. The tail should carry a plume on the last two-thirds of its length.

CHOW CHOW

Origins. It is popularly and erroneously accepted that the Chow Chow was produced as a source of food in China. In fact the Chow as we know it today is very much a product of Western breeding from Chows coming from China in the late eighteenth century, which showed the unique blue-black

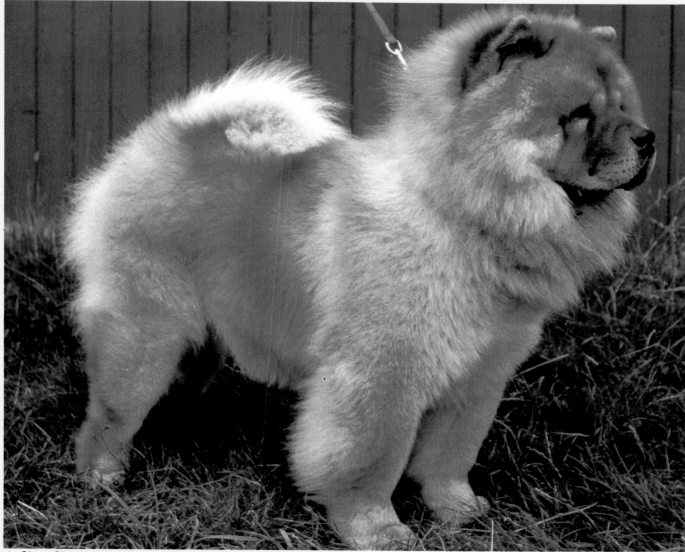

▲ **Chow Chow**

tongue and fearsome scowling expression.

Characteristics. A powerfully built dog, leonine in appearance with a proud dignified bearing, loyal yet aloof and with a stilted gait. The head is large and broad, the ears small, thick and rounded, the eyes small and dark. The body is short, compact and strong. The tail is carried well over the back. It has a reputation as a one-person dog.

Group. Non-Sporting. Utility (KC).

Size. Large.

Coat. *Color:* Solid colored black, red, blue, fawn, cream and white. *Texture:* Abundant, dense, straight and standoff. Outer coat rather coarse with a soft woolly undercoat.

CLUMBER SPANIEL

Origins. The Clumber is a very different animal from other spaniels – heavier, longer and lower to the ground – indicating that we should look for different origins. The body shape suggests some Basset Hound blood, while the heavy head is suggestive of the old Alpine Spaniel. By 1859 this breed was being shown and had achieved considerable popularity as a gundog particularly well adapted to a country with abundant game.

Characteristics. The Clumber is nothing if not distinctive: it is a dog with a thoughtful expression, very massively built but active, and moves with a rolling gait which is characteristic of the breed. The head is large, square, and massive with heavy brows. The eyes are dark amber, the ears large and vineleaf shaped, well covered with straight hair. The body is long and heavy, close to the ground; the back is straight, broad and long. The hindquarters are very powerful and well developed. The Clumber is an intelligent dog with a calm, reliable temperament.

Group. Sporting. Gundog (KC).

Size. Large; heavy body on short legs.

Coat. *Color:* Plain white with lemon markings. *Texture:* Abundant, close, silky and straight. The legs are well feathered.

COCKER SPANIEL (ENGLISH)

Origins. The Cocker Spaniel, like other spaniels, is a descendant of the dogs which, in Spain, were used to drive birds into nets. It is referred to in the prologue to Chaucer's *Wife of Bath's Tale* showing that 'Spaynels,' even as early as the fourteenth century, had attained some popularity in England. However, at this time the distinctions between spaniels of different types had not been drawn. By the eighteenth century, the breed was called the cocking-spaniel and used to flush out woodcock. Thus it came by its present name.

Characteristics. The general appearance of the Cocker is of a merry sporting dog, well balanced and compact. The head is well developed and cleanly chiseled, neither too fine nor too coarse. The eyes are full with an expression of intelligence and gentleness; the ears are long and set low, well clothed with long, silky, straight hair. The body is immensely strong and compact for the size and weight of the dog. The tail is usually docked. The Cocker makes a happy, friendly and gentle companion.

Group. Sporting. Gundog (KC).

Size. Small/Medium.

Coat. *Color:* Various. *Texture:* Flat, silky in texture.

COLLIE, ROUGH

Origins. This breed originated, like the other three Collie breeds, Smooth, Border and Bearded, in the dark-colored herding dogs of Scotland, from which

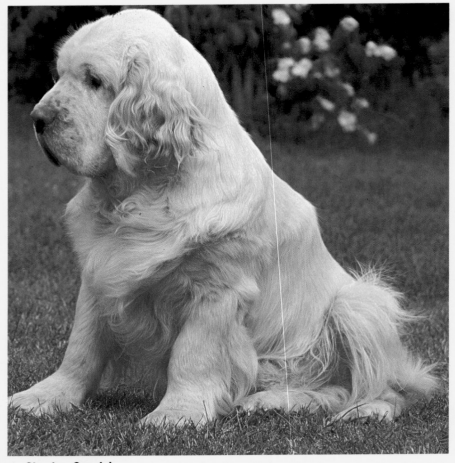

▲ **Clumber Spaniel**

▼ **Cocker Spaniel (English)**

the name is derived. 'Col' is Anglo-Saxon for black. For centuries they carried out their arduous work herding sheep on the northern hills, with only local recognition. In 1860, however, Queen Victoria visited Balmoral for the first time, saw the breed, fell in love with it and so assured its future popularity.

Characteristics. This is a strong and active dog, free from coarseness. The head is tapering, the expression alert, intelligent and inquisitive. It makes an excellent, loyal pet, responding well to training.

Group. Herding. Working (KC).

Size. Large.

Coat. *Color:* Sable and white, tricolor, and blue merle, each with white markings. *Texture:* Very dense, the outer coat straight and harsh, the undercoat soft, furry and very close. Mane and frill very abundant, legs well feathered.

COLLIE, SMOOTH

Characteristics. The Smooth Collie is similar in temperament and characteristics to the Rough Collie. As it lacks the glamour of a long coat, this dog looks rather angular.

Coat. *Texture:* Hard, dense and smooth.

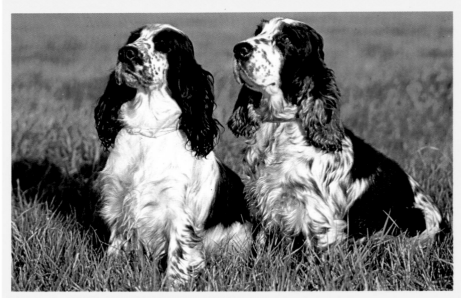

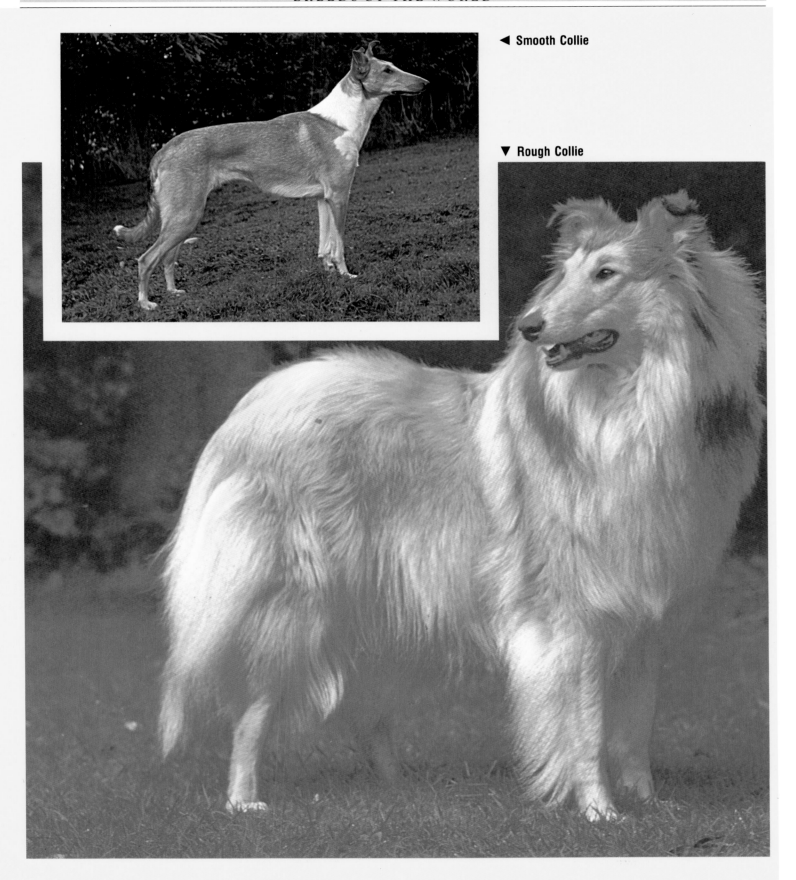

◄ Smooth Collie

▼ Rough Collie

▶ Long-haired Dachshund

▼ Curly-coated Retriever

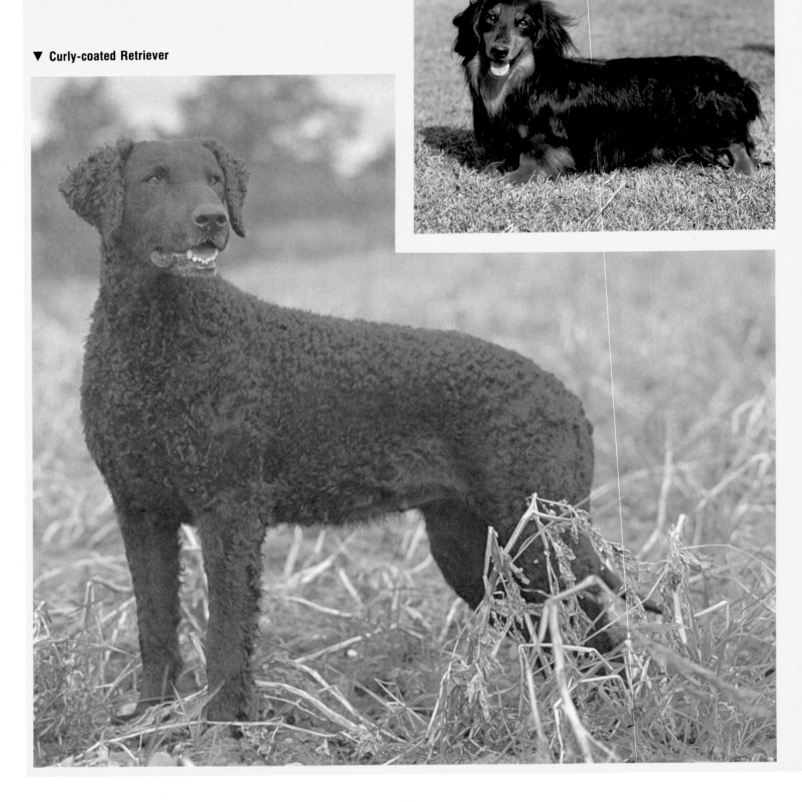

CURLY-COATED RETRIEVER

Origins. The breed was produced as a gundog superbly adapted to working in water, on a basis of the Old English Water Spaniel, with the judicious introduction of Irish and English Water Spaniels, Newfoundland and Poodle.

Characteristics. A smart upstanding dog showing activity, endurance and intelligence. The head is long and well proportioned, with black or brown eyes, and rather small, low-set ears lying close to the head. The neck is moderately long and the body strong and muscular. The tail is shortish, carried straight and covered with curls.

Group. Sporting. Gundog (KC).

Size. Large.

Coat. *Color:* Black or liver. *Texture:* The main characteristic of the breed is a mass of small, crisp curls all over the body.

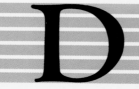

DACHSHUND

Origins. Dachshunds represent a small and distinctive subgroup within the hound group, differentiated from other hounds by their small size, the work for which they were intended and to some extent by the quarry they used to hunt. 'Dachshund' simply means 'badger dog,' but must not be taken to mean that these diminutive hounds, whose history dates back to the fifteenth century, were used exclusively for that quarry. Larger hounds, weighing 13.6 kg (30 lb) or 15.8 kg (35 lb) were used for badger, while smaller ones were kept for stoat and weasel.

Characteristics. First and foremost a sporting dog, but is equally adaptable as a house pet. The general appearance is long and low, but with a compact and well-muscled body, with a bold defiant head carriage. The head is long, the eyes are of medium size, oval and dark in color. The body is long and muscular, the chest very oval. The tail is high set, strong and tapering. There are two sizes, Standard and Miniature, and three coat varieties: Smooth-haired, Long-haired and Wire-haired.

Group. Hounds.

Size. Small. The Standard Dachshund has a heavy body on very short legs; the Miniature version weighs up to 4.9 kg (11 lb).

Coat. *Color:* Various. *Texture:* Short, dense and smooth for the Smooth-haired, soft and straight or slightly waved for the Long-haired and short, thick, hard and rough for the Wire-haired.

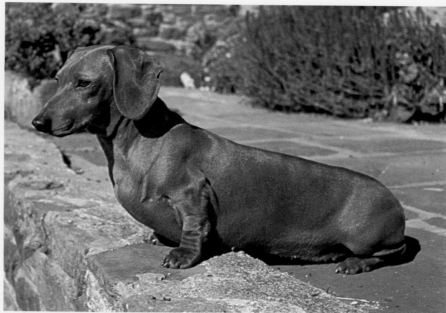

▲ **Smooth-haired Dachshund**

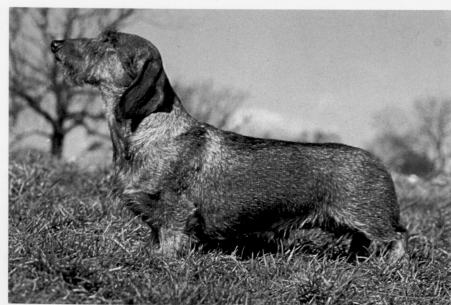

▲ **Wire-haired Dachshund**

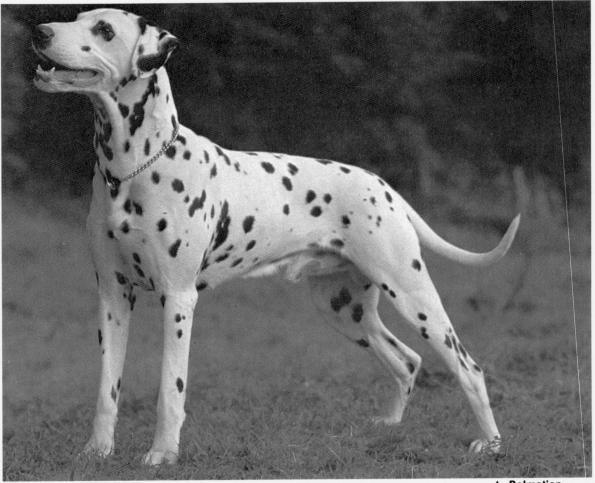

▲ Dalmatian

DALMATIAN

Origins. The breed is said to have originated in Dalmatia on the Adriatic coast, though spotted dogs are found in many parts of the world. However, the breed has been established for so long in Britain, where it was used as a carriage dog, that it can perhaps be recognized as a British breed. In America its affinity with horses and carriages earned it a place with the horsedrawn fire engines and it became the Firehouse Dog.

Characteristics. Dalmatians should be strong, muscular and active. They are graceful in outline, elegant and capable of great endurance. The most obvious characteristic is the spotted coat. Dalmatians have great freedom of movement, a smooth powerful rhythmic action with a long stride. They are good-tempered dogs, intelligent and easily trained.

Group. Non-Sporting. Utility (KC).

Size. Large.

Coat. *Color:* The ground color is pure white, evenly covered with well-defined black or liver spots. *Texture:* Short, hard and dense, sleek and glossy in appearance.

▼ **Dandie Dinmont Terrier**

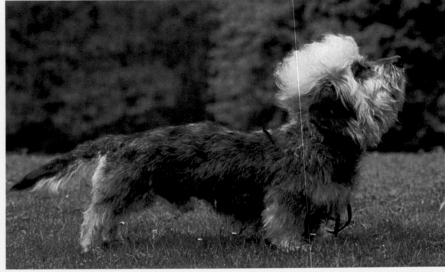

DANDIE DINMONT TERRIER

Origins. A breed which owes its present name to the character in Walter Scott's *Guy Mannering*, but which was certainly in existence in the Cheviot Hills long before the book was written. The Dandie is a close relation of both the Border and Bedlington Terriers.

Characteristics. The Dandie is a very distinctive breed with a strong and rather large head. The dark eyes, set wide apart, are full and round, the ears pendulous, falling close to the cheek. The forelegs are short with immense muscular development and bone, set wide apart. The body is long, strong and flexible, the hindquarters are set wide apart. The tail is rather short, carried a little above the level of the body. The loyal little Dandie makes a useful watchdog.

Group. Terriers.
Size. Small.
Coat. *Color:* Pepper or mustard. *Texture:* A mixture of hardish and soft hair, giving a coat that feels crisp to the touch.

DEERHOUND (SCOTTISH DEERHOUND)

Origins. The Deerhound of today is just as it has always been when, having been produced out of the hounds used by Pictish hunters, the breed was used to bring deer to bay and were the prized possessions and constant companions of their masters.

Characteristics. The general conformation is similar to that of a Greyhound, but of larger size. The head is long, the eyes are dark and moderately full, the ears set on high and folded back. The neck is long and strong. The shoulders are well sloped and the forelegs are straight. The tail is long, thick at the root and reaches almost to the ground. The Deerhound makes a delightful pet; gentle, calm and affectionate.

Group. Hounds.
Size. Large: 76 cm (30 in) or more.
Coat. *Color:* Usually gray. *Texture:* Harsh and wiry on body, neck and shoulders and about 7.6–10 cm (3–4 in) long. It should be thick, close-lying, ragged and harsh or crisp to the touch.

DOBERMAN(N) PINSCHER

Origins. This breed is of such recent origin that it can be traced to the person who first produced it, Louis Dobermann, a German tax collector. Between 1865–70 he set about producing a first-class guard dog based on the concept of a giant terrier, combining agility with strength, speed and great intelligence. So well did he succeed that the

◀ **Deerhound**

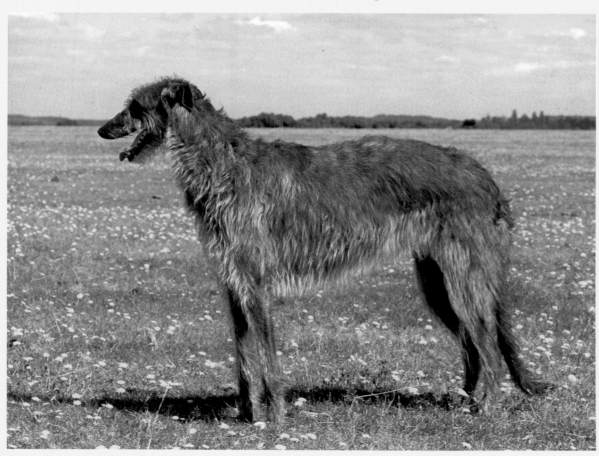

Dobermann Pinscher demands the highest standards of its handlers.

Characteristics. A medium-sized dog with a well-set body, muscular and elegant, proud carriage and bold alert temperament. The breed is compact and tough with light, elastic movement. The head is long and clean, the eyes deep and almond-shaped. Ears may be erect or dropped, cropped in countries where the operation is permitted. The body is square, the back short and firm.

Group. Working. Non-Sporting (ANKC).

Size. Large.

Coat. *Color:* Black, red, brown or blue with rust-red markings. *Texture:* Smooth-haired, short, hard, thick and close lying.

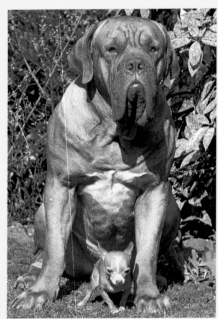

▲ **Dogue de Bordeaux**

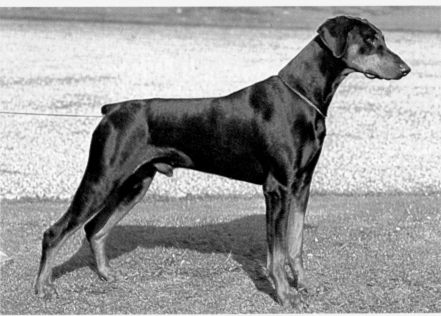

▲ **Doberman Pinscher**

DOGUE DE BORDEAUX

Origins. The Dogue de Bordeaux may lay claim to being the national dog of France.

Characteristics. In appearance the breed is very similar to the English Mastiff and is descended from the Roman mastiffs originally imported from the East. In France, the breed was developed as a fighting dog and was used as such until the beginning of the twentieth century. Nowadays, the breed makes an excellent watchdog as it is vigilant, faithful and has great strength.

Group. Working (FCI).

Size. Large.

Coat. *Color:* Apricot, silver, fawn or dark fawn-brindle with black points. *Texture:* Smooth and short.

E

ELKHOUND (NORWEGIAN ELKHOUND)

Origins. The Elkhound is another of the Scandinavian Spitz breeds. It has arrived at its present distinctive appearance as a result of selection based on its ability to hunt the elk, bringing the animal to bay while summoning the hunters with its shrill barking.

Characteristics. The Elkhound is friendly and intelligent, with great energy and independence of character. However, it requires firm handling from its owner. In general appearance it is compactly built with a short body, thick, abundant coat, pricked ears and a tail curled tightly over the back. The head is broad, the eyes dark with a fearless and friendly expression.

Group. Hounds.

Size. Large.

Coat. *Color:* Gray of various shades with black tips on the long outer coat. *Texture:* Thick and abundant, coarse and weather resistant with a longish, coarse top coat and a light colored, soft woolly undercoat.

ENGLISH SETTER

Origins. Although it is likely that the setters originally sprang from imported spaniel stock, there is evidence that by the late sixteenth century

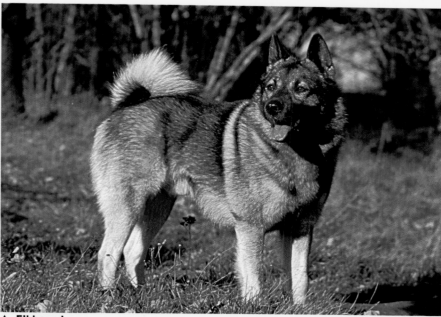

▲ Elkhound

the two groups of bird dogs were distinctly differentiated. The Setter, with its long head, curly coat and well-developed ability to find and point game, showed evidence of crosses with Pointers, the large Water Spaniel and the Springer Spaniel. The modern breed was developed by intensely selective breeding in the mid-nineteenth century.

Characteristics. The English Setter is an intensely friendly and quiet-natured dog with a keen game sense. It is clean in outline, and elegant both in appearance and movement. The head is long and rather lean, the eyes are bright, mild and intelligent and of a dark hazel color. The ears are set low and hanging close to the cheek; the tips are velvety, the upper parts clothed in fine silky hair. The tail is set almost in line with the back, the feather long, soft and silky.

Group. Sporting. Gundog (KC).

Size. Large.

Coat. *Color:* Black and white, lemon and white, liver and white or tricolor. *Texture:* Slightly wavy, long and silky, the breeches and forelegs well feathered.

ENGLISH SPRINGER SPANIEL

Origins. In the early seventeenth century there was a tendency to refer to the larger spaniels, which were

▼ English Setter

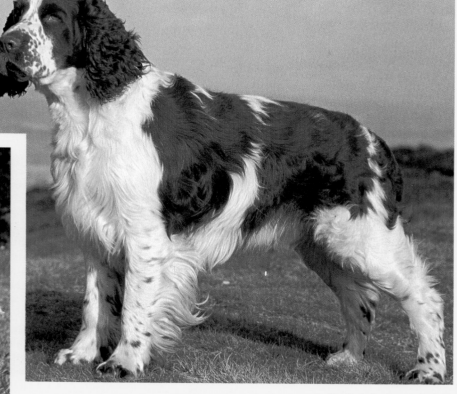

▲ English Springer Spaniel

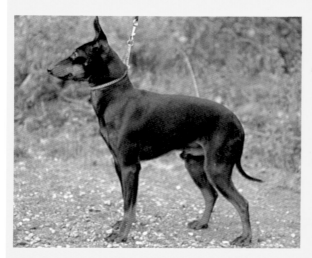

▲ English Toy Terrier

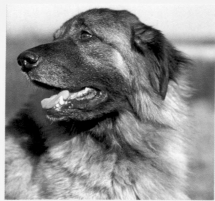

▲ Estrela Mountain Dog

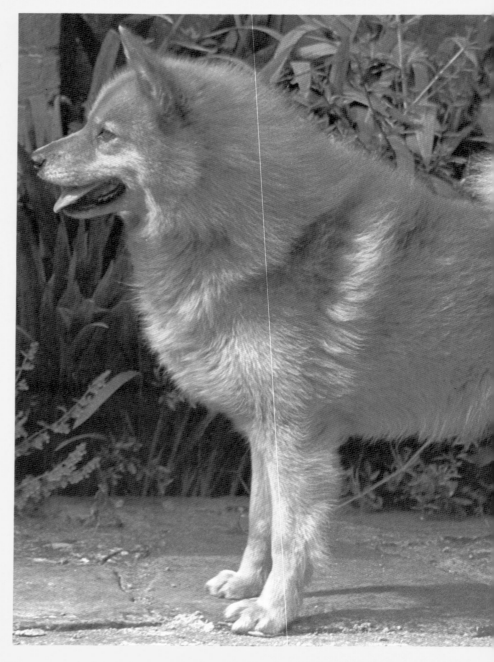

used to startle game so that it sprang into the air, as Starter or Springer Spaniels. With the advent of quick-firing guns which increased their popularity, these early Springers were divided into the lighter Welsh Springers and the heavier English.

Characteristics. The general appearance of the modern Springer is that of a compact, strong, upstanding, merry and active dog, built for endurance and activity. The skull is fairly broad, the eyes dark hazel and the ears are lobular in shape, set close to the head. The neck is long and muscular, the body strong and the chest deep with well-sprung ribs. The tail is set low, well feathered and has a lively action.

Group. Sporting. Gundog (KC).

Size. Large.

Coat. *Color:* Usually liver and white or black and white. *Texture:* Close, straight and weather-resistant, without being coarse.

ENGLISH TOY TERRIER (TOY MANCHESTER TERRIER)

Origins. The English Toy Terriers, formally called Toy Black and Tan Terriers or Toy Manchester

Terriers, made their reputation in the rat pit in the nineteenth century. Often weighing no more than 2.7 kg (6 lb), they were matched either to kill a certain number of rats against the clock, or in competition with another dog.

Characteristics. A well-balanced, elegant and compact Toy dog with a terrier temperament and characteristics. The head is long and narrow, the ears 'candle flame' shaped, thin and erect, and the eyes very dark, small and almond-shaped. The neck is long and graceful and slightly arched, the chest narrow and deep. Front movement is akin to the 'extended trot'; a hackney action is undesirable. This dog makes an affectionate pet.

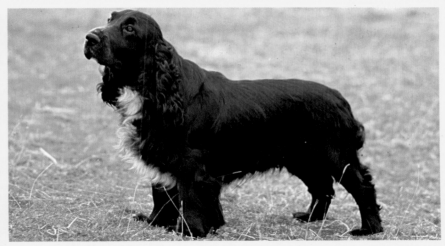

◄ **Field Spaniel**

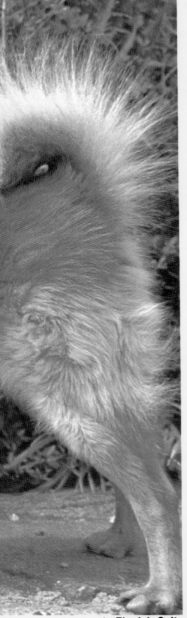

▲ **Finnish Spitz**

Group. Toys.
Size. Small.
Coat. *Color:* Black and tan. *Texture:* Thick, close, smooth and glossy.

ESTRELA MOUNTAIN DOG

Origins. The Estrela Mountain Dog from Portugal, like so many of the European dual-purpose herding and guard breeds, is a large and very powerful dog with great courage and stamina. It is independent by nature and needs careful training.

Characteristics. The head is massive, broad and moderately long. The skull is slightly domed with a strong muzzle. The eyes are almond-shaped, dark and wide-set. The ears are small and carried folded back. The body is rather longer than it is tall with a broad, muscular back and deep chest. The tail is long and carried low.

Group. Working. (KC).
Size. Large.
Coat. *Color:* Gray, tawny and red, red or light tan. *Texture:* Short, thick and rather coarse, smooth and very slightly wavy.

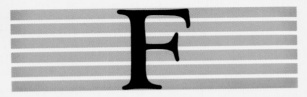

FIELD SPANIEL

Origins. During its early career in the show ring the Field Spaniel was classified with Cocker Spaniels and the breeds were only separated in 1892.

Characteristics. A well-balanced dog, noble, upstanding and sporting, built for activity and endurance and combining beauty with utility and unusual docility. The muzzle is long and lean, the eyes dark hazel in color with a grave expression. The neck is long, strong and muscular set into long and sloping shoulders which give great activity and speed. The body is of moderate length, the chest deep, the back and loins strong and muscular. The tail is carried level with the back or below it.

Group. Sporting. Gundog (KC).
Size. Medium.
Coat. *Color:* Black, liver, golden liver, mahogany red, roan, or any of these colors with tan over eyes, on feet. *Texture:* Flat or slightly waved, silky and appears glossy and refined.

FINNISH SPITZ

Origins. In its own country this breed is very popular indeed. Originally these dogs were used to track down and mark with their piercing bark the position of a variety of game in the Finnish woodland; now they are principally regarded as bird dogs. In 1927, the breed was introduced into Britain where it is admired by a few enthusiasts.

Characteristics. The general outline is square, the head – with its keen eyes, erect pointed ears and pointed muzzle – is distinctly foxlike. The back is short and straight, the chest deep. Forelegs are straight, hindquarters strong, and the bushy tail, in the typical Spitz manner, is carried over the back. The breed is loyal and useful as a watchdog but needs firm, gentle training.

Group. Miscellaneous. Hound (KC).
Size. Medium.
Coat. *Color:* Reddish brown or yellowish red. *Texture:* Short and close on the head and legs, longer on the body, with a mane of coarser hair.

FLAT-COATED RETRIEVER

Origins. The breed is a subtle mixture of the St John's Newfoundland (a smaller version of the Newfoundland) with setters, sheepdogs and spaniels, and is a first-class retriever of water fowl. The breed was first shown in Britain in 1859 under a

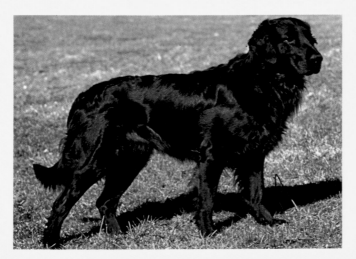

► **Flat-coated Retriever**

FOXHOUND (ENGLISH)

Origins. A breed which has been developed exclusively for a single purpose and which in Britain has not been diverted from its original purpose by popularity either as a pet or as a show dog, for in neither role has it achieved a place.

Characteristics. The skull is broad, the neck long and not thick, the body has plenty of heart room. The hindquarters are full and muscular. The Foxhound is bred as a pack animal and is unsuitable as a pet.

Group. Hounds.

Size. Large.

Coat. *Color*: A good 'hound color' – black, tan, white in any combination. *Texture*: Weather-resistant, short, dense, hard and glossy.

classification which included curly coats, wavy or smooth-coated Retrievers, but had to wait until 1873 when Mr E. Shirley, founder of the Kennel Club, took an interest in it and stabilized type.

Characteristics. A bright, active dog of medium size with an intelligent expression, showing power and raciness. The head is long and nicely molded, the jaw long and strong. The eyes are dark brown or hazel of medium size and the ears small and fitting close to the side of the head. The neck is long, the chest deep and fairly broad, the back short. The tail is short, straight and carried gaily. The dog is intelligent and trainable.

Group. Sporting. Gundog (KC).

Size. Large.

Coat. *Color*: Black or liver. *Texture*: Dense, of fine quality and texture, and as flat as possible.

FOX TERRIER, SMOOTH

Origins. The Smooth Fox Terrier is undoubtedly the aristocrat of the terrier group, able to look back over a long history of work with hounds. At the beginning of the century, it was among the most popular of companions and show dogs. This early popularity has left a considerable literature devoted to the breed and a mass of carefully drawn illustrations which demonstrate that the breed has changed very little since, for example, the publication of Daniel's *Rural Sports* in 1801.

Characteristics. The dog must present a gay and active appearance and is compactly built. It has a short back but stands like a Foxhound, covering a lot of ground. It is intelligent and trainable but needs firm handling.

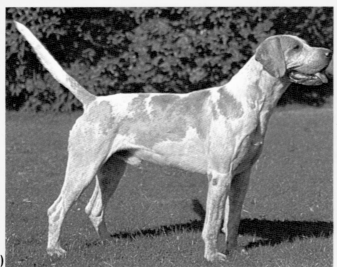

► **Foxhound (English)**

▲ **French Bulldog**

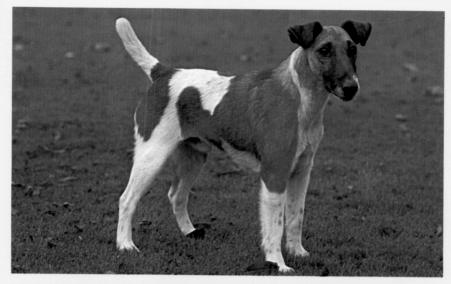

◄ **Smooth Fox Terrier**

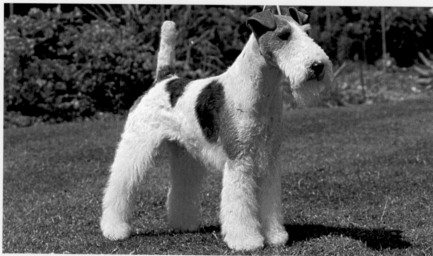

◄ **Wire Fox Terrier**

Group. Terriers.
Size. Small/Medium.
Coat. *Color:* White predominates. *Texture:* Straight, flat, smooth, hard, dense and abundant.

FOX TERRIER, WIRE

Origins. The early Fox Terrier breeders did not differentiate between smooth and broken-coated dogs. Both coats appeared in the same litter but for companions and show dogs the smarter smooth coats were at first preferred. The wire coats followed them into the show ring about twenty-five years after their debut. Nowadays, with better skills in trimming and presentation, it is the Wire which takes the high prizes.

Characteristics. Similar to the Smooth in temperament and conformation, except for the coat. The texture is dense and wiry, like coconut matting and the face has plenty of whiskers.

FRENCH BULLDOG

Origins. This breed has descended from Bulldogs introduced from Britain into France, probably at the end of the nineteenth century. This stylish miniature Bulldog speedily swept to popularity among the fashion-conscious French, who called them the Boule-Dog Français even though the breed's British ancestry was obvious.

Characteristics. A French Bulldog should be sound, active and intelligent, of compact build. The head is massive, square and broad, with a domed forehead and loose skin forming symmetrical wrinkles. The bat ears are distinctively different from the ears of other Bulldog breeds. It is a very affectionate dog and a bit of a clown.

Group. Non-Sporting. Utility (KC).
Size. Small.
Coat. *Color:* Brindle, pied and fawn. *Texture:* Fine, smooth, lustrous, short and close.

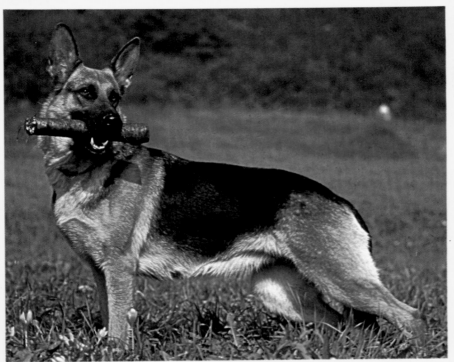

▲ **German Shepherd Dog**

G

GERMAN SHEPHERD DOG (ALSATIAN)

Origins. A breed with origins and uses as indicated by its name. The first breed club was formed in 1899. By 1926 it was the most popular dog in Britain, where it was called the Alsatian Wolf Dog. Thoughtless breeding and ignorant handling gave the breed a dubious reputation which only the worst deserve. The best are intelligent, resourceful and eager to please but all these virtues must be in the hands of an owner able to develop them.

Characteristics. The characteristic expression of the German Shepherd Dog gives the impression of perpetual vigilance, fidelity, liveliness and watchfulness; fearless, but with a decided suspiciousness of strangers. It is a well-proportioned dog, with a long strongly boned body, obviously capable of endurance and speed and of quick, sudden movement.

Group. Herding. Working (KC).

Size. Large.

Coat. *Color:* Usually black and a sandy tan. *Texture:* Smooth and double texture with a thick, close, woolly undercoat and a close, hard, straight, weather-resistant outercoat.

GERMAN SHORTHAIRED POINTER

Origins. There are few records of the breed before the Klub Kurzhaar stud book was started in the 1870s, but it had long been established among those who appreciated its working qualities. The breed probably has its origins in the dogs introduced by homecoming crusaders intermingled with indigenous bird dogs and the Spanish Pointer, with style and elegance being largely dependent on the blood of the English Pointer. Nowadays the breed has a high reputation as a general purpose gundog.

Characteristics. An aristocratic, well-balanced, symmetrical animal displaying power, endurance and agility. Its expression shows enthusiasm for work. The head is clean cut, the shoulders sloping, the chest deep and the back short and powerful. This is an obedient dog with a good temperament.

Group. Sporting. Gundog (KC).

Size. Large.

Coat. *Color:* Solid liver or any combination of liver and white. *Texture:* The skin is close and tight, the hair short and thick.

GERMAN WIREHAIRED POINTER

Origins. This dog was developed by selectively crossing several indigenous gundog breeds – the

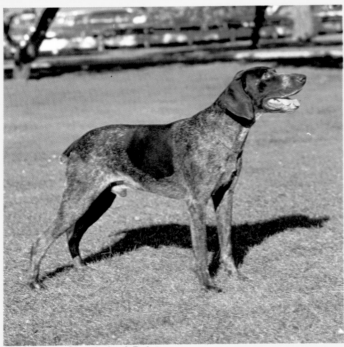

▲ **German Shorthaired Pointer**

wirehaired Pointing Griffon, the Stichelhaar, the Puderpointer and the German Shorthair which, apart from the coat, it very closely resembles. The breed has been slow to gain recognition outside Germany, but now has a growing band of enthusiastic followers who appreciate the breed's outstanding abilities as an all-purpose gundog.

Characteristics. Essentially a dog of the Pointer type, of sturdy build, lively manner and with an intelligent, determined expression. In disposition the breed has been described as energetic, rather aloof, but not unfriendly. The head is moderately long with a broad skull, the ears are rounded but not too broad and hang close to the sides of the head. The body is a little longer than it is high, the back short, straight and strong.

Group. Sporting. Gundog (KC).

Size. Large.

Coat. *Color:* Liver and white. *Texture:* Weather-resistant and to some extent water-repellant. Outer coat straight, harsh, wiry, lying flat, 2.5–5 cm (1–2 in) in length; the undercoat is dense in winter, thinner in summer.

GLEN OF IMAAL TERRIER

Origins. Very few of this breed are seen in the show ring or as companions outside their native Wicklow Mountains where their qualities as badger and fox hunters are highly prized among a select band of enthusiasts. The breed first appeared in the show ring in 1934, but has not taken to its new career with enthusiasm.

Characteristics. The Glen of Imaal Terrier is gentle with children and a lovable pet which usually abstains from fighting. Like all terriers of Ireland it loves water, it is silent in its work and about the house. The skull is strong, the ears pendulous, the eyes brown and placed well apart. The forelegs are short and bowed, the chest is wide and strong.

Group. Terrier (KC).

Size. Small.

Coat. *Color:* Blue and tan, wheaten. *Texture:* Long and coarse.

GOLDEN RETRIEVER

Origins. This breed originated when, in 1865, Lord Tweedsmouth mated a yellow wavy-coated

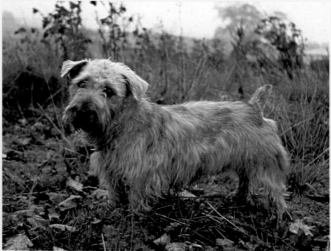

◄ **Glen of Imaal Terrier**

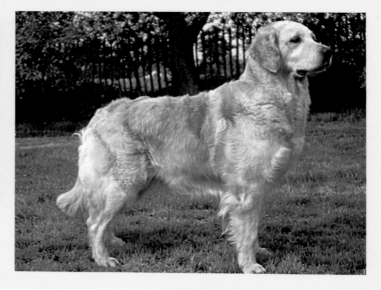

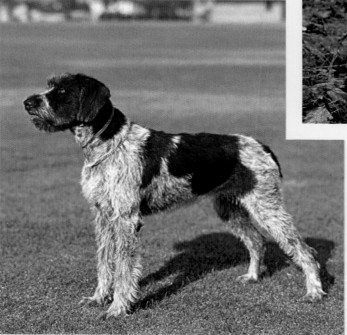

▲ **German Wirehaired Pointer**

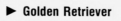

► **Golden Retriever**

▼ Gordon Setter

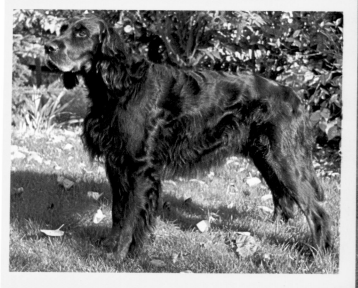

Retriever to a Tweed Water Spaniel, a breed from Scotland, and then bred on to further crosses with Tweed Water Spaniels, black Retrievers, an Irish Setter and a Bloodhound, so that by 1913 the Kennel Club was able to recognize the result as a separate breed.

Characteristics. The Golden Retriever is well-proportioned, active and powerful. The head is broad, the expression kindly, the eyes dark. The neck is muscular, the body well balanced. Feet are round and catlike and the tail is well-feathered.

Group. Sporting. Gundog (KC).

Size. Large.

Coat. *Color:* Any shade of gold or cream. *Texture:* Flat or wavy with good feathering and dense, with a water-resistant undercoat.

GORDON SETTER

Origins. As early as 1620 Markham, a contemporary writer, was able to remark that the 'black and fallow setting dog' was the 'hardest to endure labor.'

But it was not until the end of the eighteenth century, when the fourth Duke of Gordon's kennel of Setters had made the breed famous, that the Gordon Castle Setters began to achieve fame outside Scotland. The Gordon Setter has never achieved the popularity of the Irish or. English Setters and so has avoided some of the worst effects of popular demand and remains an honest, basically sensible gundog.

Characteristics. The breed is stylish, built on galloping lines, with a thoroughbred appearance. The back is strong, fairly short and level, the tail shortish and the head fairly long, with an intelligent expression. Eyes are of a fair size, dark brown and bright; ears are medium-sized and rather thin, set low and hanging close to the head. This stylish dog has a happy disposition and a strong will.

Group. Sporting. Gundog (KC).

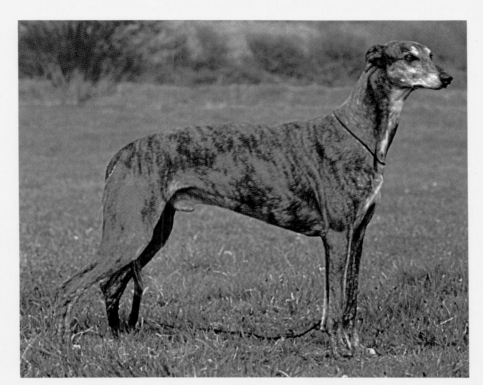

◄ **Greyhound**

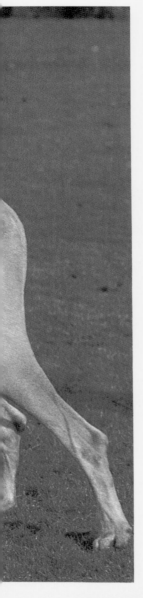

◄ **Great Dane**

Size. Large.

Coat. *Color:* Deep shining coal-black with tan markings of a rich chestnut red. *Texture:* Soft and shining, straight or slightly waved. Long hair on ears, under stomach and on chest, back of fore and hindlegs and under the tail.

GREAT DANE

Origins. In spite of its name the breed has no close association with Denmark. Indeed because drawings of very similar dogs were found on Fourth Dynasty tomb walls, some people might put its origins in Egypt, but it was in Germany that the breed was developed and achieved popularity. The breed was the one favored by Bismarck and used to hunt wild boar.

Characteristics. Great Danes should be very large, very muscular, strongly though elegantly built. Their heads are carried high and they have a clean-cut, impressive look. They are loyal, easily-trained dogs that make good pets.

Group. Working. Non-Sporting (ANKC).

Size. Large: 76.2 cm (30 in) upwards.

Coat. *Color:* Brindle, fawn, steel blue, black or white patched with black or blue. *Texture:* Very short and thick, smooth and glossy.

GREYHOUND

Origins. There can be no doubt that Greyhounds are of very ancient origin. As early as 1016 Canute's law forbade 'mean persons' from keeping Greyhounds and, in 1408, Dame Juliana Berners used an older description of the breed in her Book of St Albans.

Characteristics. The Greyhound possesses remarkable stamina and its long-reaching movement enables it to move at great speed; indeed the Greyhound over a measured sprint is probably the fastest of all dogs. The head is long and elegant, the eyes bright and intelligent, the neck long and muscular. The chest is deep, the legs are strong, well boned and powerfully muscled. Though Greyhounds are usually kept for racing, they also make clean, affectionate companions.

Group. Hounds.

Size. Large: average 74 cm (29 in).

Coat. *Color:* Black, white, red, blue, fawn, fallow, brindle or any of the colors broken with white. *Texture:* Fine and close.

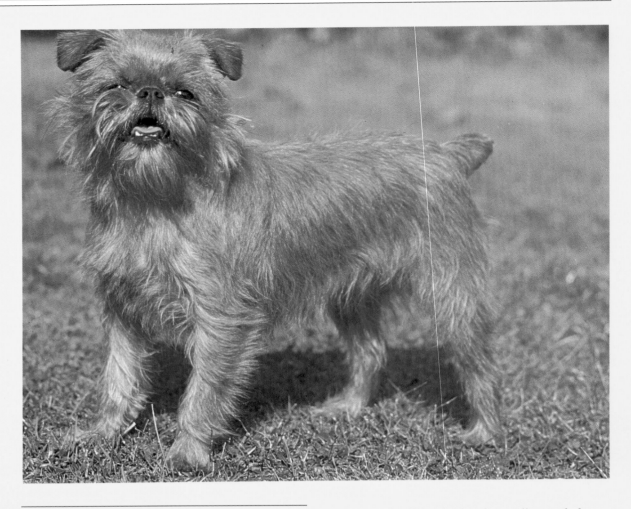

► Griffon Bruxellois

GRIFFON BRUXELLOIS (BRUSSELS GRIFFON)

Origins. Originally the Griffon was a humble adjunct of stables, used to keep down vermin and as an effective early warning system of unauthorized intrusion. Probably the breed has origins in the more ancient Affenpinscher.

Characteristics. The Griffon is a smart little dog with a pert monkeylike expression. It is well balanced, square in outline, lively and alert. The head is large and rounded, the eyes also large and round. Ears are small, semi-erect and high set. The chest is wide and deep, the back short, the hind-quarters are well muscled. The tail is short, docked and carried high.

Group. Toys.
Size. Small.
Coat. *Color:* Red, black or black and rich tan. *Texture:* Harsh and wiry.

GRIFFON VENDÉEN, GRAND

Origins. This dog is a descendant of the white variety of the ancient St Hubert hound of France.

Characteristics. The Griffon Vendéen is an intelligent dog, sure of itself and distinguished in physique and gait. The head is well rounded, not too broad, and the eyebrows bushy. The eyes are large, dark and vivacious, and the pendulous ears are soft, fine, narrow and covered with long hair.

Group. Hounds for big game (FCI).
Size. Large.
Coat. *Color:* Fawn, white and orange; white and gray; tricolor. *Texture:* Long, bushy, heavy and hard.

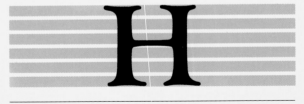

HAMILTONSTÖVARE

Origins. The Hamiltonstövare is a breed produced by crosses between the Holstein, Hanover and Kurland Beagles and the Foxhound made by Adolf Patrick Hamilton, hence the breed's name.

Characteristics. The appearance is very much that of a small and lightly built Foxhound. It is a strong and willing hunter but does not make a

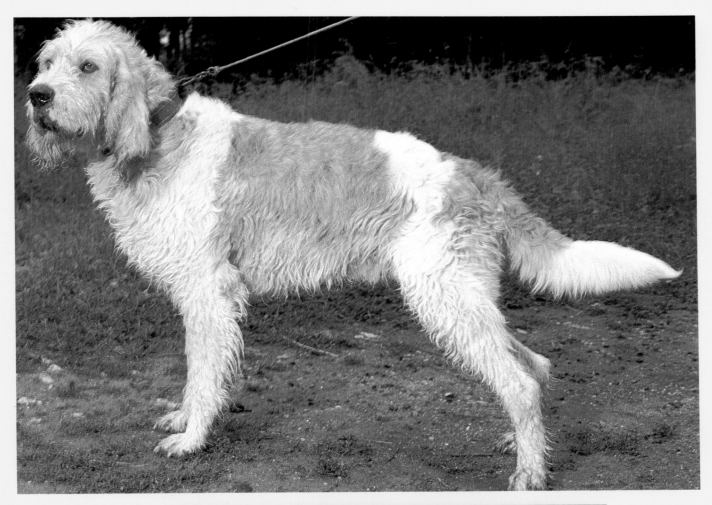

▲ Grand Griffon Vendéen

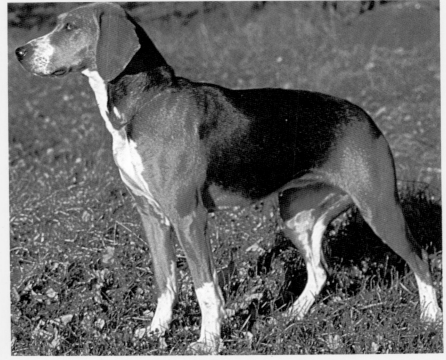

► Hamiltonstövare

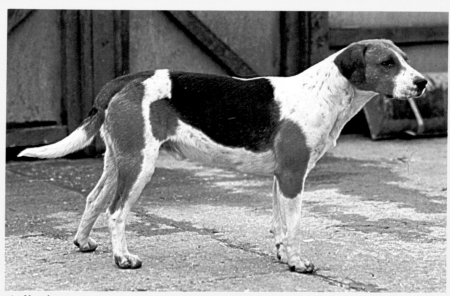

▲ Harrier

▼ Short-haired Hungarian Vizsla

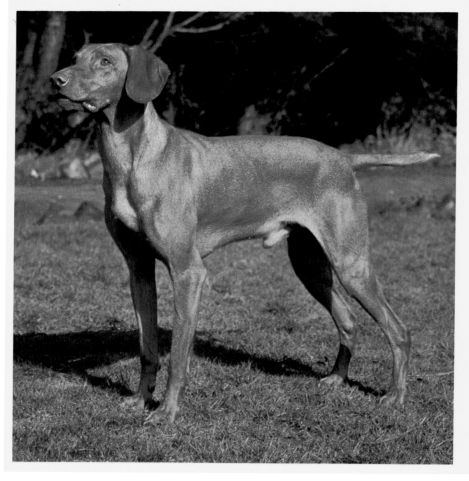

suitable pet.

Group. Hound (KC).

Size. Medium.

Coat. *Color:* The back black, shading to brown on the head and legs, with white on the muzzle, chest and legs. *Texture:* Short and dense.

HARRIER

Origins. In 400 BC Xenophon was able to describe two types of hounds, the Castorean and the fox-breed said to be the product of a fox-dog cross. Xenophon listed the qualities necessary in hare hounds, qualities which were still relevant when Sir Elias de Midhope of Penistone gathered the first pack of Harriers together in 1260.

Characteristics. In every respect a small Foxhound. This is a hunting dog, not a domestic pet.

Group. Hounds.

Size. Medium.

Coat. *Color:* Any hound color. *Texture:* Short, smooth and dense.

HUNGARIAN VIZSLA

Origins. The breed is sometimes called the Hungarian Pointer, which gives clues to its origins. Drawings dating from the Magyar invasions 1000 years ago show Vizsla-like dogs being used in conjunction with falcons.

Characteristics. The breed is robust yet lightly built, showing power and drive in the field, but with a tractable and affectionate nature in the home. The head is lean and muscular, moderately wide between the ears, which are thin and silky, hanging close to the cheeks. The neck is strong, smooth and muscular, the back is short and the chest moderately broad and deep. The tail is docked and set just below the level of the back. The gait is light-footed, graceful and smooth. There is a Short-haired and a Wire-haired version of the Vizsla; both are intelligent, loyal dogs.

Group. Sporting. Gundog (KC).

Size. Large.

Coat. *Color:* Solid, rusty gold or dark sandy yellow in different shades. *Texture:* Short, smooth, dense and close-lying, without evidence of a woolly undercoat. The wire-haired version has a wiry coat.

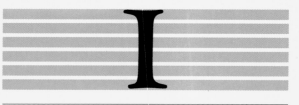

IBIZAN HOUND

Origins. One of the ancient sight hound breeds with origins in the lands around the Mediterranean and with a history which reaches back into ancient Egypt and the courts of the Pharaohs. In the tomb of Hemako a carved dish was found which carries the image of an Ibizan Hound; this dish was made during the 1st Dynasty between 3100 and 2700 BC. The tombs of Tutankhamen and the Ptolemies also provide evidence of the breed's ancient origin. Probably the hounds were first taken to Ibiza by Phoenician traders, where selection based on survival of the fittest produced a breed capable of hunting with skill, endurance and tenacity and with an exceptional jumping ability.

Characteristics. The head is long and narrow, the eyes small and ranging in color from amber to caramel. The neck is long, slender and slightly arched and the dog has an elegant look. It has a friendly disposition but is only obedient when it feels so inclined.

Group. Hounds.

Size. Large.

Coat. *Color:* Red and white, or solid red. *Texture:* Short-coated hounds have a short hard coat; wirehaired hounds have a hard coat from 2.5–7.6 cm (1–3 in) in length.

IRISH SETTER

Origins. Ireland is the home of two breeds of setter, the Red and White and the Red. The former never achieved popular recognition and now survives only in the kennels of a few enthusiasts. The Red Setter, however, has achieved a degree of popularity

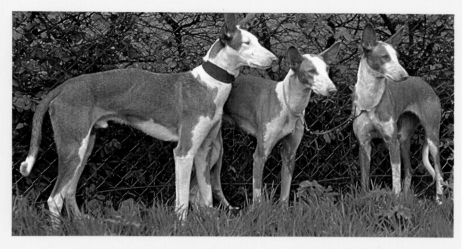

▲ **Ibizan Hound**

which may not always have been to its benefit as it has led to the breed being carelessly bred.

Characteristics. Irish Setters are attractive, lively dogs with a kindly expression. The head is long and lean, the eyes are dark hazel or dark brown; the ears are of moderate size and fine texture and hang close to the head. The neck is moderately long, very muscular and slightly arched. The shoulders are deep and sloping, the chest is rather narrow in front and fairly deep. This is a loyal, affectionate dog with plenty of energy.

Group. Sporting. Gundog (KC).

Size. Large.

Coat. *Color:* Rich chestnut. *Texture:* Flat and sleek; long and silky on the ears, legs and tail.

▼ **Irish Setter**

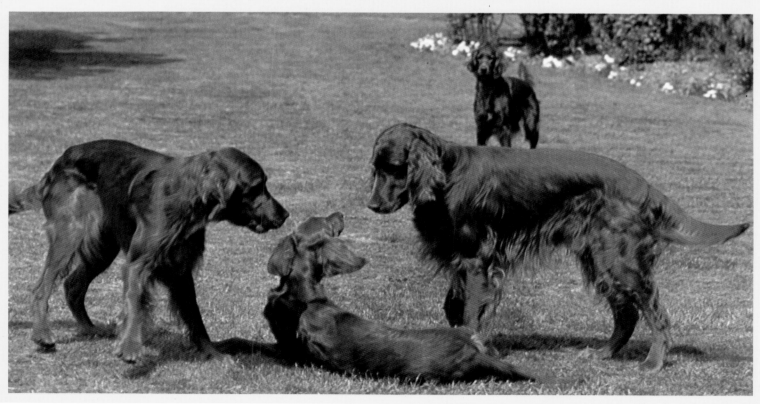

IRISH WATER SPANIEL

Origins. The Irish Water Spaniel represents a very old type of dog whose remains have been found in archaeological sites throughout Europe and which had emerged in Ireland as a distinct breed probably as early as the twelfth century. Nowadays, the Irish Water Spaniel is a gundog bred to work in shooting.

Characteristics. This is an intelligent dog, easily trained and very loyal to its owner. Its head is of good size, the muzzle long, strong and somewhat square, the face covered with characteristic curls and the topknot formed of longer curls. The eyes are small and dark, the ears very long and lobular, again covered with long curls. The neck is powerful, long and arched, set into sloping and powerful shoulders. The tail is distinctive, short and straight, set low and partly covered with curls, partly with straight hair.

Group. Sporting. Gundog (KC).

Size. Large.

Coat. *Color:* A rich dark liver. *Texture:* Dense, tight, crisp ringlets with a natural oiliness.

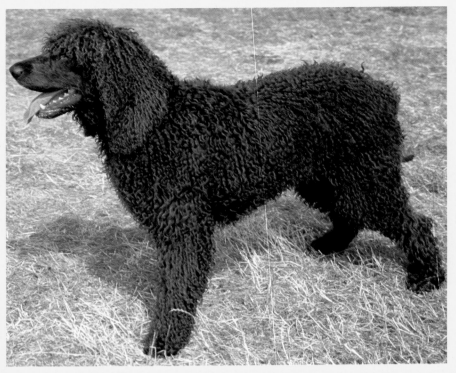

▲ **Irish Water Spaniel**

IRISH TERRIER

Origins. The Irish Terrier shares much the same origins as the Kerry Blue and made its debut in the show ring in 1879. The breed is hardy and adaptable like so many of the terriers: it is loyal, and makes an excellent guard.

Characteristics. The Irish Terrier is even-tempered especially with people, though sometimes fiery with other dogs. The dog is active, lively, lithe and wiry in appearance. The head is long, the skull flat, the eyes dark, the ears small and V-shaped. The neck of fair length, the shoulders fine, long and sloping, the body moderately long. The tail is generally docked.

Group. Terriers.

Size. Medium.

Coat. *Color:* Various shades of red. *Texture:* Hard and wiry.

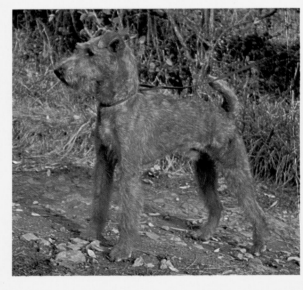

◀ **Irish Terrier**

IRISH WOLFHOUND

Origins. In AD 391 Consul Quintus Aurelius recorded that a gift of seven wolfhounds had filled 'all Rome with wonder.' The breed was obviously already well established, but the extinction of the wolf led to the breed's decline, so that by the mid-nineteenth century the breed was almost extinct. However, in the 1860s the breed was recreated by Captain George Graham, a Scot living in Gloucestershire.

Characteristics. The breed's most obvious characteristics are its commanding appearance and the impression of considerable strength it conveys. The head is long, the skull not too broad, the ears small and Greyhound-like in carriage. The neck is rather long, and very strong and muscular. The chest is very deep, the back rather long, and the hindquarters long and strong as in the Greyhound. It has large, round feet. This gentle, dignified dog needs sympathetic training.

Group. Hounds.

Size. Large and heavy: 78.7 cm (31 in) and 54.5 kg (120 lb).

Coat. *Color:* Gray, brindle, red, black, white or fawn. *Texture:* Rough and hard on the body, wiry and long over eyes and underjaw.

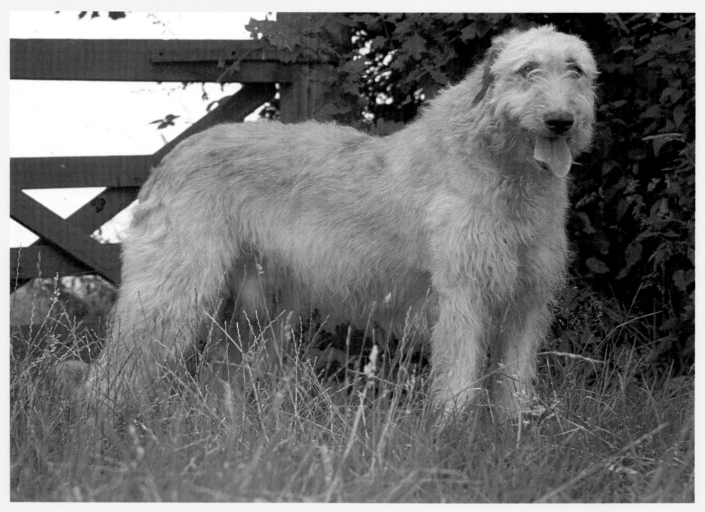

▲ **Irish Wolfhound**

ITALIAN GREYHOUND

▼ **Italian Greyhound**

Origins. A breed of ancient origin which was certainly widely known and admired among the civilizations around the Mediterranean 2000 years ago, but which probably achieved its peak of popularity in sixteenth century Italy and in the courts of James I, Frederick the Great and Catherine the Great. The Italian Greyhound is prized today as it always has been for its elegance, its sweet nature and its beauty.

Characteristics. A miniature Greyhound, slender and elegant, with a high-stepping and free action. The skull is long, flat and narrow, the muzzle very fine, the eyes rather large, bright and full of expression and the ears are rose-shaped, soft and delicate. The neck is long, gracefully arched and set into long, sloping shoulders.

Group. Toys.

Size. Small.

Coat. *Color:* All shades of fawn, white, cream, blue. *Texture:* Thin and glossy, like satin.

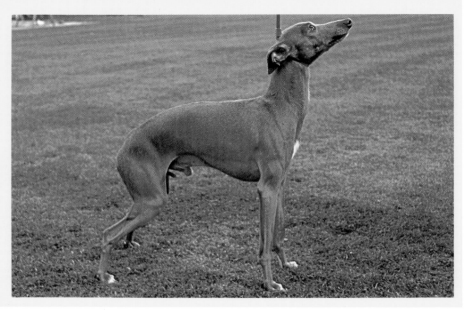

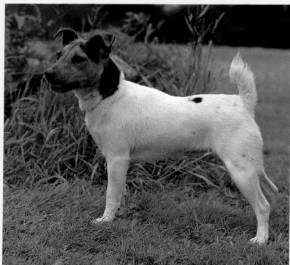

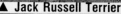
▲ **Jack Russell Terrier**

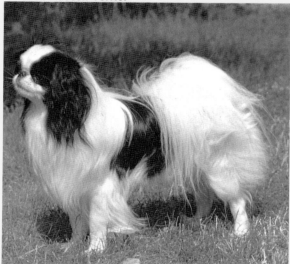
▲ **Japanese Chin**

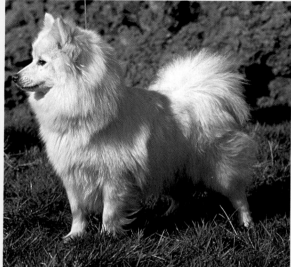
▲ **Japanese Spitz**

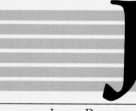

J

JACK RUSSELL TERRIER

Origins. These terriers were originally bred in the nineteenth century by a sporting parson from Devon, and his pack of working terriers became known as 'Parson Jack Russells.' They are not recognized by the Kennel Club but are very popular in Britain, especially among owners who feel that some other terriers have been overbred and lost their working character.

Characteristics. These tough, sporty little dogs are full of confidence and enthusiasm. As there is no breed standard, looks vary considerably and Jack Russells can be long or short-legged, prick or drop-eared. Their ears are dark brown and almond-shaped and the tail, usually docked, is carried high.

Size. Small.

Coat. *Color:* Usually white with tan or black markings. *Texture:* May be short and smooth or longer and rougher.

JAPANESE CHIN

Origins. Like so many of the toy breeds which originated in the Orient, the Japanese Chin, sometimes called the Japanese Spaniel, has long been associated with the Royal courts. The breed's ancestors probably arrived in Japan as gifts from the Chinese Emperor to his Japanese counterpart. The breed makes an excellent companion, but one with a mind of its own.

Characteristics. The Japanese Chin is a lively little dog of dainty appearance, smart compact carriage and with a profuse coat. It is stylish in movement, lifting the feet high, and carries its plumed tail over the back. The head is large in proportion to the size of the dog, with a broad and rounded skull, and the muzzle very short. The dark eyes are large and set wide apart, the ears small, V-shaped and carried slightly forward. The body is squarely and compactly built, and cobby in shape.

Group. Toys.

Size. Small.

Coat. *Color:* Black and white or red and white. *Texture:* Profuse, long, soft and straight, and silky.

JAPANESE SPITZ

Origins. This dog was bred from Spitz breeds taken to Japan which were used to form a breed with similarities to the Pomeranian.

Characteristics. The muzzle is pointed, the ears are erect and pointed. The tail, richly fringed, falls

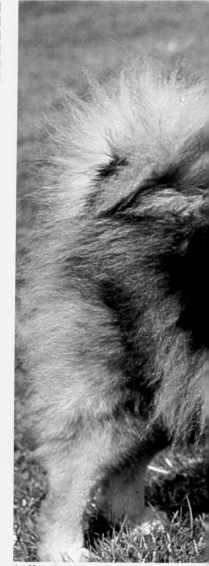
▲ **Keeshond**

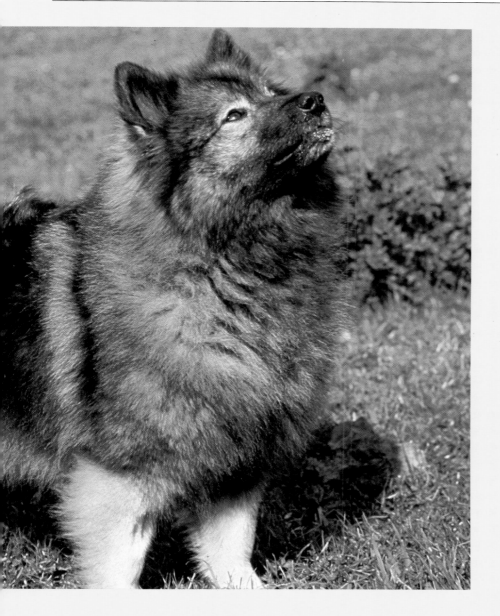

KEESHOND

Origins. For centuries this breed was used as a watchdog on the barges of Holland, but it has its origins among other more northerly Spitz breeds. Since its rise to popular recognition some two centuries ago, the breed has changed little.

Characteristics. The Keeshond has a short, compact body, alert carriage and foxlike head. It carries its well-feathered tail curled over its back in the typical Spitz manner. It is a vigilant watchdog with a sturdy, independent character.

Group. Non-Sporting. Utility (KC).

Size. Medium.

Coat. *Color:* Wolf or ash gray. *Texture:* Dense and harsh, standing away from the body with a thick soft undercoat.

KERRY BLUE TERRIER

Origins. The Kerry Blue shares a common ancestry with the Soft-Coated Wheaten Terrier and shares, too, a common birthplace among the mountains of Kerry, where it was developed to provide sport, security and companionship for the sporting farmers of that area. Nowadays, by careful breeding, skillful trimming and painstaking presentation, it has been transformed into a very successful show dog, to a far greater degree than other Irish Terriers.

Characteristics. The Kerry Blue is a compact, powerful terrier with an attitude of alert determination. It is well proportioned, with a well-developed and muscular body. The head is long and lean, the jaw strong and deep, the eyes dark and the ears small and V-shaped. The tail is set high and carried erect. The Kerry Blue makes an excellent watchdog

► **Kerry Blue Terrier**

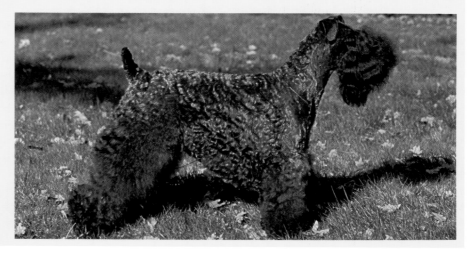

on the back. The body is compact and the general appearance handsome. The Japanese Spitz is characterized by great courage and its intelligent and cheerful disposition.

Group. Utility (KC).

Size. Medium.

Coat. *Color:* Pure white. *Texture:* Straight and standing away from the body. The undercoat is short, soft and abundant.

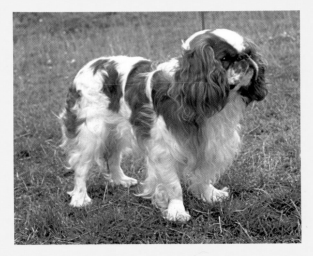

▶ **King Charles Spaniel**

▼ **Komondor**

KING CHARLES SPANIEL (ENGLISH TOY SPANIEL)

Origins. A toy spaniel which derives its name from its popularity in the court of King Charles II, which was so great that few portraits of the period seem to be without the customary King Charles Spaniel reclining on milady's lap, or peeping from behind a chair. Though it was Charles II who gave his name to the breed, toy spaniels had been popular for some time before. Mary, Queen of Scots was fond of them and one even accompanied her to her death.

Characteristics. The King Charles has a massive head with large dark eyes full of expression, a short snub muzzle and long, pendulous, well-feathered ears, set low and lying close to the cheeks. The body proportions should be those of a miniature spaniel. It is a quiet, friendly little dog.

Group. Toys.

Size. Small.

Coat. *Color:* Black and tan, white and chestnut, chestnut red, and tricolor. *Texture:* Long, silky and straight.

but is over-keen to fight with other dogs.

Group. Terriers.

Size. Medium.

Coat. *Color:* Shades of blue. *Texture:* Soft, silky, plentiful and wavy.

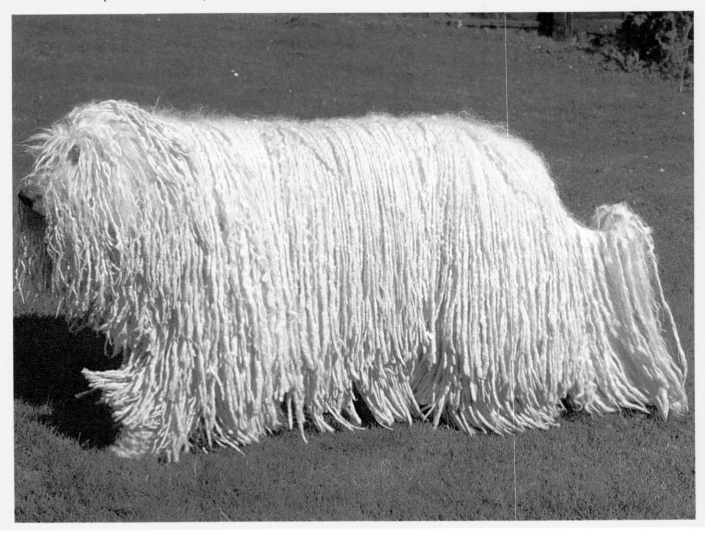

KOMONDOR

Origins. The herding breeds of Hungary and Russia form a loose family group; many are probably descended from the Aftschowka, an ancient breed from Eastern Europe. The Komondor probably has retained the closest resemblance to this breed which the Magyars have bred for more than a thousand years as guards to the flocks of sheep which graze the Puszta.

Characteristics. The Komondor is characterized by imposing strength and courageous demeanor. In general it is a big muscular dog with an unusual heavy white coat. The breed make excellent guards, being wary of strangers, earnest, courageous and loyal. The head is short and wide with a powerful muzzle, the ears are pendulous, the neck of moderate length and arched. The powerful deep chest is wide and muscular. Feet are strong and rather large with close arched toes.

Group. Working.

Size. Large and heavy: average 54.5 kg (120 lb).

Coat. *Color:* White. *Texture:* Dense, weather-resisting and very soft in the puppy, but growing into heavy tassel-like cords in the mature dog; these cords form naturally.

KUVASZ

Origins. The breed is said to have been introduced into Hungary in the twelfth century by the Kurds, its name being a corruption of the Turkish 'Kawasz', meaning 'the protector.' Originally it was used to protect farm stock from marauding wolves and bears, but was also used, though purely as a side line, as a hunting dog.

Characteristics. A strongly boned dog, big and powerfully built, the head is noble with an intelligent expression, the chest deep and powerful. Forelegs are straight and well boned, hindquarters powerful. The Kuvasz makes an affectionate pet but is suspicious of strangers, so it makes a good watchdog.

Group. Working.

Size. Large and heavy: 73.5 cm (29 in) and 50 kg (110 lb).

Coat. *Color:* Pure white. *Texture:* Long, straight or slightly wavy.

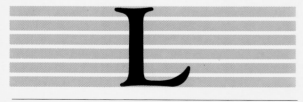

LABRADOR RETRIEVER

Origins. In 1822 reports of 'small water dogs . . . admirably trained as retrievers in fowling and are

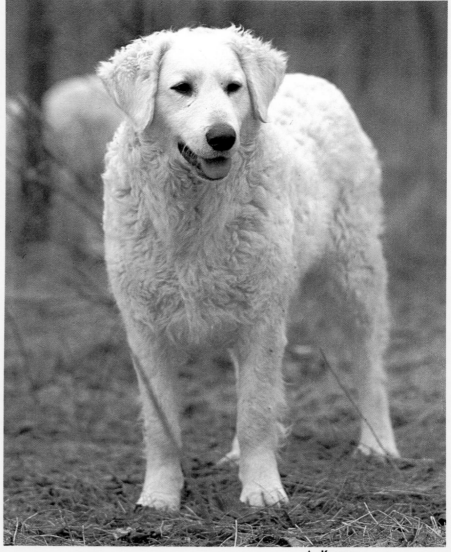

▲ **Kuvasz**

▼ **Labrador Retriever**

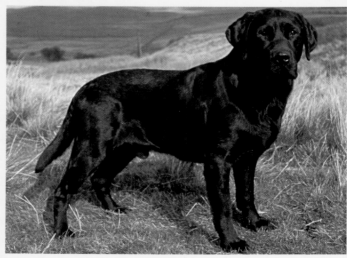

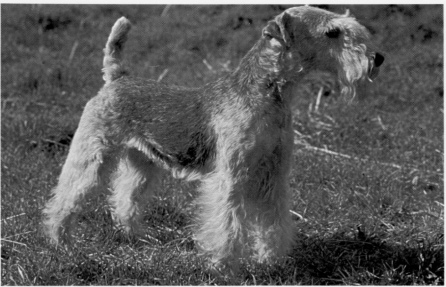

▲ **Lakeland Terrier**

▼ **Large Munsterlander**

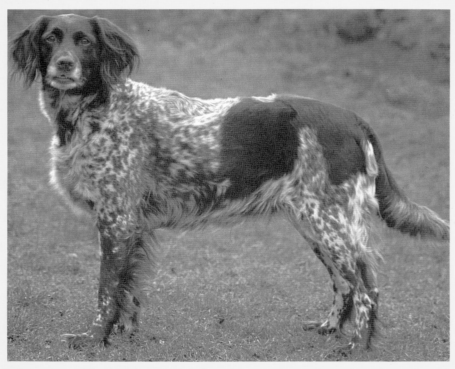

otherwise useful' indicated that there existed in Newfoundland a breed of gundog which British sportsmen were quick to recognize as being first class and imported into Britain. Today Labradors make excellent pets; they have a reliable temperament and get on well with children.

Characteristics. The general appearance is that of a strongly built, very active dog, with a broad skull, broad and deep through the chest and ribs, with powerful hindquarters. The tail is a distinctive feature of the breed and is very thick at the base gradually tapering towards the tip and giving that peculiar rounded appearance which has been described as the 'otter' tail.

Group. Sporting. Gundog (KC).

Size. Large.

Coat. *Color:* Generally black or yellow, sometimes chocolate. *Texture:* The coat is short and dense and without wave, with a weather-resistant undercoat, and should be fairly hard.

LAKELAND TERRIER

Origins. The Lakeland was developed as a working terrier with the packs of hounds which hunt the rugged country in England's Lake District. Nowadays the breed has split to produce two distinct types: those which are still used for work and a refined type seen at shows.

Characteristics. The breed has a smart, workmanlike appearance with a gay, fearless demeanor. The skull is flat and refined, the eyes dark and the ears moderately small, V-shaped, and carried alertly. The chest is narrow, the back strong and fairly short. The hindquarters are strong and muscular. The Lakeland Terrier is active, exuberant and fearless, but needs firm handling.

Group. Terriers.

Size. Small.

Coat. *Color:* Usually black and tan or red. *Texture:* Dense and weather-resisting, harsh with good undercoat.

LARGE MUNSTERLANDER

Origins. Known as a good working dog in Germany for centuries, this breed was originally classed as a German Longhaired Pointer.

Characteristics. The Munsterlander is a working gundog with sharp intelligence, vigor and fidelity, able to adapt quickly to any type of terrain or quarry. At home it is an excellent guard and a good-natured companion. The head is lean and distinguished, the nose brown, the muzzle is long. The eyes are dark, the ears light and pointed with good feathering. The neck is slightly arched and very muscular, the chest deep and broad. The tail is carried straight out.

Group. Gundog (KC).

Size. Large.

Coat. *Color:* Usually black and white. *Texture:* Smooth and slightly wavy.

LHASA APSO

Origins. In Tibet, the Lhaso Apso's homeland, the breed is known as Abso Seng Kye, the Bark Lion Sentinel Dog, a name which sums up its function. The Apso is one of four breeds now justly popular in the West which for very many years acted as guards within the precincts of the lamaseries in and around the sacred city of Lhasa.

Characteristics. The Apso is a solid dog with a gay and assertive character, yet chary of strangers. The head is narrow, with hair completely covering the face. The ears are pendant and heavily feathered. The tail is high-set and carried over the back. The Apso carries a considerable abundance of coat. It is an affectionate dog that needs plenty of company.

Group. Non-Sporting. Utility (KC).

Size. Small.

Coat. *Color:* Golden honey, also various other colors. *Texture:* Straight and hard, long and with dense undercoat.

LÖWCHEN

Origins. From the Middle Ages, dogs very like the modern breed of Löwchen appeared in paintings and Lion Dogs are described by Bewick. Whether the modern Löwchen is the same as these dogs is a matter for conjecture, since it seems unlikely that these dogs had to be clipped in order to produce their lionlike appearance.

Characteristics. A small intelligent dog with an affectionate and lively disposition combining all the good qualities of a companion dog. The body is clipped in the traditional lion clip.

Group. Toys (KC).

Size. Small.

Coat. *Color:* Various. *Texture:* Fairly long and wavy.

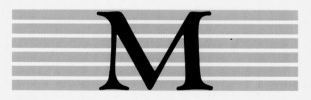

M

MALTESE

Origins. This breed has been known in the Mediterranean islands probably since the time of the Phoenicians. Certainly the breed existed very much in its present form since, at the time of the Apostle Paul, Publius, the Roman Governor of Malta, owned a Maltese.

Characteristics. The breed is sweet tempered and very intelligent, smart, lively and alert. The

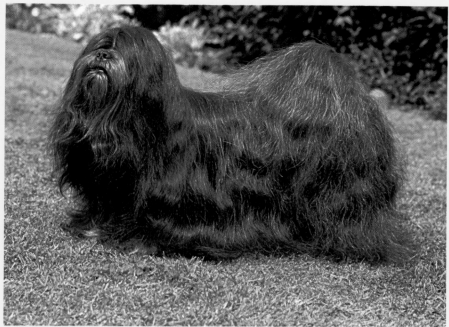

▲ **Lhasa Apso**

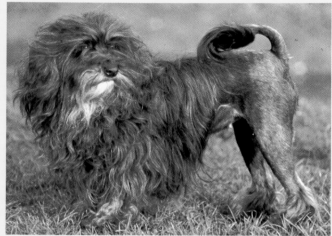

▲ **Löwchen**

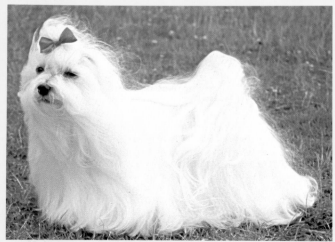

▲ **Maltese**

profuse white coat covers a well-made little dog with dark brown eyes and long pendant ears. The body is short and cobby and the tail is well arched over the back and feathered.

Group. Toys.
Size. Small.
Coat. *Color:* Pure white, sometimes with slight lemon markings. *Texture:* Straight and silky.

MANCHESTER TERRIER

Origins. Old prints show that a great many of the old terriers of different types were black and tan. The Manchester Terrier was developed for sport by the working people of Lancashire, people who looked to a day's ratting or rabbiting with their terriers to provide recreation. The Manchester Terrier makes an ideal house dog, being clean, and a good guard.

Characteristics. The dog is compact, with a long head, narrow in skull, with small, dark, sparkling eyes, and small V-shaped ears carried above the top line of the head. The neck is fairly long and the forelegs quite straight and set well under the short body. The tail is naturally short.

Group. Terriers.
Size. Small.
Coat. *Color:* Black with rich tan markings. *Texture:* Close, smooth, short and glossy; of a firm texture.

MAREMMA

Origins. The Maremma is a large, heavy-coated herding dog from Italy, very much in the pattern of other European herding breeds to which it is undoubtedly closely related. It was first imported and recognized in England in 1935.

Characteristics. The breed is large and strongly built, majestic in appearance, distinguished, robust and courageous. In general appearance the breed much resembles the Pyrenean Mountain Dog, with a strong build and large head.

Group. Working (KC).
Size. Large.
Coat. *Color:* Usually solid white. *Texture:* Very abundant, long and rather harsh with a soft undercoat.

MASTIFF

Origins. One of the ancient mastiff breeds of Europe with origins in the war dogs of Europe, which fought alongside their masters to repel the invasion of Britain by the Roman legions in 55 BC. The Romans recognized their great courage and imported them to Rome to take part in gladiatorial contests against bulls, bears, lions and tigers. The breed was so greatly admired that mastiff-like dogs, generally called 'dogues,' eventually were to give

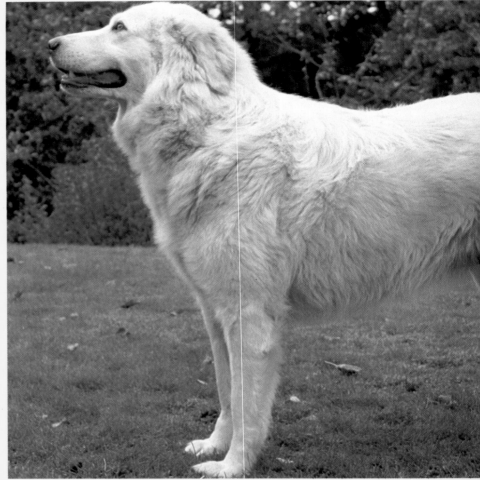

▲ **Maremma**

▼ **Manchester Terrier**

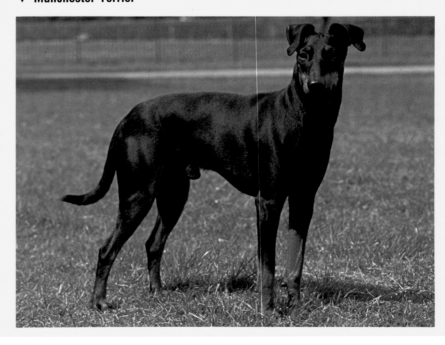

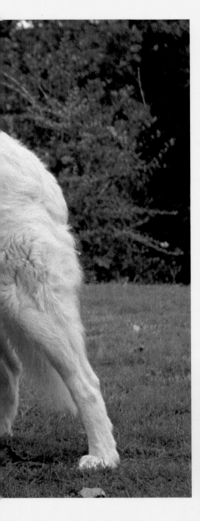

their particular name to all domestic dogs.

Characteristics. A massive and powerful dog, combining grandeur with good nature and courage with docility. The head is square in appearance, the muzzle short and broad. The eyes are small, dark, and set wide apart. The ears are small and thin, lying flat and close to the cheek. The neck is very muscular, set into heavy, slightly sloping shoulders. The forelegs are heavily boned, straight and strong, the hindquarters broad, wide and muscular.

Group. Working. Non-Sporting (ANKC).
Size. Large: 76 cm (30 in) upwards.
Coat. *Color:* Apricot or silver, fawn or dark fawn, brindle with black on the muzzle, ears and nose and between the eyes. *Texture:* Short and close-lying.

MINIATURE PINSCHER

Origins. Contrary to popular misconception the Miniature Pinscher is not a small Doberman; its original name 'Reh Pinscher' referred to the breed's resemblance to small forest deer. It has existed for several centuries in Germany and Scandinavia, where it is valued as a very alert watchdog.

Characteristics. The Miniature Pinscher is structurally a sturdy, compact toy dog, naturally well groomed, proud, vigorous and alert. Its natural high-stepping gait, complete self-possession and its spirited presence differentiate the breed from other toy dogs. The head is narrow, the ears upstanding, cropped in countries where the operation is still allowed. The body is compact and muscular, the tail set high and docked short.

Group. Toys.
Size. Small.
Coat. *Color:* Red or black with tan markings, solid brown or chocolate. *Texture:* Smooth, hard and short, straight and lustrous.

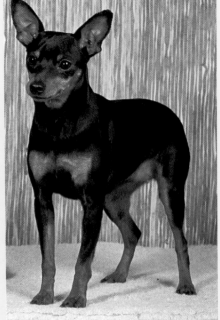

▲ **Miniature Pinscher**

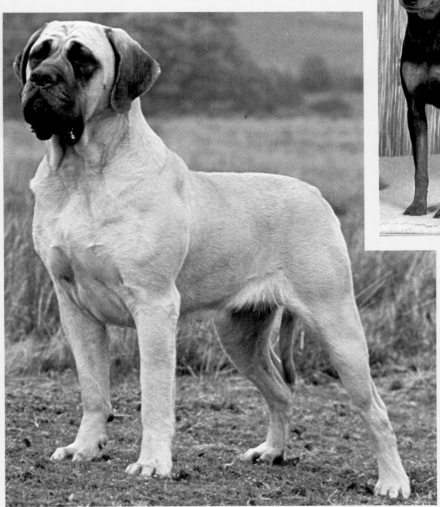

◄ **Mastiff**

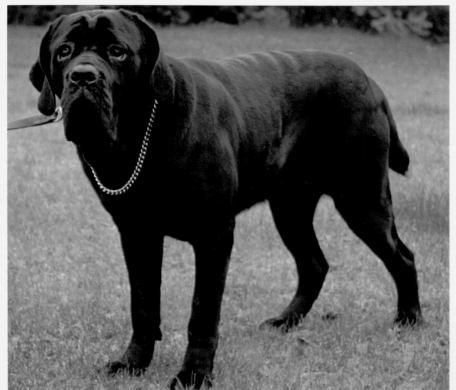

▲ **Neapolitan Mastiff**

N

NEAPOLITAN MASTIFF

Origins. Many of the European Mastiff breeds are of ancient origin and the Neapolitan Mastiff is no exception for, although it made its appearance in the show ring only after World War II, it is descended from the Roman fighting dogs.

Characteristics. The Neapolitan Mastiff is a first-rate guard dog but can make a docile and friendly pet. Its head is massive, its body deep and powerful. Its eyes are dark, its nostrils wide and its nose broad.

Group. Working (KC).

Size. Large.

Coat. *Color:* Black, or lead or mouse gray. *Texture:* Dense and smooth.

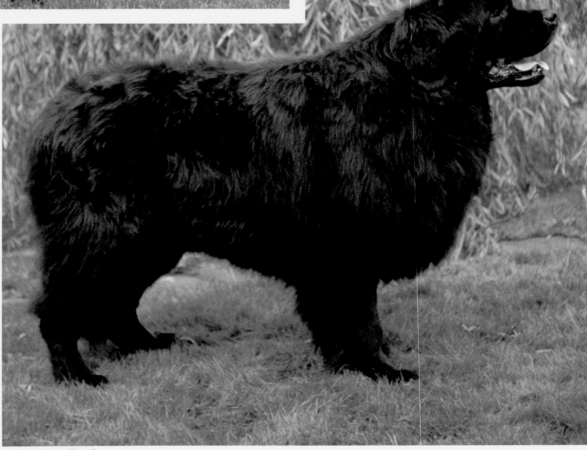

▲ **Newfoundland**

NEWFOUNDLAND

Origins. The Newfoundland breed was primarily developed not, as is often suggested, as a canine lifeguard, but as a draught dog, big and strong enough to pull carts or carry heavy loads. However, its affinity with the fishermen of Newfoundland made it a superb water dog. Early prints suggest that the breed has its origins among the Huskies of northern Canada.

Characteristics. The Newfoundland has an exceptionally gentle and docile nature and should be strong and active. The head is broad and massive, the eyes small and dark, the ears small, set well back and falling close to the head. The chest is deep and fairly broad, the forelegs are straight and well feathered, the hindquarters very strong. It becomes devoted to its owner.

Group. Working. Non-Sporting (ANKC).

Size. Large and heavy: average 59 kg (130 lb).

Coat. *Color:* Dull jet black, black with white markings, and solid bronze. *Texture:* Flat and dense, with a fairly coarse texture and oily nature, and water-resistant.

NORFOLK TERRIER

Origins. One of the smallest of the terriers, but one which retains all its sporting instincts. Until 1964, the breed could have either drop or prick ears, but at that time the two types were separated and the prick-eared variety became Norwich Terriers. (Both types are known as Norwich Terriers in the USA.)

Characteristics. The Norfolk Terrier has a lovable disposition, is not quarrelsome, has a hardy constitution and is alert and fearless. It is a small, low, keen dog, compact and strong with a short back. The skull is wide and slightly rounded, the muzzle wedge-shaped and strong, the eyes oval, deep set and dark, giving an alert, keen and intelligent expression. The ears are V-shaped and drop forward, close to the cheek. The tail is docked.

Group. Terriers.

Size. Small.

Coat. *Color:* Usually red. *Texture:* Hard, wiry and straight, lying close to the body.

NORWEGIAN BUHUND

Origins. A typical Spitz breed, used as a general farm dog and guard. The breed formed the basis for the Icelandic Dog which was bred from stock taken to Iceland in AD 874. The ancient origin of the breed is thus established.

Characteristics. The breed is fearless, brave and

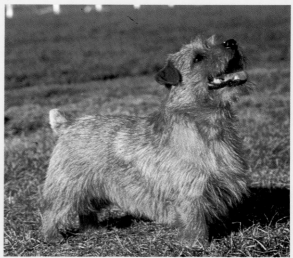

▲ **Norfolk Terrier**

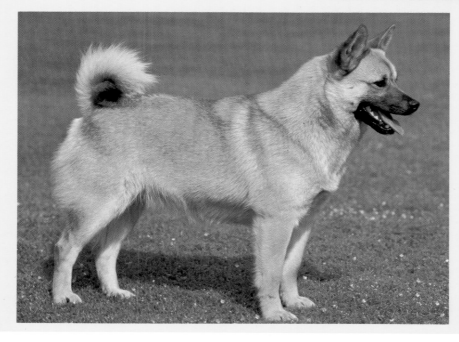

◄ **Norwegian Buhund**

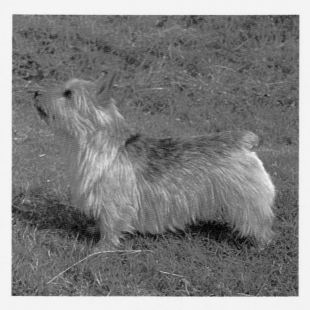

▶ **Norwich Terrier**

energetic, of medium size, lightly built with a short compact body. It is adaptable and makes a good watchdog.

Group. Working (KC).

Size. Medium.

Coat. *Color:* Biscuit, ripe wheat, light red, sable, black. *Texture:* Close and harsh with soft undercoat.

NORWICH TERRIER

Origins. The breed dates from the early years of the century when it was known as the Jones Terrier and shares its short history up to 1964 with the Norfolk Terrier.

Characteristics. Similar to those of the Norfolk Terrier, except for its pricked ears.

Group. Terrier.

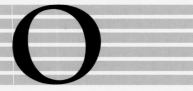

OLD ENGLISH SHEEPDOG

Origins. The breed was probably developed, if it did not originate, in western England. The Old English Sheepdog was a drover's dog used for driving sheep and cattle to market. Drover's dogs were exempt from taxes if they were docked, hence the tailless outline of the Old English Sheepdog; hence also its popular nickname of 'Bobtail.'

Characteristics. A strong compact-looking dog, profusely coated all over, very elastic in a gallop, but

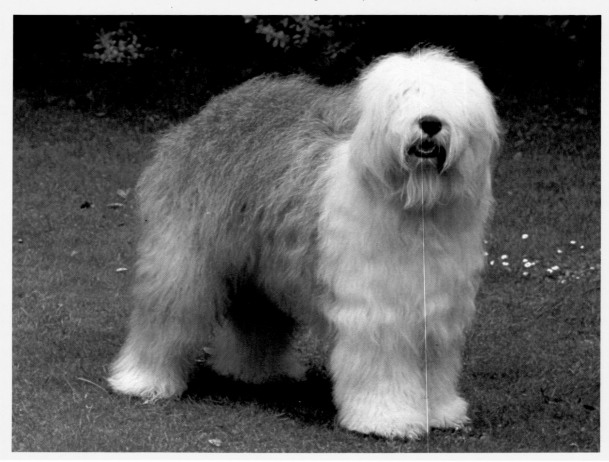

▶ **Old English Sheepdog**

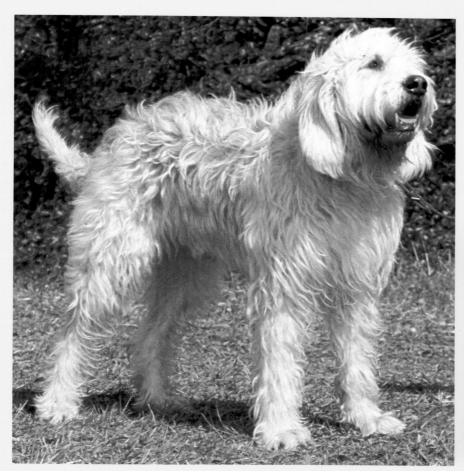

◀ Otter Hound

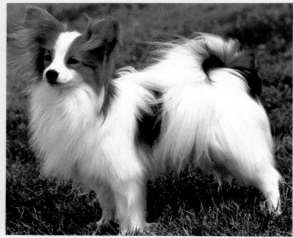

▲ Papillon

when walking or trotting has a characteristic ambling movement. The bark is loud with a 'bell-like' ring to it. The head is large and rather squarely formed, the jaw fairly long and strong; the ears are small and carried close to the head. The body is short and very compact. The tail in puppies born with tails is docked short. The 'Bobtail' has a good temperament and gets on very well with children and other pets.

Group. Herding. Working (KC).

Size. Large.

Coat. *Color:* Any shade of gray, with or without white markings. *Texture:* Profuse and of good hard texture, shaggy and free from curl.

OTTER HOUND

Origins. Although otter hunting in England dates back to the early twelfth century, it was not until the reign of Edward II (1307–27) that a description of hounds which fits the modern breed was set down. Otter Hounds have been shown in the USA since 1907; in England only since 1977.

Characteristics. The Otter Hound is a large, rough-coated, squarely built hound, with an exceptionally good nose and deep musical voice. The head is large and narrow, the chest deep, the legs are heavy-boned. The feet are large, broad, compact and webbed. Movement is smooth and effortless, with the feet only just coming off the ground, and the dog has great strength and stamina. The Otter Hound is basically a pack animal, rather than a pet, but is friendly and good with children.

Group. Hounds.

Size. Large.

Coat. *Color:* Various. *Texture:* The rough outer coat is hard and 7.6–15 cm (3–6 in) long; the weather-resistant inner coat is short and woolly.

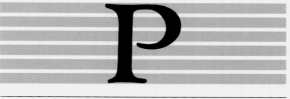

PAPILLON

Origins. Arguably Papillons or their Miniature Spaniel progenitors appear in more paintings by artists, such as Rubens, Watteau, Boucher and Fragonard, than any other breed of dog. As companions to the ladies of the courts of Europe, these elegant little creatures led a noble existence.

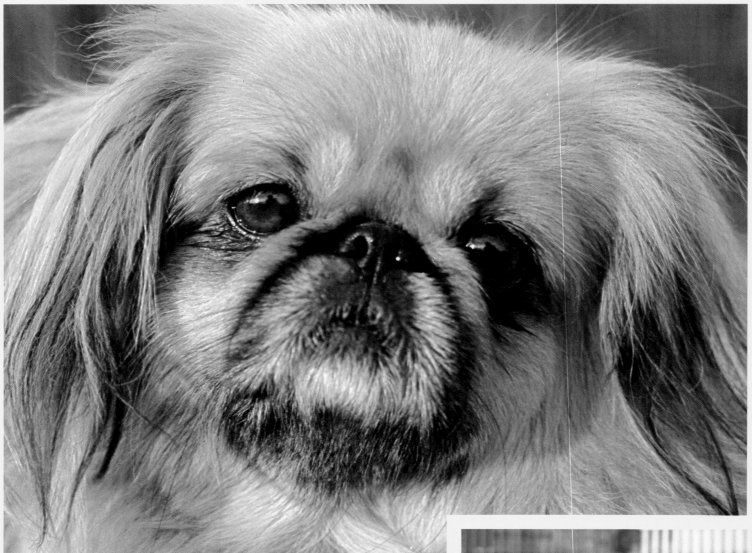

▲ **Pekingese**

Today they have lost none of their elegance or their great charm and vivacity. They have also to a large degree retained much of the toughness inherited from gundog ancestors.

Characteristics. A dainty, balanced toy dog with an attractive, slightly rounded head with finely pointed muzzle and round, dark eyes showing an alert, lively expression. The bearing is alert, movement sound, light and free. The ears are large, rounded at the tips, heavily fringed and carried like the spread wings of a butterfly, hence the name Papillon. It is very affectionate towards its owners and can become possessive.

Group. Toys.

Size. Small.

Coat. *Color:* White with colored patches. *Texture:* Abundant and flowing, long, fine and silky, with a profuse frill on the chest.

PEKINGESE

Origins. In ancient times the Pekingese was the sacred dog of China. Certainly during the Tang Dynasty in the eighth century these dogs were already highly prized, carefully bred and jealously guarded. Their introduction into the West came after the Imperial Palace in Peking had been looted, part of this loot was a fawn and white Pekingese which was given to Queen Victoria.

Characteristics. This is a well-balanced, thick-set dog with great dignity, a fearless carriage and an alert, intelligent expression. The head is massive, the skull broad, wide and flat between the ears and eyes. The nose is very short and broad, well wrinkled with a firm underjaw, giving a flat profile. The eyes are large, clear, dark and lustrous, the ears heart-shaped and carried close to the head, with long profuse feathering. The body is short with a broad chest, the forelegs are short, thick and bowed. The Pekingese is a determined, independent little dog.

Group. Toys.

Size. Small; heavy for its size.

Coat. *Color:* Various. *Texture:* Long and straight with a profuse mane forming a frill around the neck, and profuse feathering on ears, legs, thighs, toes and tail, which is carried over the back. The top coat is rather coarse with a thick undercoat.

PHARAOH HOUND

Origins. This dog originated in Egypt and North Africa. The Pharaoh Hound or Balearic Greyhound was much admired by Phoenician traders who introduced the breed throughout the Mediterranean countries.

Characteristics. Much the same in type as the Greyhound, but distinguished from it by its triangular head and large erect ears, unique among gaze hounds. The eyes are quite small and deep set, amber or light brown, the neck slender. The ears are large and erect. The Pharoah is a fast, agile and playful dog.

Group. Hounds.

Size. Large.

Coat. *Color:* White with chestnut or rich tan or yellow tan markings. *Texture:* Short, fine and glossy, with a soft skin.

◀ **Pharaoh Hound**

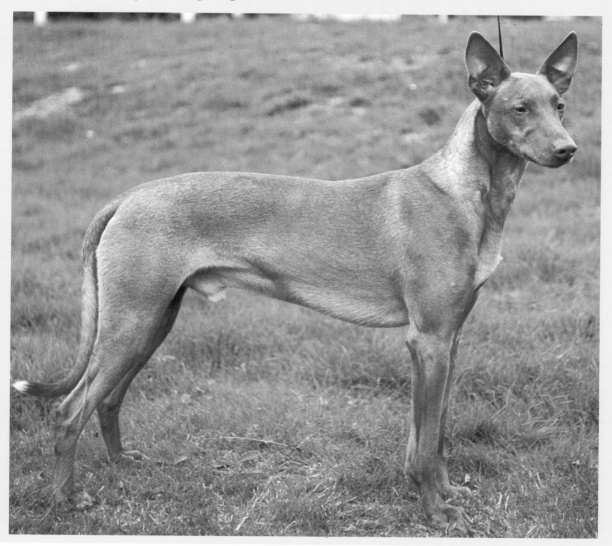

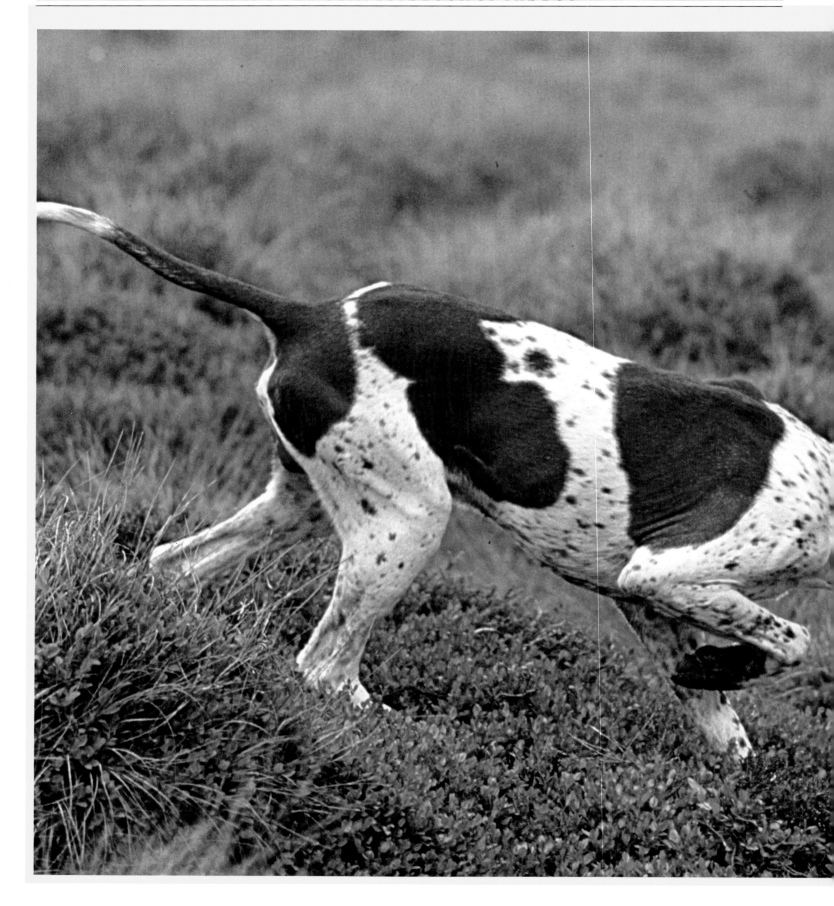

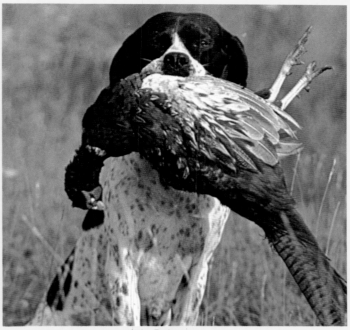

◄ ▲ **Pointer**

POINTER

Origins. Pointers have been used in Britain since the mid-seventeenth century to indicate by pointing just where game was hidden. Early in the eighteenth century, when guns came into use, the Pointer began to function as a gundog. The breed's distinctive appearance owes something to the Foxhound and something to the Greyhound; other ancestors include the Bloodhound and, of course, the 'setting' spaniel.

Characteristics. The Pointer is bred for work in the field and gives an impression of compact power and agile grace allied to intelligence and alertness. The head is aristocratic with an unusual dish-shaped muzzle, the ears pendulous, the eyes rounded and dark. The neck is long, clean, muscular, and slightly arched, the shoulders long and sloping. Forelegs are straight, hindquarters muscular and powerful with great propelling leverage. The gait is smooth and powerful with the head carried high. The Pointer makes an obedient and devoted pet.

Group. Sporting. Gundog (KC).
Size. Large.
Coat. *Color:* Liver, lemon, black, orange; either a solid color or with white. *Texture:* Short, dense, smooth with a sheen.

POMERANIAN

Origins. Originally sled dogs from Iceland and Lapland, the Pomeranian is possibly the smallest of the Spitz breeds, but one which retains all the courage and character of its larger cousins. During the last century the Pomeranian has been reduced in size and it is no longer used to herd sheep, but it remains an alert housedog, capable of giving warning of intruders with a surprisingly deep bark.

Characteristics. The Pomeranian is a compact dog with a head foxlike in shape and expression, eyes bright and dark in color, ears small and erect.

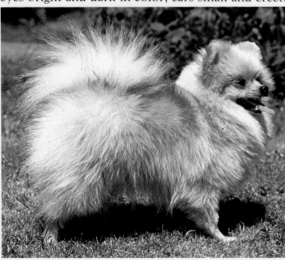

► **Pomeranian**

▶ Standard Poodle, unclipped

▼ Standard Poodle, with lion clip

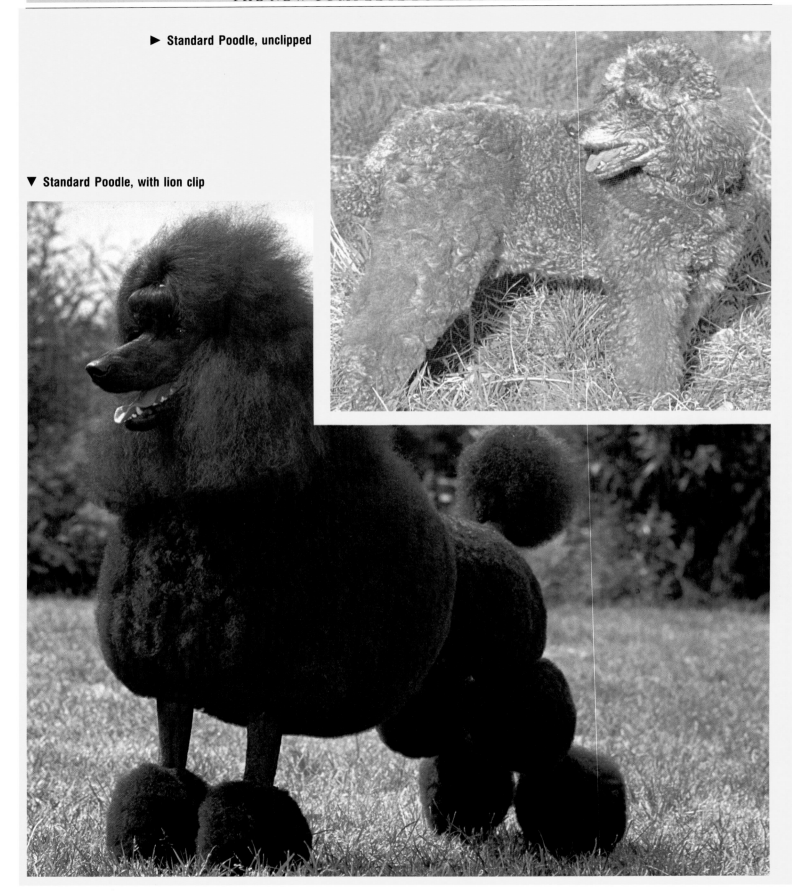

The neck is rather short, a shortness which is accentuated by the characteristic Spitz ruff. The tail is curled back over the body, nearly reaching the head.

Group. Toys.

Size. Small.

Coat. *Color:* Usually orange. *Texture:* Double-coated: a short, soft thick undercoat with a longer, coarse, harsh-textured outer coat.

POODLE

Origins. Originating in France, the poodle was used as a gundog over a wide area, including France, Germany and Russia. Its adaptability, intelligence and unusual appearance soon led to its use for a wide variety of purposes, as well as in the production of other gundog breeds.

Characteristics. A very active and elegant dog, carrying itself proudly. The head is long and fine with almond-shaped eyes, the chest deep and moderately wide, the back is short and strong. The tail is docked. The Miniature and Toy versions have overtaken the Standard Poodle in popularity.

Group. Non-Sporting. Miniature version: Toys. Utility (KC).

Size. Medium (Standard) or Small (Miniature and Toy).

Coat. *Color:* All solid colors, clear colors preferred. *Texture:* Very profuse and dense and of harsh texture. The coat has the advantage that it does not shed like most other breeds and lacks the distinctive and sometimes objectionable doggy smell. The distinctive appearance is achieved by careful and laborious clipping and grooming.

PUG

Origins. The Pug is another of the toy breeds with roots in ancient China, where it has flourished for the past 2000 years. Although very much a toy dog,

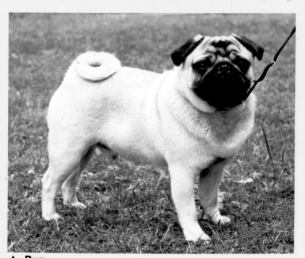

▲ **Pug**

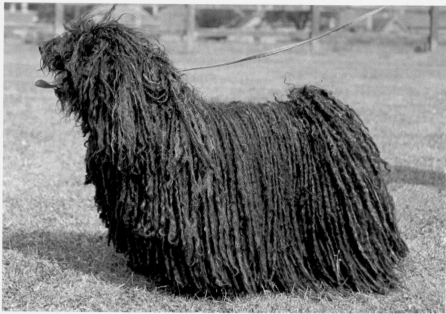

▲ **Puli**

the Pug has all the characteristics of some of the Eastern mastiff breeds which it so closely resembles.

Characteristics. The Pug is a square and cobby little dog, giving an impression of considerable substance packed into small size. The head is round, massive, and deeply wrinkled. The muzzle short and blunt, the eyes very large, bold and dark. The body is short and wide in the chest. The forelegs are strong and straight, the hindquarters muscular. The tail is curled tightly. Pugs are affectionate dogs with charming dispositions.

Group. Toys.

Size. Small.

Coat. *Color:* Usually black or fawn with a black mask and black ears. *Texture:* Fine, smooth, soft, short and glossy.

PULI

Origins. This breed is a working partner of the Komondor and the Kuvasz and shares the same origins among the herding dogs which invading Magyars brought into Hungary. The Puli was used to herd and drive sheep.

Characteristics. A vigorous, alert and extremely active breed. By nature Pulis are affectionate and loyal, but being excellent guards are suspicious of strangers. The construction of the Puli is not exaggerated in any way, the head is of medium size, the neck strong and muscular. The chest is deep and fairly broad and the body of medium length, straight and level. The tail is never docked and is carried over the back.

Group. Herding. Working (KC).

Size. Medium.

Coat. *Color:* Usually rusty black. *Texture:* The coat hangs in tight, even cords.

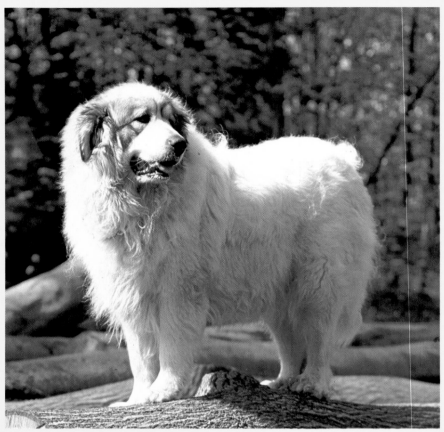

▲ Pyrenean Mountain Dog

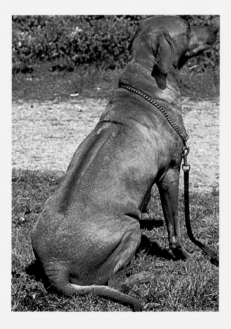

▲ Rhodesian Ridgeback

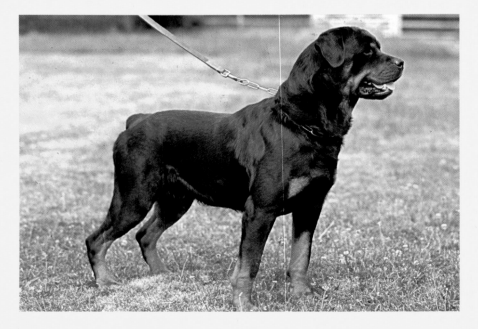

▲ Rottweiler

PYRENEAN MOUNTAIN DOG (GREAT PYRENEES)

Origins. This dog is a descendant of the South European herding and guard breeds, originating in the mountains on the borders of France and Spain. It was the guard dog of the region.

Characteristics. The dog is serious in play and at work, gentle and docile to the point of self-sacrifice. A dog of great majesty, keen intelligence and kindly expression. The head is large, the neck short and muscular. The dog's protective instincts need careful training.

Group. Working. Non-Sporting (ANKC).

Size. Large and heavy: 71 cm (28 in) upwards, 54.5 kg (120 lb).

Coat. *Color:* All white or principally white, with markings of badger, gray or shades of tan. *Texture:* Fine undercoat and thick overcoat of coarser hair.

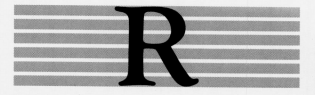

RHODESIAN RIDGEBACK

Origins. The European farmers, who in the sixteenth and seventeenth centuries settled in South Africa, developed a hound suitable for the conditions and game encountered in South Africa, and which was also willing to act as a guard. They did this by crossing their dogs with a native hunting dog which had a ridge on its back. The dog had to be tough to withstand hard work in extremes of temperature, sufficiently versatile to either retrieve a partridge or put down a wounded buck, had to be easily kept and fit well into the family. The breed, which was developed by the Boer farmers, was introduced into Rhodesia in 1877.

Characteristics. The peculiarity of the breed is the ridge on the back formed by hair growing against the nap of the rest of the coat. The Ridgeback is a strong, muscular and active dog. The head is of fair length, flat and broad between the ears. The eyes are bright and colored to harmonize with the color of the dog. The chest is deep and capacious, the back powerful. The tail is carried with a slight upward curve.

Group. Hounds.

Size. Large.

Coat. *Color:* Light wheaten to red wheaten, with a little white on the chest and toes. *Texture:* Short and dense with a sleek, glossy appearance.

ROTTWEILER

Origins. Yet another of the European mastiff breeds which probably have their origins among the dogs which guarded and helped drive the herds of cattle which accompanied the Roman armies. The breed's courage, strength and forbidding aspect make it a marvelous guard for those able to control it. Good training is essential.

Characteristics. The Rottweiler is a compact dog, well proportioned and powerfully built to permit great strength, maneuverability and endurance. The bearing displays boldness and courage. The head is distinctive, broad, of medium length, with well-muscled cheeks and moderately wrinkled. The neck is strong, round and very muscular, set into long and sloping shoulders. The body is broad and deep, the back straight and strong.

Group. Working. Non-Sporting (ANKC).

Size. Large.

Coat. *Color:* Black with clearly defined tan markings on cheeks, muzzle, chest and legs, as well as over the eyes and under the tail. *Texture:* Coarse and flat, with a medium-length topcoat.

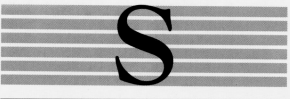

ST BERNARD

Origins. The St Bernard's ancestors were probably brought to Switzerland by invading Roman armies. These dogs were crossed with native dogs to produce the Talhund and Bauernhund which, by the eleventh century, were in common use on Swiss

▼ **St Bernard**

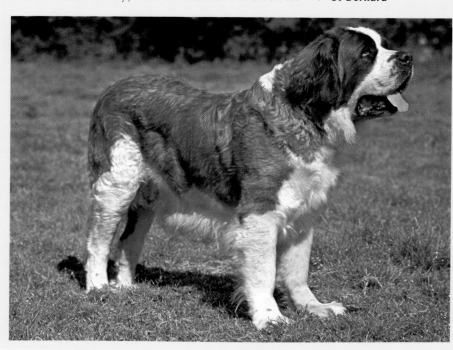

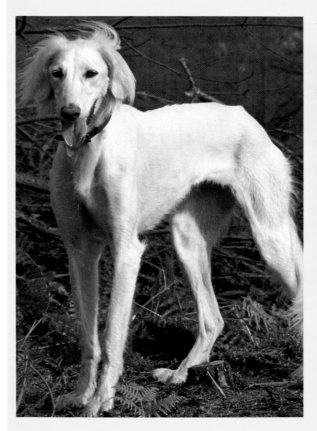

◀ **Saluki**

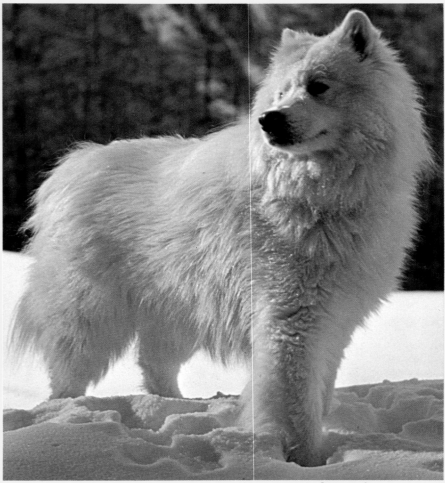

▲ **Samoyed**

farms. In the seventeenth century they became known for their rescue work in the Alps.

Characteristics. The head of the St Bernard is massive and round with an expression of benevolence, dignity and intelligence. The neck is long, thick and muscular, and slightly arched. Forelegs are perfectly straight, shoulders are broad and sloping. The back is broad and straight, the chest wide and deep. Hindquarters should be heavy in bone with well-bent hocks. As a pet, this huge dog is gentle, docile and easily trained.

Group. Working. Non-Sporting (ANKC).

Size. Large.

Coat. *Color:* Orange, mahogany-brindle, red-brindle, white with patches on body of these colors. *Texture:* Long, dense and flat; there is a smooth-haired variety.

SALUKI

Origins. The breed existed when Alexander the Great invaded India, four centuries before the birth of Christ, and carvings on Sumerian and Egyptian tombs dating from 7000 BC are recognizable as Salukis.

Characteristics. The appearance of the breed is one of grace together with speed and endurance. The head is long and narrow, the eyes dark to hazel and bright. The ears are long and mobile and covered with long silky hair. The neck, too, is long,

supple and well muscled, set into sloping shoulders. The chest is deep and moderately narrow, the back is muscular and slightly arched. The tail is long, low set and carried in a graceful curve, well feathered with long silky hair. The Saluki has an independent and sensitive nature.

Group. Hounds.

Size. Large.

Coat. *Color:* White, cream, fawn, golden red and other colors. *Texture:* Smooth and silky, with elegant silky feathering on ears, legs and tail, except in the breed's smooth variety.

SAMOYED

Origins. Just as the Saluki may lay claim to being the oldest of the Mediterranean sight hounds, so the Samoyed may claim to be the oldest of the northern Spitz breeds. Originally bred as a guard for herds of reindeer, the breed also acted as companion, guard and sledge dog, in which capacity it accompanied polar expeditions. The breed's strength, stamina and hardiness are belied by its childlike good nature and fairy-tale and soft appearance.

Characteristics. The Samoyed is intelligent, alert and full of action. The breed should be strong, active and graceful, with a muscular back of medium length allowing liberty of movement. The head is powerful and wedge-shaped, the eyes almond-shaped with an intelligent expression. The ears are erect and thick, covered inside with hair. The tail is long and profusely coated, carried over the back when alert.

Group. Working. Non-Sporting. (ANKC).

Size. Large.

Coat. *Color:* Pure white, white and biscuit, cream. *Texture:* A thick, close, soft and short undercoat, covered with an outer coat of straight harsh hair, which grows straight away from the body providing protection against extreme cold.

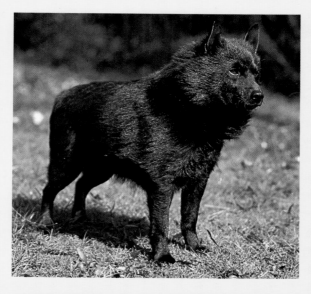

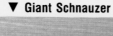
◀ **Schipperke**

SCHIPPERKE

Origins. The Schipperke is descended from the same herding dogs which produced the Belgian Shepherd Dog (Groenendael), the latter remaining as herders and Schipperkes becoming smaller watchdogs. It was not until 1888 that their name was changed to Schipperke, which in Flemish means 'little captain,' a reference as much to the breed's air of self-importance as to their association with the barges of the Flemish canals.

Characteristics. The general appearance is of a small, cobby animal with a sharp expression, intensely lively and alert. The head is distinctly foxy with small, rather oval, dark brown eyes and sharply pointed, stiffly erect ears. The neck is strong and rather short, the shoulders muscular and sloping. The rump is tailless and rounded; the feet small and catlike. Apart from making a useful watchdog, the Schipperke is a perky, affectionate pet.

Group. Non-Sporting. Utility (KC).

Size. Small/Medium.

Coat. *Color:* Black. *Texture:* Abundant, dense and harsh, smooth on the head, ears and legs, but erect and thick around the neck, forming a mane and frill, and with a good culotte on the back of the thighs.

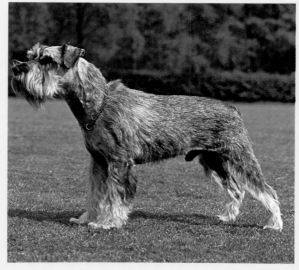
◀ **Standard Schnauzer**

SCHNAUZER

Origins. The Standard Schnauzer may be regarded as the forerunner of the three Schnauzer breeds: Miniature, Standard and Giant. The Schnauzer is a German breed with a long history dating back to the fifteenth and sixteenth centuries. It has been used in its various sizes as a vermin killer, a yard dog and a most effective guard.

Characteristics. The Schnauzer is a robust, sinewy, nearly square dog with a temperament that combines high spirits, reliability, strength, endurance and vigor. The head is strong, the eyes dark and

▼ **Giant Schnauzer**

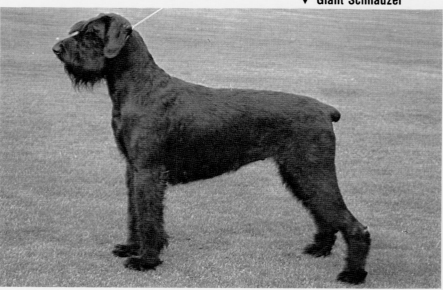

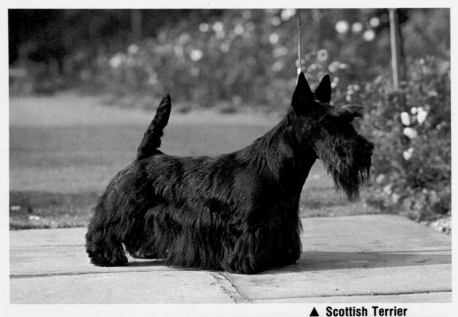

▲ **Scottish Terrier**

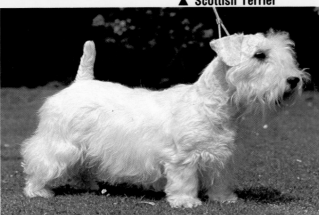

▲ **Sealyham Terrier**

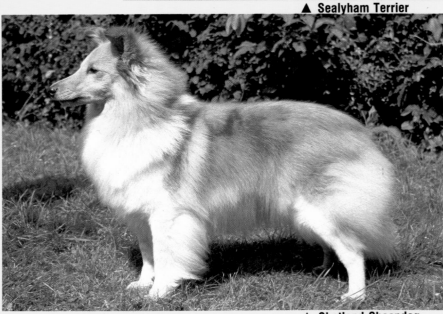

▲ **Shetland Sheepdog**

oval, the ears V-shaped, neat and dropping forward or cropped in countries where the operation is permitted. The tail is carried high and docked to three joints. The Schnauzers are loyal, stubborn and responsive to training.

Group. Working. Miniature Schnauzer: Terriers. Utility (KC). Non-Sporting (ANKC).

Size. Large (Giant Schnauzer) Medium (Standard Schnauzer) and Small (Miniature Schnauzer).

Coat. *Color:* Pure black or pepper and salt. *Texture:* Hard and wiry, with a good undercoat.

SCOTTISH TERRIER

Origins. It is difficult to be precise about the history of the Scottish Terrier because the name has long and variously been used to describe any one of several terrier breeds which originate in Scotland. Certainly the terriers of Scotland have a long history dating back to the fourteenth century. Rawdon Lee writing at the end of the nineteenth century claimed that the Scottish Terrier was the original Skye Terrier.

Characteristics. The Scottish Terrier is a sturdy thick-set dog set on short legs, alert in carriage. The head gives the impression of being long for the size of dog, the almond-shaped eyes are dark brown, the ears neat, pointed and erect. The muscular neck is of moderate length set into long sloping shoulders. The back is short and very muscular, the hindquarters are remarkably powerful with big and wide buttocks. This dog is a stubborn individualist.

Group. Terriers.

Size. Small.

Coat. *Color:* Black, wheaten or brindle of any color. *Texture:* The undercoat is short, dense and soft, the outer coat harsh, dense and wiry.

SEALYHAM TERRIER

Origins. This is one of the very few breeds which owe their development to the work and inspiration of one man. Between 1850 and 1891 Captain John Edwardes of Sealyham in Haverfordwest, Wales, set out to develop a strain of terrier which would be able to hunt fox, otter or even badger. By 1910 the breed was appearing in the show ring.

Characteristics. The general appearance should be of a free-moving sturdy little dog. The eyes are dark and round, and the ears falling at the side of the cheeks are rounded. The neck is fairly long, thick and muscular, the forelegs short, strong and straight. The body is of medium length, the hindquarters are powerful, and the tail is carried erect. The Sealyham can be devoted to its owner but has an obstinate streak.

Group. Terriers.

Size. Small.

Coat. *Color:* Usually white. *Texture:* Long, hard and wiry.

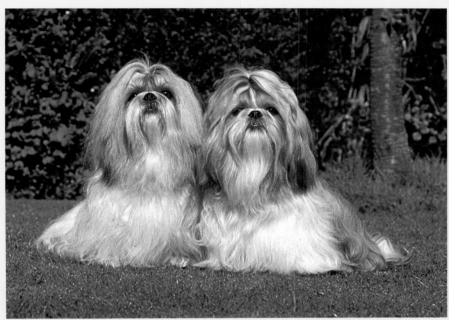

▲ **Shih Tzu**

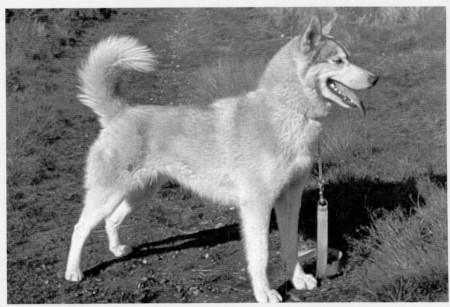

▲ **Siberian Husky**

refined, a long blunt wedge tapering from ear to nose; the eyes dark brown and almond-shaped. The ears are small and carried semi-erect with the tips dropping forward. The neck is muscular, the chest is deep, the hindquarters broad.

Group. Herding. Working (KC).

Size. Small.

Coat. *Color:* Tricolor, sable, silvery blue-gray, black and white or black and tan. *Texture:* The outer coat is long, harsh and straight, the undercoat short and close. The mane and frill should be abundant.

SHIH TZU

Origins. Records dating from AD 624 show that dogs were given as tribute to the Tang Emperor by K'iu T'ai; paintings and carvings show these dogs and others offered in later tributes to have been very like the modern Shih Tzu. Whether these dogs originated in Tibet or in some part of the Byzantine Empire is not known, but the centuries of careful breeding which the Chinese have devoted to the breed must be regarded as sufficient to regard the breed as Chinese.

Characteristics. The Shih Tzu is a very active, lively and alert dog with a distinctly arrogant carriage. The head is broad and round, wide between the eyes with a short square muzzle. The eyes are large, dark and round and the ears are pendulous. The tail is heavily plumed and carried well over the back. The Shih Tzu makes a busily important housedog, friendly and affectionate.

Group. Toys. Utility (KC). Non-Sporting (ANKC).

Size. Small.

Coat. *Color:* Various. *Texture:* Long and dense but not curly, with a good undercoat.

SIBERIAN HUSKY

Origins. This is a breed forged in the hardest imaginable environment among the Chukchi people who inhabited the frozen wastelands of north-eastern Asia. The Chukchi were nomadic hunters who depended for their survival on the strength, speed, courage, intelligence and toughness of the breed they had developed by rigorous selection.

Characteristics. The general appearance is of a medium-sized working dog, quick and light on its feet and graceful in action. The moderately compact and well-furred body, erect ears and brash tail suggest its northern heritage. Its characteristic gait is smooth and seemingly effortless. The dog adapts well as a pet and companion.

Group. Working. Non-Sporting (ANKC).

Size. Large.

Coat. *Color:* All colors, from black to pure white. *Texture:* Double, of medium length; the undercoat dense and soft, the overcoat straight and smooth-lying.

SHETLAND SHEEPDOG

Origins. The Shetland Sheepdog is a distinctive breed produced in response to the peculiar demands made by the hard climate and terrain of the isolated northerly islands of Scotland. The breed is undoubtably of ancient origin but, due to lack of records, we know little of its history before it achieved the distinction of being recognized as a breed by the Kennel Club in 1914.

Characteristics. The Shetland is a dog of great beauty, intelligence and alertness. It should be affectionate and responsive towards its owner, but may be reserved towards strangers. The head is

SKYE TERRIER

Origins. Some authorities argue that the Skye Terrier and the present Scottish Terrier share common origins and that the modern Skye, with its extraordinary appearance, is a fairly recent development.

Characteristics. The Skye Terrier is a one man

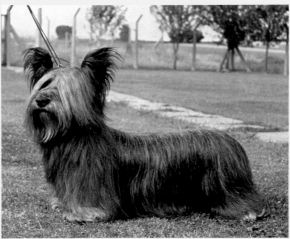

▶ **Skye Terrier**

dog, distrustful of strangers, but not vicious. The head is long with powerful jaws, the dark eyes are close set and full of expression. Ears may be prick or drop and should be fringed with hair. The neck is long and slightly crested, the shoulders are broad, the chest deep and the forelegs short and muscular. The body is long and low to the ground, the hindquarters well developed and muscular.

Group. Terriers.
Size. Small.
Coat. *Color:* Dark or light gray, fawn, cream, black, all with black points. *Texture:* A soft, short, woolly, close undercoat is hidden by the long, hard, straight, flat topcoat which is such a characteristic feature of the breed.

SLOUGHI

Origins. Although the Arab races are not particularly fond of dogs, they treat the Sloughi as if it were one of the family. The nomadic tribes of North Africa value the Sloughi as a hunter and as a guard. Much of their hunting takes place at night to avoid the heat of the sun and when the quarry is active. As a consequence of this the breed has itself a tendency to be nocturnal in its habits.

▼ **Sloughi**

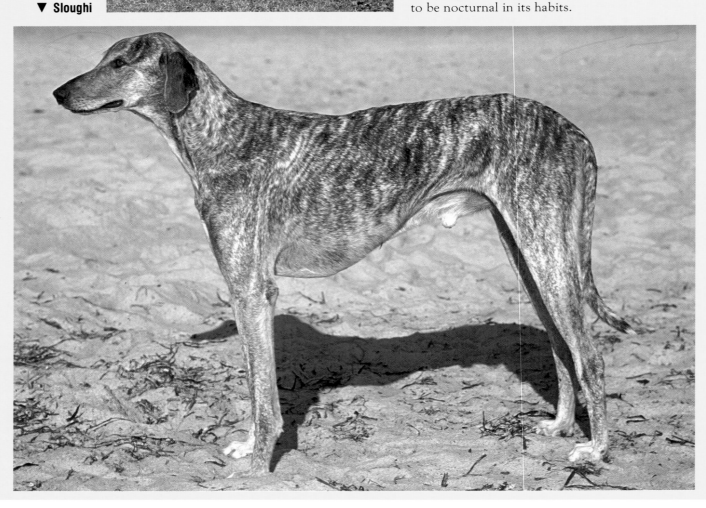

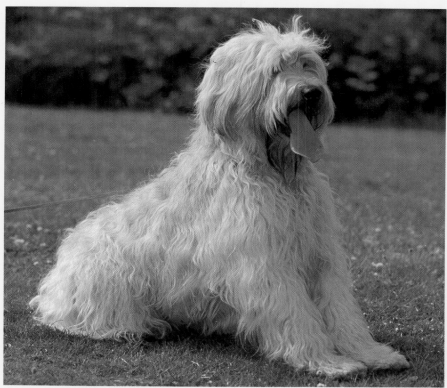

▲ **Soft-coated Wheaten Terrier**

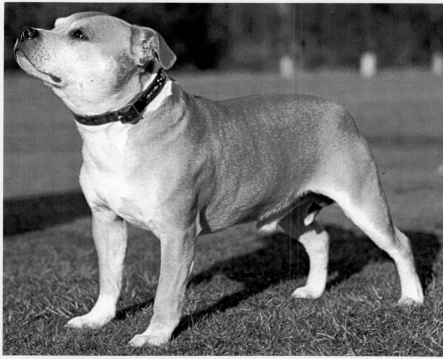

▲ **Staffordshire Bull Terrier**

Characteristics. The general appearance of the Sloughi is of a very racy dog, with a frame impressive for its muscular leanness and delicacy. In outline the breed closely resembles a racing Greyhound. This dog makes a good reliable pet.

Group. Hound (KC).

Size. Large.

Coat. *Color:* Sable or all shades of fawn with or without a black mask. *Texture:* Smooth and close.

SOFT-COATED WHEATEN TERRIER

Origins. The breed shares much the same origins and original purpose in life as the Kerry Blue Terrier; indeed it could almost be argued that the two are but color varieties of the same breed, their different appearance owing more to the hairdresser's art than to any basic differences. Legend has it that terriers the color of ripe wheat existed in Ireland before dogs from the wrecked ships of the Armada introduced the color which produced the Kerry Blue.

Characteristics. The soft wheaten-colored coat is the most obvious characteristic of the breed. In Ireland and in America the coat is trimmed, in Britain trimming is objected to by many breeders. The breed should be good tempered, spirited and game, full of confidence and humor; they make delightful, affectionate companions. Wheatens are of medium size, compact, strong and well built, standing foursquare with head and tail up. A good Wheaten makes a very attractive sight.

Group. Terriers.

Size. Medium.

Coat. *Color:* Wheaten. *Texture:* Soft and silky, loosely waved or curled.

STAFFORDSHIRE BULL TERRIER

Origins. One of the two gladiatorial members of the terrier group evolved to fight with other dogs or to bait bull, bear or badger. The old breeds used for these savage sports were mastiffs or Bulldogs and a dash of terrier blood was introduced to give speed and agility and so laid the foundations of the 'Bull and Terrier' breed. The breed still enjoys a good fight, but with people, particularly children, it is a most faithful companion and an excellent and fearless guard.

Characteristics. The Staffordshire has great strength for its size and, although very muscular, should be active and agile. The head is short, the skull broad, the foreface short and powerful. The eyes are round and look straight ahead. The neck is short and muscular, set into wide, strong shoulders. The tail is low set and carried like an old-fashioned pump handle. This dog needs firm training.

Group. Terriers.

Size. Medium.

Coat. *Color:* Red, fawn, white, black or blue, or

any of these colors with white. Brindle or brindle and white. *Texture:* Smooth, short and close to the skin.

SUSSEX SPANIEL

Origins. This distinctive spaniel has been bred since the eighteenth century, when breeding was organized in a very different way, utilizing large numbers of sturdy well-trained dogs. Conditions have now changed and spaniels with a greater turn of speed and able to cover more ground have become more popular.

Characteristics. The Sussex Spaniel is massive and strongly built, with a characteristic rolling movement quite unlike that of any other spaniel. The skull is broad, the eyes are fairly large, hazel colored with a soft expression. Ears are thick, fairly large and lobular. The neck is long, strong and slightly arched, not carrying the head much above the level of the back. The shoulders are sloping, the chest is deep and wide, the back wide and fairly long. Hindquarters are strongly developed. This dog is very loyal and may attach itself to one person.

Group. Sporting. Gundog (KC).
Size. Medium.
Coat. *Color:* Rich golden liver. *Texture:* Abundant and flat, with ample undercoat.

SWEDISH VALLHUND

Origins. Both the resemblance and the similar function in life argue some shared ancestor between the Väsgötaspitz and the Corgi. The fact that both have distinct Spitz characteristics seems to indicate origins in Scandinavia. This Swedish breed has only recently been recognized, in 1948.

Characteristics. The breed is low slung, long in the body, small and muscular. The carriage and expression indicate vigilance, courage and energy. The tail is naturally short, not docked. The Vallhund is an intelligent, loyal dog.

Group. Working (KC).
Size. Small.
Coat. *Color:* Gray. *Texture:* Of fair length, hard and dense, the undercoat fine and tight.

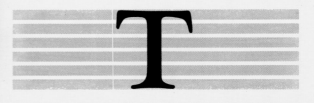

TIBETAN SPANIEL

Origins. Throughout ancient history the rulers of China, Tibet and neighboring countries showed

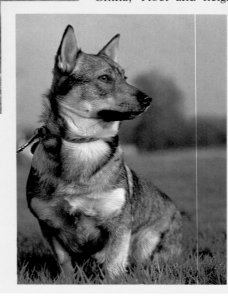

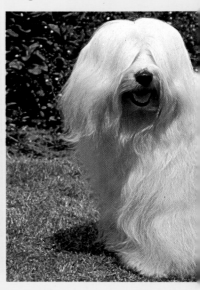

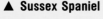
▲ Sussex Spaniel

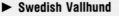
▶ Swedish Vallhund

great interest in the small breeds of dogs which they kept at their courts and which were their constant companions. These dogs were exchanged between the courts, dogs from Tibet moving to China with possibly the Happa becoming the ancestor of the Pekingese and the Carla becoming the ancestor of the Tibetan Spaniel.

Characteristics. The breed is gay, intelligent and aloof with strangers. The head is small in proportion to the body and proudly carried. The ears are of medium size and pendulous. The neck is moderately short, the body fairly long. The forelegs are slightly bowed, the feet small and neat. The tail is set high, richly plumed and carried in a gay curl over the back when moving.

Group. Non-Sporting. Utility (KC).

Size. Small.

Coat. *Color:* Various. *Texture:* Double coat, silky in texture.

TIBETAN TERRIER

Origins. Legend places the Tibetan Terrier's origins in the Lost Valley of Tibet and, with a breed whose history stretches back 2000 years, legend may be as reliable as supposed fact. In Tibet they are called 'Luck Bringers' or 'Holy Dogs' and were kept purely as companions and symbols of status. The breed is healthy, tough and affectionate, an ideal companion.

Characteristics. The general appearance is rather like that of an Old English Sheepdog in miniature. The head is of medium length and slightly domed, the eyes are large and dark, the ears V-shaped and pendant. The forelegs are straight, the hind legs slightly longer. The body is compact and powerful for its size. The tail is of medium length, set fairly high and carried in a gay curl over the back; it is very well feathered and often has a kink near the end.

Group. Non-Sporting. Utility (KC).

Size. Small.

Coat. *Color:* Any color except chocolate or liver. *Texture:* Double-coated, the undercoat of fine wool and the top coat profuse, long and either straight or waved.

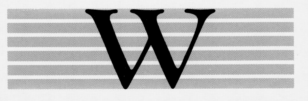

W

WEIMARANER

Origins. The breed has a history which only goes back to the beginning of the nineteenth century when it was produced by crossing Bloodhounds

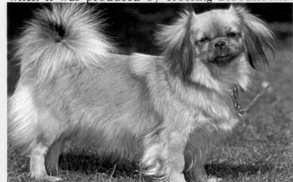

◄ **Tibetan Spaniel**

▼ **Weimaraner**

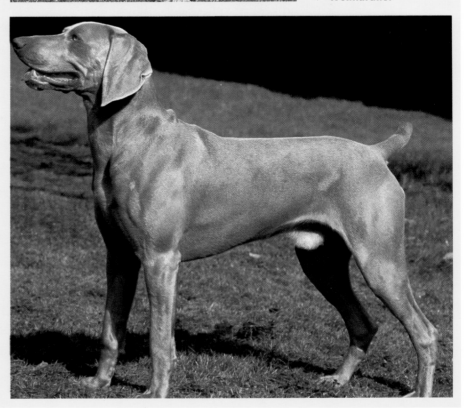

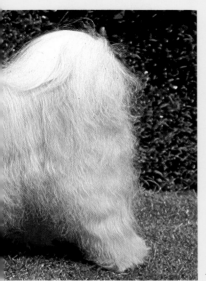

◄ **Tibetan Terrier**

with native German hunting breeds, such as the Red Schweisshund, and became known simply as the Weimar Pointer. In its early days the Weimaraner was used to hunt Europe's larger game, boar and deer, but is now very much at home fulfilling the duties of a gundog accompanying modern sportsmen. The Weimaraner is not a kennel dog, being happier and working better when living as part of the family. The breed's distinctive gray color, silent and effortless movement have earned it the popular name of 'Gray Ghost.'

Characteristics. The Weimaraner is fearless, friendly, protective and obedient. It is a large dog with considerable presence. Its head is moderately long and aristocratic; the eyes are unusually light, amber or blue-gray, and the ears long and lobular. The forelegs are straight and strong, the hindquarters powerful. The body is square in outline and the tail is docked.

Group. Sporting. Gundog (KC).

Size. Large.

Coat. *Color:* Silver gray or shades of mouse. *Texture:* Short, smooth and sleek. In the long-haired Weimaraner the coat is 2.5–5.8 cm (1–2 in) long on the body and the limbs are feathered.

WELSH CORGI (CARDIGAN)

Origins. The breed shares a common heritage with its more popular cousin from Pembrokeshire. (See below).

Characteristics. Apart from the fact that Pembrokes are without tails and Cardigans have good full ones, the two share considerable and obvious similarities. The tail in the Cardigan is moderately long and set in line with the body, closely resembling the brush of a fox. The Cardigan is also slightly larger, with not such a sharp head, and larger ears.

Group. Herding. Working (KC).

Size. Small.

Coat. *Color:* Any color except white. Blue merles may be wall-eyed. *Texture:* Short or medium, and of hard texture.

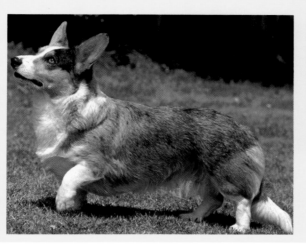

◀ **Welsh Corgi, Cardigan**

WELSH CORGI (PEMBROKE)

Origins. The two breeds of Corgi, the Pembroke and the Cardigan, and the as yet unrecognized Lancashire Heeler, were developed as specialist cattle dogs sometime during the twelfth century. The Corgi is said to have been brought over from Holland by Flemish weavers who settled around Haverfordwest in west Wales. Certainly such a history would do much to explain the distinct Spitz characteristics carried by the Corgi and which may have produced, crossed with the Old Black and Tan Terriers, the lighter built Black and Tan Heelers.

Characteristics. The Corgi is low set, strong, sturdily built and active, giving an impression of substance and stamina in small space. The head in all respects is foxy, the neck and body fairly long. The legs are short, the tail is docked as short as possible, though some puppies are born without a tail.

Group. Herding. Working (KC).

Size. Small.

Coat. *Color:* Red, sable, fawn, black and tan or with white markings on legs, chest and neck. *Texture:* Short or medium length and of hard texture.

WELSH SPRINGER SPANIEL

Origins. History does not record the advent of the Welsh Springer Spaniel as a distinctive breed, though it is certain that red and white spaniels very similar to the modern Welsh have been in existence for very many years since they are to be seen in many old sporting drawings and paintings. The Welsh Springer is a first-class gundog and makes an excellent companion as well as an eye-catching show dog.

Characteristics. The head is of moderate length

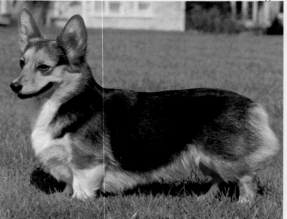

▲ **Welsh Corgi, Pembroke**

and slightly domed. The eyes are hazel or dark, the ears set moderately low and comparatively small. The neck is long and muscular, neatly set into long, sloping shoulders. Forelegs are of medium length, straight, and moderately feathered; quarters are strong and muscular. The Welsh Springer is a happy, active and willing dog.

Group. Sporting. Gundog (KC).

Size. Medium.

Coat. *Color:* Dark rich red and white. *Texture:* Straight and thick and silky.

WELSH TERRIER

Origins. The Welsh Terrier is the counterpart of the Lakeland which in some ways it resembles. It was used to accompany the hunts in Wales in order to drive fox or otter from places of refuge. Until the turn of the century there appears to have been little distinction made between the Welsh and the Old English Black and Tan Terrier.

Characteristics. The Welsh Terrier has a gay, volatile disposition and is only rarely shy. It is affectionate, obedient and biddable. The head is flat and rather wider between the ears than a Fox Terrier, the jaw is powerful. The eyes are small and dark, the ears are V-shaped and carried forward and close to the cheek. The neck is slightly arched and slopes gracefully into long shoulders. The body is short, the forelegs straight and muscular, the hindquarters strong with muscular thighs.

Group. Terriers.

Size. Small.

Coat. *Color:* Black and tan. *Texture:* Wiry, hard, very close and abundant.

WEST HIGHLAND WHITE TERRIER

Origins. According to the Malcolm family, the breed has its origins in Poltallock, Scotland, where for three generations the family bred these white terriers. Certainly the breed was called the Poltallock Terrier and the Roseneath Terrier, but it is likely that these places only concentrated on devel-

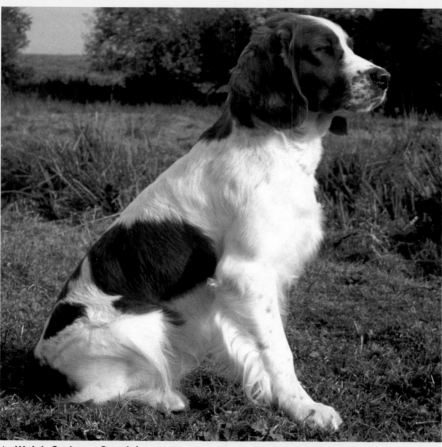

▲ **Welsh Springer Spaniel**

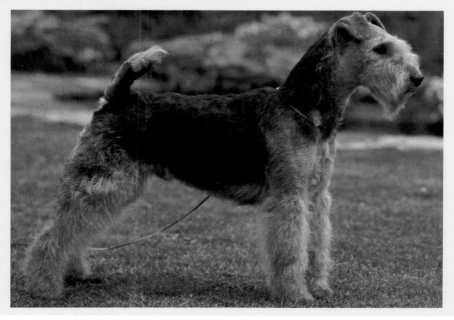

◄ **Welsh Terrier**

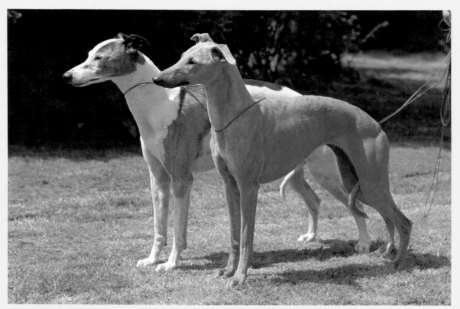

▲ **Whippet**

WHIPPET

Origins. The Whippet is not, in spite of obvious similarities, a miniature Greyhound. It is the working man's sight hound, intended for coursing small ground game and for racing against its fellows. The breed came into existence in the early nineteenth century and the breed's speed over a furlong made exciting racing, a sport which predates the more commercially organized Greyhound races that take place today.

Characteristics. Whippets convey an impression of balanced muscular power and strength allied to elegance; the dog is built for speed. The skull is long and lean, the expression bright and alert, the ears fine and rose-shaped. The neck is long, muscular and slightly arched, the chest is very deep, the back broad. The tail is long and tapering. The breed is gentle and affectionate.

Group. Hounds.

Size. Medium.

Coat. *Color:* Various. *Texture:* Fine, short, as close as possible.

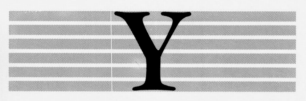

YORKSHIRE TERRIER

Origins. Although by Victoria's reign the Yorkshire Terrier, because of its diminutive size and glamorous coat, had been taken up as a fashionable pet, its origins are much more humble. Originating among the Scottish Terriers, the breed was taken up in the 1840s by Yorkshire weavers who wanted a sporting little terrier for ratting expeditions or for competition in the rat pits. The breed in those days weighed anything up to 9 kg (20 lb) with 4.5 kg (10 lb) being regarded as an ideal but, when killing rats ceased to be part of the breed's purpose in life, the size was even further reduced.

Characteristics. The Yorkshire Terrier is very compact and neat, its carriage conveying an air of importance. It is a brave, intelligent and affectionate little dog. The head is rather small and flat, the eyes dark and sparkling and the ears small, V-shaped and carried erect or semi-erect. The forelegs are straight, the body very compact with a good loin and level topline. The color and length of the coat is very important for a show dog.

Group. Toys.

Size. Small.

Coat. *Color:* A dark steel blue, with rich bright tan markings. *Texture:* Long and perfectly straight, glossy and of a fine silky texture.

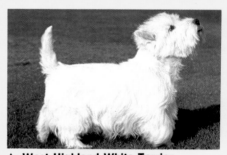

▲ **West Highland White Terrier**

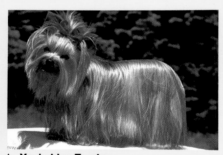

▲ **Yorkshire Terrier**

oping and refining a white strain of the old Scottish Terriers. In so doing, they produced a smart, courageous and hardy little sporting dog, which is now much valued as a companion and has achieved considerable success in the show ring.

Characteristics. The general appearance is that of a small, game and hardy terrier, with plenty of self-esteem. The breed is strongly built, deep in the chest and back ribs, the back level and the quarters powerful. The head is slightly domed, the eyes are set wide apart and are dark in color giving a sharp and intelligent look. The ears are small and carried erect. The tail is 12.7–15 cm (5–6 in) long, not docked and is carried jauntily.

Group. Terriers.

Size. Small.

Coat. *Color:* Pure white. *Texture:* Outer coat hard and free from curl, undercoat short, soft and close.

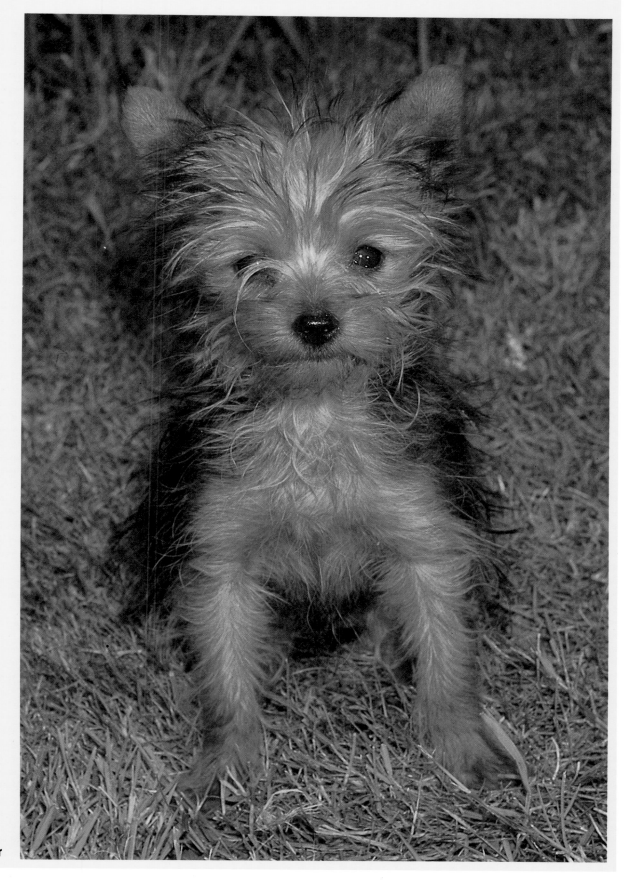

► **Yorkshire Terrier**

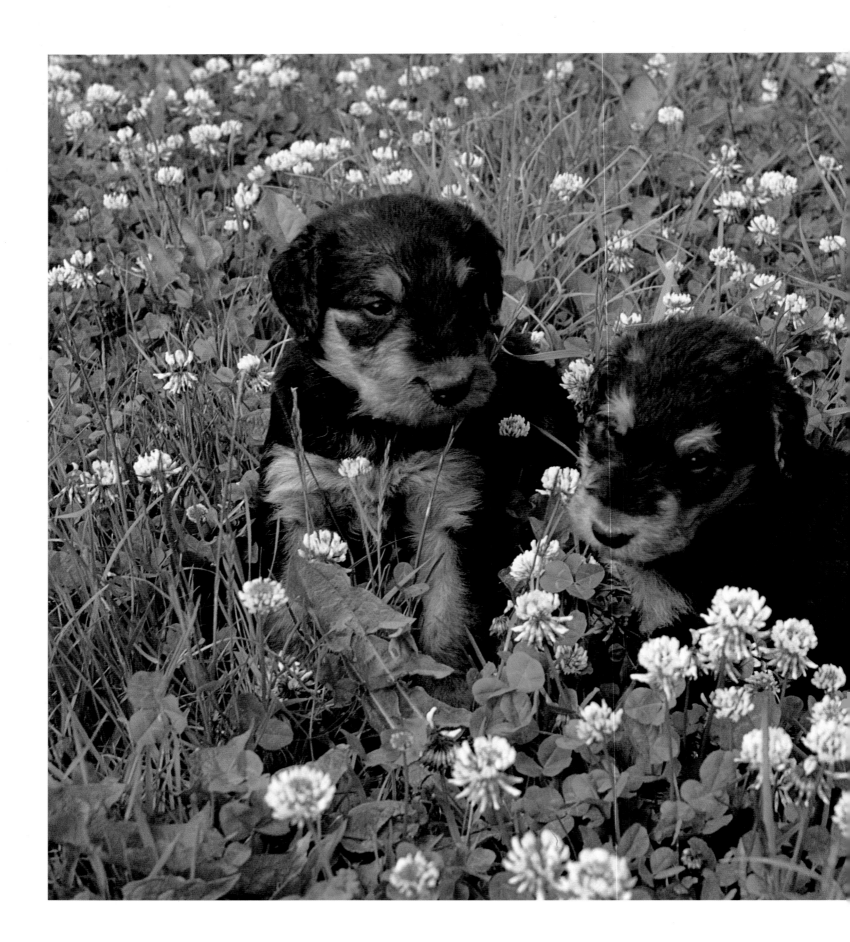

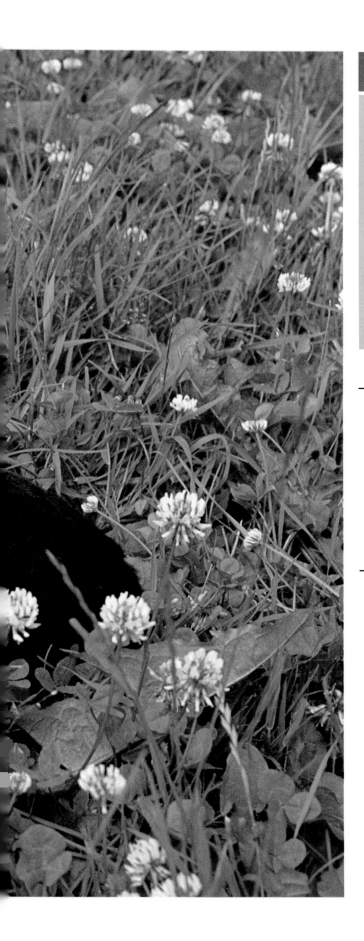

THE
NEW PUPPY

A new puppy is a delight but it needs special care to ensure that it grows into a healthy, well-adjusted dog. As a responsible owner, you will want to smooth its first days with its new family and make sure that it has a comfortable place to sleep, a suitable diet and plenty of love and attention. The puppy will need to be housetrained, to get used to a collar and lead and to learn the rules it is expected to live by. The way that you handle these early lessons can make all the difference to your dog's behavior in the future.

You will probably be collecting your puppy at about seven weeks old, when it is fully weaned and at an age when it should adapt well to a change of ownership. Remember that going to its new home is one of the most unsettling and frightening experiences of its life. Its family and safe, familiar surroundings are left behind and it is being subjected to a bewildering variety of new scents, sights and sounds. A young puppy is still a baby and, like a baby, needs a great deal of affection. A bitch constantly licks, caresses and pushes her puppies about in play and 'talks' to them in soft tones, usually inaudible to humans. You will find that a tense or worried puppy will relax at the touch of a sensitive and sympathetic hand and a quiet, reassuring tone of voice.

Every dog should be trained in basic obedience and a well-behaved pet will fit better into your family life, to the benefit of everyone concerned. However, your new puppy will have no notion of the way it is expected to behave. You can indicate what you consider acceptable house manners from the beginning by making sure that the puppy knows which parts of the house and which items of furniture are out of bounds, that slippers are not for chewing and that begging at the table is not allowed. However, these early lessons must be taught with gentleness and patience. If you shout or smack, the puppy is more likely to associate the punishment with its new owner and the new home in general rather than with the 'wrongdoing'. This kind of treatment can turn a bold, friendly puppy into a timid, nervous creature within a matter of days, leaving the puzzled owners wondering what has gone wrong.

DOGPROOFING YOUR HOME

A young puppy will chew everything within reach so you will need to keep slippers, gloves, children's toys and houseplants well out of reach and loop up any trailing electrical cord. Think how you would behave with an active toddler in the house and follow the same regime: make sure that the puppy cannot get into your stores of household disinfectant, dry cleaning fluid, pesticides, antifreeze or even mothballs. You may need to fix a wire netting guard on the underside of an open tread staircase or over a stairwell, to prevent any damaging fall. One way of keeping the puppy out of trouble is to partition the area around the puppy's bed. You can use a pen with wire mesh panels and wooden frames specially made for the job and obtainable through pet shops, or improvize with a fireguard or a baby's discarded playpen, with wire mesh attached to the sides to prevent a tiny puppy from squeezing through the bars.

You will also need to guard against hazards out in the garden or yard; cover swimming pools and ponds until the puppy has been taught to keep away

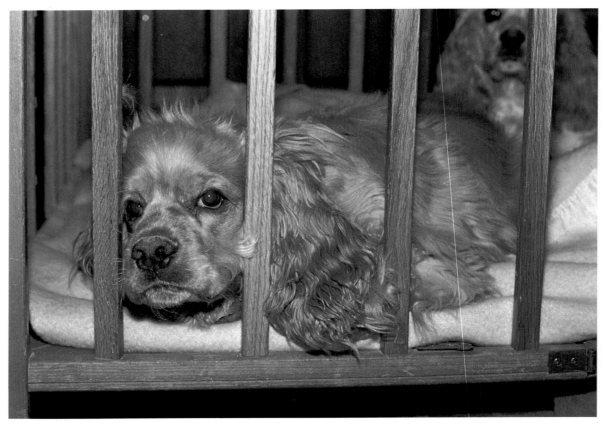

A child's crib, lined with a washable blanket, can make a useful bed for puppies in the early weeks, keeping them out of danger and mischief when you are not there to supervise.

from them. Although most dogs can swim naturally, they cannot clamber out up steep sides and might drown through panic or exhaustion. You will need to fence off an area of the yard for your puppy's use or make sure that fences and gates are escape-proof.

EQUIPMENT

The puppy will need its own bed, set in a draught-free area. Initially, a sturdy cardboard box with a piece cut out of the front to allow easy access, lined with an old sweater or blanket, is ideal. It should be just large enough for the puppy to lie on its side; this size will give enough room for comfort but will convey a feeling of security. As the box becomes chewed and soiled, it can be replaced by another. It is pointless to provide young puppies with wicker baskets as these are almost made to be chewed and in any case, this type of bed is hard to keep clean and lets in draughts. Beds made of heavy plastic are fairly resistant to chewing, light in weight and easy to wash and disinfect. Another hygienic type of bed is the one filled with polystyrene beads that take on the shape of the dog, making a warm nest; these have removable, washable covers.

Your dog must have its own bowls and dishes of a design suitable for its breed so that it can eat and drink comfortably without getting its nose or ears submerged; these should be kept separate from the crockery used by the rest of the family. Plastic and aluminum dishes are too light and will frequently be upended, so a heavy pottery bowl may be more suitable.

Make sure that your puppy's toys are specially made for dogs. It will enjoy rawhide chews, a hard rubber ball too large to be swallowed and a substantial toy with an exciting squeaker inside. Make sure that none of the toys is made from soft rubber, that they have no sharp edges and no bits that can be chewed off and swallowed.

COLLECTING YOUR PUPPY

Try to bring home your puppy at a time when the house is peaceful, without too much coming or going and when you will have plenty of time to spend with the little dog. Morning is the best time for collection, so that your new pet will have time to get used to its surroundings before you leave it alone for the night. If possible, take someone with you when you collect the puppy by car, so that one of you can wrap it in a warm towel or blanket and hold it on your lap. If you have to collect the puppy alone, it is wise to buy a cardboard box from the pet shop. Have plenty of newspaper and a roll of kitchen paper with you in case the puppy is sick.

If you are buying a purebred dog, the breeder will provide you with a copy of its pedigree, the record of its ancestry going back some four or five

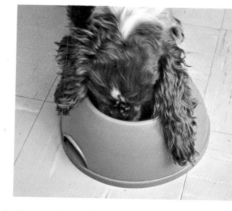

Some breeds, such as the Spaniel, need feeding bowls designed to keep their ears out of their food.

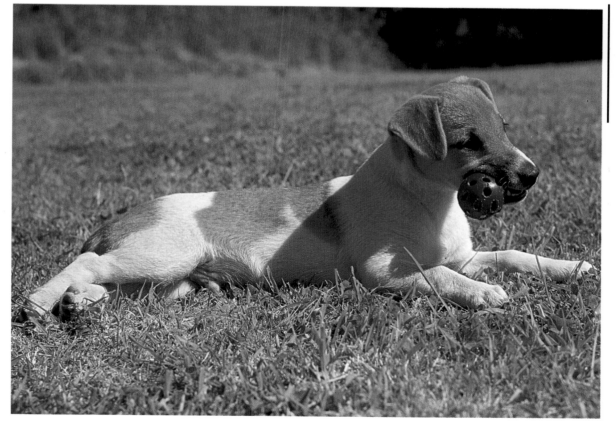

Toys will give your puppy a great deal of pleasure but they should be carefully chosen so that they cannot be swallowed or chewed into pieces.

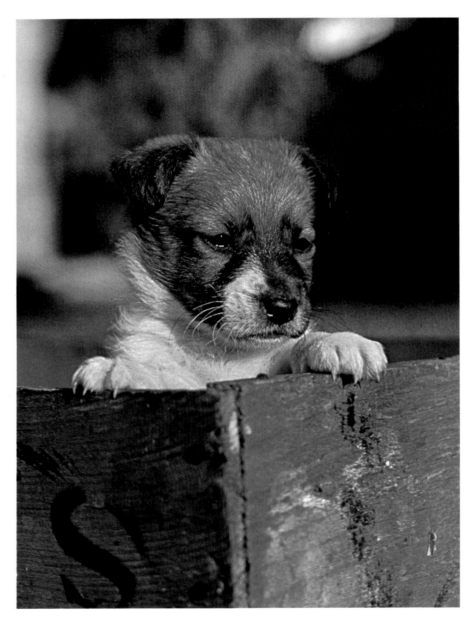

Puppies are naturally curious and love to explore, so make sure that they are in no danger, either indoors or outdoors.

A child and a puppy can spend many happy hours together but children must be taught that the little animal is not a toy and must be treated properly.

the food or it may be too nervous to eat. If it refuses the meal and whines, wrap it in its blanket and put it in its prepared bed for a nap. Puppies spend a lot of time sleeping and this is necessary for their well-being, so leave it in peace and make sure that other members of the family are not constantly petting and cuddling it. On the other hand, it should not be left completely alone for long at first. At this stage, the puppy's play periods are about half an hour long, interspersed with long sleep sessions.

At night, play with the puppy until it is sleepy, then take it outside for a final elimination. As this is the first night it has spent alone, the puppy is likely to cry and whine. A well-wrapped stone hot water bottle will give it something comforting to snuggle up to and a ticking clock in a corner of the bed, simulating the mother's heartbeat, can help. Some owners decide that ignoring any sounds of distress is the most sensible course, as the puppy will quickly adapt and realize that there is no reason for fright; others go down a couple of times during the night to soothe the new pet. If you do this, it is important to maintain a matter-of-fact approach as you do not want the puppy to learn that it only has to make a noise to bring a sympathetic person running. You may get around the problem by putting a pen in a corner of your bedroom as this will give the new arrival a much greater sense of security. You can then accustom the puppy to spending short periods shut up alone during the day before you leave it alone for a whole night.

CHILDREN AND PUPPIES

A healthy puppy is naturally playful and full of fun, so it is bound to enjoy playing with children. However, they should understand that the puppy is not a toy; they must never be allowed to smack it, pull it around on a lead or overdo the playing so that the puppy becomes too excited or exhausted. Any teasing at this stage may lead to aggressive behavior that will be difficult to cure later. They should not feed sweets and tidbits to the puppy or throw small toys for it to chase, as it may swallow them and choke.

Encourage the children to keep the puppy's bedding tidy, change the water in its bowl and help prepare its meals. They can help to groom the little dog and get it used to having its ears, mouth, paws and tail examined without fuss. They need to know that they should never pick up a puppy by the forelimbs or by the scruff of the neck. Teach them to hold it carefully with two arms encompassing both fore and hindlimbs to give control and support.

Make sure that children do not play in any area where dogs urinate or defecate, teach them that they must discourage the puppy from licking their faces and that they should wash after playing with the dog.

generations. If the puppy has been registered with the kennel club, you will also have a certificate to enable its particulars to be officially transferred to your ownership. You should check when the puppy was last wormed and when worming will be due again and whether any vaccinations have been given. Many breeders will give a detailed diet sheet but if not, find out what the puppy has been eating and follow the same diet, at least at the beginning, making any changes gradually.

Get home as quickly and smoothly as possible, holding the puppy close for comfort and talking to it in a soothing voice. At the end of the journey, the first thing the puppy will need to do is to relieve itself, so take it outside first and give it plenty of praise when it performs. After that, take it indoors and offer a small milk and cereal feed. It may accept

INTRODUCTION TO OTHER PETS

When introducing a new puppy to established pets, you need to ensure that the older animal has no cause for jealousy. Arrange the meeting between a puppy and an older dog in the garden. Hold the older dog on its lead, giving it plenty of attention and fuss as you bring the new puppy forward. They will probably sniff one another thoroughly, then may begin some excited form of play, but do not let the games get out of hand; the older dog may become exhausted or it may hurt the puppy unintentionally. If they get along reasonably well, then let the older dog loose and encourage them both to follow you into the house. In this way, the dog will feel that it has made the decision to bring the puppy into the family. Feed the dogs separately at first and keep the puppy in a pen whenever you leave the two alone together. So long as the older dog is given no cause for resentment, the two should become inseparable pals.

If the ruse does not work, you will have to spend a good deal of time with the dogs while they get used to one another. Do not allow growling and praise any sign of friendly behavior. Do not leave them alone together but have them in the same room as often as possible when you are there to supervise. It is rare for two dogs to be completely incompatible and they will usually make friends eventually.

Before introducing a puppy to the family cat, trim the cat's front claws. The dog's first instinct is to rush forward and try to sniff the cat all over; the cat will resent this and try to claw the dog's nose and if the claws are sharp, the puppy will be hurt and upset. Most cats know exactly how to put a cheeky puppy in its place but it is important that they have a high shelf as a safe haven. The cat may spend a good deal of time away from home over the first few days, or even weeks, but it is important to give it a good welcome every time it comes in and show it that its place has not been usurped. Some cats end up sharing the dog's basket; others remain aloof.

DIET

From weaning until four months, a puppy needs four meals daily, two of meat and biscuit and two of milk and cereal. The biscuit should be good quality wheatmeal; the meat can be fresh meat, cooked and minced, or a canned meat specially prepared for puppies. If you use fresh meat, add a little bone meal for extra calcium. Cow's milk or diluted evaporated milk can be thickened by adding fine cereal of the sort made for human babies. Give a milky meal first thing in the morning and late afternoon, and meat meals at noon and dinner time.

When the puppy reaches four months, discontinue the first of the milk meals and bring the times of the other meals forward slightly, increasing the amounts as necessary. Observation will tell you if

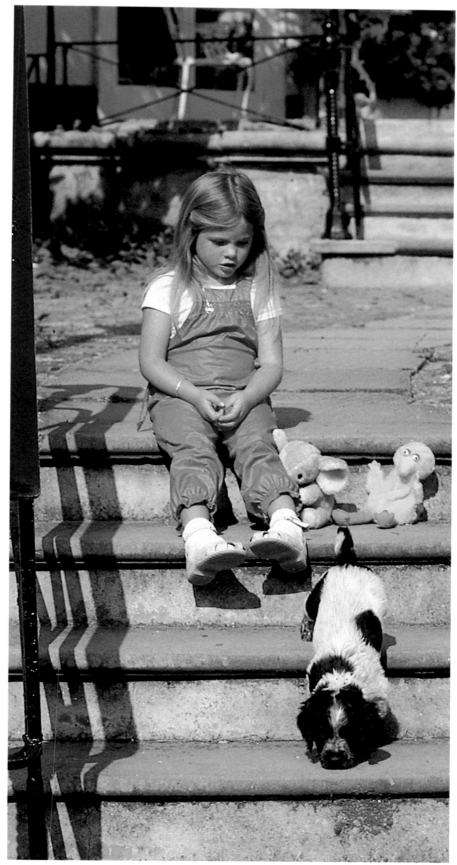

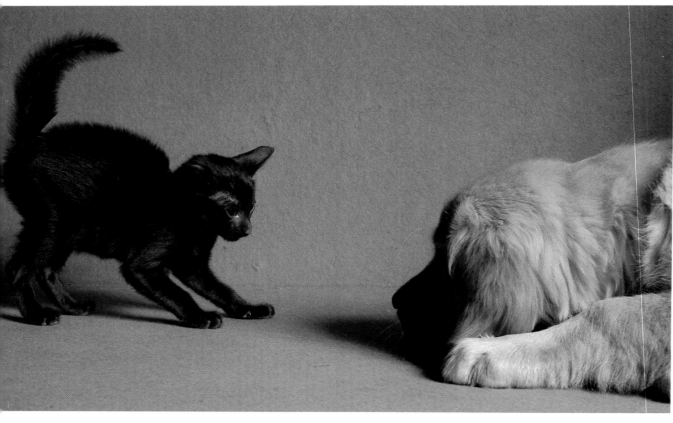

The new puppy should be carefully introduced to other pets, though the family cat will soon put the newcomer in its place if it becomes over-familiar. It is a good idea to trim the cat's claws in advance.

your puppy is getting the right amount of food. If you are overfeeding, the puppy will be lethargic, with thickening around the waist and neck. If your puppy's ribs are showing through its skin, you are not giving enough food. At six months, feed two meals a day, both meat and meal; from nine months, you can feed one meal a day. This is sufficient for most dogs but you can split this into two meals a day if you prefer. Very small dogs, giant breeds and old dogs will probably benefit from two meals a day; this ensures that the stomach is not overloaded and makes digestion easier.

PUPPY HEALTH

Vaccination. Your dog needs vaccination to protect against the major canine diseases. An unvaccinated dog can easily become infected when playing in parks or sniffing around lampposts, staying in boarding kennels, taking part in dog shows or anywhere that it mixes with other dogs. Puppies are particularly susceptible to infection and should not be taken out of their home and yard until their vaccination program is complete. They should receive a combined first vaccination against distemper, hepatitis and the two forms of leptospirosis at 6–8 weeks of age, with the second half of the course at about 12 weeks. Vaccination against canine parvovirus, a comparatively new disease, can be given on the same schedule. Booster injections

should be given regularly throughout the dog's life.

Rabies vaccine, given at 9 weeks with a second dose a year later, is essential in countries where the disease is present. Subsequent vaccinations will be at one or three year intervals, depending on the vaccine used.

Worming. Most vets will advise routine twice-monthly worming of puppies up to three months of age. A well-reared puppy will have been wormed by the breeder as a matter of course. Your vet will prescribe a suitable product; proprietary medicines bought from a pet shop may not be suitable.

Teething. At about four months old, the puppy teeth are pushed out by the growth of the adult set. Most puppies teethe without any trouble, though occasionally sore gums will put them off their food for a day or two. If a puppy does go off its food, keep a sharp eye on it to make sure that teething is the cause and that it is not sickening for some reason.

LEARNING ITS NAME

One of the first things a puppy needs to know is its own name. Choose a name as soon as you acquire your pet and stick to it; changing names after the first couple of weeks because you think of something better or using 'Pup' some of the time, will leave the animal thoroughly confused and basic

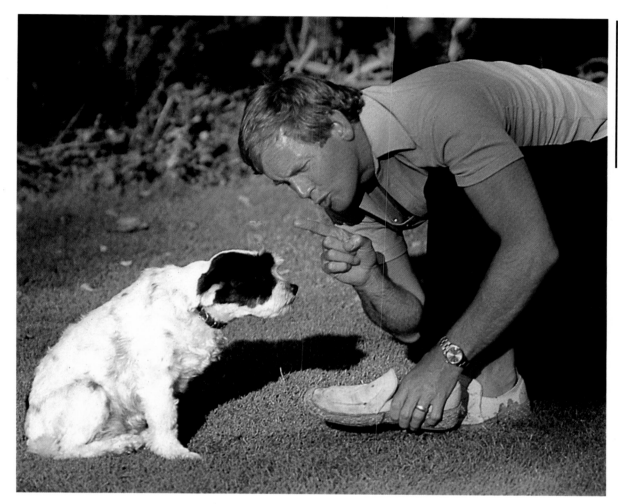

A puppy that chews its owner's shoes must learn the meaning of the word 'No!', reinforced with a reproving index finger. Always give the puppy a suitable chewy toy as a substitute.

training will be more difficult. A short one-syllable or a simple, flowing two-syllable name is best and it should not sound too much like the command words used in training; 'No', 'Come', 'Sit', 'Stay', 'Wait', 'Down', 'Leave' and 'Heel'. You could hardly blame a dog called Kit for bounding towards you every time you told it to 'Sit' and if you call your dog Joe you may have to invent a different word for forbidding bad behavior.

The puppy should associate its name with pleasure, so that it will always answer to it willingly. Call it by name when giving food, offering a tidbit, a game or plenty of fuss. Do not use its name when you are scolding. Call your puppy in a coaxing tone of voice. Attract its attention by clapping your hands, slapping your leg or something else that indicates that a game is possible. If your puppy ignores you, wait until it has finished what it is doing and try again when it is more likely to respond. Giving a command when it is unlikely to be obeyed only reinforces disobedience at this stage. Wait until the puppy looks as though it might come to you, then call it and when it comes, make a big fuss of it. If your pup is willful and still fails to come, try turning and walking away slowly. This will often bring it bounding to your side, then you can pet and praise it.

EARLY LESSONS

You will need to lay down rules for your puppy from the beginning and keep them. It is important to be consistent and every member of the family should help in teaching early lessons. No puppy will understand if it is allowed to snuggle into the best armchair one day and is shooed out of it the next. If you can prevent bad habits from forming in the first place – for instance, by making sure the puppy is always supervised when in the living room and not allowed to climb into the forbidden chair in the first place – you will find the whole training process much easier. Puppies are naturally lively and mischievous but you can often distract them from behavior you consider unacceptable by giving them something else to do.

The puppy must learn the meaning of 'No,' which should be said firmly, perhaps in a gruff voice like a growl, but not shouted. Dogs are very sensitive to nuances of tone and you can make use of this by the amount of enthusiasm or displeasure you show in

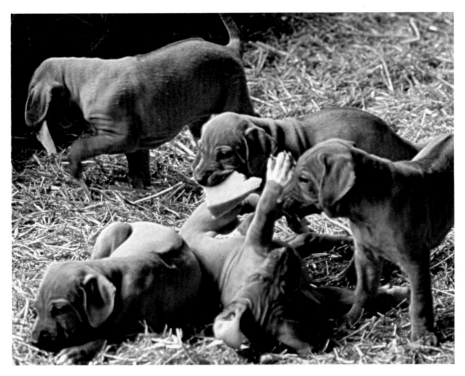

Play is very important in a puppy's life and this litter of Rhodesian Ridgebacks is learning the rough and tumble of family life. When you take a puppy into your home, you should continue the games it has learned to enjoy.

your voice. 'No' can be reinforced by a raised, reproving finger and if the puppy ignores this command, repeat it and physically stop the dog from its misdeed, perhaps emphasizing your displeasure with a little shake. Never accept behavior from your puppy that will be unacceptable in a full-grown dog. Make it clear that growling, for instance, is not allowed; give a little shake, hold the puppy up level with your eyes and rebuke it, even showing your teeth a little.

You will need to give plenty of praise and encouragement to compensate for the many times that you need to say 'No' and even the most willful pet prefers petting to the stern chastisement of 'No.' Puppies vary in their need for encouragement; some are delighted with just a pat and a word of praise but others need a great deal of fuss to encourage good behavior. Some dog trainers suggest using a rolled-up newspaper as a training aid and with some dogs this may help but it is a risky tool. Extrovert dogs sometimes look on the waving newspaper as an invitation to a game rather than a mild punishment. The use of a newspaper may upset a nervous or introvert puppy and could engender resentment or aggressiveness.

Once the vaccination program is complete, the puppy should be encouraged to mix with plenty of people outside the family circle and to become used to crowded situations and strange noises. If for instance, there is no man in the house, enlist the help of neighbors and friends to make sure that the dog does not build up a fear of men. It should also get used to children, even if there are none in your household, so that it will not behave unpredictably when confronted by children at some time in the future.

PLAY

The importance of play cannot be overemphasized. It is vital in preparing the young puppy both physically and mentally for adult life. When a puppy is taken from its canine family and made a part of your own, you will need to continue some of the games the young dog has come to enjoy. The commonest form of puppy play is the mock fight in which puppies in a litter engage in rough-and-tumble battles with each other. You can play such a game with your puppy. Taking care not to be too rough, push and roll it around on the floor, grasping the loose skin of the neck from time to time and giving it a little shake. The puppy will back off, then growl and pounce on your hand and arm and thoroughly enjoy the game. Never pull your hand sharply back, however, or the pup's sharp teeth could snag your skin. The puppy will snap, chew, and gnaw at your hand, but it will never close its jaws because the threats are all bluff. This form of play is designed to build up muscles and develop the reflexes. Another puppy game is 'tag', when young dogs take turns to chase one another. Here again you, as owner, can take the place of a litter mate and establish an excellent relationship with your dog.

It is imperative that your dog should both respect and really love you if you are to achieve good results from later training. The close relationship that develops from the early sharing of games gives an excellent start. When playing doggy games try to think and act like a dog yourself. Do not let the puppy become overexcited. The 'No!' command can be given to restrain its exuberance followed by praise and reward when the little dog relaxes.

COLLARS AND LEADS

A puppy can be taught to wear a collar from a very early age. The first collar can be of a cheap quality and must be very light in weight. It should be buckled around the neck, tight enough to stay on when the puppy lowers its head but loose enough for you to be able to insert two fingers between collar and neck. The collar must be checked at least every week; it is surprising how quickly puppies grow, and a tight collar can be dangerous. The puppy will soon accept its collar, and it may be left on all day if you wish. It is best to take it off at night, however, to prevent the puppy's neck from becoming marked.

Every dog should bear its owner's name and address on an engraved disc attached to the collar by means of a small split ring; it can then be transferred to each successive collar as the pup grows. Never add the dog's own name to the disc, as this could help anyone who tried to entice your dog away.

It is not necessary to lead-walk a young puppy, which gets all the exercise it needs by romping and playing in the house and yard. Indeed, long tiring walks can cause physical damage in the young dog. Nevertheless, you may begin lead training the puppy if you wish. Clip a light lead to the collar and allow the puppy to pull it around. After a few days hold the end of the lead and encourage the puppy to follow you. Always keep the puppy on your left-hand side; this will help with heelwork training later on. Praise the little dog when it walks eagerly alongside you. Never drag the puppy along by its lead, nor use it to tie him up or to smack him. The sight of the lead should fill a dog with excitement and anticipation of a training session or a walk; it should not be regarded as an instrument of punishment.

Never put a choke collar or slip collar on a very young puppy. Such a collar could choke the little animal and the terrifying experience could make the puppy head-shy for many months afterwards.

When the puppy approaches six months serious training can begin. It is important to select the correct collars, leads, and other equipment according to the dog's size and breed. Short-necked and toy breeds often feel more comfortable wearing harnesses rather than collars, but harnesses are not recommended for a boisterous young puppy

because continued pulling and romping could damage the animal's shoulders and forelegs. Rolled leather collars are comfortable to wear and are easy to keep in good condition. They need a weekly wash followed by an application of saddle soap, worked well in and then polished off and allowed to dry before the collar is put back on the dog.

Small dogs need long, light leads; short but strong dogs need long, tough leads and large dogs need short but strong leads. Avoid all leads with spring-clip attachments which can get caught in the fur, or snap shut on lips, ear flaps, and paws, causing pain and distress; sometimes they have to be removed by the veterinarian. The best leads have clips which open and close with a sliding metal button. These are completely safe in use and are kept in good working order by applying one drop of fine machine oil to the sliding part whenever the lead is washed and cleaned.

Some owners delight in dressing up their dogs and there are many designs available in both collars and leads. Heavily studded collars are quite unsuitable for a young dog. Others, in brightly colored leather, are inclined to shed their dye if they get wet, tinting the dog's neck and sometimes giving rise to allergic reactions that cause irritation and distress. By visiting dog shows and training classes you will soon discover the sort of equipment knowledgeable dog handlers prefer to use.

Your dog should not be allowed to mix with animals outside the family until its vaccination program is complete and even then, it should never be allowed to roam unsupervised.

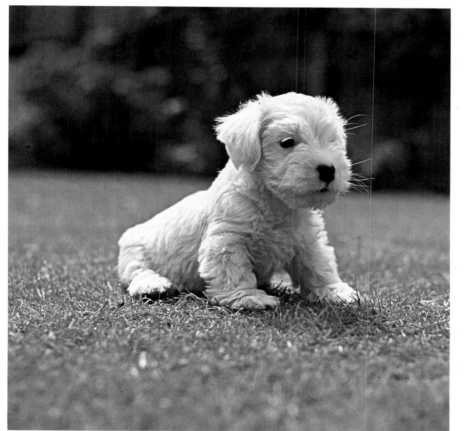

GROOMING

If you establish a regular grooming routine from the earliest days with your puppy, it will grow up to enjoy the experience and the act of grooming will reinforce your dog's affection and trust. Grooming removes old dead hair and prevents the formation of felting or matting in long-coated breeds. It stimulates the blood supply to the skin, and this in turn improves the condition of the coat, giving the dog a healthier appearance. Correct grooming can also improve muscle tone in the dog's back and limbs and leads to a general sense of well-being.

Each type of coat requires its own set of grooming equipment. It is best to seek advice from the breeder at the outset in order to avoid buying expensive brushes and combs that turn out to be unsuitable.

Pure-bristle hairbrushes are needed for toy dogs and some of the smooth-coated breeds. Most types of dog require a good quality steel comb. Cheap combs are a false economy as the nickel plating soon wears through and peels off. Good combs have teeth with rounded ends so that they are not sharp enough to scratch the dog's skin. Choose a comb with correctly spaced teeth for your dog's coat type. Remember that the longer and thicker the coat, the wider the teeth should be spaced. Short satinlike coats are best rubbed down with a grooming mitten, and for short hard coats you can buy an excellent glove.

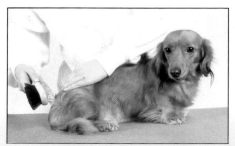

1 The top coat is lifted forward so that the undercoat may be thoroughly brushed.

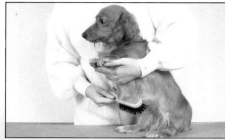

5 In using the wire brush, care must be taken to avoid scratching the dog's skin.

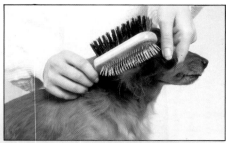

8 The bristle brush is used to groom the long, fine hair behind the dog's ears.

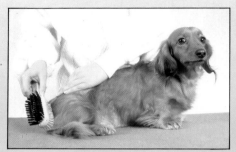

2 The hind legs are dealt with first of all and groomed down to the pads.

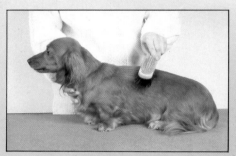

6 After dealing with the undercoat, each layer of top coat is smoothed into place.

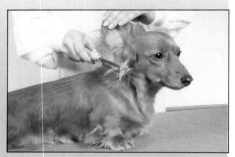

9 Careful combings of all soft areas can help to prevent the formation of mats.

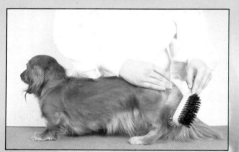

3 The dog may be sensitive in this area and any knots should be teased out.

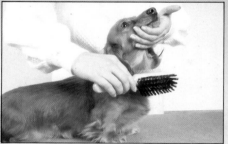

7 The brush is then used down the throat and between the forelegs.

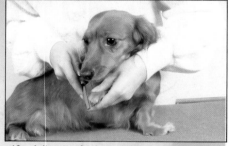

10 A fine-toothed comb removes grit, dirt and dust from the hair between the toes.

4 The tail must be treated gently, paying extra attention to the fine feathering.

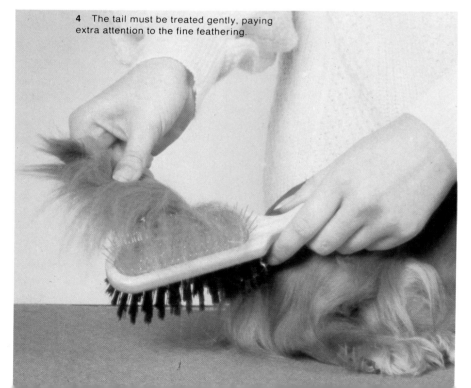

The coat. Generally speaking, the long-coated dogs need the most attention. A good wire brush is the best tool for separating the hairs. It should be of very good quality and have wire teeth that are neither too harsh nor too soft and are firmly set into a wooden base with a comfortable handle. The wire brush must always be used gently and with care, so that the teeth do not scratch the animal's skin.

When brushing out the long-coated varieties it is best to have the dog standing comfortably and relaxed on a bench or table. This is for your benefit rather than the dog's, for it will take some time to go right through the coat, and it can be a backbreaking job if you have to bend down to do it. If the dog is inclined to be restless, tie it up with a fairly short chain on its collar and talk soothingly to it throughout the grooming. Learning to stand still for grooming is an important feature of the dog's training and should be taught as thoroughly as any other part of the training program.

Start at the rear end with one of the hind legs. Lift

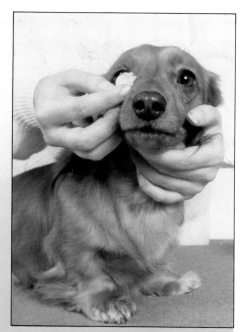

11 A fresh pad of dampened cotton is used carefully to clean each eye.

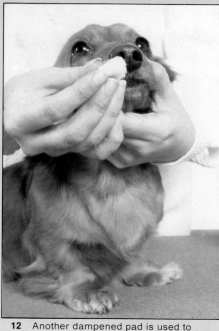

12 Another dampened pad is used to remove any discharge from the nostrils.

Grooming equipment

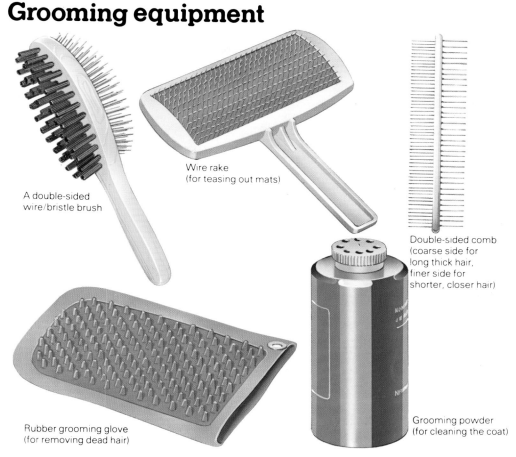

A double-sided wire/bristle brush

Wire rake (for teasing out mats)

Double-sided comb (coarse side for long thick hair, finer side for shorter, closer hair)

Rubber grooming glove (for removing dead hair)

Grooming powder (for cleaning the coat)

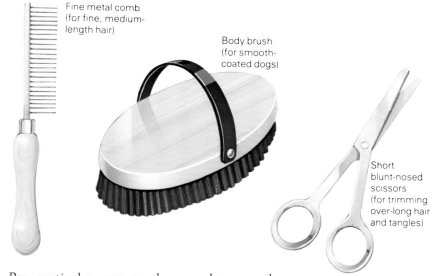

Fine metal comb (for fine, medium-length hair)

Body brush (for smooth-coated dogs)

Short blunt-nosed scissors (for trimming over-long hair and tangles)

up the long outer hair and use the wire brush to go through all the undercoat of the thigh and down the lower leg. Brush carefully down the inner side of the thigh where the skin may be sensitive, then groom the top coat smoothly back into place. Repeat this procedure for the other hind leg, then thoroughly groom the rump and down the entire length of the tail. Brush out the front legs next, again lifting the top coat and grooming the undercoat first.

Pay particular care to the area between the forelimbs and along the belly; bear in mind that these parts can be ticklish and tender, and it will be necessary to tease out any small tangles or knots. In this area the hair can be extremely soft and fine, and easily mats together. Grass seeds and prickles get caught up in this soft hair and cause tangles which may have to be clipped out with blunt-nosed scissors if they are not promptly removed by brushing.

Groom the body hair from the shoulders back over the ribs to the hips. Brush down the neck and chest, then deal with any long hair on the face and the ears if they have long furnishings. After you have gone all over the dog with the wire brush and are certain that no areas have been missed, use a metal comb to deal with any feathering or extra long hair around the head, ears, legs or tail.

Follow the same general pattern for grooming short-coated breeds, starting at the hind legs, progressing to the body and finishing with the head. Most dogs benefit from a final polish with a soft, clean chamois leather or a silk or velvet pad to bring up a gloss on the coat. White legs and feet can be rubbed with powdered chalk to remove any trace of discoloration, and grooming powder will help to keep the hair from matting too quickly in fine, soft coats.

The feet. The dog's feet need careful attention, especially if there is long hair between the toes. All sorts of things can get caught here, like small stones or seeds which embed themselves into the soft skin and cause intense irritation. Feel between the toes with your fingers, then use a small comb to separate the hairs. The pads can receive a lot of punishment, especially when the animal gets a type of exercise outside the normal pattern. A dog which normally exercises on grass but has a day out involving lots of roads may damage its pads quite severely. A day at the beach may be an unusual and enjoyable experience for the dog but could possibly harm its feet. Take time during the daily grooming to examine the pads. Apply a little vegetable oil and work it well into the skin if they look dry or cracked, and pack in some antiseptic ointment if they are bruised or lacerated.

The face. Finish the grooming procedure by cleaning the dog's eyes and nostrils. Use a fresh piece of damp cotton to wipe out each eye and another piece for the nostrils. If the nose is inclined to dry up or become caked with dirt, try softening it with petroleum jelly rubbed well into the skin. The ears must be kept clean at all times. Use dry cotton buds to wipe away accumulated dust and wax from the complicated folds inside the ear flaps. Never use

Dalmatians should have a glossy look to their coats and this can be achieved by a daily rubbing down with a grooming glove to remove dead hairs and the dust collected from outdoor romping, and an occasional shampoo.

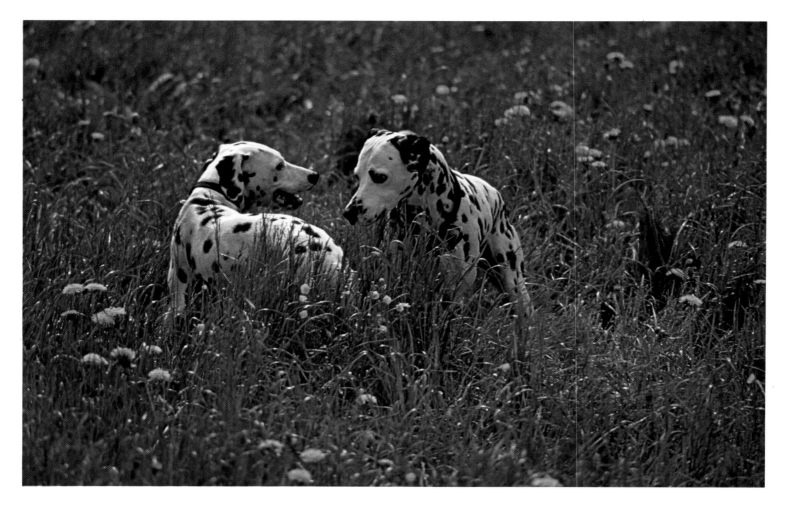

these buds to poke around within the ear, however. If you do so you may easily damage the ear's delicate structures.

HOUSETRAINING

Housetraining a puppy takes care, understanding and patience and you should use the puppy's built-in behavior patterns as an aid to training. If you watch your puppy carefully you will see that after it wakes from a deep sleep it will start to play, then after 5 or 10 minutes it circles backwards before defecating. Play resumes for 15 or 20 minutes more, and is followed by an hour's sleep before the cycle starts again. Defecation also occurs about five minutes after each meal. It is not difficult, therefore, to guess when the puppy needs to be taken into the yard.

Prepare a section of the yard, preferably screened, for use by the dog. It is unsatisfactory to allow your dog to soil random areas of the lawn and flowerbeds; furthermore, the urine of the female dog soon patterns grassed areas with round brown patches. The chosen area of yard should be well drained and spread with a fairly thick layer of coarse sand ballast, gravel, or ashes topped by dry garden peat. Urine will filter through the top layers and droppings will soon dry out, when they can be removed and disposed of. A supply of fresh peat is useful for raking over the area from time to time.

During housetraining the young puppy must be lifted and put on this chosen spot whenever you think it is likely to produce results. Remember to choose the most favorable times, five minutes after feeding or after the start of play. Say 'Be good!' or 'Hurry up!' and repeat it in a friendly but brisk tone. When your timing produces a successful result, be lavish in your praise of the puppy and rub its ears or pat its chest. Suitable praise words include 'Very good!', 'Good boy!' or 'Good girl!', as the case may be, with the emphasis always given to the first word. Only after several successes should you begin to punish errors; even then you must be satisfied that they are the fault of the puppy and not the consequence of your lack of attention.

On no account must you slap or smack a puppy at this stage; neither must you indulge in the old-fashioned and barbaric practice of rubbing the pup's nose in its puddles or messes. Any punishment must be given within 30 seconds of the misdeed, otherwise the puppy will not relate the action to the deed. The most effective punishment that you can give closely resembles the sort that would be given by the puppy's mother. A gruff 'No!' sounds very like a bitch's remonstrative growl and is quickly understood. Taking hold of the loose skin at the scruff of the puppy's neck and giving it a shake also works well and simulates canine behavior, for a bitch will often shake her puppies in this way if they misbehave.

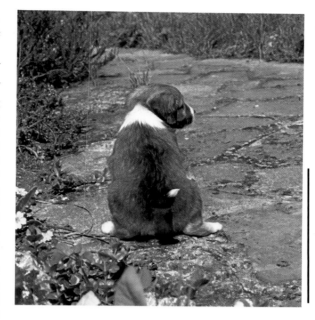

Always ensure that your puppy has a chance to relieve itself last thing at night and first thing in the morning as this will help to reinforce a good training regime.

Early failures in housetraining are generally due to lack of surveillance. Dogs rarely bark to ask to go out but they do indicate their needs in many ways. During housetraining you must be constantly attentive to the pup's needs.

Bladder control at night is slow to develop, so you should make sure that the puppy has the chance to relieve itself before settling down for the night, then get up early in the morning and take it outside at the first opportunity. The little dog will urinate as soon as it wakens, a routine that is quickly established. It will help to reinforce a successful training pattern. If your puppy persistently defecates at night, alter the feeding time by providing the last meal much earlier. This will give the puppy a chance to empty itself before bedtime. Replacing a milk and cereal feed with a smaller meat feed, or vice versa, sometimes helps, but as each puppy is different it is really a matter of trial and error with your own dog.

The kitchen with its washable floor is generally chosen as a young dog's first base. Any accidents should be wiped away with absorbent kitchen paper, the area washed with a mild solution of domestic bleach, then dried with more kitchen paper to prevent the puppy's pads from coming in contact with the chemical. Strong-smelling disinfectants could contain ingredients that are harmful to the young dog's health, but bleach is nontoxic and effectively kills all germs.

If you keep a small dog in an apartment, you may prefer paper-training, which involves spreading several thicknesses of newspaper on a washable floor and putting the puppy on this, instead of outside, for the purposes of elimination. The great disadvantage of this method of training is that the puppy may come to regard any newspaper as an invitation.

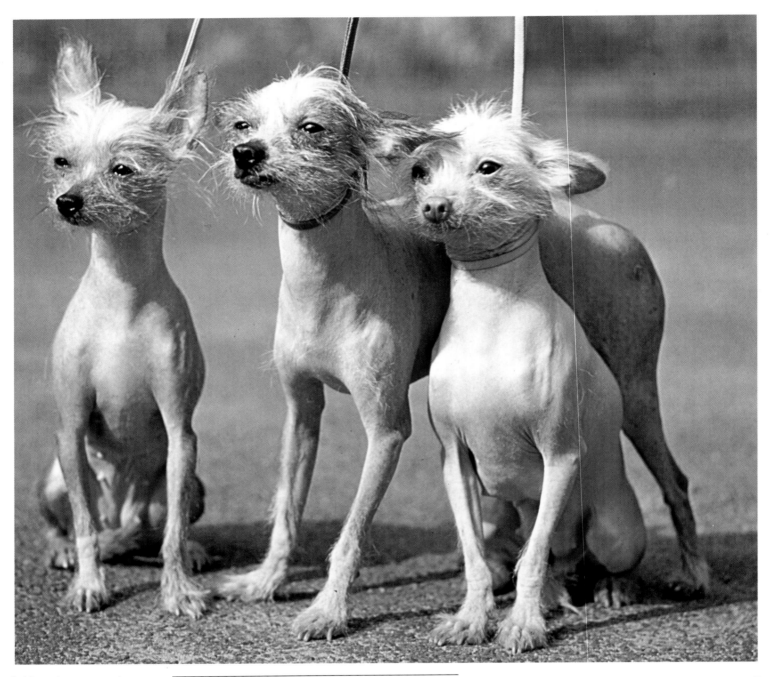

Keeping your dog on a lead at all times when out in the street is safer for the dog and for other people; these Chinese Crested Dogs look happy enough under restraint.

CAR TRAVEL

The sooner your puppy gets used to car travel, the better. The animal's first trip in a car has probably taken it away from familiar surroundings to a new home; all too often the next trip is to the vet for injections. If you allow the dog to associate car travel with frightening or unpleasant experiences, the journeys will always be a problem. Instead, take the puppy along when you take the children to school, so that they can play with it on the way, then feed it when you get home. Once the vaccinations are complete, take the puppy a short distance in the car, then take it out for a romp, so that it will associate the car with enjoyable events. If the puppy is obviously nervous of riding in the car, try feeding it inside when the vehicle is stationary and see that it has its own blanket and a favorite toy to play with.

Your dog must never be allowed to ride along with its head hanging out of the window, as this can cause serious inflammation of the eyes. You will need to train it to sit quietly on the lead and wait patiently until told to get into the car. It is even more important to train the dog to keep sitting quietly inside the car when the door is opened and to wait calmly until it is allowed to get out. It is very dangerous indeed if a boisterous dog leaps out in an uncontrolled way every time the car door opens.

Many puppies are carsick to begin with, so cover the seats with newspapers or old towels at first. Always allow at least three hours to elapse after the last meal before setting out on a journey and give the puppy a chance to exercise and empty itself before departure. Most dogs will grow out of travel sickness and the best way to cure them is to take them for frequent short runs so that they become accustomed to the car's motion.

If you leave a dog in the car at any time, make sure that it has adequate ventilation and that the car is parked in the shade on hot days. You should always see that the dog has a bowl of water on the floor.

DOGS AND THE LAW

Every country has its own laws governing dogs and in countries like Australia or the United States, these can vary from state to state, so owners should check carefully on the regulations in their own area. In most parts of the United States dogs must be licensed once they reach four months of age and the license is conditional on proof of vaccination against rabies. Some states have reduced license fees for spayed or neutered dogs. 'Leash laws' and the strictness with which they are enforced vary widely. In one city dogs may have to be muzzled on the streets or on the lead at all times when away from home; in others, they merely need a collar with a license attached to be within the law.

In Britain, dog licenses have been abolished but the law requires that every dog in a public place must wear a collar with an identity disc giving the owner's name and address. Owners can find themselves subject to heavy penalties if they allow their dogs to chase farm animals and farmers are within their rights to shoot a dog found worrying sheep. You are likely to be held responsible if your dog causes injury or damage to property or person and there are a number of insurance schemes covering this eventuality.

RESPONSIBLE DOG OWNERSHIP

It is up to you, as an owner, to ensure that your dog does not cause annoyance to other people. First and foremost, you should train it to eliminate in the correct place, preferably in a suitably prepared corner of your own yard. Some parks have specially created 'dog lavatories' but dogs should never be allowed to use areas where children may play as toilets. If a city street is the only place where your pet can defecate, use a disposable scoop and bag to remove the mess immediately. Dogs get a bad name through fouling sidewalks but the owners, not the pets, are to blame.

When out in the street dogs should be on the lead at all times and your dog should never be allowed out alone. A loose dog may chase a cat across a road, causing an accident; it may be teased by children and react by biting; it may find and eat some poisonous substance. It is far safer, both for your dog and society at large, if you keep your pet at home except for its supervised exercise.

Gnawing at a large bone will keep a puppy happy for long periods and is good for its teeth but be sure that you never give the type of bone that will splinter.

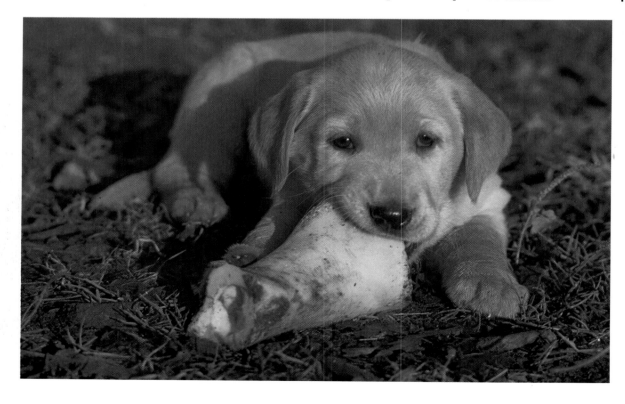

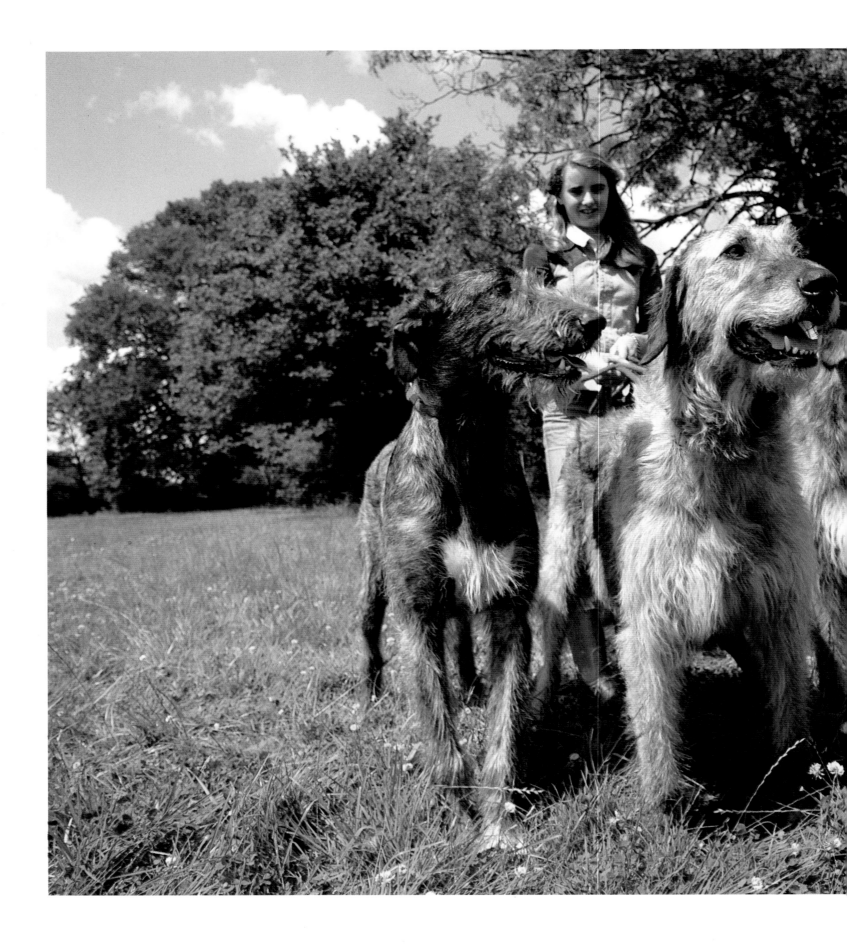

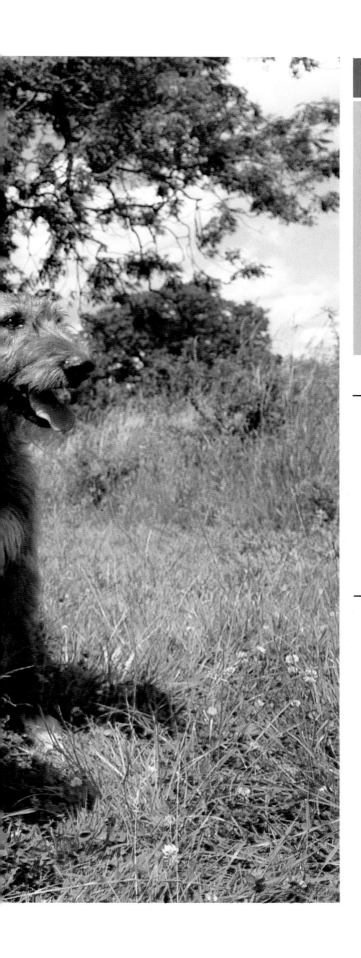

TRAINING
AND OBEDIENCE

Firm and sensitive training will turn a boisterous and uncontrolled animal into a tractable and obedient pet. A good grounding in obedience work means that you can control your dog under all circumstances so that you can keep it out of trouble and protect it from danger. Even if your dog already has a collection of bad habits – chewing your slippers, attacking your visitors, stealing food from the table or barking incessantly whenever you leave it alone – a suitable training regime, plus the right attitude and tone of voice, can achieve a transformation.

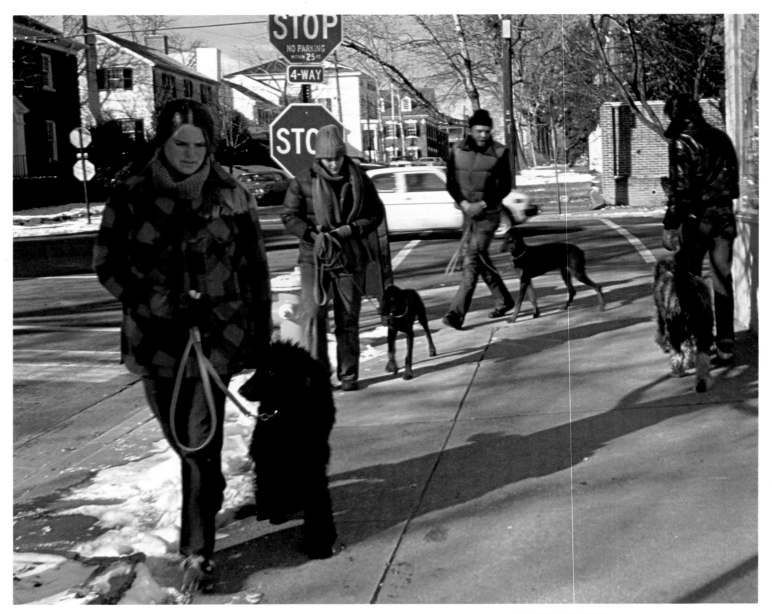

Training a dog in obedience takes a great deal of time and patience and the will to succeed but the results are well worth it. A spoiled dog easily becomes a neurotic dog; it will be happier and more settled if it leads the secure, structured life of a well-trained pet. Any dog can be trained and a mongrel may prove just as responsive as a pedigree animal. Some breeds do learn more easily than others but it is a mistake to think that the most intelligent dog will be the most trainable. A highly intelligent dog may be more resentful of new exercises, needing to be convinced that there is some point in performing them before it will respond to commands. A bold dog with an equable temperament is the best subject for training and may achieve high standards in obedience work while a shy, nervous dog may be able to master only basic exercises.

JOINING A CLASS

Many owners feel that they need help in training their dogs and there are dog training classes and courses in most areas. Most people enroll dogs from the age of six months onwards but do not be discouraged if your dog is well beyond puppyhood and disobeys your every command. The old saying that 'you can't teach an old dog new tricks' is untrue; good training can do a great deal to remedy the situation. Training classes will teach you how to train your own dog and give the animal the chance to socialize with other dogs in a controlled setting. If possible, arrange to go along to a session as an observer before you enroll. You will then know what to expect and you will be able to see how other owners behave, so that you can avoid the more

Training classes can be useful in educating both dogs and owners; after initial training indoors, the class takes to the street, where obedience and good behavior is essential.

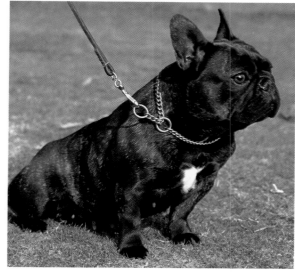

Choke collars can be invaluable in training but must be correctly fitted, as shown here, otherwise they can cause great discomfort.

Use the choke collar only during training sessions and remember to remove the dog's normal collar beforehand. You will not be able to use the choke collar correctly if it is impeded by the normal one. Always remove it after training as a choke collar can be dangerous if left on an unsupervised dog; the ring may catch on something and strangle the animal. Your pet will soon understand that the training collar means lesson time and if the sessions are as enjoyable as they should be, it will show keen excitement when the choke collar is produced.

TRAINING SESSIONS

Proper training should begin when your puppy is between six and eight months old. By this time it should know its name and it should be used to going out wearing collar and lead, even if it does leap about and tug you along. Fit a good quality choke collar of the right size and put this on just before you start the daily lesson. All early training should be carried out on the lead, so that you can reinforce any command you give to the puppy.

Whether the lesson is at home or at training class, make sure that your dog has a good romp beforehand to get rid of excess energy and has every opportunity to relieve itself. Three or four hours should elapse between the dog's last meal and the lesson. Never begin a training session if you are short of time or feeling tired or tense; if you end up snapping at your dog or jerking at its collar impatiently, you may undo a great deal of good work. Lessons need only be about 20 minutes long and shorter lessons of five minutes or so can be worked in with other things, such as playtime.

You must be calm and consistent at all times. A firm, authoritative tone will indicate to your dog that you mean business. Once you have given a command, you must be prepared to persevere until your dog has obeyed. Never shout or attempt to bribe an unwilling dog with tidbits and never, never allow yourself to lose your temper; your dog will only become worried and confused and do even worse. It is a good idea to begin each lesson by repeating exercises that the dog has learned already, so that you can give plenty of praise and the lesson begins on a happy note. You can use the same ploy at the end of the session and at any time during the lesson if things are not going well. The dog should never be allowed to feel a failure; repetition and praise are the keys to training success.

obvious mistakes when you arrive with your own dog. Remember that not all teachers running classes are equally able; note how the teacher handles both dogs and owners and watch the dogs which have been coming to the class for some time. If they behave in the way you wish your dog to behave, then that is the class for you.

Preliminary classes cover all the basic commands; the more advanced classes are for those who wish to progress to the higher levels of obedience work required at competition standard. The classes can teach you valuable lessons but the success of training is up to you. You may need to modify the knowledge you receive to suit your dog's temperament and you will certainly need to reinforce the message of the lessons with daily practice. Many owners claim that the classes have failed, when the fault lies with them because they have not bothered to carry on with the necessary 'homework' between sessions.

CHOKE COLLARS

A choke collar is a very useful training aid. This is a chain with an equal-sized ring at either end; the lead is attached to one ring and the chain slips through the other ring to form a loop. Fitted correctly, the loop will hang loose around the dog's neck but a slight tug on the lead will tighten it so that you can attract the dog's attention or check undesirable behavior. Remember when choosing a choke collar that large curb links that twist to lie flat are the most comfortable. Although narrow chains may look very elegant, they can hurt the dog unduly, cutting into the neck whenever a corrective jerk is given on the lead. To find the correct length of chain collar for your dog, measure around the neck midway between the head and shoulders and add 50 mm (2 in) to the measurement; this is the length of chain your dog will need.

'COME!'

This simple exercise, to teach your puppy to come when called, can be used at the start of each lesson. Have your dog at your left-hand side. Walk smartly forward and allow the dog to walk or trot ahead of you. Call its name and say 'Come!' invitingly, at the same time walking backwards and pulling the slack lead towards you. The first two or three times you do this, you may need to give the lead a smart jerk to attract the dog's attention and to encourage it to follow you; but very soon the dog will come to enjoy this almost as a game, and will bound towards you with pleasure. Give it lots of praise.

THE RELEASE WORD

Before you continue with true training, you need to decide on a 'release' word or phrase which you can use every time you wish to release your dog from the position in which you have left it. Some trainers say 'Okay!', some prefer 'Paid For!' or 'Free Now!'; but whatever you choose, make sure that it cannot be confused with any of the command words that you intend to use during training. The release word may be accompanied by a physical release gesture,

and the well-trained adult dog can be taught to respond to either the word, the gesture, or a combination of the two. The release word is used when you feel that the dog has performed well during training and you have praised or rewarded it. When it is praised or rewarded the dog must not relax its position; but the release word indicates that it may now romp or play.

It is now time to teach the basic 'Sit!', 'Stay!', 'Down!', and 'Wait!' commands as well as correct walking at heel. Keep the lessons short and well structured. Make all the lessons enjoyable; never continue with an exercise when your dog is tired, bored, or distracted by circumstances beyond your control. Try to use the same training lead for every lesson. Your dog should enjoy learning and show signs of excitement when the training equipment is produced.

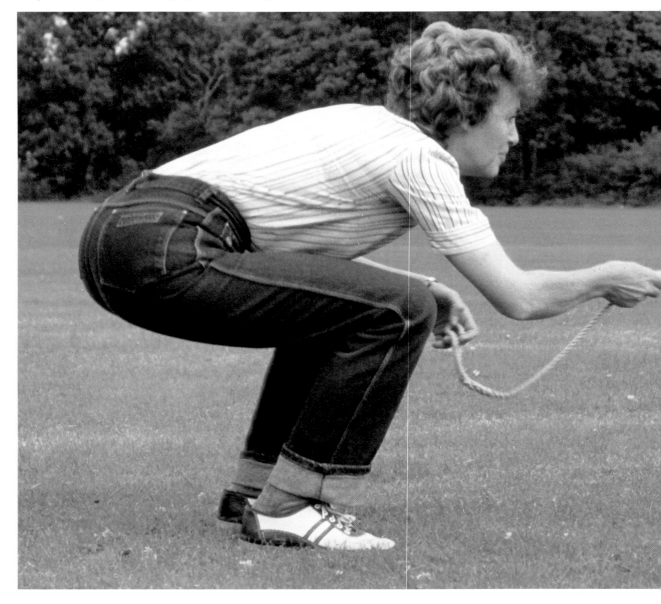

'HEEL!' AND 'SIT!'

In teaching your dog to walk at heel you want it to stride eagerly along on your left-hand side with its right shoulder about even with your left knee. Fit the choke collar correctly so that it can be tightened or slackened at will. Attach it to the training lead. Hold the spare length of lead in your right hand and level with your waist. It should have a slight loop in it so that no tension is exerted on the choke collar. To start the exercise, give the command 'Heel!' in a firm and businesslike manner, jerk the lead very slightly and move off with the left foot. Your stride should be short and bouncy and the pace fairly brisk. Keep your left hand free of the lead and use it to encourage the dog to keep close by tapping your left thigh or clicking your fingers. You may find it helpful to carry a small article in your left hand to keep your dog interested – one of its favorite squeaky toys, perhaps, or a biscuit. Avoid grabbing at your dog as this could make it hand-shy, which is difficult to cure.

Start by walking in straight lines. If your dog is inclined to pull to the left, walk close to a fence or wall. Repeat the command 'Heel!' from time to time, using a pleasant tone and chat to your dog while it walks along. Keep the dog constantly alert and do not let its attention wander from the lesson. If it drags behind, give the lead a short sharp jerk to bring the dog forward, repeat 'Heel!' and keep on walking. You may need to repeat this once or twice. When the dog comes forward to the correct position, give it verbal praise.

Some dogs persistently pull forward on the lead during heelwork training but it is a great mistake to try to counteract this by pulling on the lead. If you

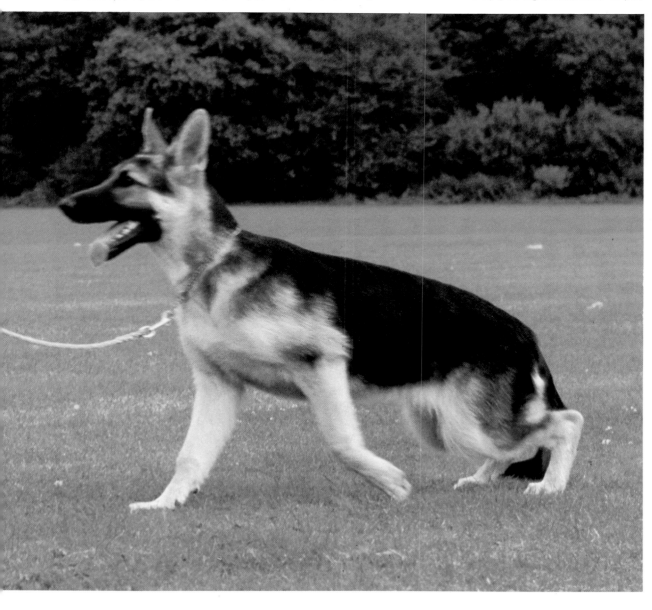

It is essential to teach a young dog to come to you whenever you call. This exercise is taught by having the dog on a long training lead and encouraging it to come forward eagerly when it is asked to do so.

do this, the walk will become a trial of strength with you and the dog pulling against each other. When the dog is walking correctly, the lead will be slightly slack; as soon as the dog pulls forward, give a reminder on the choke collar by taking the slack of the lead in the left hand and jerking it sharply backwards. Your dog will soon learn that it is most comfortable to trot along at your side, and that pulling forward or hanging back results in an unpleasant jerk on its neck.

Every time you decide to stop, put your dog into a sitting position on your left side, facing forward, and with its right shoulder still near your left knee. To encourage it to sit from the walk, give the 'Sit!' command, raise your right hand to keep the dog's head high and lean over and use your left hand to push down on the dog's rump. The 'Sit!' command should be given in a firm voice and slightly drawn out, emphasizing the 't'. Insist on instant reaction from your dog in this exercise. Do not accept sloppy results with the dog swiveling around to sit sideways, half sitting, going right down or rolling over. Repeat the 'Heel!' and walk for a few paces, then repeat the 'Sit!'. Try to avoid giving the commands at the same points in the yard as it is important to prevent your dog from connecting landmarks with commands.

When the dog sits correctly and you have praised it, wait a moment, and then give your release word in a pleased voice along with your chosen release gesture, best given with a gentle tap of the foot to a small dog or a nudge with the knee. Using hand gestures for release is not a good idea, as you use your hands for praise and reward and the dog could misunderstand your wishes. Most dogs enjoy being released and leap around excitedly like small boys let out of school.

When your dog walks well to heel on straight lines, start teaching it right-hand and left-hand circles. Begin by walking in a fairly large circle to the right. Encourage the dog to keep close to your left knee by giving slight jerks with the lead in your right hand, slapping your thigh with your left as an encouragement, and continually repeating the 'Heel!' command. Continue to reinforce the 'Sit' exercise while working on the circle, give lots of praise when the work goes well, but stop and start again if it seems to be going badly.

Try not to scold for poor results at first. It is better to ignore bad work and immediately praise the dog when it gets something right. Never let the lesson go on until the dog becomes bored. If things have gone badly, go back to an earlier exercise such as walk to heel on a straight line, put the dog in the sit position, give it praise, and release it for the day.

Walking in a left-hand circle is more difficult, and it is all too easy to fall over your dog until it understands just what is required. It helps if there is some sort of guiding line around which you can steer the dog; your parked car would do, or some

When the dog is walking to heel (below left) it should follow the handler's changes of direction while maintaining its position, with the shoulder alongside the handler's left knee.

When teaching the 'Sit!' command (below right), hold the dog's head in position with the lead, and at the same time press down on the hindquarters. The dog will soon get the idea.

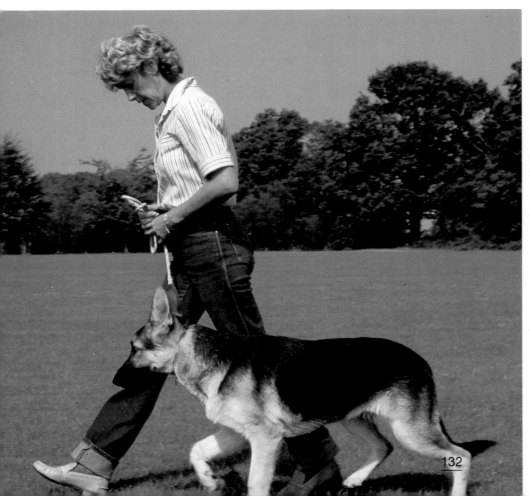

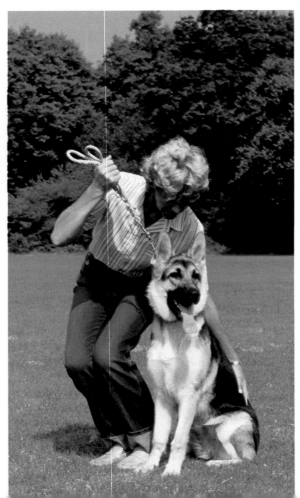

chairs arranged in a circle. Start with the dog sitting at your side in the usual manner. Give the 'Heel!' command and move off with your left foot. Raise the lead slightly with your left hand to guide the dog over to the left if necessary; take longer strides than normal and use your left leg to ease the dog's head and neck into the left-handed circle you require. As soon as you achieve a satisfactory result, praise the dog and end the lesson. Repeat it at the start of the next day's session. Be sure to add lots of sit exercises on these circles, and remember to give the commands at different places each time.

At about this stage in the training, your dog may be getting lax about its sitting position and slow in assuming it. It is important to expect accurate and instant responses at all times, and if you praise the dog for a movement that it has not performed well you will have reinforced the error. Once made and allowed to pass, mistakes are hard to erase; if they are also rewarded with a pat, they may never be erased. If your dog does get lazy about the 'Sit!' command, some stern effort is required to put it right. Walk briskly forward with the dog at heel, give it the order to 'Sit!', jerk up the head slightly with the choke collar and press down the dog's rump; ensure that the dog is pressed well up against your left leg. Walk on and repeat this several times, giving praise when the exercise is well performed. The first time it is done perfectly, praise the dog and release it.

Practice heelwork daily, and prevent boredom by varying your pace, walking in zigzags, serpentines and figures-of-eight as well as in straight lines, squares with sharp corners, and alternate circles. It might seem difficult at first, but with correctly given praise words and the proper use of the choke collar, both you and your dog will become extremely proficient.

'SIT AND STAY'

When your dog sits well on a verbal command and no longer needs the additional aids of lead and hands, proceed to the 'Sit and Stay' exercise. Tell the dog to 'Sit!' in the normal way, then let the slack of the lead loop down to the ground and change the end of the lead from your right to your left hand. Show the dog the palm of your right hand: hold it near its face and give a firm and slightly drawn-out command 'Stay!'. Repeat the word, hold the hand towards the dog and take a long slow step to your right. Extend the left arm so that the lead does not pull the dog towards you. The dog should remain sitting and watching you. Repeat the word 'Stay!' and reverse your step until you are next to your dog once more. If the dog does not move, praise it and repeat the exercise once or twice more, but keep this first lesson quite short. If the dog does move, either to lie down or to follow you to the right, put it back in position and try again. Punish movement with a

stern 'No!' before repositioning the dog with the 'Sit!' command. Repeat this exercise daily; when the dog seems really steady, develop the movement.

This is done in stages. The first progression is carried out by looping the end of the long training lead onto the thumb of your left hand. Sit the dog in the usual position, give the 'Stay!' command and take the long step to your right. Fully extend your left arm so that your hand is virtually over the dog's head. Using your left thumb as a pivot point, slowly walk anticlockwise right around your dog until you are back in the normal training position once more. The dog must not move. If it does, start again from the beginning and revert to the original Sit and Stay exercise if necessary until you achieve a positive result, then praise profusely and release the dog. Work the Sit and Stay exercise in with daily heelwork and random sits so that the dog has variety in its exercises.

When you are confident that the dog will stay in the Sit position while you circle around, try the Stay without the lead. Practice first of all by putting the end of the lead on the ground while you ask for the 'Stay!' and take your long step to the right. If this is successful, walk in a circle around your dog and return to the training position. If your work is progressing satisfactorily the dog will remain motionless; if you are rushing things or have a slow or willful dog, go back to a previous stage and work up to the 'Stay!' once more.

The next stage is to remove the lead while the dog is at Sit and Stay and to walk away. Always take the side step first before moving forward so your dog does not think it should go forward at heel. Your dog should, by now, connect your sideways step with remaining motionless, and your left-foot-forward step with going to heel.

Walk only a few paces away from your dog at first and keep repeating the 'Stay!' command in a calm and steadying manner. Always return to the training position before praising the dog, then either continue with a new exercise or give the release. Vary your procedure so that the dog never anticipates the release and waits for your next instruction at all times. When you and your pet have mastered this exercise, you will have reached an important stage in training, and your dog will realize that 'Stay!' always means that you are going to return to its side.

'WAIT!' AND 'COME!'

When you want the dog to remain in its position initially and then to come to you when you call, you must teach a different word to avoid confusion in the animal's mind. 'Wait!' is a very important command, and must be thoroughly and correctly taught from the outset. The easiest way to start this exercise is to sit the dog in the normal way, praise it a little, then move quietly around in front of it. Place your right hand in front of the dog's nose, showing the palm, and say 'Wait!' in a low and drawn-out way. Holding the end of the slackened training lead in your left hand, take small steps backwards away from your dog, repeating the command, until you get to the end of the lead. If the dog remains motionless, call its name and say 'Come!' in a pleased and welcoming way. Give a little pull on the lead if it seems reluctant to obey. When the dog reaches you, praise it and try to get it to sit facing you.

If all goes well, the 'Wait!' command can be given again while you move back once more to reinforce the lesson. If the dog moves forward as you start to reverse, you must begin again, taking one small step at a time. This exercise must be taken very slowly

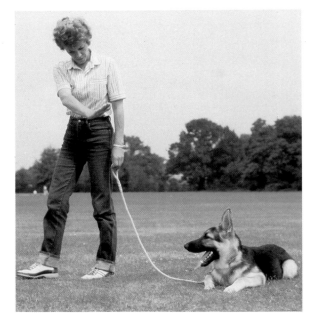

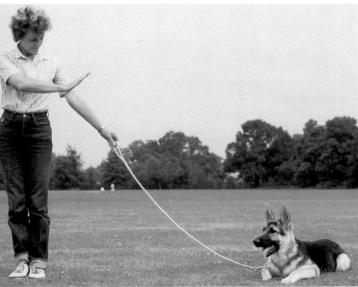

and built into the previous program without letting your dog get bored. Only when it is completely mastered should you go on to the next stage.

Replace the training lead with a long thin cord so that you can extend your distance from your dog while remaining in control if it moves away from its sitting position. Always make your 'Come!' command as welcoming as possible, and fuss your dog in its favorite way whenever it responds correctly. A tidbit encourages some dogs, especially those of willful or scatterbrained breeds which are easily distracted. Keep a favorite biscuit or liver treat in the palm of your hand and make sure your dog knows that it is there. In the 'Come!' exercise, recall your dog and add an arm gesture by holding your hand up to your chest or by extending your arms. If the hand with the tidbit is held up to your chest, the dog is likely to race towards you and sit immediately, looking up at your face expectantly, hoping for the tidbit. Do not give a tidbit every time; vary the reward so that your dog does not require constant food bribes in order to perform correctly.

When you are certain that the dog will come to you from the Wait position when you recall it, remove the cord. If you have some failures and your dog runs off or will not come right up to you, revert to more controlled methods for a while.

At this stage, your young dog should be giving you a great deal of satisfaction, walking to heel at all paces, sitting when told and staying on command until your return.

'DOWN AND STAY'

Once your dog reaches this point in training, you are ready to teach the 'Down!' command. If your dog was apt to collapse in a heap every time you wanted it to sit, you may find that it is slightly bewildered to find that you now want it to take up that previously unacceptable position. Teach your dog to lie down on command by pulling the lead forward, giving the command 'Down!' in a low voice and, if necessary, getting down on the ground with the dog. With a large dog you may gently pull its forelegs forward and press down on its shoulder blades until it is in the desired position. Praise the dog when it is down correctly. If it persists in getting up, persevere until you are successful. Take several days perfecting this exercise. Only when your dog goes into the down position promptly and without any fuss should you progress to the 'Down and Stay' exercise.

This is taught in exactly the same way as the Sit and Stay. Use a loosely looped lead and step away to the dog's right then walk slowly around in a circle. Praise the dog only when it remains in the down position; if it deviates from this, start from the beginning again. End the lesson as soon as you achieve the desired result. Never recall your dog from the Down position. It should be fixed in its

1 Having given the command and shown the dog the flat of her hand, the handler takes a side step to the right before moving smoothly and slowly away.

2 The stay command is constantly repeated and reinforced by the hand signal until the handler has reached the limit of the training lead's length.

mind as a stationary posture, so that it always remains in position until you return and give the release signal.

If your dog has successfully performed all these exercises it will have reached an acceptable level for a family dog. Try and perfect these simple exercises until your dog happily responds both on and off the lead. The Down exercise should be practiced frequently and at length, until your dog immediately drops down at your command, no matter what it is doing. This training can save a dog's life, as you can control it from a distance, even in a hazardous situation.

'LEAVE!'

The command 'Leave!' can also be a lifesaver. The object of the exercise is to teach your dog to leave an object alone until you release it with another simple command.

A good way of teaching the lesson is to show the dog a favorite treat, like a tasty biscuit, but make the animal leave it alone until you give permission. Put the dog on its choke collar and lead, and hold it in check with your left hand. Start at the Sit position, as this makes control easier. Show the dog the biscuit and say 'Leave!' in a very commanding voice. Put the treat on the ground just out of the animal's reach. The dog will naturally go to take the biscuit but you must pull it back with a short jerk, repeating the 'Leave!' command. When you wish the dog to take the biscuit use a different release word. If 'Okay!' is your normal release, use 'Paid For!' or 'Fetch it!'. Dogs quickly learn this exercise and before long you will be able to add refinements such as rolling the biscuit past your dog, or even throwing it, and the dog will not pounce on it until you indicate that it is allowed to do so.

The exercise can be expanded to include all sorts of things. Dogs can be prevented from being destructive by learning this command. You can shout 'Leave!' from your bedroom window when you notice your pet digging up a rose bush or about to chase the neighbor's cat. It can prevent the inquisitive dog from being stung by bees or wasps and stealing cake from the tea table. As usual, it is important that your dog obeys the command instantly and without question, knowing that it will eventually receive a reward.

THE RETRIEVE

Many dogs have a natural instinct to retrieve objects. It presumably dates back to their ancestors' wild state when food was carried to the den. Some gundogs are bred for their propensity to retrieve, and such breeds can be trained very easily. A young puppy should be encouraged to carry its toys around in its mouth; if it has been scolded for doing so, it will be more difficult to teach this exercise.

Train the retrieve by having your dog on a long line or cord and sitting at your left-hand side. Throw a suitable article, either a proper training dumbbell or a piece of wood of similar size, and give the 'Fetch!' command in an encouraging manner. The dog should run and pick up the article. Once this has occurred, gently pull the line and give the 'Come!' command. When the dog responds, ask it to sit in front of you and praise it for holding the article well. Take the dumbbell or wood in both hands, give a command such as 'Drop it!', and gently remove the article from the dog's jaws. Take care not to hurt your pet's mouth in removing the object, and praise it profusely for a job well done. It is a short progression to working off the lead, and then to training the dog to fetch any article you point to. If a young dog races about excitedly with the object retrieved, you must go back to an earlier stage of the exercise.

TRICKS

If your dog proved to be a good learner you might like to try teaching it a few party tricks. This should only be attempted after your dog has completely

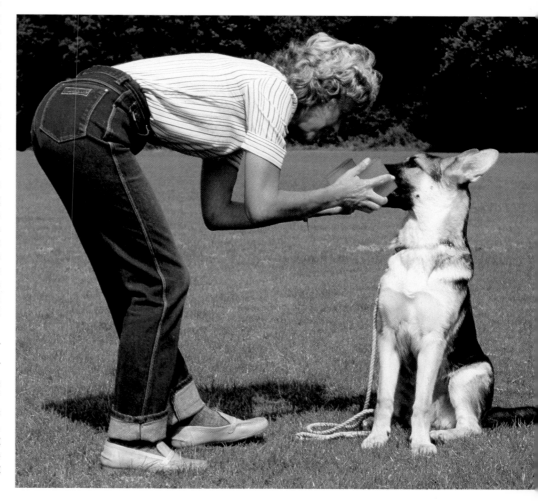

3 After a successful retrieve, the dumbbell should be taken gently from the dog's mouth, with plenty of praise for a job well done.

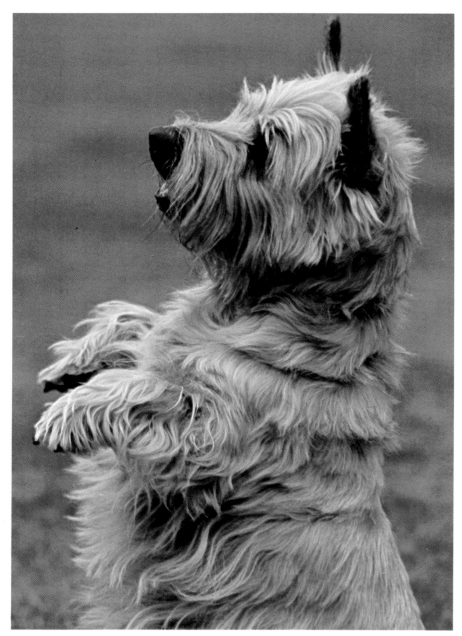

haunches and it is unkind to try to teach them to do so. Short-legged, stocky dogs like Pugs or Sealyhams find this trick very easy and hardly need any teaching. Wait until your puppy is at least six months old, then start by holding a tempting tidbit just out of reach over its head. Say 'Beg!' or 'Up!' in a pleasant but firm manner and gently lift up the front end of the pup. Find the point of balance and repeat the command, simultaneously giving the reward. Repeat the process, encouraging the dog to balance itself. Take plenty of time or it may panic, and be ready with a steadying hand at the first sign of a wobble. If the dog is very unsteady, try practicing in a corner, so that the walls give support and a feeling of security. A perceptive puppy grasps this trick very quickly and soon your puppy will be sitting up appealingly at every opportunity. Never reward this behavior when the family is eating or your dog will become a mealtime pest that has to be banished from the room. Reward sitting up only after you have given the command and not when the dog does it voluntarily, trying to scrounge an extra tidbit.

As your dog grows up, you may notice little habits which can be developed naturally into its own particular tricks. Some dogs are able to throw objects; some, particularly the retrieving breeds, enjoy carrying articles in their mouths; others learn to lift a rug and hide an article underneath. These actions are variations of normal canine behavior and can be expanded by encouragement and reward, as well as a command or signal to indicate when they should be carried out.

One of these tricks is 'shaking hands'. Tiny puppies instinctively knead at the bitch to stimulate the milk supply, so kneading becomes an action associated with pleasure. As they grow up, the puppies often feed off the bitch as she is standing up and as they would topple over if they tried to knead, they sit down and reach up with one paw. This is why so many dogs seem to teach themselves to shake hands. To teach a dog to shake hands on command, sit or kneel and have the dog sitting in front of you. Give the command 'Shake hands!' and

This little Cairn Terrier cheerfully begs for a tidbit but this trick should not be taught too early as the puppy's back may not be strong enough.

Some dogs love to carry things in their mouths (right) but it may mean that your newspaper arrives slightly damp.

mastered its basic training and can be relied upon to be obedient and well-behaved in all situations. It would be unfair to encourage your pet to perform in a way that makes it appear foolish or to let the dog feel a failure if it does not master a particular trick. Tricks are taught by encouraging the desired behavior in easy stages and giving rewards when they are properly performed. Though in basic training the rewards may be a pat and verbal praise, tricks are usually rewarded with a tidbit.

One of the favorite tricks is having the dog sit up and beg. It is only suitable for small to medium-sized dogs of the right conformation. Dogs with very long backs or long legs find it virtually impossible to balance while sitting up on their

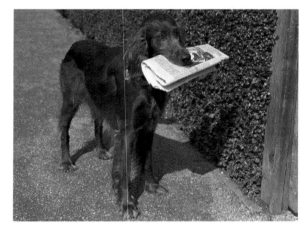

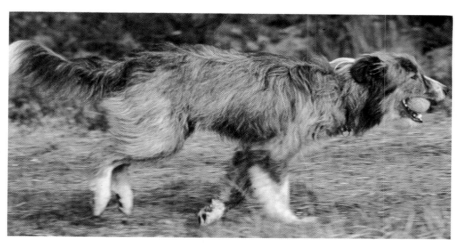

It is part of the dog's hunting instinct to chase and carry a ball, so this is a very easy form of behavior to teach; some dogs find it just as easy to catch a ball thrown by the owner.

at the same time press against its right shoulder with your left hand. This will make the dog move its paw off the ground, so take the paw in your other hand and praise the dog well. Gradually ease the left hand pressure, simply giving the command and holding out your other hand. Once the dog has grasped the idea, repeat the process with the other paw, saying 'Now the other one'.

To play 'dead' or 'die for your country' is a little more difficult. Assuming that you have taught your dog to lie down on command, the next step is to teach it to lie on one side: give a command such as 'On your side!', gently push the dog into position and hold it there. Once the dog will do this on its own and remain steady, give the command 'Dead!' in a harsh tone of voice that will tend to make it 'freeze'. Try to keep your dog quite still even for a few seconds at the beginning. Once the dog understands the command and responds, encourage it to go straight into the 'dead dog' position from standing, pushing it down gently with your hand. Do not praise or reward too soon or the dog will not stay in position long enough.

It can be useful, as well as entertaining, if a dog can bark on command. To begin with, give the command 'Speak!' every time the dog barks of its own accord. As it begins associating the word with the action, offer a tidbit and say 'Speak!'. When the dog gets the idea and barks, give the tidbit and plenty of praise. Practice often enough and the dog will soon be barking each time you give the command.

Some dogs are naturals at learning to catch on command but others seem to miss every time at first. Put your dog on the lead and have it sitting or standing in front of you. Have a pocketful of small biscuits and show it the food in your hand. When it is watching, give the command 'Catch!'. At first, throw the biscuit towards the dog from a very short distance. If it misses, check it with the lead, pick up the biscuit yourself and try again. If you are lucky and the dog catches a piece fairly soon, praise it and finish the training for the day. If the dog does not

seem to be making any progress, finish for the day by dropping a piece of biscuit into its mouth and praising it well. Each lesson must finish with a success, no matter how small it may be, so that the dog feels happy and will be pleased when the next session starts.

CURING BAD HABITS

Many dogs grow up with bad habits – leaping uncontrollably at every visitor who steps into the house, barking when left alone, growling when you try to push them off your best bedspread and so on. If your dog exhibits bad behavior, it may be due to nervousness, insecurity, loneliness or overexcitement but whatever the cause, bad habits can be cured if you adopt the right strategy and persevere until you are successful.

The overall rules are much the same as those used in initial training but there are several important 'don't's' for owners of problem dogs:

● Don't take the easy way out. If you give a command, work to see that it is obeyed; otherwise your dog will not see any reason to change its ways.

● Don't threaten your dog. You may frighten it into obedience in the short term, but it will learn nothing – except, perhaps, to keep out of your way at the crucial time.

● Don't punish bad behavior unless you catch the dog in the act. Any punishment or reprimand must be given within 30 seconds of the offense, otherwise the animal will not link the two events.

● Don't rush. Bad habits will not be cured overnight. You will need to consolidate each small advance before going on to the next lesson.

● Don't give a dog that is apt to misbehave when you are out of the house a stiff lecture just before you leave. It will not understand and you may leave it so anxious or excited that its bad behavior becomes even worse.

AGGRESSION

Never allow your dog to growl, snap or show its teeth at you. When a dog shows aggression within the home, it may be trying to dominate the family members and needs to be shown its proper place in the hierarchy. Increasing the standard exercises of obedience training to several short sessions a day will help to establish your place as pack leader. Make sure that you are in control at all times. If your dog gives out any aggressive signals, ignore it completely; when it comes to you for a pat, brings its ball for a game or puts its head on your lap, simply walk away without speaking. Then when you are ready, give it the command 'Down!' and when it obeys, give it the petting or the game it was seeking. If your dog only growls when it is in a particular position, such as under the table, on the bed or in a favorite chair, then wrap heavy plastic

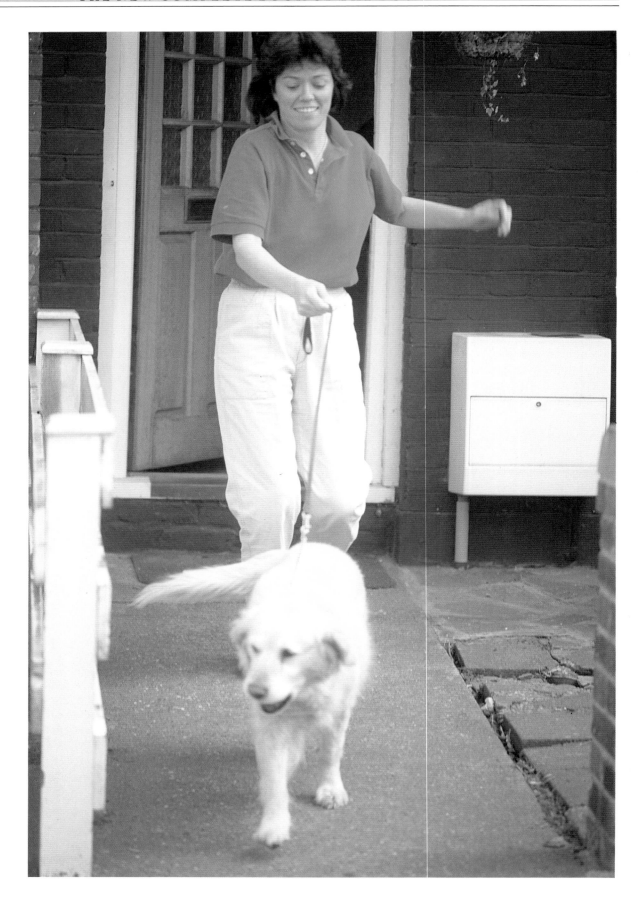

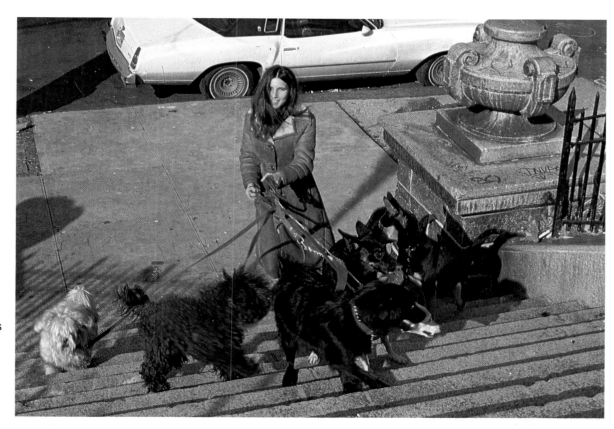

This American dog-walker has her hands full, coping with a bunch of dogs that have not been well-trained in walking to heel and obeying commands.

around the table legs to block off the area, close the bedroom door to keep the dog out or remove the chair altogether. If this is impractical because your dog has so many little 'territories' that it guards aggressively then keep it on the lead while in the house and use the lead to move it from place to place, so that you can be dominant without putting your hand near the bared teeth. If the dog is only aggressive towards one particular member of the family, then that person should practice obedience training with the dog, when it is restrained on its choke collar and lead. Otherwise you might try putting that person in charge of feeding the dog; if it is very aggressive, you might need to keep it on the lead during feeding times at first, punishing any show of aggression with a sharp jerk, so that the dog learns that this behavior will not be tolerated.

CLIMBING ON FURNITURE

Most dogs have an unerring instinct for finding the most comfortable piece of furniture in the living room and, if allowed, will monopolize the best armchair or spread themselves over the sofa. If you do not want your dog to sit on the furniture, you should train it from its first days in your household. Alternatively, you might allow it to sit on one chair but not another; with attentive training, the dog will quickly grasp the difference. If you find that the dog sneaks onto the forbidden furniture when there is

no one to see, then either exclude it from the room altogether when there is nobody to supervise or stand the seat cushions on end when you are out of the room for a time. If you allow your pet to sit on a particular chair, it is wise to train the dog to vacate it instantly when ordered to do so. Make sure that the command you use will not be confused with 'Down!' or any other command used in basic training. 'Off' or 'Go' might be suitable, if you do not use them for different activities.

PULLING ON THE LEAD

If your dog pulls on the lead, the worst thing you can do is to let yourself be pulled along faster and faster. This simply tells the dog that this is a delightful pastime. Sufficient attention to heelwork should cure the problem but if a normally obedient dog is a habitual puller, try giving the 'Heel' command as soon as the dog starts pulling, then to turn smartly and walk in the opposite direction, so that the dog follows you, not the other way around. It may be difficult to make these methods work with large, strong dogs capable of pulling their owners off their feet. This is one of the few occasions when a rolled-up newspaper may come into its own. Begin walking with your dog at your side and every time it tries to pass you to pull ahead, tap its nose with the newspaper. The dog will try to avoid this, so practice alongside a fence or wall. Many large dogs

Never allow yourself to be hauled along by a dog that pulls on the lead or the dog will take a delight in pulling you faster and faster.

get very excited when they know that they will soon be going for a walk. A quick run around the yard off the lead helps to take the edge off this excitement.

WANDERING

If your dog persistently jumps over the fence and runs away for the day you must take action. No dog should be allowed to roam free, for no matter how well-behaved it may be at home, you have no means of knowing what it would do in an unusual situation, and it could cause injury to itself or others. Make the fence higher if your dog is able to jump over it, or keep your pet on an extendable running line when it is left alone in the yard. Such lines can easily be fastened onto a hook on an outside wall, or looped around a gatepost. The end is clipped onto the dog's collar and the line pulls out of the holder as the dog runs around. Any slack is drawn back in, so that there is no chance of the animal becoming entangled. However, keeping a dog on a running line should not be used as a substitute for proper exercise and playtimes, and it should not be left alone out of doors for long periods, as loneliness and boredom will only encourage other bad behavior, such as barking or digging in the flower bed.

MOUNTING

Owners become very worried when their young dogs begin mounting table legs, or other male dogs, convinced that their pet is oversexed. Though many dogs do stop this behavior when they become adult, it is better to put a stop to it as early as possible, before it becomes a habit – a dog that is continually trying to mount a visitor's leg is an embarrassment. If the object of unwanted affection is always the same, such as a cushion or a child's cuddly toy, the answer may be as simple as shutting it away where the dog cannot find it. Otherwise, watch the dog closely and, the moment the mounting begins, issue a firm 'No!'. If necessary, take the dog by the scruff of the neck and give a little shake. Then ignore it completely for a few minutes. If there are particular occasions when this behavior happens, such as the exciting few moments when a visitor arrives, then preempt it by calling the dog to 'Sit!' before the visitor enters. Of course, this will only work if your dog is trained in basic obedience already. If your dog is mounting anything and everything and nothing that you do has any effect, consult your vet. A short course of hormone injections may improve matters; otherwise castration may be the answer.

PHOBIAS

Some dogs become terrified of certain noises: fireworks send many pets into a panic but everyday noises like the vacuum cleaner or the ringing of the phone can have the same effect on some animals and others cower in terror whenever a visitor arrives at the door. This behavior will not cure itself and will probably get worse if neglected. It may be worth asking the vet to prescribe tranquilizers for a scheduled fireworks party and tranquilizers may also be useful for calming the dog while you retrain it, but they are not a long-term solution. Instead you will need to spend time 'desensitizing' the dog, in a process similar to that used for human phobia sufferers. If, for instance, your pet cowers shivering in a corner or runs in frenzied circles every time the phone rings, enlist the aid of a friend who will make a series of calls on schedule. Muffle the phone with a blanket and take your dog to the part of the house furthest from the instrument. At first your friend should let the phone ring four or five times; while it is ringing, stay with the dog, talk soothingly and feed it tidbits. Once your dog can remain calm under these circumstances, progress in easy stages until the phone is in the same room. Organize two or three rings on a muffled phone to begin with, still petting and soothing your dog, then progress to longer calls, then remove the blanket from the phone. Follow the same pattern if, for instance, your dog is afraid of visitors. First ask someone to walk up the path without coming to the door, then to walk up the path and stand on the step, then to ring the doorbell without coming in, and so on. Never try to speed up the process or you will undo all your good work. The more patient you can be, the better the final results.

DESTRUCTIVE DOGS

The puppy naturally chews things to help in the cutting of its second teeth, and because of this, it may well cause damage in the home. A young dog should never be left alone where it can spoil valuable property or furnishings. It should be confined within a playpen while you are out of the house and given its own toys and rawhide chews to play with. Some adult dogs resent being left alone and become distressed, scratching at doors and carpet. Unless checked, this behavior may develop into determined tearing and chewing. It is pointless to punish such misdeeds as soon as you arrive home, because the dog will be so pleased to see you that the punishment will seem to the dog to be linked with the exuberance of its greeting. If you expect to leave your dog alone for long periods, you should prevent the onset of destructive behavior by early training.

If the problem has become ingrained you have several alternative solutions. The first and most obvious is never to leave your dog alone. You may have the sort of job which enables you to take your pet to work. Other dogs give up destructive behavior if they are allowed the complete run of the house, but it may be impracticable to try this out for

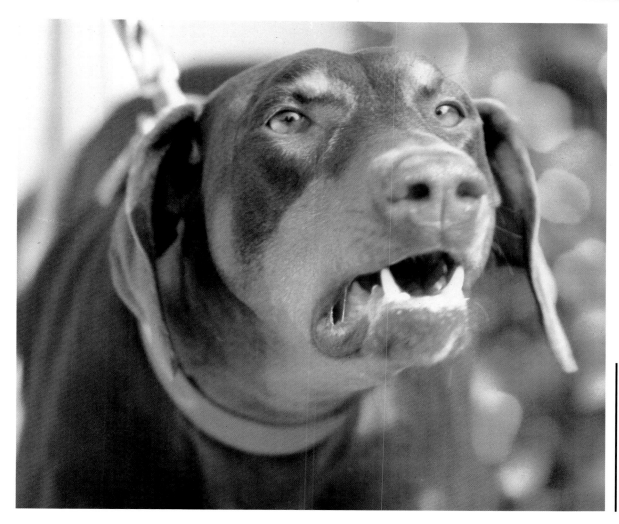

Most owners find it useful to have a dog that will bark to warn of approaching strangers, but if it barks at every sound, or goes on barking for long periods, it is a nuisance to the whole neighborhood.

the first few days, especially if you have valuable belongings. The third alternative is to buy a second dog. When the two animals become friends you will probably find that all destructive behavior ceases completely.

Positive action is needed to retrain a destructive dog. Start by leaving the room and closing the door. Return a minute later and check for damage; if there is none, praise the dog. If some damage has been caused, make a point of examining it but totally ignore your dog. Do not punish the dog as that will not help matters. Sooner or later – and you may need a lot of patience – the dog will be left for a short period without doing any damage. This is the breakthrough point. Take care to extend the periods of isolation very, very gradually until the dog is retrained and may confidently be left alone. Some dogs are less troublesome if the television is left on for company.

BARKING

A dog that barks incessantly for no apparent reason is a nuisance to owners and neighbors and such

behavior must be stopped at once. Young puppies are unable to bark at all, and when they first learn to do so they often look surprised at the noise they manage to produce. Although it can be tempting to encourage the puppy to bark it is a mistake to do so and is difficult to correct later on. A dog will learn to bark aggressively when it feels that either itself or its property is being threatened. If the dog learns this naturally, barking will likely be kept to the minimum and you will know that a bark from your dog really does mean that a stranger is around and not that the animal is merely feeling a bit bored and wants some action. While you must accept the fact that your dog will bark when visitors arrive at your door, the animal must be trained to stop barking when you have let them into the house. The best way to do this is to slip the choke collar and lead onto your dog while it is barking and the doorbell is ringing. Praise the dog, take it to the door and tell it to 'Sit!'. Open the door and invite your guests in while restraining the dog in the Sit position. Punish further barks with a stern 'No!', then allow your dog to meet and greet the visitors.

A dog that persistently barks when left alone in a

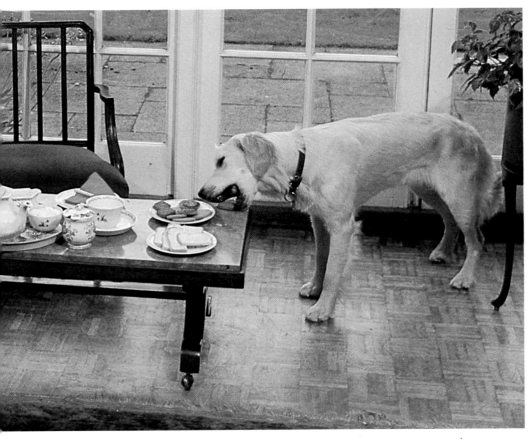

Some dogs cannot resist stealing food at any opportunity. This is unhygienic, as well as annoying, and should be stopped by use of aversion therapy.

times, but in most cases the dog will quickly learn acceptable manners.

If your dog runs up to you and jumps up, the choke collar will be of little use. The easiest way to stop this behavior is to bring your knee up into the dog's chest at the moment it jumps forward. While it is still bewildered by this unkindness, give the 'Sit!' command, then praise the dog. Here again the younger dog should learn very quickly. The lesson, once learned, should never be relaxed, and no one should be allowed to encourage your dog to go onto its hind legs.

STEALING FOOD

It is asking rather a lot of the dog to expect it to sit patiently alone in a room where lots of tempting food is set out and not to steal any. It is a different matter, however, when your dog habitually takes tidbits from your kitchen work surface or dining table when your attention is elsewhere for a moment or two. Teach your dog the 'Leave!' command and get it used to staying away from items of food when you have told it to do so. This behavior can be reinforced by aversion therapy. Fill a soft chocolate or similar delicacy with a teaspoon of mustard and put it on the table. Give the 'Leave!' command, then go out of the room for a moment. If the dog has left the decoy well alone, praise it profusely upon your return. If it has eaten the bait it will have had punishment enough. Some dogs swallow tidbits so fast that they might not taste the mustard, in which case you should offer larger baits that need to be chewed. Repeat this process until your dog is convinced that all stolen food tastes awful. The mustard should deter your dog from stealing, but is not harmful when swallowed.

room can be difficult to retrain. You must shut it in the room then creep away. Immediately when it starts to bark, scold it with a series of severe 'No!' commands. This can be reinforced by clapping your hands as you give the commands. If it still has no effect you may have to punish the dog physically by shaking the scruff of its neck or even giving the animal a short sharp slap. Only do this while the dog is still barking, not after the barking has ceased.

JUMPING UP

An exuberant dog will often run up to visitors and friends and jump up against them, trying to get its mouth as close as possible to the visitor's face. While this is natural behavior for the dog, it is usually unacceptable to people, particularly if the dog has been romping in the yard and has muddy paws. Jumping up is easily corrected in any dog, but the sooner it is done the better. Have the dog on a choke collar and a long training lead or length of line and set up the situation beforehand with an assistant. The assistant should walk naturally in through the front gate, for example, or through a door. The dog will run forward as usual in greeting. Just as the dog starts to jump up, jerk the lead hard and command a very stern 'No!' Give the 'Sit!' command, and if it is obeyed the assistant can make a fuss of the dog. This may have to be repeated a few

CHASING CATS

Curing a dog of cat-chasing can be quite difficult. The best way undoubtedly is to have a dog-proof cat – a really tough and fearless animal which, instead of running away from the dog, fluffs up and gives it a good scratch across the sensitive end of its nose. If your dog chases your own cat you will need to work hard at trying to make them friends. Have your dog on the choke collar and lead; every time the cat makes off and the dog leaps up in pursuit, jerk the lead and give a stern 'No!' command. Never encourage your dog to chase anything except a ball or toy that you have thrown for it, and scold it whenever it shows signs of running after birds in the yard.

CHASING VEHICLES

Chasing cars and bicycles is a bad habit which should be stopped promptly before a serious accident occurs. Dogs should never be allowed to

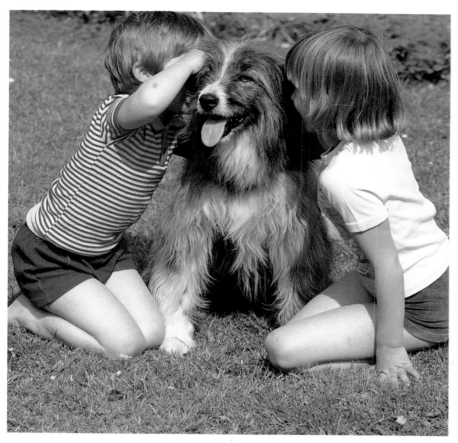

Plenty of petting and handling from puppyhood is the best way to ensure that a dog will allow examination of any part of its head and body.

roam the streets freely, and it is also dangerous if a dog on its lead tries to leap at passing vehicles. To break this aggressive habit, attach a training collar and lead and take the dog to a stretch of road where the traffic is fairly heavy, where there are few pedestrians and the sidewalk is reasonably wide. Make your dog sit correctly on your left side and wait quietly for the first car to pass. As the dog starts to leap forward or bark, jerk it back on the choke collar and give a severe 'No!' command. When this has had some effect, try walking with the dog at heel with traffic coming from behind. Correct impulsive forward moves by the dog until success is achieved. Finish the lesson on a positive note and take the dog home. Repeated and regular lessons are required until your dog is calm with all traffic. It is useful to have a friend ride past you on a bicycle each day while you train the dog to accept this experience in a similar way.

CHASING SHEEP

Sheep have an excitable effect on most dogs. They look vulnerable and run away in an inviting sort of way, often turning to look back at the dog. A great deal of harm can be done to such valuable livestock when they are chased around: pregnant ewes drop premature lambs, for example, and other sheep become so distressed that they may die of heart

failure. Dogs sometimes gang up and methodically hunt down a sheep before savaging it to death – an example of ancient instincts coming to the fore despite centuries of domestication. It is virtually impossible to teach an ordinary family dog not to chase farm animals so you must therefore ensure that your dog always remains under your control. Keep it on a lead during country walks, and if it likes to lope around and explore, use a long cord or line in place of the normal lead.

DIGGING HOLES

All dogs love to dig. This innate behavior dates back to the days when dogs buried the uneaten portion of their kill to hide it from other predators. Nowadays, bitches dig burrows in which to whelp, and over-heated dogs dig earthy pits in which to cool off from the sun. As digging is a natural part of canine behavior, it is very difficult to stop when it is done in an unacceptable place, like the middle of the lawn or around the prize rose bushes. Try to distract the digging dog and give it some other exhausting exercise for a while. Give a firm 'No!' command every time it looks as if it is going to start on another excavation. If these ruses are not effective, you will have to confine your dog to unimportant areas of the yard or invest in a running chain or portable run.

RESENTMENT OF HANDLING

Your dog may show resentment or even aggression when you attempt to touch a particular part of its body. If it has a coat that demands a lot of grooming and it has suffered at your hands through tugging at knots and tangles, this is quite understandable. It is up to you to undo the harm by gentle and careful retraining. It is extremely important for an owner to be able to handle his or her dog under any circumstances and at any time. At the scene of an accident, for example, ease of handling could mean the difference between life and death for your pet. If a puppy shows any resentment when a certain area is touched you will need to begin a familiarization program. Stroke or groom the sensitive part, talk soothingly to the puppy and praise it the moment it ceases to resist. Older dogs take a little longer to retrain, but with plenty of patience success can be achieved.

If a dog tends to snap during this type of training you may have to use a muzzle at first. Properly-made leather muzzles are available in all sizes and the one you choose should fit snugly. If it is too large the muzzle may slip off at the crucial moment; if it is too small it will hurt the dog and cause more resentment. If a muzzle is used, put it on the dog from time to time during normal playtime and exercise. Never let the dog connect the fitting of the muzzle with an unpleasant aspect of training.

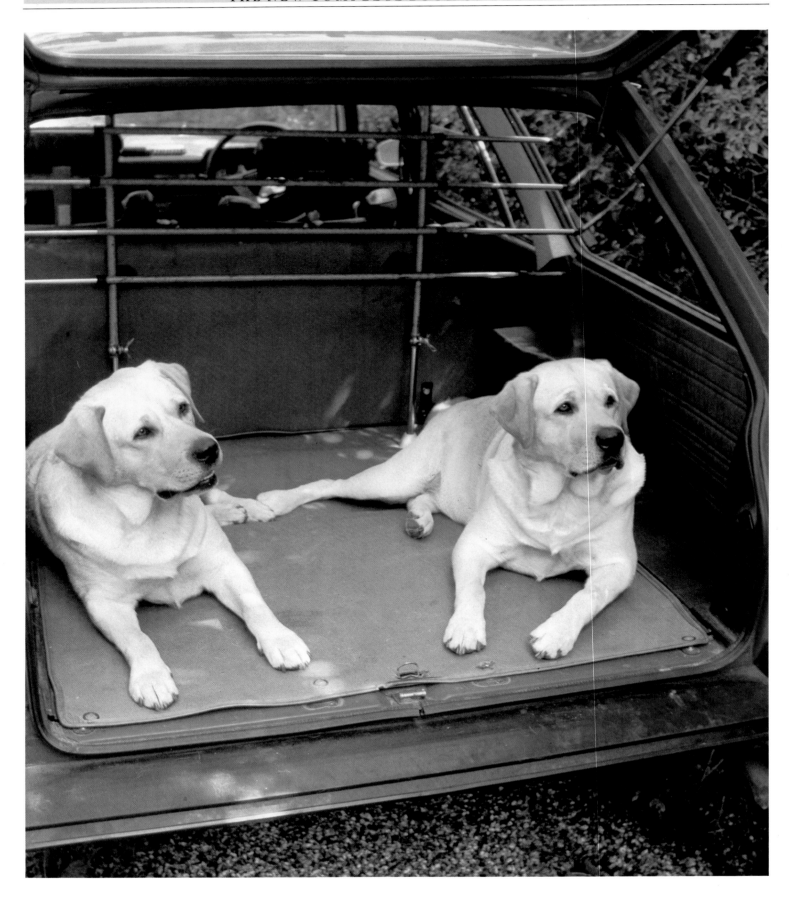

A dog-guard fitted behind the back seats of his station wagon ensures that the dogs cannot jump over the seats and distract the driver.

URINATING INDOORS

If your pet urinates indoors, it may be an extension of the territorial marking that normally goes on outside. This may happen when another dog or a human visitor arrives in the house and the visit stimulates it to mark out its ownership. Your best defense is vigilance: noticing the danger times and moving quickly to prevent the behavior. Dogs usually have favorite spots for territorial marking and you may be able to rearrange furniture or close doors to make the spot unavailable. Clean up the spots very thoroughly with bleach or biological stain remover.

Some dogs urinate when they are overexcited and an owner who then gets angry and shouts or smacks the dog is only raising the excitement level and compounding the problem. Instead, you should ignore the dog if it wets the floor and concentrate on keeping its life as calm as possible. If your dog is so excited about your return home that it loses control of its bladder, stop greeting it with enthusiasm and open arms; instead greet it coolly without looking at it and save the petting until later when the dog is calmer. If it tends to urinate when it gets overexcited while playing, try to make sure that you only initiate games where urinating will not cause a problem.

Submissive urination happens when a dog, particularly a puppy, feels insecure or intimidated. If you find that your dog tends to urinate a little when you greet it, then try not to tower over the dog; squat down for your greeting, don't look the dog straight in the eye and speak softly. Make sure that visitors do not swoop on the dog but wait until they are sitting down before they take any notice of it.

COPROPHAGIA
(eating feces)

For wild dogs, the eating of the droppings of large herbivores probably provides essential roughage and minerals, as well as quantities of the B group of vitamins, so what seems to us a revolting habit has its roots in natural behavior. Members of a dog pack often eat part of each others feces and also wash one another's anal regions. This may help to ensure that all the pack members have the same microorganisms living within their intestines, so lessening the likelihood of outbreaks of disease within the group. Most dogs grow out of coprophagia, especially when they find that it displeases their owners. You can help to break the habit by disposing of feces promptly and by distracting your dog by some other activity if it is tempted while you are out walking. The family cat's litter tray may be a problem area; if your dog is large, then a covered tray with a small entrance for the cat may be the answer, otherwise you may need to put the litter tray out of the dog's reach. The cat will adapt easily to a tray on a high surface and will probably welcome the peace and privacy.

CAR TRAVEL PROBLEMS

If your dog refuses to stay still when traveling in the car, you may be a danger to other road users; if you are distracted at a crucial moment, a serious accident could result. If you travel regularly, it is a good idea to fit a dog grille, so that the dog is confined to its own area of the car and cannot jump over the seats. Alternatively, you will need to work at extending obedience training to the car. Work on the basic 'Down!' and 'Stay!' commands until your dog will lie down when told and stay there until released. Then have your dog maintain this position in a stationary car with the doors open. Make sure that you always practice with the dog lying where you want it to travel, whether this is on the seat or the floor. Once this is accomplished satisfactorily, ask a friend to drive so that you can make sure that the dog stays in position; then begin by making very short journeys, then lengthening them.

DOG FIGHTS

Play fighting is first seen in young puppies of four to five weeks of age and it is these competitive trials of strength that lead to the formation of a social hierarchy. Most adult dogs avoid actual fights: males establish their territorial rights by urine marking whenever possible and simply threaten other dogs by assuming various body postures like walking stiff-legged, holding the tail rigid, and perhaps giving a few warning growls.

When a serious fight breaks out between two dogs, most owners dive into the midst of the battle and try to separate their pets. This is foolish in the extreme and usually results in injuries to all those involved. Each owner should simultaneously pull his dog away by gripping it at the root of its tail. This must not be done however, if one dog has a firm grip with its teeth or else the other dog could suffer extensive damage. To make a dog release its hold, insert a forefinger into its rectum. The dog will react immediately to this and relax its grip. It should then be smartly pulled away from its adversary and prevented from returning to the attack. A bucket of cold water poured over two fighting dogs might force them apart, but they need to be quickly caught and controlled before they fall upon each other once more.

When two neighboring dogs constantly threaten one another and are always spoiling for a fight, it is sometimes thought wise to let them sort out their battle for dominance once and for all. This used to be the practice on farms when it was considered preferable to allowing feuds to continue. Once two dogs have settled the matter they need never fight again.

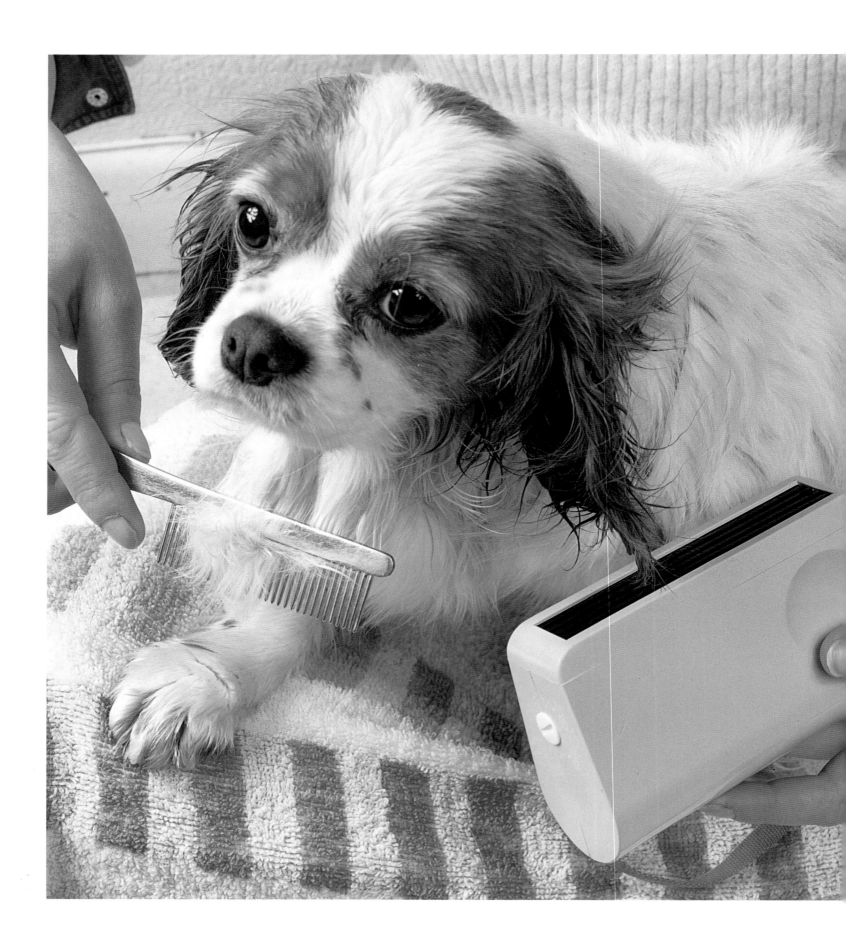

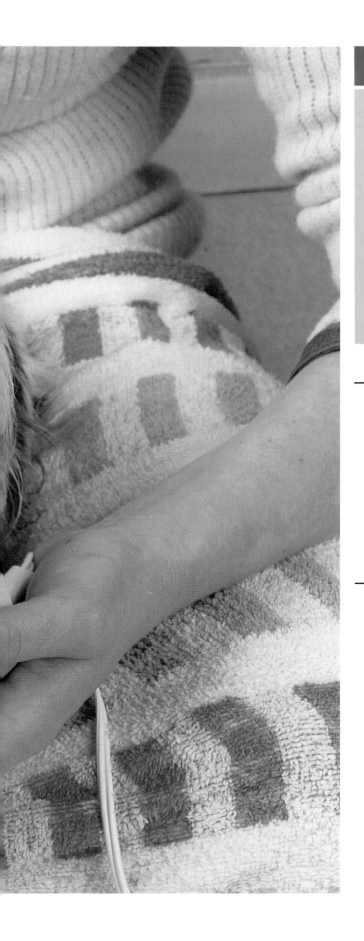

CARE OF THE DOG

From youth to old age, your dog will be dependent on you for loving care and its health and well-being will show in its bright eyes, its shining coat and alert reactions. As it grows old, it will need and deserve special consideration. Your dog may go through its whole life without accident or illness but it is very important to know how to administer first aid and how to detect the first signs and symptoms of disease. There are times when recognizing a developing problem and taking veterinary advice quickly can make all the difference between a quick recovery and a serious illness.

The amount of food needed by individual dogs varies considerably; a sporting dog like this Welsh Springer Spaniel needs much more than a pet leading a sedentary life.

Many breeders maintain that 'half the pedigree goes in at the mouth'; in other words, correct feeding from the beginning will make a great difference to the dog's future condition and well-being. Though adult dogs are adaptable and will eat a wide variety of foods with enjoyment, any dog will be healthier and happier if fed a well-balanced diet. In past generations, pet dogs were fed on table scraps and leftovers but today so much of our food is processed, pasteurized, dehydrated, preserved and so on, that a diet of scraps would probably be lacking in some essential ingredients.

In the wild, dogs would eat other animals and consume the whole carcass, which would provide them with proteins, carbohydrates, fats, minerals and vitamins. Breeding and domestication do not seem to have had any marked effect on the dog's digestive functions so domestic dogs should be fed on meat and plenty of roughage.

FOOD AND FEEDING HABITS

There are three main types of prepared proprietary dog food:

Canned food is usually cooked meat in various forms. Better quality products have more meat than gravy and as meat is 75 per cent water, make sure that you buy this type, otherwise your dog may end up with a meaty drink rather than a filling meal. It makes very little difference what meat is in the cans so if you find that your dog prefers liver, chicken, rabbit or beef, serve what it likes best. Most of these foods are supplemented with vitamins and minerals and they may or may not have cereal added. It is important to check whether the canned food you buy is intended as a complete diet or whether you must also buy biscuits to supply carbohydrate.

Dried food may take the form of flakes or pellets and is specially formulated to give all the necessary nutrients, so long as it is given with plenty of water. The flaked type of food has the advantage that it can be fed moist if the dog prefers, though some manufacturers claim that the pellet form is more easily digested. It is important to remember that dried foods have only a water content of 8 per cent, as against the high water content of meat, so that the success of the diet depends on fresh water being available to the dog at all times.

Semi-moist foods are popular with many dogs. They are softer in texture than dried foods and may be more convenient to store than cans. The product keeps well until opened but must then be used up fairly quickly.

Foods produced by reputable firms will contain all the essentials but dogs, like people, are individuals and what suits one may not suit another. If your dog is not enjoying its dried food, try canned and so on. When switching to another food, make the change gradually or gastric upsets may result.

It is almost impossible to give advice on the amount of food to give an individual dog. Like people, some dogs are good food converters, some are not. Some of the very lively toy breeds and the small energetic terriers will need more food in proportion to their body weight than larger, slow-moving dogs. The amount of food required also varies widely according to the dog's lifestyle. For example, a German Shepherd working as a police dog may need 750 g (1½ lbs) of meat and the same quantity of biscuits daily. A similar animal leading a

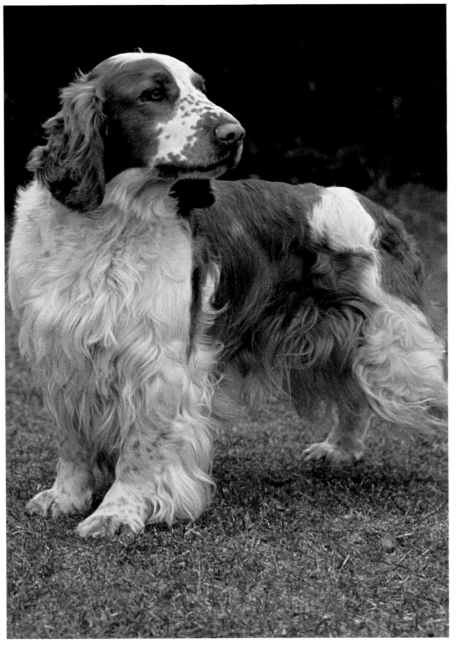

sedentary life as a pet would probably need only half this quantity, while a bitch of a similar size nursing three- to four-week-old puppies will need at least three times as much. An adequate diet is one that leaves the dog looking neither fat nor thin, lively and alert, with its coat in good condition. In our society, there are probably more overfed than underfed dogs and overweight owners tend to have overweight dogs. Overfeeding a dog is no kindness as it will become lazy and lethargic, its coat will shed constantly and its life may be shortened.

Food should be served at room temperature; if it is given straight from the refrigerator it can cause gastric upsets. Always put the food in a clean bowl of the right size and shape for the breed. A healthy dog fed a suitable amount will eat its food very quickly and lick the bowl clean. Never leave a dish of uneaten food on the floor; it will only attract flies and can lead to infection and disease. Feed your dog at regular times but do not give it a heavy meal just before taking it for a run. Make sure it has access to clean water, always keep the water bowl in the same place and wash it every morning before refilling it.

Avoid giving your dog tidbits at the table; it encourages begging and greed. Special chocolate drops or other candy do no harm if they are given in moderation, as an aid to training or for some special reward. Give your young dog an extra biscuit at bedtime. Chewing the biscuit prevents the boredom that often leads to destructive behavior at night and the biscuit also helps to remove tartar from the teeth. A large raw marrowbone is excellent for your dog but cooked bones, especially poultry or chop bones, are very dangerous. Cooking makes them brittle and they can splinter and pierce the dog's intestines with disastrous results.

If your dog has a well-balanced diet it will not need extra vitamins or tonics. You may find, however, that a little margarine or vegetable oil added to the food will help to counteract a dull or scurfy coat at molting time and the occasional egg or dish of liver or fish will benefit the dog's general health.

SPECIAL GROOMING

Some breeds require specialist trimming or clipping to keep their coats in order and you should make sure that you know what is necessary for your particular breed. It is only possible here to give a general idea of the grooming needed by some popular breeds:

Yorkshire Terrier. Brush with, then against and finally with the growth of hair. The coat parts in the middle of the back and falls straight to the ground. After grooming, trim the coat in a straight line to prevent it from trailing along the floor. Many pets have their coat trimmed to 10 cm (4 ins) above the ground so that it is easier to look after. Trim around

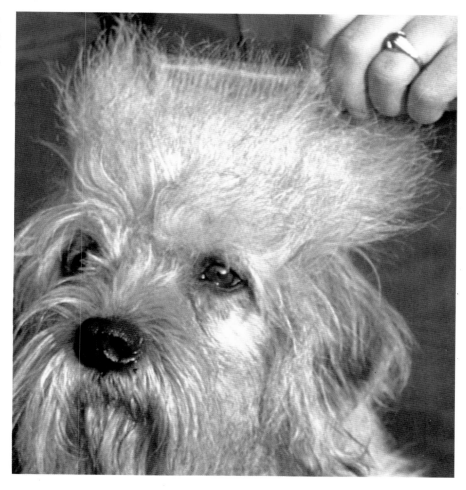

the feet in the shape of the paw and trim the hair between the toes. Gather up the topknot and fasten with wool or ribbon; take care never to tug as this can break the hair. In a pet, the topknot can be trimmed into a fringe. Trim the hair from the top of the ears, scissoring from the tips to where the ears widen out.

Shih Tzu. It is important to brush the coat regularly to remove mats and give a glossy sheen. Again, make a central parting and tie up the hair on the head. Keep the body hair underneath scissored in a straight line and clean the hair between the pads of the feet.

Poodle. The adult Poodle will need its coat clipping and bathing every six to eight weeks, and it is usual for the dog to go to a beauty parlor for this to be done. Puppies need to have only their feet and tail trimmed and this should be done at about four months. There are a multitude of different pet trims or clips for you to choose from, all aimed at keeping the coat within manageable proportions. Show dogs are kept in the puppy clip up to the age of one year and then have to be shown in either lion or continental clip. In the lion clip, the face and body

Each breed has its special grooming needs: this Dandie Dinmont has its topknot combed upwards to give it a 'woolly' appearance.

This poodle is obviously accustomed to having its beard trimmed and waits patiently for the job to be completed.

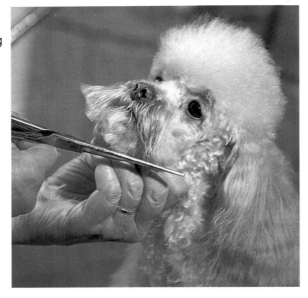

of the dog are shaved, leaving a luxurious mane of hair over the shoulders and part of the rib cage. The hair is shaved off the front legs leaving two bracelets of hair on each leg. A pompom of hair is left on the end of the tail. The continental clip is similar, but leaves patterns of hair on the hindquarters.

Good diet, a healthy lifestyle and regular grooming all show in the general appearance of the dog; these Irish Setters are obviously fit, happy and in the peak of condition.

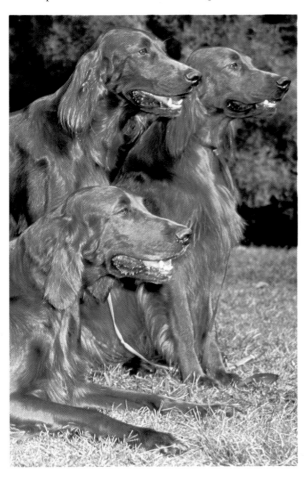

Cocker Spaniel. It is important to brush vigorously and particularly important to get out the dead hair so that the coat looks flat and gleaming. The feet should be neatened by trimming around them with blunt-ended scissors and the hair should also be snipped from between the toes. This helps to keep the foot compact and prevents the dog from bringing too much mud indoors. Thinning scissors should be used on the feathering down the back of the legs and on the tops of the ears to prevent it from becoming too profuse. The show presentation of a Cocker Spaniel is a job for the specialists.

Pekingese. The Pekingese needs a great deal of brushing with a good quality bristle brush. The hair should be brushed out from the sides of the body and the brush then taken upwards in a lifting motion; this gives the impression of fullness. Ears are groomed towards the face and the coat between the ears is brushed outwards to give a ruff-like effect. The tail is parted down the middle and the hair brushed to fall either side of the body in a fan shape. Combing should be done sparingly as in time it will reduce the density of the coat by taking out too much hair. Some Pekingese grow a great deal of hair on their feet and this should be trimmed for their own comfort. Great care must be taken when grooming around the eyes as even a slight knock or scratch on the eye can lead to ulceration.

Afghan. When grooming an Afghan as a family pet, your main concern will be keeping the long flowing coat free from tangles. You can help this by scissoring between the pads of the feet, being careful not to nick the skin. Trim around the feet to give a clublike appearance. Taper the tail feathering carefully. The Afghan's coat is parted from head to tail and the hair must be brushed downwards from the parting. The long, lean face should be kept free from straggling hairs by carefully plucking them out with the fingers; the same technique should be used with odd hairs appearing along the center parting. Stripping combs or knives should never be used on Afghans.

Old English Sheepdog. Trimming establishments do not have time to cope with the great thick coat so they usually run clippers down the body from head to toe. The typical look of the Old English Sheepdog should be preserved by regular brushing and careful removal of mats. Hair around the eyes should be trimmed into a squarish shape to reveal the eyes. Scissor around the paws and clean hair from between the pads of the feet. When brushing, work in layers. Begin at ankle level, part the hair a few inches up and across the leg, brush the lower hair down then comb. Take a section above and repeat the procedure. With the dog lying on its side, part the hair on the body from neck to tail and proceed as for the legs.

NAILS

If your dog is regularly exercised on hard surfaces its nails are unlikely to need any attention as they will naturally wear down to the correct length. The nails of dogs confined to grassy areas, or walked only in the park, can grow excessively long, however, and must be clipped back to enable the animal to walk properly. Always use guillotine-type nail clippers to cut your dog's nails, and ask your veterinarian to show you how to use them correctly. Dogs dislike having their nails cut at any time so it is doubly important for you to know the correct point at which the nail should be shortened to avoid cutting the sensitive quick. If you cut too close to the quick you will hurt your dog; and if the nail is cut too short it will bleed profusely.

ANAL SACS AND GLANDS

The dog has a pair of sacs lying inside the body cavity just below and on either side of its anus. These sacs store a distinctively and powerfully pungent gray-brown fluid produced by the anal glands. A small duct leads from each sac to the opening of the anus. Each time the dog defecates, a little of the fluid passes up the tube and is smeared on the stool, giving it its characteristic doggy odor. This scent is important in the wild dog, acting as a territorial marking agent.

The anal sacs sometimes present problems in the domestic dog, becoming impacted and failing to drain adequately. An affected dog may drag its seat across the ground in an attempt to relieve the irritation, or it will try to bite the area. If neglected the anal sacs will become infected and antibiotic treatment will be required. The veterinarian can empty the sacs manually whenever necessary and will show you how to do this yourself if you wish to do it yourself.

To empty the sacs, put on rubber gloves and take a large piece of cotton in one hand. Hold the dog by the root of its tail with the other hand, place the cotton over the region of the anal sacs and press inwards and upwards with your thumb and forefinger. This action does not hurt the dog and the offensive matter will pass out into the cotton pad.

Fed a good diet and given adequate exercise, some dogs never have any trouble with their anal sacs while others seem to spend a good part of their lives going to and from the veterinarian's office. If the problem is persistent it is advisable to have the sacs and glands removed surgically, which does not seem to affect the dog adversely.

BATHING YOUR DOG

It is not necessary to bathe your dog as long as it is kept clean and sweet-smelling with normal grooming. Bathing removes the coat's natural oils which

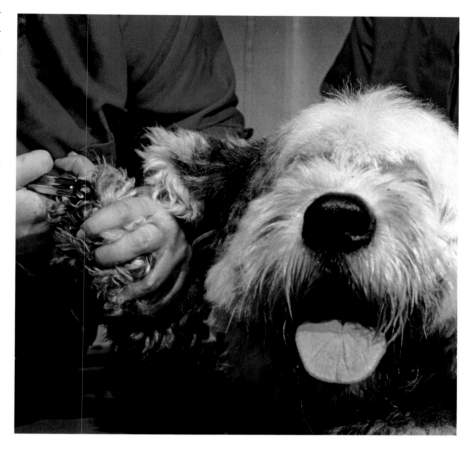

act as weatherproofing agents, so that a dog living in the open could be detrimentally affected by too-frequent tubbings. Pet dogs living in centrally heated homes often shed a lot of hair and may need fairly frequent baths to keep fresh, clean and tidy. Apart from removing the coat's oils, bathing is not otherwise detrimental to the dog's health so long as it is carried out correctly and the animal is thoroughly dried before it can catch a chill.

Some short-coated dogs may go their entire lives without ever needing a bath. Others which need regular stripping, clipping or trimming are often bathed at these times as the freshly washed coat is then easier to handle. Long-coated breeds, and those which are regularly shown, may have quite frequent bathing sessions. Bathing a smallish, short-coated dog is comparatively easy, but bathing a large, long-coated dog may take time and a great deal of patience especially if the animal is uncooperative.

Small breeds can be bathed in an old baby bath, or a large bowl; larger breeds will need the family bath tub or may be placed near a drain outlet, preferably on concrete, and have warm water poured over them from a bucket or tub. If it is necessary to bath a dog outdoors, it must be done on a warm day. If the bath or sink is used, place a small rubber mat at the bottom to help the animal feel more secure. Every dog must be thoroughly

When nail clipping is needed, it must be carefully done with special clippers but it should seldom be necessary for a dog taking plenty of exercise on hard surfaces.

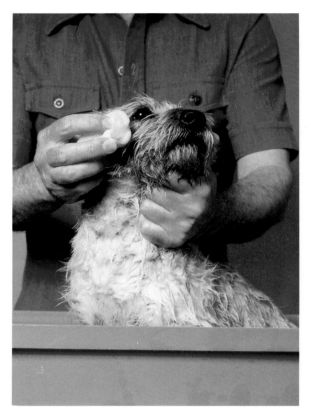

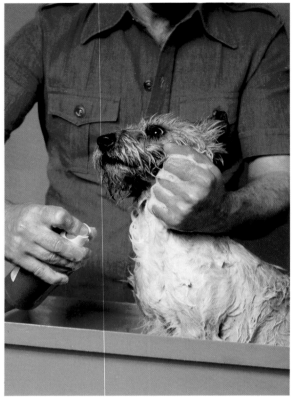

1. When bathing a dog, wash the face first, using clean water to wipe the eyes and nostrils and to wash any soiled areas around the mouth and lips.

2. When the entire coat is thoroughly wet, apply a dog shampoo, rubbing it well into the coat, following the manufacturer's instructions.

groomed before bathing, with any matted hair being teased or clipped out. Make sure the dog has a chance to relieve itself before you begin.

A hand spray is useful for wetting the coat and giving the final rinse; alternatively, you can use a jug or large sponge for the purpose. A large plastic apron or a plastic raincoat worn back to front will help to keep you dry. Remove everything from the bathing area before you begin in case the dog slips through your wet hands, and firmly shut the door.

Take off the dog's collar and sit the animal in the bowl or tub. Wash its face carefully and wipe out the ears; put a smear of Vaseline along the eyelids and plug the ears with non-absorbent cotton, also smeared with Vaseline. Thoroughly wet the coat from the neck downwards, then apply the dog shampoo, following the manufacturer's directions, and work up a lather. Wash the dog's coat thoroughly and pay particular attention to the underparts, around the tail and between the toes. Use fresh water to rinse every trace of shampoo from the coat. Take care to keep the shampoo and rinsing water out of the dog's eyes, nose and ears and use tepid water only throughout the whole of the bathing process.

When you rinse the dog, squeeze as much of the surplus water as possible out of the coat and down the legs, envelop it in a large towel and place on the floor. Encourage it to give a really good shake. Towel as much moisture as you can from the coat, then use a drier or another dry towel to finish the job. If you have a breed that needs regular bathing, it would be wise to invest in a drier specially made for dogs. Long straight coats should be groomed into place during drying. You will need one hand for the brush and one hand for the drier, so tie the dog up or have it held throughout this rather long and tedious process. If you do have to tie up your dog, be sure to use a metal choke chain collar because a leather collar may shed dye onto the coat around the dog's neck when it gets wet.

HEALTH AND SICKNESS

Many owners can tell almost instinctively when something is not quite right with their dogs but many illnesses are not detected quickly enough. Disease may be acute or chronic: acute disease develops rapidly and the signs of illness will be obvious but chronic disease is insidious and may remain unnoticed until the illness is far advanced. The ability to tell whether or not a dog is healthy comes from a combination of observation and experience and a concerned owner takes notice of

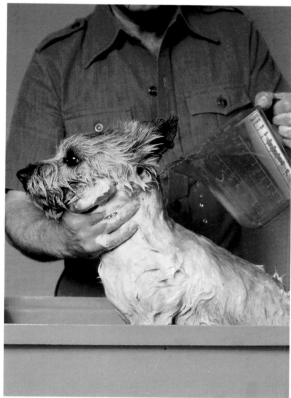

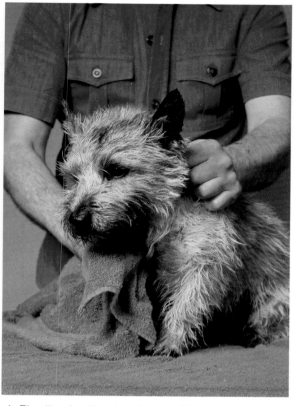

3. Make sure that you rinse all traces of shampoo from the dog's coat, using tepid water. Do not let the water get into the ears or eyes.

4. Finally, dry the dog thoroughly using a rough towel. Some dogs will allow you to finish off the drying process with a hair dryer, set at cool.

any change in normal behavior as this may be the sign of a developing problem. Knowing the normal signs of health in a dog is the first essential and a methodical check of your dog's body and assessment of any change in behavior patterns will often help to confirm the suspicion that the dog is not well and can be a great help in describing the problem to your veterinarian.

SIGNS OF A HEALTHY DOG

Appetite. Healthy dogs usually have a good appetite but a sick dog may eat less than usual. Acute disease is often accompanied by a complete refusal to eat but even a slight loss of appetite may indicate chronic illness. Never ignore excessive thirst as this may be the first sign of certain diseases. Make sure that you know the normal weight for the age and breed of your dog and never neglect any gradual, prolonged loss of weight.

Sleep and waking. All dogs sleep a good deal but should be alert and lively when they are awake. Sluggishness may result from a variety of causes, from old age or obesity to a serious disease like acute anemia. If a dog becomes slow and lethargic, it should be a cause for concern.

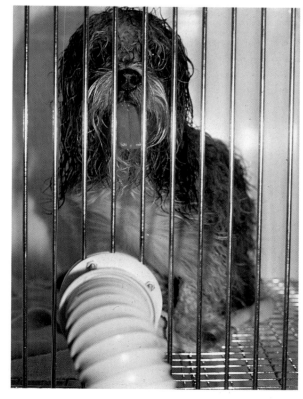

Show dogs need bathing far more often than pets and may be dried with a hot air blower.

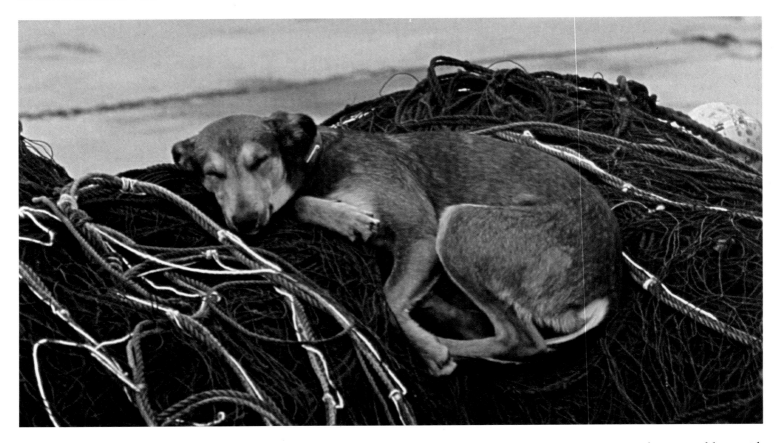

Healthy dogs sleep a lot but when awake should be alert and lively.

A dog's temperature should be taken with a snub-nosed rectal thermometer.

Eyes. The eyes should be bright, the whites clear looking, with no sign of swollen veins or discharge, but not excessively pale. The lower part of the eyeball should be bright pink.

Ears. The inside of healthy ears look clean and pink. They should be smooth, with no signs of wax, no black or gray deposits and no unpleasant smell.

Matted hair in the ears is often a problem with Poodles as this can lead to a more serious ear infection.

Nose. This should be smooth and free from any discharge or encrusted material. If a normally cold, moist nose feels hot and dry, it may be wise to check the dog's temperature.

Skin. This should be elastic and spring back into place rapidly after it is lifted away from the animal's body. The feel of the skin may vary from breed to breed. A Labrador puppy's skin, for instance, always feels several sizes too large but it still has that healthy elasticity.

Body. Careful owners will make a regular check of head, limbs and trunk for unusual swellings or skin wounds, any sign of hair loss or sore inflamed patches. Standing or moving, the dog should appear comfortable: a haunched stance or lameness always indicates that something is wrong.

Temperature. The most popular guide to determining health is the dog's temperature, which is normally between 38° and 39°C (100.5° and 101.5°F). Excited or nervous dogs may run temperatures up to two degrees higher and a bitch's temperature may fall two or three degrees before whelping.

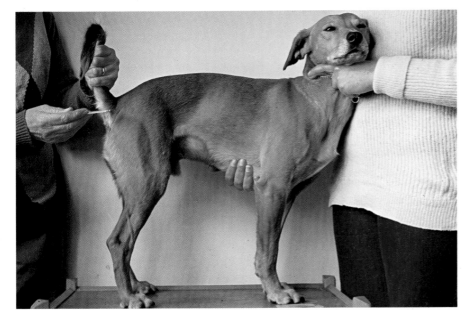

There is no reason why a careful owner should not take a dog's temperature. Use a snub-nosed rectal thermometer and grease the end. Shake down the mercury, then hold the dog in a standing position, talking soothingly, while you insert and hold it in the dog's rectum for approximately half the thermometer length, applying slight sideways pressure to hold the bulb against the wall of the rectum. Hold it in place for a full minute. Wipe it before reading and wash it afterwards in cold water and disinfectant.

GIVING MEDICATION

Medication prescribed for your dog should never be mixed with food. The correct dosage is important and your dog may detect the substance in the food and spit out half of it, or may leave the food untouched. It might be too ill to eat its food or only take a mouthful before walking away. With all but the fiercest dogs, however, giving liquid medication or pills is a fairly simple matter.

Liquid medication. Liquid medication is usually in 5 ml (one teaspoon) doses. You can give them by means of a plastic measuring spoon, which may be provided with the medication, or with a plastic syringe obtained from your vet. Have the dog sitting comfortably by your side and measure the dose. Hold the dog's jaws closed, tilt the head well back, then pull out the flap of the lip on one side of the mouth. This forms a natural funnel down which the liquid can be poured. Keep holding the dog's head and do not release it until you have seen it swallow. Rub its throat gently to help the process along.

Powdered medication. Medication supplied in powder form should never be poured into the dog's mouth because the fine particles can cause choking. Instead, mix powders with honey or margarine and smear the resulting paste on the dog's tongue with the handle of a spoon. Dogs usually enjoy the taste and look forward to the next dose.

Pills. The technique for giving tablets, pills and capsules requires a little practice. Sit your dog in front of you so that it looks towards your right. Place your left hand over its muzzle, just in front of the eyes, and gently press its lips inwards onto the teeth. With your right hand, open the mouth by pressing the front of the lower jaw downwards. At the same time, close your left hand slightly so that the dog's lips cover its teeth. This effectively prevents the dog from closing its mouth, but make sure that you do not hold the mouth so tightly that your pet is hurt, struggles or whines. Take the pill or tablet in your right hand and place it at the back of the dog's tongue. Allow its mouth to shut, hold the jaws closed and the nose pointing upwards and use the right hand to rub the dog's throat until you see it

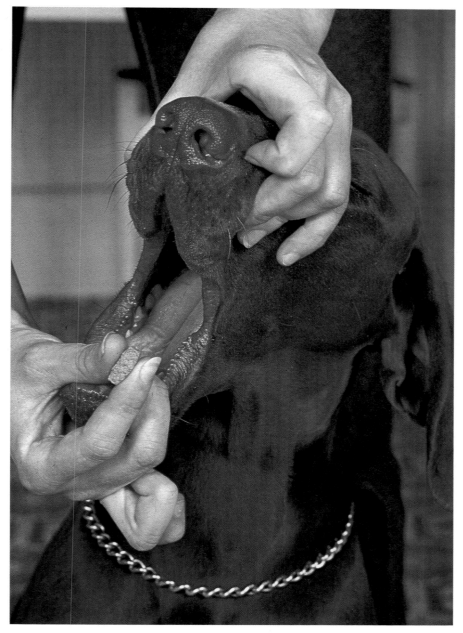

swallow. Once the pill is swallowed, pet and praise your dog. These instructions are for the right-handed owner, so left-handed owners should reverse them.

Ear drops. The dog's ear is a delicate organ and you should never put anything into the ear canal unless advised by your vet. Owners often puff or pour patent canker powders into a dog's ears with all the best intentions but they only clog the ear and cause the dog a great deal of irritation and discomfort, only relieved by syringing by the vet. Veterinary ear drops, however, are specially formulated and individually prescribed and your vet will show you how to administer them.

When giving a dog a pill, hold the mouth open gently while you put the pill on the back of the tongue, then close the mouth and stroke the throat to encourage swallowing.

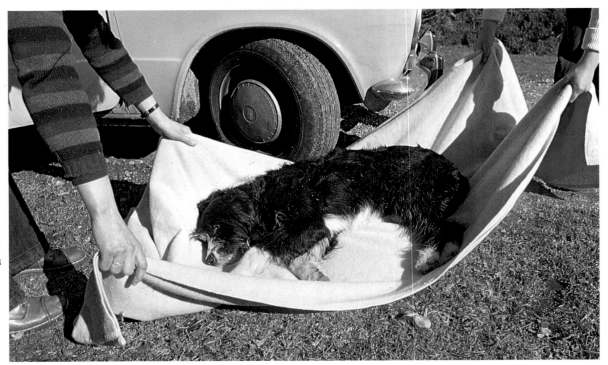

Though an injured dog should be moved as little as possible, a dog hurt in a road accident can be lifted gently onto a blanket and taken immediately to the veterinary hospital.

Eye ointments. Dogs suffer from inflamed and sore eyes for a variety of reasons but two main causes are dusty bedding and traveling by car with the head sticking out of the window. The dog's eyes are very delicate and must be handled carefully. If the whites of the eye look bloodshot or there is a discharge, clean each eye with a separate piece of cotton dipped in saline solution or a mild eyewash made for human use. Saline solution is made by dissolving one level tablespoonful of common salt in one pint of boiling water, allowing it to cool, and storing it in a spotlessly clean, sealed bottle.

Persistent eye trouble must receive veterinary attention. If you are given ointment to apply at home, it is very important to apply it exactly as shown by your vet and to continue using it for the full length of time. Even if the eyes appear better, always continue the treatment until it is completed: the trouble may only be masked and could return.

FIRST AID

Road accidents. Move a dog injured in a road accident as little as possible, as it is likely to be suffering from shock and may have internal injuries. Try to stop any excessive bleeding right away. First check that there is nothing in the wound, then apply a pad of gauze if any is available (if not, use a clean handkerchief, torn sheet or the most suitable clean covering you can find). Then bandage firmly over the pad. If blood seeps through, rebandage on top and take the dog to the vet immediately. To move a large injured dog with the least possible disturbance, use a blanket and enlist a helper. Slide the

blanket gently under the dog and, with one person at each end holding two corners, gently lift the dog into a car.

If the dog is suffering from internal bleeding, its breathing will be rapid and shallow, its skin will feel clammy, its pulse will be rapid and it may be unconscious. If this is the case, simply get the animal to the vet as fast as you can.

Burns. Extensive burns are very dangerous. The only recommended first aid is to immerse the burned area in cold water and get professional help immediately.

Heat stroke. In very hot weather, or when shut in a closed car on a sunny day, dogs can suffer badly from heat stroke. The dog will probably be panting, weak and near to collapse. It might be vomiting and its temperature will be very high. Lower the temperature as soon as you can – if you are indoors, immerse the dog in a cold bath; outdoors you may be able to find a hose or fill a bucket with water to pour over it. Once the dog shows signs of recovery, dry it off, keep it in a cool place and encourage it to drink.

Drowning. Not all dogs are able to swim and even a normally good swimmer may fall into water and injure itself or get trapped in a steep-sided pond. Once you have pulled the dog out, place its head lower than its body, pull out its tongue, try to drain out any excess water from its mouth and apply artificial respiration. Place the dog on its right side, tongue out and head forward, put your hand over its ribs behind the shoulder blade, press down on its ribs and release the pressure immediately. Repeat at intervals of about five seconds with short, sharp movements until the dog starts breathing normally.

Bites. If your dog has been involved in a fight, it is wise to examine it for wounds. These may be very minor but frequently become infected so that an abscess forms. Bathe any wound with cotton and warm water immediately to clean the area, then take the dog to the vet who will decide if antibiotic treatment is necessary.

Choking. Small rubber balls are the most usual cause of choking in dogs. The dog will be in great distress and, although able to breathe, will be unable to swallow and will salivate profusely. You will probably be able to feel the ball in its throat. The dog should be seen as soon as possible by a vet, who may have to anesthetize it before removing the object.

Dogs sometimes get a rubber ball stuck behind their molar teeth, causing an obstruction. If possible try to remove the ball but be careful not to push it further down. Bones, pieces of stick and even stones can become lodged in the back of the mouth and cause a nasty wound. A dog with something wedged in its mouth usually paws frantically at its mouth or rubs it along the ground, slobbering profusely. Open its mouth carefully, taking care not to get bitten, and try to pull out the offending object. If you cannot get hold of it, take the dog to the vet, who will give it an anesthetic before removing the object and treating the wound.

Prevention is better than cure so try to keep your dog safe from accidental injury by observing commonsense precautions. Never let it run loose on the streets and never leave it shut in a closed car. Keep your dog away from toxic substances, cooking stoves, needles and sharp bones. If, in spite of your precautions, your dog does suffer an accident, you may need to apply suitable first aid, then get veterinary treatment as soon as possible.

Remember that any dog in pain after an accident is likely to bite in fear and it is only commonsense to protect yourself by putting an emergency muzzle on your pet. You can use a large handkerchief, soft belt, panty hose, tie or scarf. Make a loop, slip it over the dog's nose and pull the knot tight under its chin; take both ends back and tie them firmly behind its ears. You should then be able to handle the dog safely.

CONSULTING A VETERINARIAN

All pet-owners should be familiar with the consulting hours of their vet and keep the phone number and out-of-hours emergency number along with the number of the family physician. Some vets hold open practices where you simply go along with your pet and wait your turn, though you should phone in advance if the case is likely to take longer than normal to deal with or if you suspect that your pet may be suffering from an infectious disease. Other practices run an appointment system where you will need to call in advance. The receptionist will normally want your name and address, the dog's name and the reason for the visit, given as briefly as possible.

The decision to hospitalize a dog for treatment is primarily one for the vet but it will be influenced strongly by the owner's attitude and circumstances. Whenever possible, it will be better for both of you if you take the dog home again after treatment or routine operations, as care and love are very important in the recovery process. In familiar surroundings, secure with its family, the dog will be more relaxed and will get better faster. However, there may be cases where a dog which has not fully recovered from an anesthetic or is in need of specialized care will be kept in the animal hospital for a time. For instance, if an intravenous drip is needed, the equipment must be set up by trained staff and continuously monitored and adjusted. In addition, the patient needs to be restrained and every veterinary nurse knows how to cope with a

When an emergency muzzle is necessary, use a length of bandage or material; this owner has used the belt of a dressing gown.

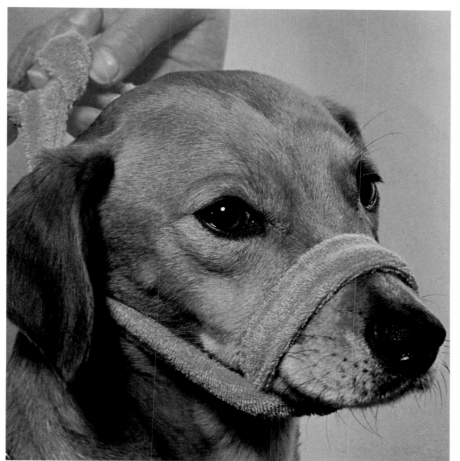

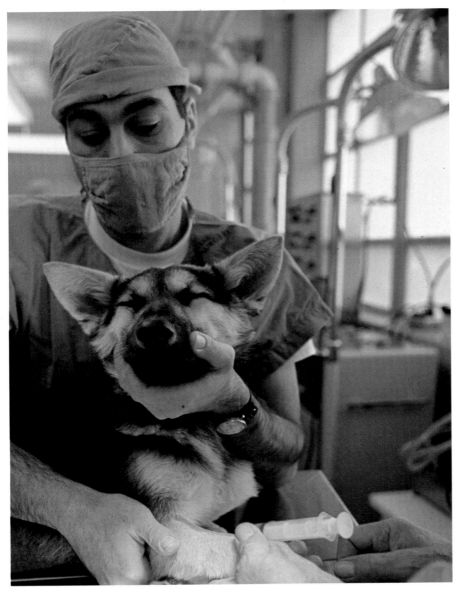

All dogs will need an occasional visit to the veterinarian to ensure that they keep in good health.

pear; otherwise desensitizing injections may be necessary.

Arthritis. Inflammatory disorders of the joints are common in dogs, particularly in the heavier breeds. Although usually associated with older animals, this disease may occur in dogs less than one year old when they are afflicted with such problems as hip dysplasia and Legge-Perthe's disease (a disorder of the hip bone). The cause of arthritis is not completely understood, but it frequently follows physical injury. Obesity tends to aggravate the condition. Signs are usually insidious, with slowly developing pain and lameness, often noticeable as stiffness in the morning which wears off with exercise. Diagnosis may require X-ray examination. Treatment is palliative, but weight reduction of obese dogs should be attempted, and the dog's bed should be warm and dry.

Bad breath. An offensive smell from a dog's mouth may result from infection in the mouth itself, either a specific bacterial infection or ulcers, from decaying teeth and associated gum disease, or from generalized disease such as chronic nephritis (See below). It may also occur when the dog appears to be in perfect health otherwise. There is no first aid treatment for bad breath caused by disease; it will be necessary to have the dog seen by a veterinarian. Foul stomach smells, if temporary, may respond to a dose of milk of magnesia. The dog with chronic bad breath, which is not caused by any apparent disease, will probably respond only temporarily to veterinary treatment but a complete change of diet may succeed. This change will probably need to be drastic, such as a diet of rice and rabbit instead of beef and biscuits.

Canker see **Ear diseases.**

Cannibalism. Bitches at whelping, even normally placid ones, may become sufficiently psychologically disturbed to attack, kill and even occasionally eat their offspring. There is no treatment, but it is essential to have as undisturbed and peaceful a situation as possible at whelping time, and to allow the bitch to whelp in surroundings with which she has become familiar, preferably over weeks rather than days. Quiet vigilance is needed rather than overanxious 'help.'

Car sickness. Some dogs have this trouble and others don't. There is no certain way of preventing it, but if a dog starts to be travel sick it is important to treat it before it becomes a habit. Depending on the puppy's size, up to half an antitravel sickness tablet may be effective, otherwise a veterinarian can prescribe something. Tablets may take a long time to work, so the dose should be given about an hour before the journey. Much of the sickness suffered

dog that suddenly decides to get up.

It may be necessary to hospitalize a recovering dog if the owner is out at work all day and unable to provide the constant observation and attention necessary, so it is important to discuss the question of care with the vet.

A TO Z OF CANINE AILMENTS

Allergy. Dogs can suffer from allergies, like their owners. The most usual symptom is an itchy skin (*see also* **Eczema**); less common is a runny nose, sneezing and watering eyes. The cause may be dusty bedding, fleas, household products such as aerosol sprays or detergent used to wash bedding, particular materials like wool or nylon, or food. It is worth experimenting to find the cause as if this can be identified and eliminated, the problems will disap-

by older puppies and grown dogs is due to nervousness from remembered previous occasions. A few trips protected by tablets may overcome the problem.

Constipation. Simple constipation occurs fairly often as a result of eating bones or indigestible matter. It may also arise from the dog's refusal to defecate because of pain from infected anal glands, or even matted hair around the anus. There are other, more fundamental causes and chronic constipation, particularly if it is associated with alternating bouts of diarrhea, needs veterinary attention. Constipation is accompanied by frequent attempts to defecate. A dog which makes no attempt to pass feces for several days is not necessarily constipated. The best first aid is probably liquid paraffin by mouth, about a dessert-spoonful for small dogs and four or five times that amount for larger dogs.

Cough. Coughing is simply a sign of irritation in the dog's throat or bronchial tubes. It must be considered with other symptoms in determining the cause. Only rarely is a foreign body such as a bone involved, but an apparent attempt to clear the throat of something is often a sign of tonsilitis or kennel cough, a highly infectious although usually not serious disease. There is now a vaccination against kennel cough. It can be given as part of the standard distemper, hepatitis and leptospirosis shot. Any persistent cough requires veterinary attention. If the cough is accompanied by distress, or refusal of food, the attention should be prompt.

Cystitis. This is an inflammation of the bladder, more common in females than males. The animal will be in pain, straining to pass small amounts of urine frequently and the urine may be blood-stained. The vet will treat cystitis with antibiotics but in some dogs the problem does tend to recur.

Deafness. This is not common in dogs, but it can occur as a congenital condition and be noticed by an observant owner while puppies are still very young. A simple handclap will usually show whether or not the puppy is reacting to noise, but hearing which is simply less acute than normal may be extremely difficult to determine. Deafness frequently accompanies old age. There is usually no treatment available. Cleansing the ears of wax is unlikely to be of more than marginal benefit.

Diabetes mellitus. Diabetes is caused when the pancreas produces insufficient insulin so that the sugar level in the body builds up and spills over into the kidneys. It occurs most frequently in overweight bitches, and is less common in males or spayed females. Particularly susceptible breeds include Dachshunds and Poodles. In spite of eating more than normal, the affected dog loses weight and it is constantly thirsty. A diabetic dog may require daily insulin injections and a strictly regulated diet. Once the condition is controlled, the dog may be able to live out its normal life. The veterinarian may recommend that diabetic bitches should be spayed.

Diarrhea. Although most attacks of simple diarrhea probably have a nutritional cause, specific diagnosis and treatment is necessary if an attack progresses to enteritis, or persists for longer than 48 hours or if any other symptoms such as vomiting or blood in the stools are present. First-aid treatment for simple diarrhea consists of removing all sources of food and drink and giving the dog a little plain boiled rice (possibly flavored with chicken stock or something similar). Allow small amounts of glucose and water, given frequently. If the dog refuses rice, give it no food for 24 hours.

Distemper and Hard pad. Both terms refer to a disease caused by a single virus that may show some variation in symptoms. The first sign of either form of the disease is a high body temperature, about 39°C (120°F). The dog refuses food and may have a cough or diarrhea; the whites of the eyes are usually inflamed. If infection progresses it will eventually affect the nervous system leading to intractable fits. The hard pad symptom occurs when the virus affects the horny layers of the pads, causing enlargement and leathery feel to the feet. Modern veterinary treatment, through the use of antibiotics, has tended to obscure the classic signs of pneumonia and enteritis in distemper. Little progress has been made in controlling the nervous involvement from which a high proportion of affected dogs die.
NB Vaccination is highly effective in preventing the disease.

Ear diseases. Head shaking, ear scratching and an unpleasant smell are usually the first signs of ear

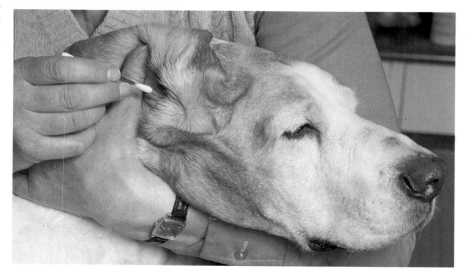

Dogs with floppy ears need their ears cleaned regularly but never probe into the inner recesses of the ear.

disease, and when this is noticed the ears should be examined. If the ear looks sore the dog needs veterinary attention. If the ears are simply dirty or contain a little clean-looking wax, clean them with liquid paraffin. Pour a small amount into the ear, work it gently from the outside and mop it with cotton. It is not safe to push pads of cotton into the ear unless you know there is nothing further down causing trouble. Acute inflammation, particularly in Spaniels, is often caused by a grass seed. More chronic infections frequently start off with ear mite infestations. Veterinary treatment depends on the cause, and in some cases may even require surgery to expose the inflamed area. Diseases of the ear are sometimes loosely referred to as 'canker' although it is a term that veterinarians rarely use.

Eczema. Most skin conditions in the dog have a considerable element of self-infliction, and a dog can turn an itchy spot into a large patch of severe moist eczema in less than an hour. The first step in preventing eczema is to stop the animal scratching or biting itself. Then try to find out what is causing the irritation. In more than 7 cases out of 10 the cause will be parasitic, probably fleas. Most other cases will be diagnosed as allergic. Treatment of parasitic skin disease, while usually straightforward, demands far longer and more determined attention than it frequently receives.

Eye troubles. Eye infections are common in the dog, usually as conjunctivitis, and prompt treatment with antibiotics usually effects a cure. Ulcerated corneas may be more serious and any indication of blueing, or damage to the surface of the eye, should be attended to without delay. An acute eye problem is usually signaled by watering of the eye and closing, partially or completely, of the eyelids. Gentle examination may reveal the cause. If it is a foreign body, such as a piece of grass and it can be removed by the fingers or the corner of a handkerchief, do so. But do not attempt greater interference than that.

Fits. The presence of intestinal worms may occasionally cause fits in young puppies. The remedy is to give a regular worm dose to puppies under six months old. Epilepsy is a common cause of repeated fits in adult dogs, often starting when the dog is between 12 months and three years old. However, loss of consciousness (usually without the typical nervous spasms of a fit) also occurs during the course of a heart attack. The best treatment for fits is to remove any object that might injure the dog; do not attempt to put anything into the animal's mouth 'to stop it choking.' This won't help and you may get bitten in the process. Then take the dog to a veterinarian.

Fleas see **Parasites.**

Fractures. Suspected broken bones can only be confirmed and treated by a veterinarian. Despite a widespread belief to the contrary, sensible movement of the dog is unlikely to make the injury worse. The animal should be carried, if necessary on a blanket, and taken as soon as possible for treatment (See page 156).

Gastric distension. Bloat, gastric torsion, or gastric distension, is a well-recognized problem in larger breeds of dog. Two to four hours after feeding the dog may show signs of obvious distress and pain. The abdomen will be distended and hard. This is a surgical emergency and must be treated immediately by a veterinarian.

Gastritis. Vomiting is the most likely indication that a dog has an inflamed stomach, or gastritis, but grass-eating without vomiting may occasionally be a sign (See below). Gastritis is often associated with simple diarrhea, as in 'diarrhea and vomiting' and in the more serious disease of gastro-enteritis. Both of these may have mechanical origins, possibly a swallowed rubber band or undigested bone, or be caused by bacterial or virus infection. *See also* **Diarrhea.**

Grass-eating. This may be a simple habit of no significance whatsoever, or it may indicate irritation in the stomach (*see* **Gastritis**). It is generally believed that a dog instinctively takes grass to induce vomiting. Grass is most effective in wrapping itself around jagged foreign bodies in the stomach, so helping to prevent damage to the bowel.

Hair loss. Shedding of hair in a seasonal pattern is normal in most breeds, other than those with a Poodle-like coat, but central heating seems to have interfered grossly with the pattern in many dogs by maintaining an average temperature. Hair loss generally occurs after whelping or regularly in an unbred bitch's cycle, again normally as part of her annual cycle. No treatment can reduce or avoid coat-shedding; but regular grooming is essential at these times to prevent matting and itchiness from the dead coat. On occasions the loss may be so heavy that skin irritation occurs. In some cases it becomes sufficiently severe to require veterinary treatment.

Hard pad *see* **Distemper and Hard pad.**

Heart disease. Heart disease is almost as common in dogs as it is in humans, and often has similar causes. The obese Labrador, for instance, is particularly at risk. Congenital heart conditions can receive effective attention. The canine 'blue baby' syndrome is recognized and can be treated by surgery, but most cases of myocardial or valvular disease are treated by drugs rather than surgery. Proper management of cardiac patients is important. Weight loss is frequently required and moderate but not excessive exercise usually desirable. Many dogs will indicate their own exercise tolerance limits quite obviously.

Hepatitis. Viral hepatitis is infectious among dogs. Adult animals may develop fever, with temperatures of up to 41°C (105°F), lose appetite and show blood-stained diarrhea and vomit. Intensive veterinary care is required, but death can result. Vaccination is a preventive measure against hepatitis, and is 99 per cent effective.

Hernia. Externally noticeable hernias in the dog are almost always congenital, and may occur at the umbilicas or in the scrotal or inguinal areas. Small hernias are not significant and are composed of fat trapped in a sac of tissue. If the bulge varies in size veterinary attention is necessary to advise on possible surgery. The rare, serious sequel to a hernia is 'strangulation' when intestines or some other vital organs become trapped in the sac. Prompt surgical treatment is required.

Hip dysplasia. This is a deformity of the hip joint caused when the joint is too shallow and the head of the femur is malformed. It occurs more often than usual in some breeds, such as St Bernards and German Shepherds. It manifests itself by pain in the area of the hip and by a swinging gait and a 'hopping' run. X-ray is needed for accurate diagnosis although there is no cure. Pain can be alleviated by drugs or through surgery. This deformity is generally considered to be hereditary, although the extent of this is unknown; in any case, no dysplastic dog should be allowed to breed.

Jaundice. Obvious jaundice with yellowing of the skin and membranes is comparatively uncommon in dogs, but the underlying causes – blood breakdown or liver disease – are regularly seen. The jaundice itself is a minor symptom but should never be ignored. Leptospirosis and viral hepatitis may both cause jaundicing of the tissues. These diseases are extremely serious. Effective vaccines are available for both and are usually included in the routine vaccinations administered to puppies.

Kidney diseases. Nephritis, inflammation of the kidneys, results from infections, including leptospirosis in particular (See below). Chronic nephritis may progress over a long period and the dog will drink more fluid and urinate more often than normal, as well as losing weight. Acute nephritis usually involves a sudden rise in temperature, pain in the abdomen and constant vomiting. The dog will be thirsty and may urinate more often, or not at all. Treatment will probably include a special diet.

Lameness. The precise location can be extremely difficult to pinpoint; it is hard to tell sometimes

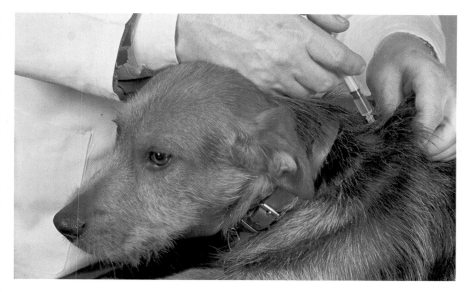

which leg is affected. It is useful to remember that the dog nods its head downwards as the sound leg touches the ground; similarly its rump will drop as the sound hind leg is put to the ground. It will help diagnosis at the veterinarian's if you notice whether, for instance, the lameness is worse first thing in the morning, or if it is intermittent. Careful observation will help. Pain on slight pressure, indicated by tensing of muscles and withdrawal of the leg, may guide you to the site of the lameness. Any lameness that is not obviously improving in 24 hours needs veterinary attention, but young puppies will often be crippled with lameness at one moment and virtually sound in half an hour.

Leptospirosis. This is a common but serious bacterial infection of dogs. Although one type of the infection can be caused by contact with rats, the most frequent transmission is by carrier dogs' urine. For this reason the infection is considered to be more common in male dogs as they are more prone to lamppost sniffing than bitches and consequently more likely to be contaminated by infected urine. In country districts carrier foxes may transmit the disease. It causes fever, marked depression, sometimes diarrhea with yellow feces, and often bright yellow urine. Visible jaundice is rarer, but both liver and kidneys are affected. Treatment is by antibiotics and effective nursing care. The disease can be prevented by annual revaccination.

Lice *see* **Parasites.**

Mites *see* **Parasites.**

Nephritis *see* **Kidney diseases.**

Paralysis. Hind-limb paralysis is frequently seen in the long-backed breeds of dog because of pressure on spinal nerves including injury caused by the protru-

The veterinarian will give injections in the loose skin at the back of the dog's neck, where they will not cause pain.

sion of intervertebral discs. Treatment may be prolonged, but should be continued while the dog has muscular tone in its hind limbs. Conscientious breeders have managed to control hind-limb paralysis in the most affected breeds such as the Dachshund. Weight control and exercise also help to prevent spinal and associated problems. Generalized muscular paralysis is sometimes a sequel to distemper, but is otherwise uncommon in dogs. Sudden paralysis of the back legs occasionally occurs through pressure caused by simple constipation. It will disappear when the constipation is treated.

Parasites. Common external parasites include fleas, which are light or dark brown, very mobile and readily visible when numerous. They are often passed back and forth between dogs and cats. Lice are also quite common. The lice or their egg cases are quite firmly attached, often around the ears; they are white in color and can be mistaken for skin scales or dandruff if not examined closely.

Sarcoptic mange is very serious and is caused by a smaller parasite that is not easily seen. It causes intense itching and skin sores.

Harvest mites are visible on careful examination. They occur usually in comparatively small numbers on the legs and lower parts of the body. They are not mobile, and cause intense local irritation.

Ticks are rarely important in Europe although they are carriers of serious diseases in Africa and parts of the United States. The sheep tick, *Ixodes*, is the common one to affect dogs in temperate climates. It looks like a small gray bladder when mature and is very firmly attached. It should either be left to fall off itself after a few days, or be removed very carefully by hand after anesthetization with spirit. The sheep tick has long mouth-parts that are difficult to remove from the skin and cause localized infection if left in place.

Tropical ticks are easily removed, but may carry the blood parasite *Babesia*, which causes tick fever.

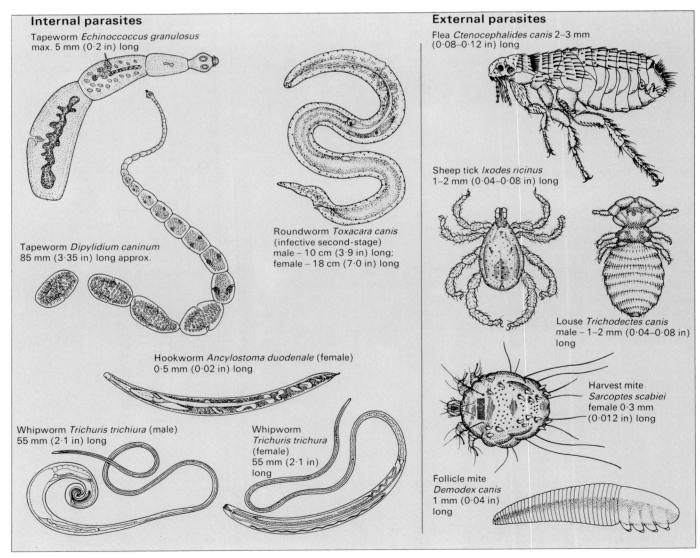

Internal parasites

Tapeworm *Echinoccoccus granulosus* max. 5 mm (0·2 in) long

Tapeworm *Dipylidium caninum* 85 mm (3·35 in) long approx.

Roundworm *Toxacara canis* (infective second-stage) male – 10 cm (3·9 in) long; female – 18 cm (7·0 in) long

Hookworm *Ancylostoma duodenale* (female) 0·5 mm (0·02 in) long

Whipworm *Trichuris trichiura* (male) 55 mm (2·1 in) long

Whipworm *Trichuris trichura* (female) 55 mm (2·1 in) long

External parasites

Flea *Ctenocephalides canis* 2–3 mm (0·08–0·12 in) long

Sheep tick *Ixodes ricinus* 1–2 mm (0·04–0·08 in) long

Louse *Trichodectes canis* male – 1–2 mm (0·04–0·08 in) long

Harvest mite *Sarcoptes scabiei* female 0·3 mm (0·012 in) long

Follicle mite *Demodex canis* 1 mm (0·04 in) long

All these parasites can be controlled by baths, powder or spray insecticides. Determined application over weeks or months may be necessary to eliminate them altogether.

'Fly Strike' occurs in untreated wounds of dogs. Certain flies lay their eggs in the dog's coat, attracted by the decaying flesh, and small white larvae hatch in a day or two. Treatment of the wound and insecticidal attack on the larvae is essential. Fly egg deposits in fecal matter caught around the anus of hairy breeds such as Old English Sheepdogs can be a serious problem also.

Internal parasites include the common intestinal worms. Roundworms infest almost all young puppies and are passed on from the dam and all puppies should be dosed from about three weeks of age. The eggs of the roundworm pass from an infected dog into its feces and develop into the infectious larval stage. If fecal material is left lying about, in parks or in the garden, where children may come into contact with it and then lick dirty fingers, the larvae may pass into the child's bloodstream. Some children have lost the sight of an eye because of the infection so it is very important that dogs are regularly wormed and that dogs are not allowed to defecate in places where children may play.

Tapeworms are common. All have a life cycle that includes a secondary host. The commonest dog tapeworm is one that has the dog flea as its secondary host. Other tapeworms have a life cycle involving sheep and are a great nuisance in sheep-farming countries. New Zealand, for example, has a compulsory treatment program for dogs.

Hookworms and whipworms are less common, but they both cause intermittent diarrhea and other symptoms.

Different drugs are effective individually against each of these worms. Some newer ones are able to combat most worms. It is worth discussing a routine with your veterinarian.

Parvovirus. This serious virus disease swept through North America, Britain and Australia in 1978. It is spread by contact with infected dogs or their feces, so it can be contracted direct or brought in on shoes or clothing. It can spread very quickly and needs immediate treatment if it is not to be fatal. The symptoms are vomiting, diarrhea (often blood-stained), depression, loss of appetite and high temperature. Every puppy should be protected by vaccination against parvovirus, and this should be renewed annually.

Peritonitis. Acute peritonitis is uncommon in dogs despite the variety of apparently dangerous objects many of them swallow. Signs include high temperature and a tense, painful abdomen. More chronic inflammation can occur with remarkably few symptoms. Take the dog to a veterinarian if you suspect peritonitis.

Pneumonia. Although bacterial pneumonia is no longer the scourge it once was it is still a serious disease. If suspected it needs prompt attention. The signs include difficult or distressed breathing and general malaise. A deep cough is usually apparent and the dog's temperature is raised. Virus infections are also involved. Apart from conventional treatment with antibiotics and nursing, the use of oxygen may be helpful.

Poisons. Poisoning in dogs is uncommon. Signs of poisoning fall into two general groups. There is nervous involvement with either heightened reactions ranging from muscular twitching to convulsions, or reduced reactions leading to coma. Modern insecticides are prominent in the poisons involving the nervous system. There is also the 'eutectic' group causing acute symptoms of gastroenteritis, with vomiting and diarrhea. Caustic poisons result in an inflamed ulcerated mouth and tongue, and the 'Warfarin' (Coumarin) type of rat poison may cause severe blood disorders in dogs. In cases of suspected poisoning do not treat the dog without reference to a veterinarian. Take any suspected container or material with you when the dog goes for treatment.

Prolapse. Rectal prolapse can sometimes occur through straining during defecation, more especially in old dogs with weak muscles. Vaginal prolapse is an even less common sequel to whelping, but prolapse of vaginal polyps, giving the appearance at first sight of vaginal tissue itself, is more often encountered. The prolapsed tissue should be kept as clean as possible and the dog prevented from licking or biting the lesion. Veterinary attention should be sought.

Rabies. All warmblooded animals can spread rabies, a disease which has horrible consequences, and once it has taken hold it is invariably fatal. In countries where rabies is present, it is frequently carried by raccoons, bats, skunks and foxes. Bites from these creatures can infect a pet dog which may then pass the infection to humans. For this reason, it is important to check your dog regularly for bites or puncture marks and if you find evidence of a bite, take the dog to the vet immediately. A person who is bitten by an animal should consult a physician as speedily as possible, as effective vaccine can be administered if action is taken in time.

If a dog has been infected with rabies it can take months for the symptoms to appear. The first sign may be a personality change with a normally gregarious dog avoiding company, a gentle dog becoming aggressive or a placid dog becoming restless. Its bark may become high pitched and it may find bright light irritating. One frequently reported symptom is a sudden and inexplicable fear of its owner. After that the dog may progress to

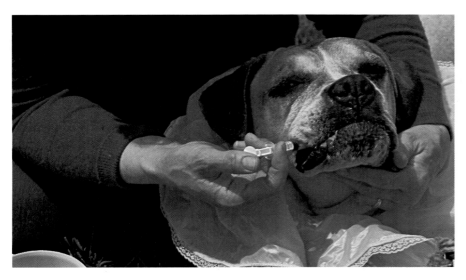

When a sick dog finds it difficult to eat or drink, it can be fed glucose through the side of its mouth with a syringe-like applicator.

'dumb' or paralytic rabies, so that paralysis sets in and it is unable to eat or drink. Some dogs may go through a 'furious' stage where they become angry and snappy, likely to bite anything that gets in their way and liable to wander off, spreading the disease over a wide area.

Quarantine regulations in a country like Britain, where rabies is not present, are aimed at preventing rabies from entering and should be strictly observed. It is highly irresponsible to try to smuggle animals into the country, however good your intentions may be. Any animal suspected of entering a rabies-free country illegally should be reported to the authorities. In countries where rabies is present, like the United States, it is essential to vaccinate pets regularly.

Rheumatism. Muscular rheumatism is common in dogs, occuring generally but not invariably, after they are six or seven years old. The signs include intermittent pain, which may be localized or in various limbs. The condition is not usually serious but demands treatment nevertheless. Drugs are usually successful in alleviating the pain. A warm and comfortable bed may help.

Rickets. Rickets is a disease of growing animals, caused by an imbalance of Vitamin D, or calcium or phosphorous. There may be lameness, but the most obvious signs are enlarged limb joints, even enlarged bone-cartilage junctions down the length of the ribs. Giant breeds are particularly prone to the disease. A well-balanced diet is the best means of prevention.

Sex play. Male or female puppies will mount each other, or humans, in apparent sex play (see page 140). In the young this is considered more as 'dominance play' than an act of overt sexual implication and should be regarded in that light. The sometimes aggressive sexual behavior of

mature male dogs to their owner may have the same origins, but it becomes actively sexual and anti-social if not curbed. It can sometimes be cured only by castration.

Shock. Shock occurs readily in dogs exposed to typical situations involving trauma, such as road accidents. The symptoms may include apparent fright or dullness, rapid shallow breathing and pale gums. Shock, rather than injury, is often the cause of death after an accident. The dog should be kept quiet and calmed until veterinary assistance is obtained.

Ticks *see* **Parasites.**

Tumors. Both benign and malignant tumors can affect dogs and you should report any lump or bump that appears on your pet's body to the vet promptly. In cases of cancerous tumors, early detection can mean a complete cure. Any moles that spread or bleed should also be reported immediately.

Vomiting. The usual cause of vomiting is some degree of gastritis but other causes include digestive upsets, bacterial infection and the presence of foreign bodies or indigestible bones. Vomiting is a symptom, not an illness in itself. Dogs can voluntarily vomit. If your dog does vomit, and this happens more than a few times in a short period, if blood is present or the dog appears to be in pain, seek veterinary help. *See also* **Gastritis.**

Warts. Older dogs of most breeds suffer from warts, but they are particularly common in Spaniels and Poodles. Surgical removal may be necessary, particularly if the warts become infected, as often happens. A vaccine may be effective in preventing their reappearance. Young puppies occasionally suffer from a crop of warts, but treatment to prevent soreness until they disappear is usually all that is necessary.

Worms *see* **Parasites.**

THE OLDER DOG

The first sign of ageing in a dog is usually graying of the muzzle. The coat may become duller and coarser and the dog may slow down in its movements. It is usually the eyes that begin to fail first, then the hearing. A dog will normally adapt quite well as its eyesight deteriorates, as scent will have played a much larger part in its life than sight, but you should make sure that its bed, food and waterbowls are always in the same place. Regular routine is important and any children in the family should be taught to approach gently, giving good warning of their presence. A dog that no longer sees or hears well may get an unpleasant shock if someone pounces suddenly, flinging loving arms around its neck and even a placid pet may react angrily. However, it should be shown plenty of gentle affection and not ignored if it spends more time sitting in its basket and fails to run to greet you.

Old dogs need quiet and warmth – though in very hot weather they should have a cool, shaded spot – and a bed large enough to allow them to stretch out, as their joints may be too stiff to allow them to curl up comfortably. The diet should be good quality, with less carbohydrates than when the dog was younger, and perhaps two smaller meals a day rather than one large one. If the dog seems to be less interested in food, it may be that its sense of smell is poor and serving liver, pilchards or perhaps a good quality cat food may help to reawaken its appetite; you might also try warming the food so that it smells more appetizing. If the dog seems to have difficulty eating, have its teeth checked for problems. In cases of constipation, add a little bran to each meal but do not serve very dry food – mixing in a little warm gravy can be a good idea.

Always let an elderly dog take life at its own pace. If it still enjoys a long walk, then there is no reason to cut down its exercise but never force it to walk further than is comfortable. If it slows down or seems to be panting, carry it home or, if this is not possible, let it lie down and rest until it feels like carrying on.

Any persistent weight loss, coughing, excessive urination or thirst should be reported to your vet without delay and in any case, six-monthly veterinary checks are advisable once a dog reaches 10 years. Diagnosis of a serious ailment does not necessarily mean that euthanasia is the only answer. With careful treatment, many dogs with kidney or heart problems can live a reasonably good life. Deciding whether or not a sick pet should be put to sleep always causes a great deal of heartache but if you are hesitating over the decision, ask yourself one important question: is the dog still enjoying life? Your vet will advise on the likely progression of any disease and if you watch your pet dog carefully, you will be able to tell if it is feeling pain.

Some families, looking ahead to the time when their pet dies and leaves an empty basket, bring in a new puppy. Though some dogs take kindly to the new arrival, which may even give them a new lease of life, it is not usually a wise course. It is natural for a puppy to get a great deal of attention and the old dog can become jealous and unhappy. This can rebound on the puppy, which finds itself snapped and snarled at so often that it becomes uncertain and shrinking.

TRAVELING

Transporting dogs abroad if, for instance, the owner is emigrating or is posted abroad for a long period is a business for the experts. It will be necessary to contact one of the agencies specializing in handling animals in transit; they will provide a traveling crate which will conform to the regulations and make sure that the dog travels comfortably. Each country has its own regulations for health tests and vaccinations and it is essential to ensure that all the documentation is correct, otherwise the dog may not be admitted on arrival.

You should accustom your dog to its traveling quarters a week or so before the journey by feeding it inside the crate, then confining it inside for a short time. Gradually increase the time until the dog will happily spend the night inside. This will lessen any anxiety the dog feels during the journey.

Most dogs will adapt well to air travel and arrive in excellent condition but a sea passage may be overlong. Special kennels are often provided but the lack of exercise and temperature changes can mean that the journey has a debilitating effect on the dog. Several countries have quarantine regulations to prevent rabies being brought into the country by an infected animal. In Britain every dog arriving from abroad, even from a rabies-free country, must spend six months in a government-approved quarantine kennel and during this period it does not come into contact with any other animal. If the dog does not develop any symptoms during this period, it is released to its owners.

BOARDING

If your dog cannot go with you on vacation and there is no one to look after it at home, you will need to leave it at a reputable boarding kennel. Anywhere with good facilities and caring staff will be booked months ahead, so be sure to make arrangements in good time. Your vet or the local canine society may be able to recommend a suitable kennel; otherwise you will have to rely on the telephone directory and personal inspection. Arrange to visit the kennel to talk to the staff. Look for spotlessly clean premises with no unpleasant smells, where the dogs are housed singly in sleeping compartments with an adjacent run. You will be able to see if the dogs look happy and come readily towards the staff when they approach.

Any responsible kennel operators will require each owner to produce a current vaccination certificate for a boarder. If they do not, then do not leave your dog there. Make sure that the kennel staff have details of your dog's normal diet to avoid any upsets caused by changing food. Ask if you can take your dog's bed and blanket to help it to settle into the new environment but do not take along the dog's feeding dishes unless you are asked to do so. Often the staff will expect you to leave your dog in reception and to collect it from the same place. This is to prevent upset and overexcitement among the other boarders.

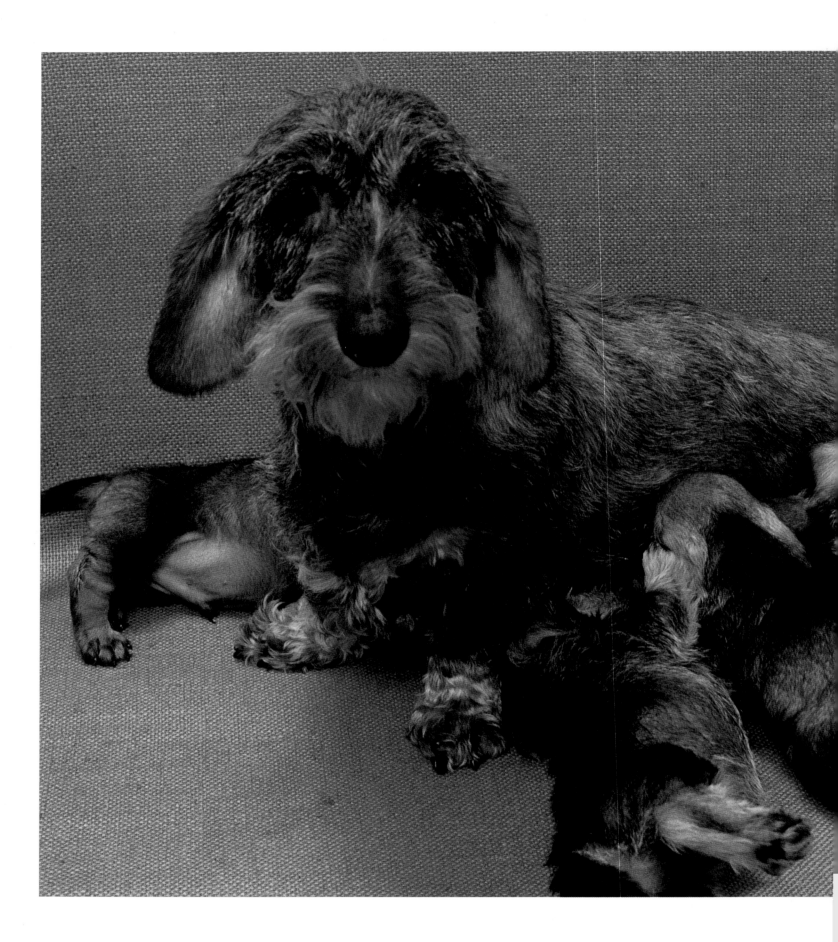

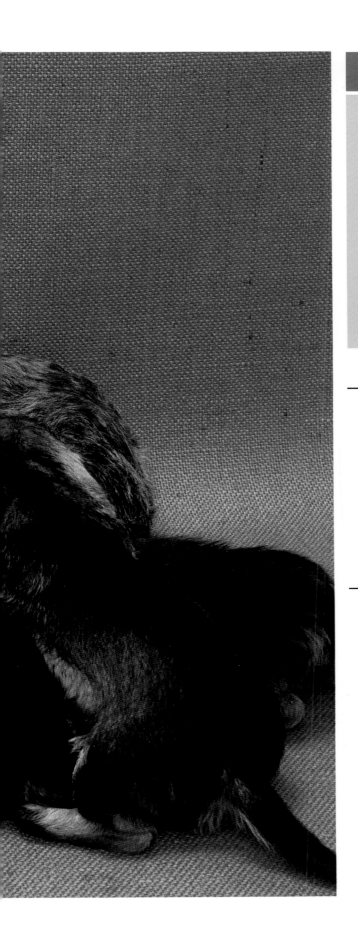

BREEDING

The process of breeding from domestic dogs needs careful management if you are to ensure a litter of good quality, healthy puppies. The stud dog, the time of mating and the whelping area must all be chosen with care. Understanding the changes in the behavior of the bitch when she is about to whelp and her instincts after the birth of the puppies will help you to take the correct action; it is also essential to watch for any signs of problems after the birth and be ready to help any puppy that is not feeding properly. Occasionally, you may even have to rear a puppy by hand.

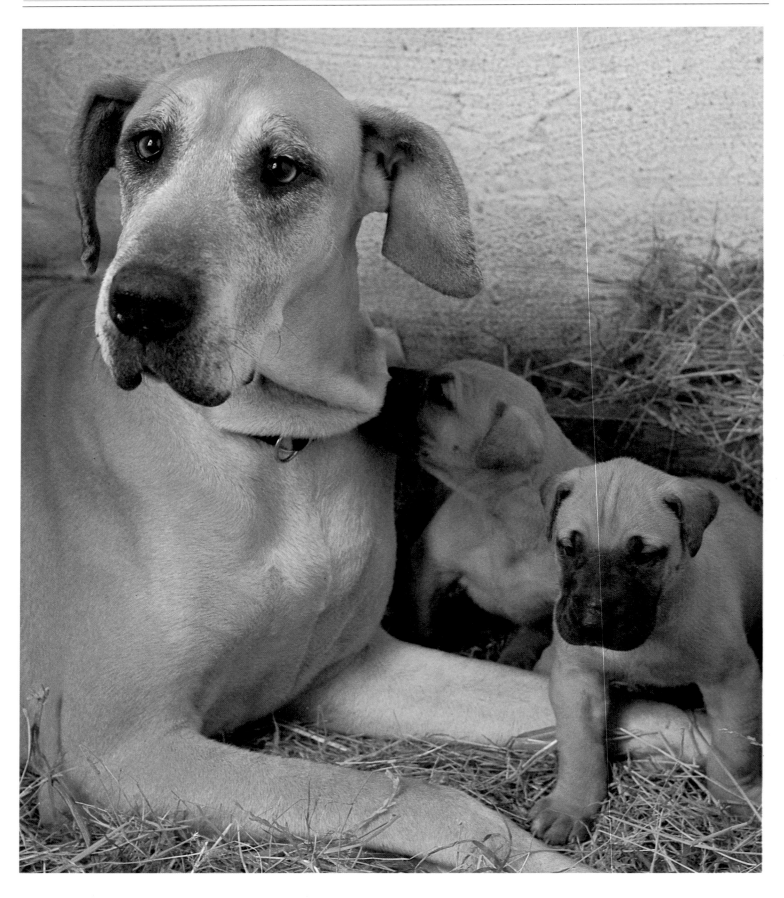

The gains you will make from breeding dogs come mainly in the pleasure of handling and raising the pups, the close relationship you will develop with your breeding bitch and the contacts and friends you will make among your customers. Dog breeding is unlikely to make money unless it is done on a large scale, in conjunction with exhibiting and perhaps a boarding kennel, so that each facet of the business feeds the others. For small-scale breeders the cost of stud fees, food, vet's bills and advertising will soon swallow up any profits from the sale of the pups.

PREPARATIONS

Your schedule should be planned so that you are available when the bitch starts whelping, and then for several days afterwards you should be on hand to resolve any problems which the dam or litter may have. After three weeks the pups will need to socialize, they must be weaned and shown to prospective owners. The next six weeks or so, before they leave for new homes, are very busy for an owner.

You will need to set aside suitable accommodation for the whelping, secluded from too much household bustle. A spare bedroom is often a good choice though many breeders like to set aside a corner of their own bedroom, so that they are on hand to attend to the pups by night as well as by day. A garage or shed is only suitable if it is warm, dry and light and if the bitch has settled in well before the event. At 21 days the pups will need to move downstairs, or indoors, so that they can get used to the sight and sound of people and you may need to fence off a corner of the kitchen or hall. An enclosed porch may be suitable, provided it is neither too hot nor too cold and the pups can be shielded from draughts. The pups may outgrow this accommodation by the time they are six weeks old and by then they will be active and lively, though not housetrained. A shed or kennel, for daytime use at least, is the best answer; in good weather an enclosure in the backyard may be suitable, providing it has some form of shelter. Puppies at this age can be very destructive if left loose in either house or yard.

MATING

Your bitch should be at the peak of condition when she is mated. Have her checked over well in advance by the veterinarian to make sure that she is in good physical condition and does not have any defects that might give problems during gestation, whelping or lactation. She should have her annual booster shots so that, being fully protected herself, she can pass on the maximum amount of antibodies against disease to her pups in the colostrum, or first milk. This protection will last the pups for about eight weeks and then they will be able to start their own vaccination program.

The breeder of your bitch may be able to advise on the choice of a stud dog. A local dog is preferable to one that lives a long distance away. A bitch in season is naturally stressed and a long, tiring journey may upset her so much that she rejects the dog's advances on arrival. For a bitch's first mating it is important to use an experienced stud. Temperament is of prime importance in choosing the sire for a litter of pet puppies: a good-tempered, cheerful dog is more likely to produce offspring with equable temperaments, who will settle well into family life with their new owners. If you are aiming to produce a litter of quality show puppies, then you may want to choose an outstanding champion as the sire. In that case, you can find advertisements in the specialist press or you can go to championship dog shows, taking your bitch's pedigree, and discuss mating with the owners of the winning dogs.

Bitches come into estrus (season or heat) for the

For the first five or six weeks after the birth of her puppies, this Great Dane bitch will be a devoted mother; after that she is less closely involved with them.

A stud dog is specially trained from a young age and his lifestyle is quite different from that of a pet.

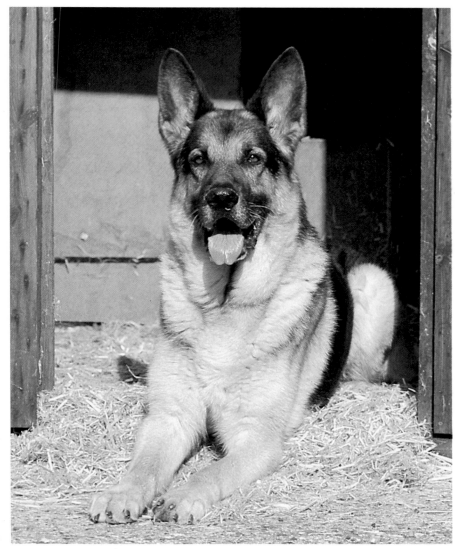

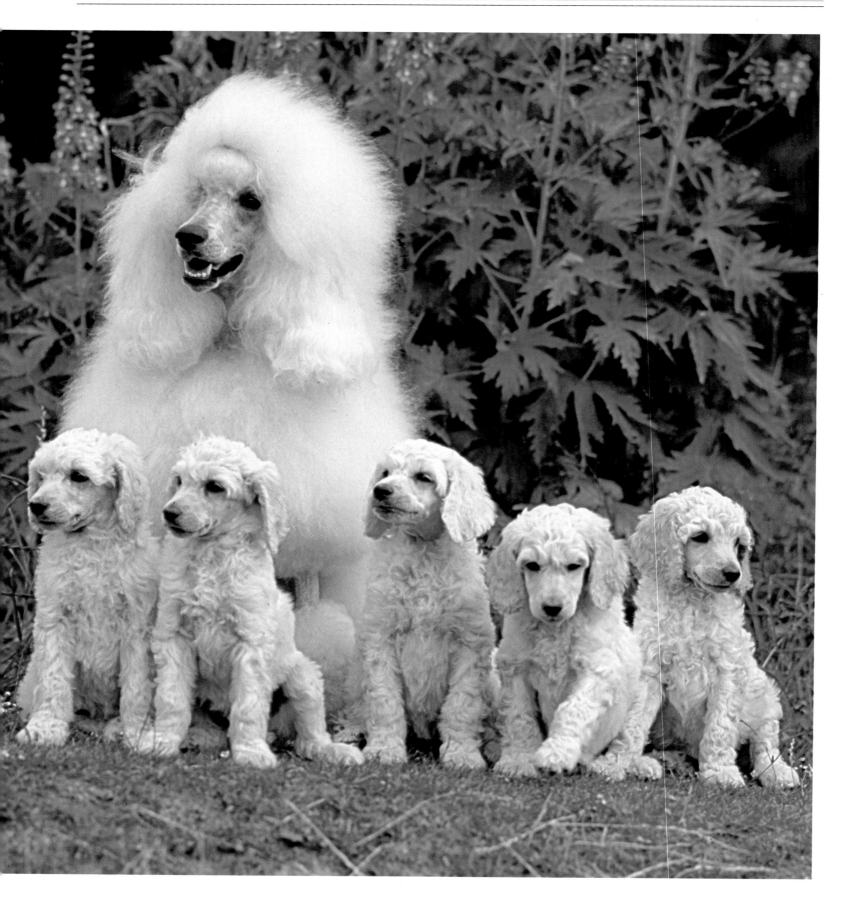

first time at about 8 months old, though this can vary from 6 to 15 months. It is not usually wise to mate a bitch at her first season as she is not yet fully mature and may make a poor mother, so most breeders will wait until the second or third season.

The usual time for mating is between the 10th and 12th day after the beginning of the red discharge. At the optimum time, the bitch will be taken to the dog. If the stud owner has the necessary facilities, it may be better to board the bitch for two or three days, so that she becomes used to the dog and they can mate at will. Otherwise two visits, not more than 48 hours apart, may be necessary, as one mating will not always do the job. The mating fee, negotiated with the stud owner, does not guarantee pregnancy but most owners will allow a free mating at the next season if no litter results.

Mating may be a brief encounter lasting 10 minutes or so, or a protracted affair of an hour or more. If the bitch is at the suitable stage in her heat, she will stand patiently while the dog mounts her and mating takes place. The anatomy of the dog is such that the mated pair are unable to separate immediately after mating. The dog gets down from the mating position and turns so that the pair stand back to back in the attitude known as the tie. Both dogs must be kept relaxed and calm at this time and under no circumstances should anyone try to separate them. After a while, the dogs will part naturally and both will clean themselves.

GESTATION

The gestation period is nine weeks, but the puppies may appear a few days earlier or later than this. During those 63 days the pups slowly develop and the bitch's abdomen increases in size in order to accommodate them. There is very little change in appearance and behavior in the first four weeks; by the fifth week, however, the mammary glands show signs of enlargement and the bitch may have slight morning sickness. By the sixth week the abdomen is definitely larger. You should now start to give an extra meal in the middle of the day.

The pregnant bitch should have high-quality and well-balanced meals throughout the gestation period. She must be kept fit and not allowed to get fat. Your veterinarian will tell you whether you should give any extra vitamin or mineral supplements. Tell him of the expected birth date in case you need to call him out. Towards the end of the pregnancy, the bitch's shape may change dramatically as the development of the puppies speeds up, and her breasts might secrete a milklike substance.

WHELPING

Loss of appetite is one of the first signs that whelping is imminent, and the bitch may go without food for 24 hours. She will also appear very restless and may repeatedly go to the whelping box and tear at the newspaper placed there. This tearing of paper harks back to the behavior of the wild dog, which would start to dig a deep burrow at this time in preparation for the birth. Just before the actual birth begins, the bitch's temperature will drop from 38.5°C to 38°C (101.3°F to 100.4°F).

Although whelping is a natural process, you may wish to call your veterinarian so that he is ready to come out to help if necessary. Most whelpings are quite normal and even the maiden bitch copes beautifully. Many novice owners are distressed by the frantic panting that the bitch often makes in the first stages of labor, but the panting subsides when whelping gets under way. Regular contractions usually produce the first puppy about an hour or so after straining begins, and the rest of the litter arrive at about 30-minute intervals. With very large litters, the bitch may tire and the last puppies will be spaced further apart.

Each puppy is born enclosed in its fetal sac, which the bitch removes by vigorous licking. This frees the youngster's head and enables it to breathe. The bitch usually cleans away the membranes and, in doing so, severs the umbilical cord. It is quite usual for her to lick up and swallow all the debris of birth, including the placentae. (In the wild, these provide the bitch with valuable nourishment while she rests and recovers from the birth of her litter.) If the bitch is unable to clean and stimulate her puppies, you must do it for her. The most important thing to remember is to quickly clear the puppies' mouths and nostrils so that they can breathe. Dry the puppies with clean, rough toweling. You do not

This white Standard Poodle has produced a fine litter of puppies.

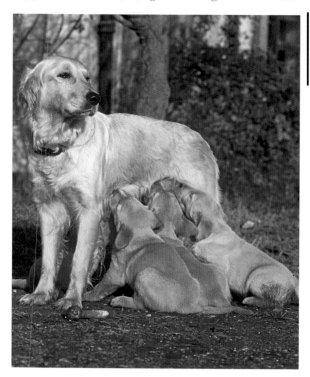

Puppies still enjoy feeding on their mother's milk, even after they have begun eating solid food.

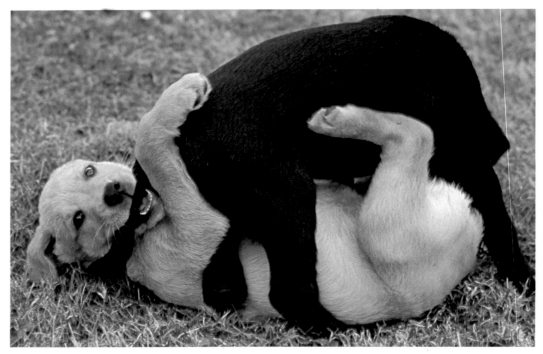

have to be in too much of a hurry to cut or break the umbilical cord.

After giving birth the bitch's instincts are to hide and protect her babies. She does not like an audience at the birth or during the first days with her litter. Take care to see that nothing happens which will cause her to be distressed or unduly disturbed.

When your bitch has produced her last puppy, she will settle down and gather them all to her. You should remove some of the soiled wet bedding and replace it with paper toweling or a blanket of the special polyester fur material made expressly for such occasions. It is important that the puppies all suckle and receive the special first-milk, or colostrum, which contains the precious maternal antibodies that protect the puppies from possible disease during the first weeks of life.

THE LITTER

Puppies are born blind and deaf but with a keen sense of smell that enables them to find the bitch's teats.

If the bitch has had a lengthy whelping or is ill, or if for some reason her milk has not developed well, you may need to give some supplementary bottle feeds to the pups; sometimes it is also necessary to do this for early arrivals during a lengthy whelping. Any pup looking thin and empty may be fed by a premature baby bottle several times a day. Give each pup as much as it will take eagerly. It is always better to bottle-feed as a supplement to the mother's milk, rather than to take some pups away from her entirely. (For more details see *Hand-*

rearing puppies, page 175) The pups should make no more than a warm humming noise, and any wailing cry or restless crawling about the box means that something is wrong.

Very few puppies are born looking like the breed standard; Dalmatians are born all white; some gray dogs are born black; brindle markings are not easily distinguishable; dogs known as 'red' look a mousy color; in all cases the proper coat color develops later. When the eyes open they are blue and this color, too, will alter later.

After the first few days following the whelping, the bitch will begin to want extra food in order to produce enough milk for her pups. This should be well balanced, served at four meals a day and generous in amount. At maximum milk production time, when the pups are three weeks old, the bitch will require three to four times as much food as normal, with vitamin and mineral supplements in proportion. By now you will find you are spending a great deal of money on your litter, but this is essential in order to rear strong and healthy puppies and to avoid the bitch 'feeding the puppies off her back' so that she becomes pitiably thin and loses all her coat.

If the puppies' tails need to be docked, this should be done when the pups are 3–4 days old, and ear cropping, in countries where this is permitted, comes at about 12 weeks of age. Toenails should be clipped soon after birth and a tiny amount taken off twice weekly thereafter in order to stop the pups scratching the bitch's teats. Navels should be inspected daily, and when the eyes open on the eighth to tenth day they should do so in a clean manner, without pus at the corners or lids.

Above left: Both yellow and black Labrador Retrievers may occur in the same litter.

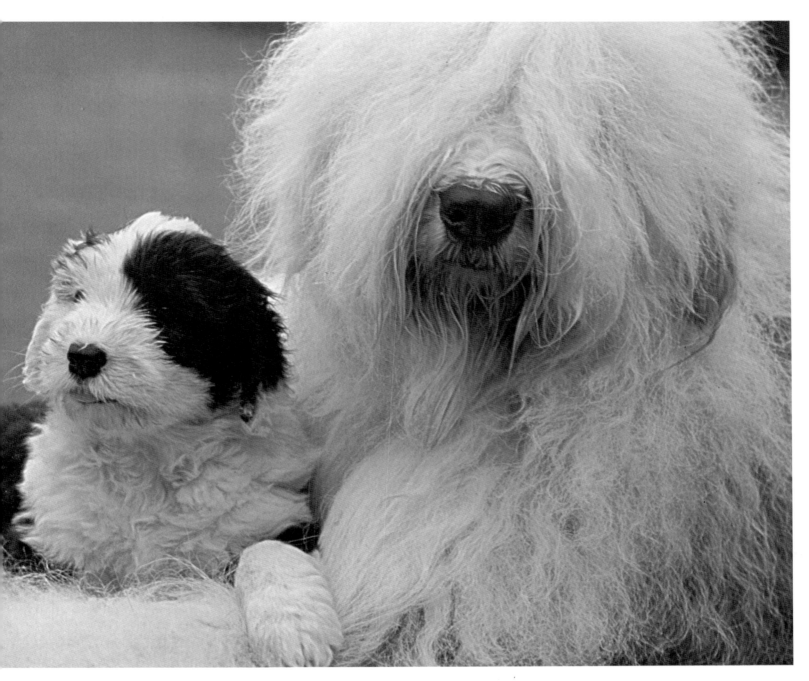

Although the ears are only just developing and hearing does not come until later, you should talk to the pups every time you see them, to accustom them to the human voice and to give them confidence. Until the pups are 20 days old, they and the bitch should remain in seclusion and not have visitors, not should the bitch go into the street for exercise. The noses of the pups will remain bright pink in most breeds. Black pigmentation begins as little dots which later fuse together to give the jet black nose desirable in all but the gray and liver breeds and the yellow Labrador Retriever.

The health of the bitch must be watched all the time she is feeding the pups as any poor appetite or refusal of food is a danger sign at this time. She should also be groomed and kept free of fleas and lice, but any powder or substance which the pups may lick must not be used. The great calamity which may overtake the bitch is eclampsia, a failure of her body to mobilize calcium which can, if neglected, lead to her death in a few hours. The symptoms are best described as 'odd behavior' – hiding under furniture, eating plaster off the walls, continually glancing at walls and ceiling, paralysis of hind-quarters, or any deranged and unnatural demon-strations. The next stage will be convulsions,

In some breeds, the coat will change color as the dog matures; for instance, this Old English Sheepdog pup will be gray and white as an adult.

Each puppy should have its own feeding bowl but it can be difficult to make sure that each gets its fair share.

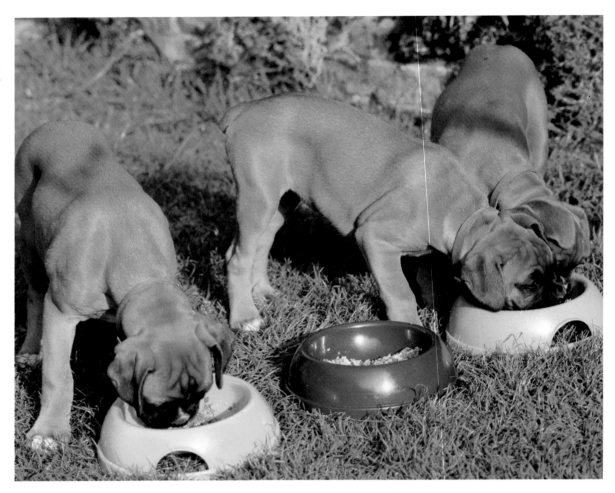

prostration and death. Immediate veterinary help, day or night, is essential from any vet if your own is not available. The reversal of the condition is quite dramatic and the bitch will be perfectly all right if you get help in time. This condition occurs most frequently when the pups are around three to four weeks old but it may come at any time, even just before the birth.

WEANING

Changing the puppy's diet from its mother's milk to a more solid diet can begin at three weeks of age or a little later. In the wild, the mother would regurgitate her own partly digested food as her milk began to dry up and breeders imitate this diet by soaking baby cereals in warm milk. You can begin by teaching the puppies to lap warm milk from a saucer. Introduce it to the puppies by wetting your finger in the milk and smearing it on their muzzles. Offer a fresh saucer of milk three times a day; first thing in the morning, at midday and in the early evening. As the puppies begin to lap, start reducing the mother's food and keep her away from the litter for periods of two or three hours.

Once the puppies are lapping freely you can introduce solid food. Soak a little baby cereal or specially prepared puppy meal in an equal volume of hot milk and allow the mixture to cool to blood heat. Offer this food two or three times a day at what you intend to be regular mealtimes. It is a good idea to feed puppies on a flat tray, large enough for all the heads to go round it, as this encourages competition. At first the pups will try to suck out the milk but in about a week they should be eating solid food. The texture should not be sticky but consist of separate, soft, moist pieces. Continue to reduce the bitch's food and remove her from the pups except at night and for one or two brief periods during the day.

After about six weeks the puppies should be fully weaned and it is now important to increase the quantity of food rapidly to keep pace with growth. Keep the midday meal small while increasing the quantity of solid food, but not of milk, at the morning and evening meals. Water must now be freely available and a little warm milk can also be offered in the late evening. The total amount of milk each day should range from about 0.15 litres ($\frac{1}{4}$ pt, $\frac{5}{8}$ cup) for very small breeds to 0.5 litres (1 pt, $2\frac{1}{2}$ cups) for giants. At this stage, the puppies should be fed in individual bowls so that each gets its share.

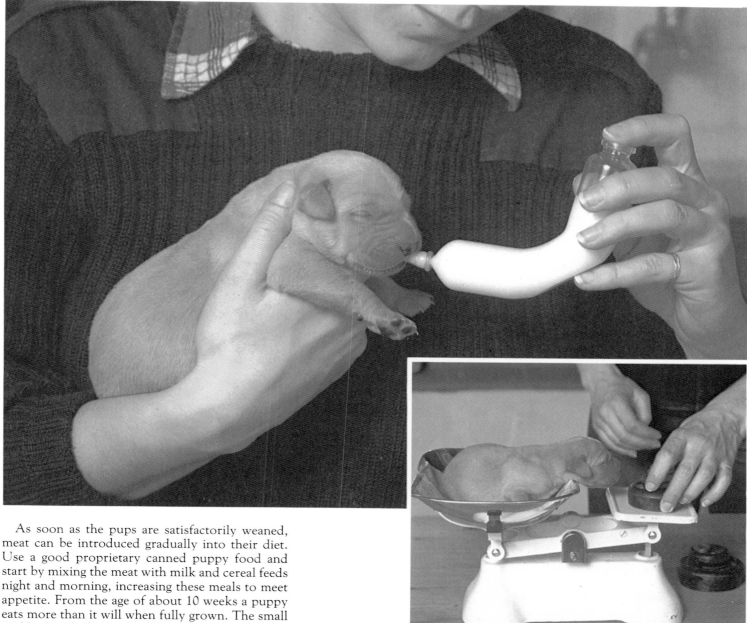

As soon as the pups are satisfactorily weaned, meat can be introduced gradually into their diet. Use a good proprietary canned puppy food and start by mixing the meat with milk and cereal feeds night and morning, increasing these meals to meet appetite. From the age of about 10 weeks a puppy eats more than it will when fully grown. The small midday meal and optional late milk can be omitted from the age of three months, if not before.

HANDREARING PUPPIES

It is sometimes necessary to handrear puppies if, for instance, they are orphaned at birth, they are rejected by the mother or she is unable to feed them. If the puppies are weak and sickly, your vet will advise on how they should be fed. If they are normally healthy, they can be fed with a proprietary canine milk substitute, mixed fresh every day and fed lukewarm. Do not feed puppies on human baby milk, as this is not rich enough for them. Use a premature baby's feeding bottle or a special animal nursing bottle; either will prevent the puppy taking in too much air. Feed at two-hourly intervals at first, lengthening to three-hourly after a couple of days, then six feeds a day within a week. After that, four feeds a day should be sufficient until weaning. Do not hold a puppy on its back while feeding, like a baby. Instead, support the puppy from underneath, with your hand under its chest, leaving its legs to move freely, as they would when feeding from its mother.

Newborn orphans must be kept warm and you will need to stimulate them to empty their bladder and bowels. You can do this by gently massaging the abdominal and anal area after each feed, using a tissue moistened with warm water or baby oil.

A puppy can be hand-reared, using a special feeding bottle and a canine milk substitute. It is advisable to keep a regular check on the puppy's weight, to ensure that it is making progress.

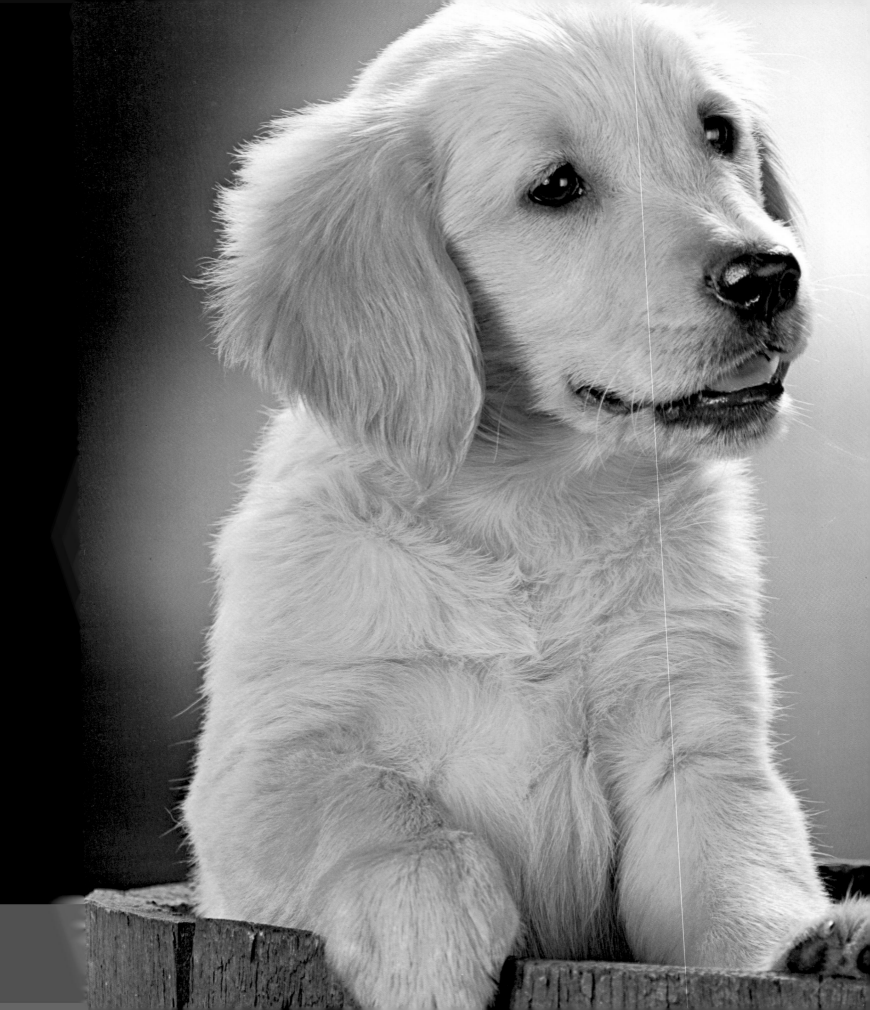

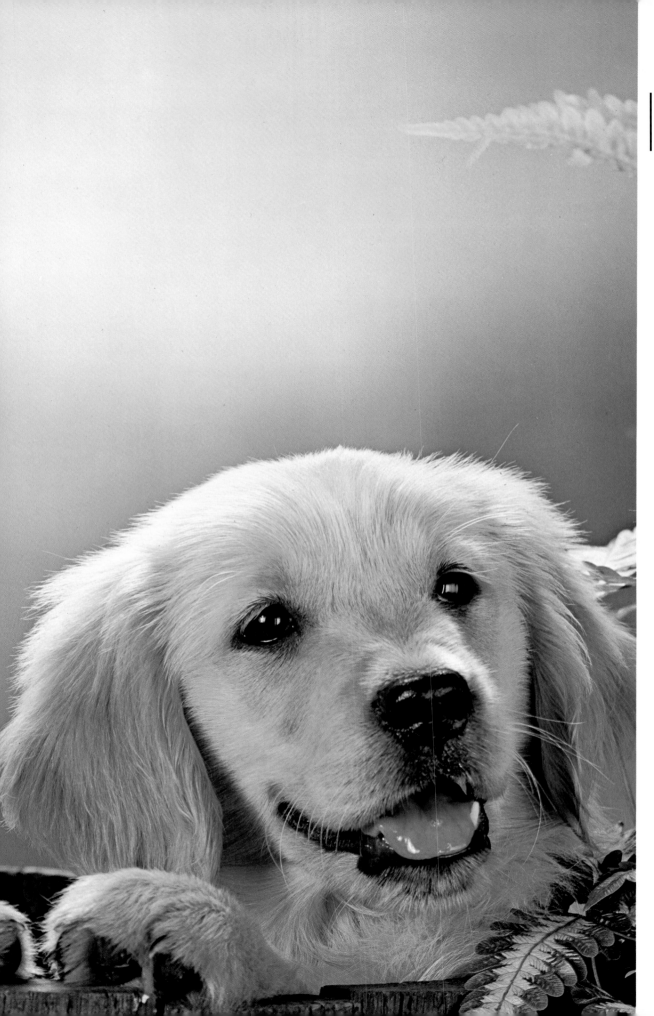

These two Golden Retriever puppies are at a most appealing stage.

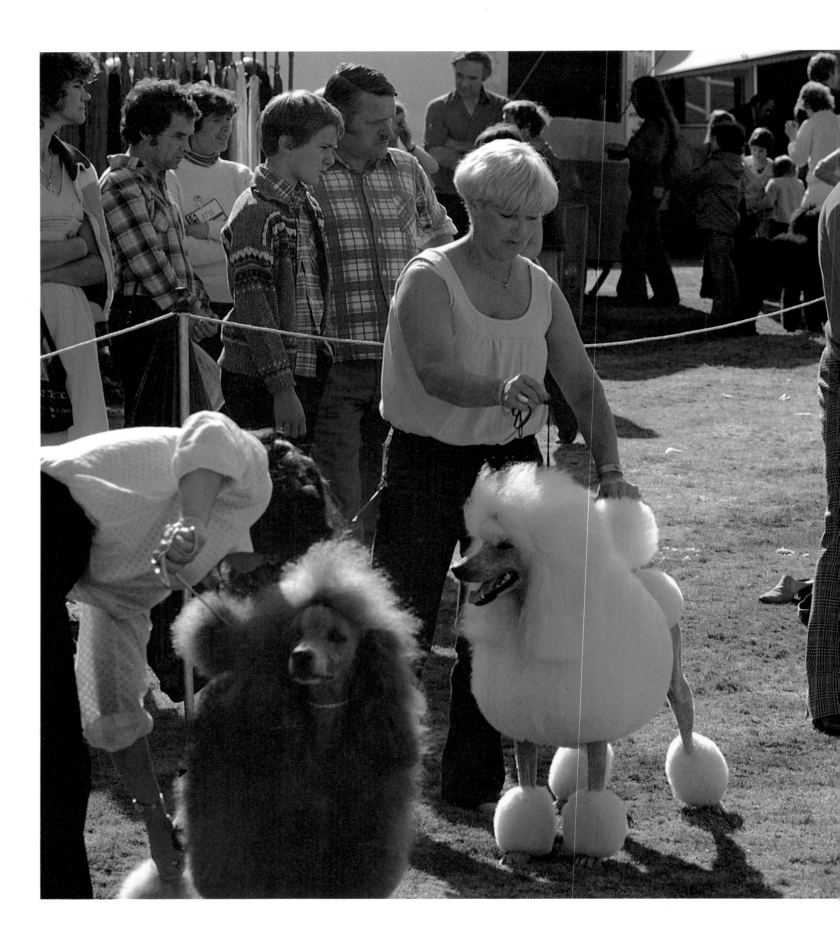

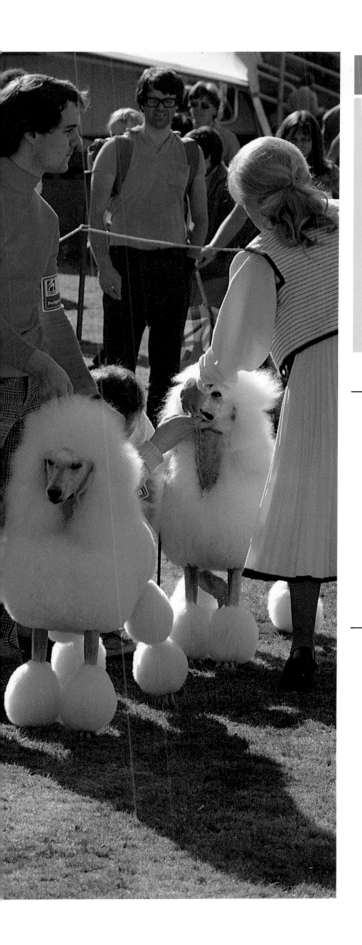

SHOWING

Every year thousands of dog shows are held all over the world, from informal local events to prestigious championship shows with only the best eligible to compete. Some shows concentrate on conformation, others include obedience trials. Apart from the opportunity to have your dog compared and assessed against others, these are social events where dog lovers can meet and share their enthusiasm and showing can become a year-round hobby for the whole family. However, presenting your dog to its best advantage is an art and you need to be prepared to spend time on preparing your dog's appearance and behavior for the show ring.

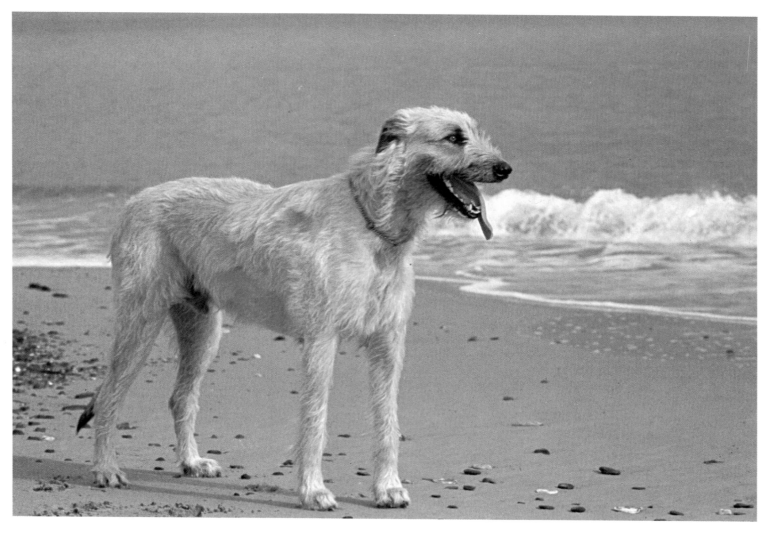

The Irish Wolfhound is one of the breeds that might have died out, but for breeding by enthusiasts for showing purposes.

In the days when dog fighting, bull- and bear-baiting were popular activities, dogs were bred for their speed, stamina and ferocity, but when these cruel sports were banned, owners began matching their dogs with one another for appearance only. The first record of an organized dog show was in Newcastle-upon-Tyne in England in June 1859, with one class for setters and one for pointers, and the following year the first 'exhibition' for all breeds was held in Birmingham. The British Kennel Club was founded in 1873 and the American Kennel Club in 1884. These kennel clubs are still recognized as the ruling bodies in their respective countries. The clubs lay down standards for the breeds, and these are the 'blueprints' against which individual dogs are judged. The breed standard covers conformation, color and type of coat, color and shape of eyes, gait and temperament. Some breeds are not universally recognized; for instance the Löwchen and the Swedish Vallhund are recognized by the Kennel Club in Britain but not by the American Kennel Club. Dogs such as the Border Collie, the Australian Kelpie and the Chinese Crested Dog, all recognized in Britain, are placed in a 'Miscellaneous' class in the United States. This means that they can compete in obedience trials or Miscellaneous classes at conformation shows but they are not eligible for championship points. Dogs in the Miscellaneous class will only be fully recognized if the American Kennel Club is convinced that there is a genuine nationwide interest in the breed.

The merits of dog shows are frequently criticized, with opposing factions maintaining that certain breeds have been either improved or ruined as a result of showing. The supporters claim that some breeds, such as the Irish Wolfhound and the Old English Mastiff, would be extinct if it were not for dog shows and that the breeding of an animal to certain standards of perfection is a never-ending source of pleasure and satisfaction. The detractors claim that breeding to supposedly desirable standards has meant that the appearance of some dogs has been exaggerated to the point where it affects their health: the Bulldog's nose is so snubbed that it has breathing problems, Basset Hounds are

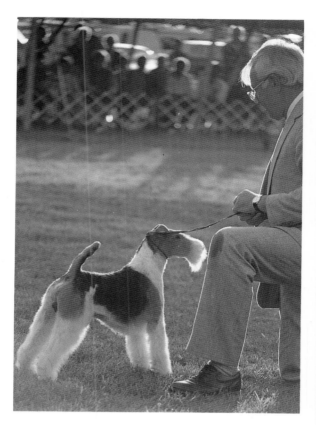

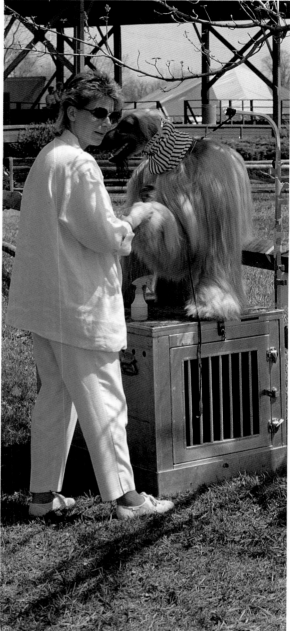

so long and heavy that they are vulnerable to back trouble and the miniaturizing of the Poodle has led to weak hip joints and slipping kneecaps.

SHOW ORGANIZATION

Dog shows fall into two main categories: those confined to a particular breed and those covering many varieties of the breeds registered with the governing kennel club. The more serious shows are run under strict rules but there are informal shows where beginners, both competitors and judges, can gain experience. In Britain these are called 'exemption' shows, because they are exempt from Kennel Club rules, and they have classes for both pedigree dogs and pets. In the United States, informal events are 'dog matches,' usually with both conformation and obedience classes.

Shows in each country have separate classes for dogs and bitches and the classes for each sex are subdivided, so that numbers do not become unwieldy.

Regular classes at an American dog show are as follows:

Puppy. This may be divided into puppies from 6 to 9 months and puppies from 9 to 12 months.

Novice. Dogs at least 6 months old which have not won other adult classes and have not won Novice more than 3 times.

Bred by exhibitor. Dogs aged 6 months or more, bred and shown by the same person or the cobreeder.

American bred. Dogs 6 months and over, bred in the US.

Open. Dogs 6 months and over, including imported dogs.

The divisions in Britain, where dog shows are some of the largest in the world, are far more complicated and details can be obtained from the Kennel Club.

For many, the highlight of a dog show is the

At a show, dogs are judged on how well they measure up to an ideal standard for the breed. Top dog handler Mr P. Green shows a Wire Fox Terrier at the Montgomery Dog Show, USA (left), while an Afghan Hound is given a final grooming before a show at Bull Run, Virginia, USA (right).

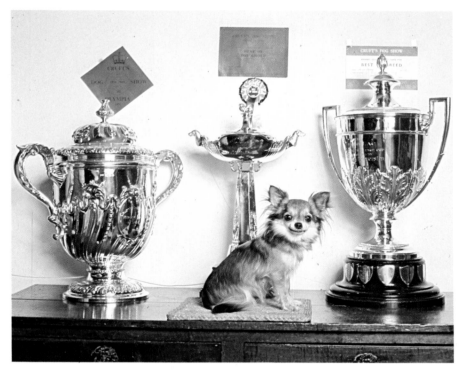

This long-coated Chihuahua has been a top winner at Crufts, Britain's most prestigious dog show.

The Yorkshire Terrier's long, silky tresses are rolled in tissue paper and secured by rubber bands to prevent them breaking or becoming matted before the show (top right).

German Shepherds are often successful in obedience trials, which include retrieving a dumbbell (below right).

selection of Best in Show. First, the best dog and the best bitch in each breed are chosen from the individual class winners. The dog and bitch then meet and one is chosen as Best of Breed. The Best of Breeds are then judged in their relevant groups (Hounds, Terriers, Working, Toys, etc) and one is chosen as Best of Group. The group winners then appear again in the ring so that the judge can choose the Best in Show.

SHOW JUDGING

Different countries use different procedures for awarding the title of champion in dog shows. The United States uses a points system. To become a champion a dog must accumulate 15 points. Points are awarded to the best of each sex in accordance with the number of dogs of the breed competing at each show. The numbers governing the points value of a show vary in different parts of the country, in an attempt to give more equal chances to the less popular breeds, or the more sparsely populated areas. The lowest rating is 1 and the highest 5. Two of the shows at which a champion has succeeded must be major shows carrying, 3, 4 or 5 points. The Canadian Kennel Club runs a similar system to the American one, though at least 10 points must be awarded by at least three different judges.

In Britain, dogs become champions when they have been awarded three Challenge Certificates by three different judges, at least one after the dog is 12 months old. Judges at Championship shows may award Challenge Certificates to the best of each sex in a breed but the award is not automatic and the

judge must consider that the animal is worthy of the title of champion. These certificates are much prized because it is considered more difficult to achieve champion status under the British system than under others. A modified form of the British system is used in Commonwealth countries, except for Canada.

The Scandinavian and west European kennel clubs, as well as some in South America and eastern Europe, operate under the auspices of the Fédération Cynologique International (FCI). This body was founded in 1911 by the French, German, Belgian, Dutch and Austrian kennel clubs to organize and control dog shows. The FCI creates champions by awarding Certificates of Aptitude, Championship International, Beauty (CACIB). The dog must win at least four of these in at least three different countries under three different judges.

The routine of judging is broadly similar in each country, though it varies slightly from one individual to another. The combination of hand and eye tells a good judge all he or she needs to know about a dog. The assessment involves looking, feeling and the study of the dog's movement. Movement is often the most searching assessment, as many blemishes can be concealed when the dog is posed by a clever handler. Toes with a tendency to turn out can be placed in the correct position and a dog with hindlegs tucked underneath can be trained to stand with them placed well out behind. Loose elbows, a badly carried head or cow hocks may not be detected when the dog is standing still but once it moves, all is revealed. The judge can assess the dog's gait, the carriage of the tail and head.

Judges measure each dog against their idea of the ideal dog in a particular breed. Judging dogs according to group involves comparing entries with the standards for each breed. A Pekingese is not compared to a Great Dane as such but the winner will be the dog which comes nearer to the judge's picture of the ideal for its breed. For instance, if the Great Dane was a fine, elegant specimen, sound in movement, with a good head and well-arched neck, while the Pekingese had a 'weak' head and protruding nose, as well as a long and oversized body, it would be easy to judge the Great Dane the winner. Working on the same principles, a skilled judge can rank 20 dogs in order.

PREPARING FOR SHOWING

Owners who are interested in showing their dogs should spend time at shows, both small local events and championship shows, observing the routine and talking to breeders and professional handlers. Watch how the experts handle their dogs and display them to the best advantage. You may hear stories about judges who 'judge the other end of the leash' from owners who have shown a dog unsuccessfully for a long time, then sold it to another owner who immediately starts winning classes. The truth is probably that the new owner has managed to present the dog to perfection, instead of dragging it around the show ring like the first owner. Presentation and showmanship may not be able to turn a bad dog into a good one but it can improve its appearance considerably.

Breeds vary so much that preparation for a show varies just as much. A book devoted to your particular breed of dog will give detailed advice on preparing the animal for the show ring and you can pick up plenty of tips by talking to experienced exhibitors. However, several general points apply to any show dog. Good condition 'goes in at the mouth' and no amount of grooming and training can make up for an incorrect diet. Adequate exercise is also essential, though 'adequate' is the key word. A showdog does not need to be as fit as a racing Greyhound; in fact, it should carry more flesh to give a more rounded appearance.

HANDLING

To win in the show ring the dog must walk well on the lead, stand to be handled by the judge and have a general air of self-possession. Training your dog to walk on the lead, adjusting to your pace and stopping when you stop, is very important; it should also be accustomed to trotting on the lead without breaking stride, holding up its head. Your pet should be used to other dogs, to noise and bustle, so training classes can be very useful and some canine societies run handling classes for 'beauty' dogs, as opposed to 'obedience' dogs.

Practice posing your dog in the correct position – head up, feet well-placed – from puppyhood. Ask friends to help by examining teeth and, on a male dog, the testicles, so that your dog is used to being handled and examined. Judges have a very short time available in which to assess a dog and the best of specimens can miss out on prizes if the animal is fidgeting and fighting the judge's hands instead of standing quietly and calmly.

Nerves will soon communicate themselves to your dog and a nervous owner will not inspire confidence in an animal. This is one of the reasons that some owners put their dog in the hands of a professional handler, who prepares and shows the dog. Professional handling is very common in America and for some breeds in Britain, with most Wire Fox Terriers and several other terriers being handled by professionals. Professional handlers often start as breeders who find that they have the knack of presenting dogs to the best advantage. Some 1000 handlers are licensed by the American Kennel Club. Some take dogs for specific shows, grooming and preparing them, then showing them in the ring; others take a number of dogs on a 'circuit', such as the Florida Circuit or the Deep South Circuit, showing them at a series of shows in

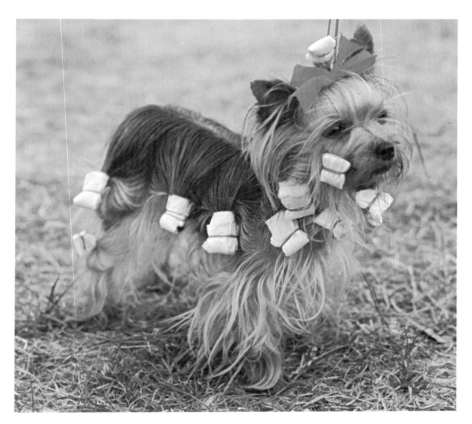

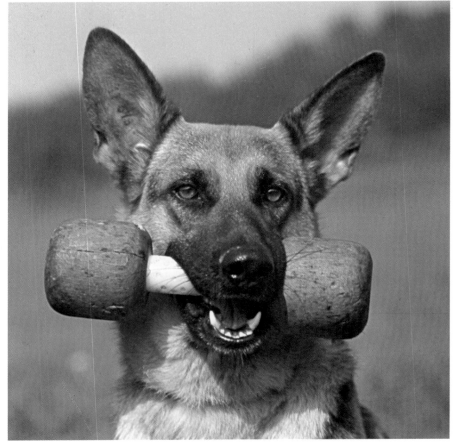

a particular area. It may be more difficult for a novice handler to win against the professional but, given a good dog and a confident owner, it does happen and the satisfaction of beating the 'experts' is enormous.

THE SHOW DAY

Necessary equipment for a day at a show includes:
* Collar and bench chain
* Show lead
* Dog food and feeding dish
* Water from the dog's usual supply and a water bowl
* Dog blanket
* Grooming equipment
* Pencil and paper to take notes
* Sensible nonfussy clothes (large pockets are useful) with nothing that jangles or flaps to distract dog or judges

Plan to arrive at the show in plenty of time so that you can exercise and play with your dog, making the outing more relaxing and enjoyable for both of you. If you arrive at the last minute, in a whirl of fuss and bother, your tension will communicate itself to your dog and it is unlikely to show at its best. Keep grooming to a minimum and allow your dog to eat and relieve itself according to its normal schedule as far as possible, though it is unwise to feed a dog just before judging as this may leave your pet sleepy and unresponsive.

Novices are often confused to find that the judge at one show will often reverse the placings of a judge at another. Though judging is according to the standard laid down for each breed, different judges may interpret the standard in different ways. One

The Terrier class at the Montgomery Dog Show.

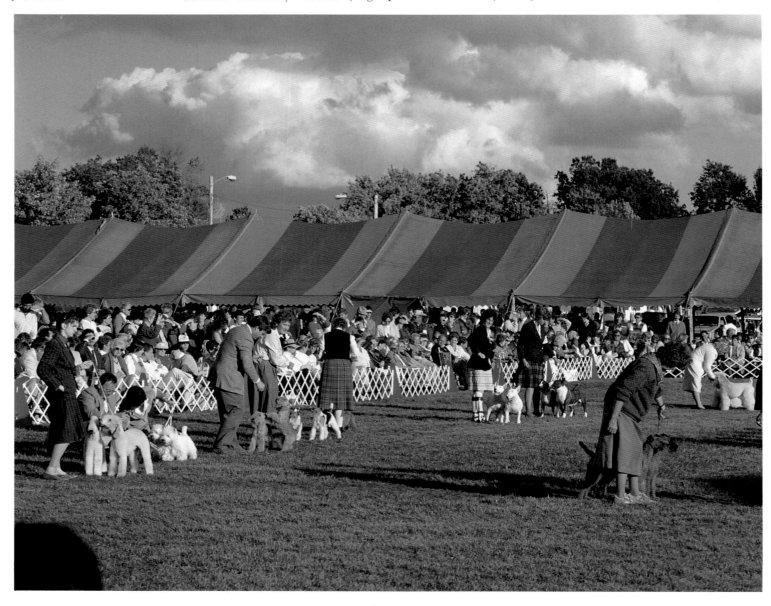

judge's idea of 'moderately wide between the ears' will differ from another's. Probably this is just as well, because if everyone could agree on the perfect dog, then that dog would win all the prizes and there would be no point in anyone else showing. Experienced exhibitors learn which judges prefer their type of dog and try to show under those judges.

OBEDIENCE COMPETITIONS

Obedience classes and competitions are often held at general dog shows, in a ring similar to that used for breed classes. However, the look of a dog and the lack of conformity with the breed standard counts for nothing in obedience competitions; what matters is the precision with which the dog carries out a series of standard exercises. Competition rules vary from country to country but novice classes include basic obedience exercises such as heel, left and right turns, sit and stay and recall. Of course, any well-trained pet can perform these exercises but this does not mean that it could hold its own in competition, where the standards will be very high and any hesitation or inexact positioning is penalized. A slight movement by the dog can make all the difference between success and failure.

In obedience competitions the aim is for the dog to work in a happy, natural manner. Although the performance of both dog and handler is judged in relation to closely defined criteria, great emphasis is placed on the dog's willingness and enjoyment of its work and on the smoothness and naturalness of the handler's control. It is very much a team effort and a nervous or overmanaging handler can cause a good dog to fail.

Long hours of work are required from both dog and handler and it is essential to enlist in a good obedience class as part of the training schedule, so that the instructor can observe your work from a distance and draw attention to any faults. Remember, however, that a class is only as good as the teacher, so it is worth making inquiries among competitors and show organizers over as wide an area as possible before enrolling.

When you feel that your dog is ready for competition, obtain a copy of the rules and regulations from your kennel club and make sure that you read them carefully; there is no point in arriving at a show to find that you have neglected one of the required exercises. Beware of overtraining your dog so that it is bored with the whole procedure. Some strong, energetic dogs may need practice on the day of the show to calm their high spirits; others will lose interest if they have to keep repeating the same exercises over and over again. Once in the show ring, listen carefully to what the judge says and

In obedience trials penalty points will be incurred by any dog breaking the line, like this Pointer.

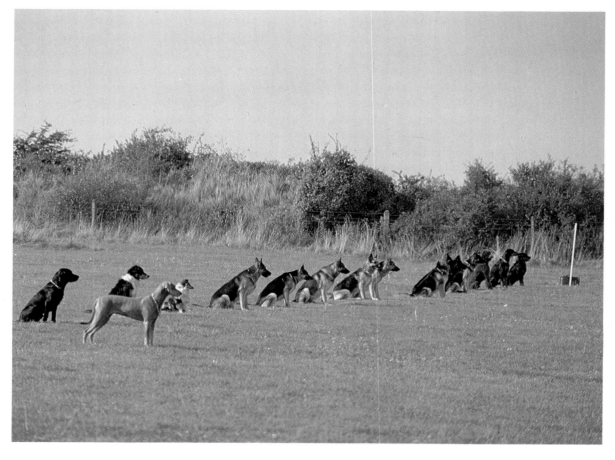

Beagle trials, where the dogs pursue cottontail rabbits or hare, are very popular in the United States.

follow it exactly. Move only when you are asked to move and do not stop until you are told to stop; a near-perfect performance can be spoiled if you anticipate instructions.

FIELD TRIALS

Field trials for gundog breeds are held in both the United States and Britain. All field trials are held in conditions as near as possible to those of an ordinary day's shooting, so anyone with an obedient, tender-mouthed, sensible dog has a chance of competing successfully. However, skilled handling is essential; many a good dog has its chances spoiled by bad handling – too much whistling, or too many confusing commands.

In Retriever trials the dog must walk to heel and wait with its handler, remaining quiet at all times.

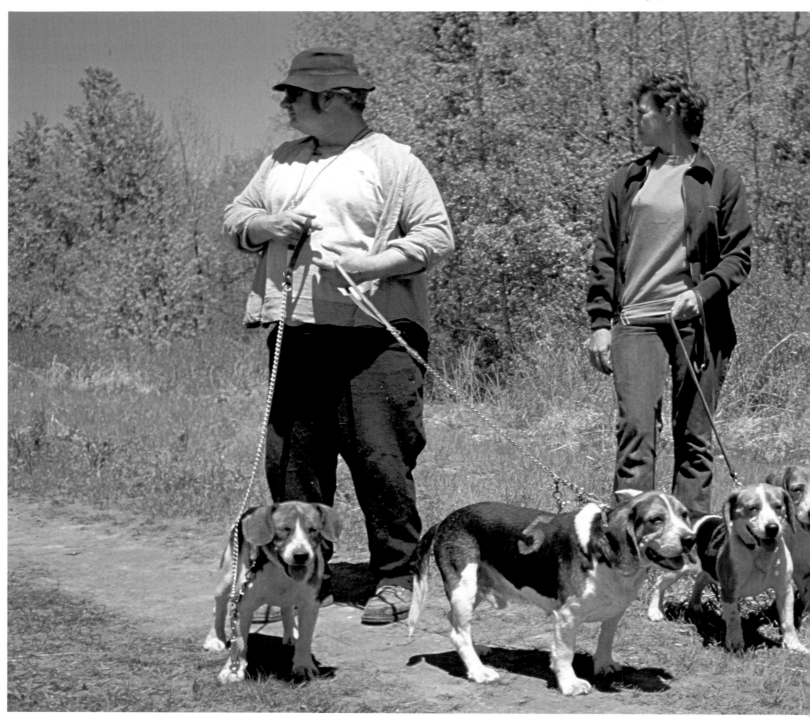

When a bird is shot it must go out on command and retrieve it, either from land or water. Dogs are assessed for their steadiness, ability to mark the fall of game, their drive and style while retrieving and their nose work. The degree of control required by the handler is also noted.

In Spaniel trials the dogs are assessed for their questing and quartering, game finding and flushing as well as for their ability to retrieve and deliver.

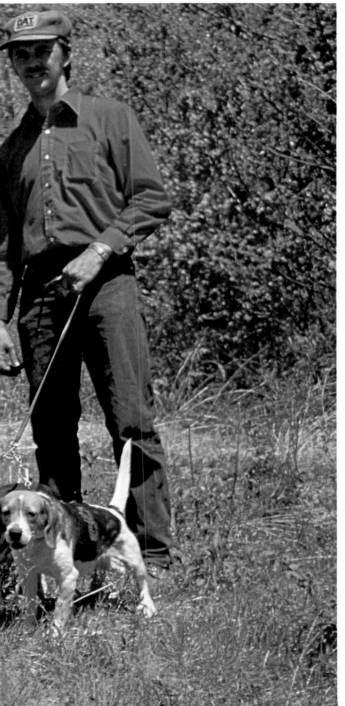

The dog must stay within gunshot range as it hunts for game, respond to directions and enter any cover, whether gorse, bramble or thorn bushes. The Spaniel's training should be geared to having the dog completely under control while still keeping it working stylishly and enthusiastically.

The task of the Pointers is to quarter the ground ahead of the guns and when game is found to come to a 'point' to indicate its whereabouts. After coming to a point the dog is usually sent ahead to flush the birds for the following guns and it must drop immediately when the birds rise and remain steady until receiving further commands.

The United States also has trials for hounds – Beagles, Dachshunds and Bassets – which compete by trailing cottontail rabbits. The hounds must be fast and tough, neither running mute, nor behaving as 'babblers' (giving tongue for no good reason). A good nose is, of course, essential. Beagle trials are particularly popular with hounds run as a brace on rabbit, as small packs on rabbit and hare and as large packs on hare. American Foxhounds also have their own trials, usually run at night. These Foxhounds need tremendous stamina and excellent noses as they may have to trail a fox for as long as 12 hours. Coonhound trials are mostly run at night with the hounds working in swampy country where they have to find and 'tree' a raccoon. Judges take a lot of notice of their 'voices' and owners identify their own hound by its individual voice. There are also Coonhound races in the daytime, when hounds have to swim across wide, fast rivers and 'tree' a raccoon on the other side.

This Pointer, on an American hunt, is alert and ready for a day's hard work.

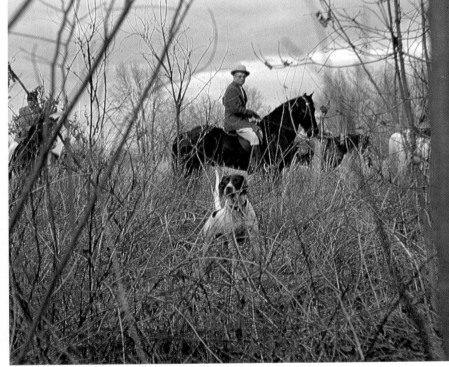

INDEX

Page numbers in *italic* refer to the illustrations

accidents, first aid, 156–7
Affenpinscher, *34*, 35
Afghan Hound, 12, 25, 26, 27, *34*, 35, 150, *181*
ageing, 164–5
aggression, *19*, 22, 137–9, 143
ailments, 158–64
Airedale Terrier, 28, 35–6, *35*
Alaskan Malamute, 36, *36*
allergies, 158
Alsatian, 68, *68*
American Foxhound, *36*, 37, 187
American Kennel Club, 34, 180, 183–4
American Staffordshire Terrier, 37, *37*
anal sacs and glands, 14, 151
Anatolian Karabash Dog, 37–8, *37*
anatomy, 14–18
appetite, healthy dogs, 153
arthritis, 158
artificial respiration, 156–7
Assyria, 12
Australia, 125
Australian Cattle Dog, 38, *38*
Australian Kelpie, 38, *38*, 180
Australian National Kennel Club, 34
Australian Silky Terrier, 39, *39*
Australian Terrier, 39, *39*

Babesia, 162
bad breath, 158
bad habits, 137–45
barking, 14, 137, 140, 141–2, *141*
Basenji, 26, 28, 40, *40*
baskets, 113
Basset Griffon Vendéen, 40–1, *40*
Basset Hound, 16, 25, 26, 27, 28, 40, 41, 180–1, 187
bathing, 151–2, *152–3*
Bayeux Tapestry, *13*
Beagle, 25, 26, 27, 41, *41*, 187
Bearded Collie, 41–2, *41*
Bedlington Terrier 27, 42, *42*
beds, puppies, *112*, 113
begging, 136, *136*
behavior, 18–19
    bad habits, 137–45
Belgian Sheepdog: Groenendael, 42, *42*
    Malinois, 43, *43*
    Tervueren, 43, *43*
Bernese Mountain Dog, 44, *44*
Bichon Frise, 44, *44*
bicycles, chasing, 142–3
biscuits, 115, 149
bitches: cannibalism, 158
    choosing a dog, 22
    eclampsia, 173–4
    feeding after whelping, 172
    mating, 169–71
    pregnancy, 171

season, 18, 22
spaying, 22
weaning puppies, 174–5
whelping, 171–2
bites, 19, 157, 163
Black and Tan Coonhound, 44–5, *44*, 187
bladder control, 123
bleach, 123
bloat, 160
Bloodhound, 26, 45–6, *45*
boarding kennels, 165
body, healthy dogs, 154
body signals, 13
bone meal, 115
bones, 14–16, *15*
    broken, 160
    gnawing, *125*, 149
Border Collie, 19, 27, 28, 46, *46*, 180
Border Terrier, 26, 27, 46–7, *46*
boredom, 140, 149
Borzoi, 47–8, *47*
Boston Terrier, 26, 47, 48–9
bottle feeding, 172, 175
Bouvier des Flandres, 48, 49
bowls, 113, *113*
Boxer, 26, 28, 48, 49
brain, 16
breathing, 16
breed standard, 180
breeding, 167–75
    development of, 12
    handrearing puppies, 175
    the litter, 172–4
    mating, 169–71
    preparations for, 169
    weaning, 174–5
    whelping, 171–2
breeds: buying, 29
    choosing a dog, 25–8
    descriptions, 33–108
    drawbacks, 28
Briard, 49, *49*
Brittany, 49–50, *49*
brushes, 119, 120
Brussels Griffon, 72, *72*
Bull Terrier, 26, 50–1, *51*
Bulldog, 15, *25*, 26, 50, *50*, 180
Bullmastiff, 50, *50*
burns, first aid, 156
buying a dog, 29

Cairn Terrier, 52, *52*, *136*
calcium, 115, 173
Canadian Kennel Club, 182
canidae, 10
canine parvovirus, vaccination, 116
canis familiaris, 10
canker *see* ear diseases
canned food, 148
cannibalism, 158
car sickness, 158–9
Cardigan Corgi, 106, *106*
care of the dog, 147-65
cars: chasing, 142–3
    travel in, 124–5, 145

castration, 22
catching, 137, *137*
cats: chasing, 142
    introducing puppies to, 115, *116*
    litter trays, 145
Cavalier King Charles Spaniel, 27, 52, *52*
cereal, 148, 174
cervix, 18
chalk, grooming with, 122
Chesapeake Bay Retriever, 52, *52*
chewing, 140–1
Chien Français, 53, *53*
Chihuahua, 14, 27, 28, 54, *54*, *182*
children: dog bites, 19
    family dogs, 27
    and puppies, 114
China, 12
Chinese Crested Dog, 28, 54, *54*, *124*, 180
choke chains, 119, 129, *129*, 131
choking, 157
choosing a dog, 21–31
Chow Chow, 54–5, *55*
circles, walking in, 132–3
classes, obedience, 128–9, *128*
clippers, nail, 151
clipping, Poodles, 149–50, *150*
Clumber Spaniel, 55–6, *56*
coat: ageing dogs, 164
    choosing a dog, 26–7
    diet and, 149
    grooming, 26, 119–23, *120–2*, 143
    hair loss, 160
    molting, 27, 149
    puppies, 172
Cocker Spaniel, 27, 150
    English, *31*, 56, *56*
    American, 36–7, *36*
collars, 118–19, 125
    choke chains, 129, *129*, 131
Collie: Rough, 26, 28, 56, *57*
    Smooth, 56–9, *57*
color-blindness, 13
colostrum, 172
combs, 119, 122
'come!', training, 129–30, *131*, 133-4
communication, 13–14
constipation, 159, 165
coprophagia, 145
Corgi, 26, 106, *106*
coughs, 159
coyotes, 10
Curly-coated Retriever, 58, 59
Cynodictus, 10
cystitis, 159

Dachshund, 16, 26, 58, 59, *59*, 187
Dalmatian, 26, 28, 60, *60*, *122*, 172
Dandie Dinmont Terrier, 60, 61, *149*
Darwin, Charles, 10
'dead', playing, 137
deafness, 159
dealers, 29
Deerhound, 16, 61, *61*
defecation, 123, 151
destructive dogs, 140–1

diabetes mellitus, 159
diarrhea, 31, 159
'die for your country', 137
diet *see* feeding
digestive system, 16–18
digging holes, 143
discipline, housetraining puppies, 123
diseases, 152, 158–64
disinfectants, 123
distemper, 159
   vaccination, 116
Doberman Pinscher, 26, 27–8, 61–2, *62*
dogproofing the home, 112–13
Dogue de Bordeaux, 62, *62*
domestication, 11–12
'down and stay', training, 134–5
dried food, 148
drops, ear, 155
drowning, 156–7
drying dogs, 152

ears: care of, 122–3, *159*
   cropping, 172
   diseases, 159–60
   drops, 155
   healthy dogs, 154
   puppies, 173
eclampsia, 173–4
eczema, 160
Egypt, *11*, 12
Elkhound, 62, *63*
English Foxhound, 66, *66*
English Setter, 27, 62–3, *63*
English Springer Spaniel, *26*, 63–4, *63*
English Toy Spaniel, 28, 80, *80*
English Toy Terrier, 64–5, *64*
epilepsy, 160
equipment, for puppies, 113
Estrela Mountain Dog, 64, *65*
estrus *see* season
evolution, 10
exercise, 28, *28*
eyes, 13
   ageing 164–5
   ailments, 160
   cleaning, *121*, 122
   healthy dogs, 154
   ointments, 156
   puppies, 172

face, grooming, 122–3
family dogs, 27
farm animals, 125, 143
fear, 19, 140
feces, 17, 145
Fédération Cynologique Internationale (FCI), 34, 182
feeding, 148–9
   diet sheets, 114
   lactating bitches, 172
   older dogs, 165
   pregnant bitches, 171
   puppies, 114, 115–6, 172, *174*
   weaning puppies, 174–5

feet, grooming, 122
'fetch!', training, 135
Field Spaniel, 65, *65*
field trials, 186–7
fighting, 145
Finnish Spitz, 27, 65, *65*
first aid, 156–7
fits, 160
Flat-coated Retriever, 65–6, *66*
fleas, 31, 162, *162*, 173
'fly strike', 163
follicle mites, 162
food, stealing, 142, *142*
foreign bodies, in the mouth, 157
fossils, 11
Fox Terrier, 28
   Smooth, 66–7, *67*
   Wire, 67, *67*, *181*, 183
Foxhound, 66, *66*
fractures, 160
French Bulldog, 66, *67*
furniture, bad habits, 139

gastric distension, 160
gastritis, 160
genitals, 18, *18*
German Shepherd Dog, *14*, 27–8, 68, *68*, 148, *148*, *182*
German Shorthaired Pointer, 68, *68*
German Wirehaired Pointer, 68–9, *69*
gestation, 171
gestures, release, 130, *132*
Glen of Imaal Terrier, 69, *69*
gloves, grooming, 119, *122*
gnawing bones, *125*, 149
Golden Retriever, *19*, 22, 27, 69–70, *69*, *177*
Gordon Setter, 70–1, *70*
grass-eating, 160
Great Dane, 22, 28, 71, *71*, 169, *182*
Great Pyrenees *see* Pyrenean Mountain Dog
Greece, 12
Greyhound, 12, 15, *16*, 25, 71, *71*
Griffon, 28
Griffon Bruxellois, 72, *72*
Griffon Vendéen, Grand, 72, *73*
Groenendael, 42, *42*
grooming, 26, 143
   bathing, 151–2, *152–3*
   nails, 151, *151*
   puppies, 119–23, *120–2*
   special grooming, 149–50, *149*
grooming powder, 122
growling, 137
guard dogs, 11–12, 19, 27–8
gundogs, 12, 25, 135, 186–7

hair *see* coat
hairbrushes, 119
Hamiltonstövare, 72–4, *73*
handrearing puppies, 175, *175*
handling, show dogs, 183–4
hard pad, 159
harnesses, 119
Harrier, 74, *74*

harvest mites, 162, *162*
health, 26
   puppies, 116
   signs of, 152–4
hearing, 13
   ageing, 164–5
   puppies, 173
heart disease, 160–1
heat, 18, 22, 169–71
heat stroke, 156
'heel!', training, 131–3, *132*
hepatitis, 161
   vaccination, 116
herding instinct, 19
hernias, 31, 161
hip dysplasia, 161
holes, digging, 143
hookworms, 162, *163*
housetraining puppies, 123, *123*
howling, 14
Hungarian Vizsla, 74, *74*
hunting instinct, 19
Husky, Siberian, 101, *101*

Ibizan Hound, 12, 74–5, *75*
identity discs, 118, 125
illness, 152, 158–64
injections, *161*
instincts, 18–19, *19*
insurance, 125
intestines, 17
Irish Setter, 75, *75*, *150*
Irish Terrier, 28, 76, *76*
Irish Water Spaniel, 76, *76*
Irish Wolfhound, 28, 76, *77*, 180, *180*
Italian Greyhound, 77, *77*
Ixodes, 162, *162*

Jack Russell Terrier, 78, *78*
jackals, 10
Japanese Chin, 78, *78*
Japanese Spitz, 78–9, *78*
jaundice, 161
jaws, 14–15
judging, shows, 182
jumping up, 142

Keeshond, *78*, 79
Kennel Club, 12, 29, 34, 114, 180, 181
kennels, boarding, 165
Kerry Blue Terrier, 27, 28, 79–80, *79*
kidneys, 18
   diseases, 161
King Charles Spaniel, 28, 80, *80*
Komondor, 80, *81*
Kuvasz, 81, *81*

Labrador Retriever, 26, 27, 28, *29*, 81–2, *81*, *172*, 173
Lakeland Terrier, 28, 82, *82*
lameness, 161

Large Munsterlander, 82–3, 82
laws, 125
leads: lead training, 119
    pulling on, 139–40, 139
    walking at heel, 131
'leave!', training, 135
legs, 15–16
    lameness, 161
leptospirosis, 161
    vaccination, 116
Lhasa Apso, 28, 83, 83
lice, 162, 162, 173
licenses, dog, 125
liquid medication, 155
liver, 17-18
longhaired dogs: bathing, 151
    breeds, 26–7
    grooming, 120–1
Löwchen, 83, 83, 180

male dogs: choosing, 22–4
    stud dogs, 22, 169–71, 169
Malinois, 43, 43
Maltese, 12, 28, 83–4, 83
Manchester Terrier, 84, 84
mange, 162
Maremma, 84, 84
marking, territorial, 145
marrowbones, 149
Mastiff, 12, 84–5, 85
mating, 18, 22, 169–71
meat, 115
medication, 155–6
Miacis, 10
Middle East, 12
milk, 115, 174
milk teeth, 16
minerals, 148
Miniature Pinscher, 26, 28, 85, 85
mites, 162, 162
mittens, grooming, 119
Molussus dog, 12
mongrels, 25, 128
molting, 27, 149
mounting, 140, 164
muscles, 16, 16
muzzles, 143, 157, 157

nails, care of, 151, 151, 172
names, learning, 116–7
Neapolitan Mastiff, 86, 86
neck, vertebrae, 15
nerves, 16
nervousness, 19
Newfoundland, 86, 87
Norfolk Terrier, 26, 87, 87
Norwegian Buhund, 87–88, 87
Norwegian Elkhound, 62
Norwich Terrier, 88, 88
nose: care of, 121, 122
    healthy dogs, 154
    puppies, 173
novice shows, 181

obedience: competitions, 185–6, 185
    training, 127–37
ointments, eye, 156
Old English Mastiff, 180
Old English Sheepdog, 26, 88–9, 88, 150, 163, 173
older dogs, 164–5
Otter Hound, 89, 89
ovaries, 18
overfeeding, 149
overseas travel, 165

pack instinct, 18–19
pads, care of, 122
panting, 16, 16
paper-training, puppies, 123
Papillon, 26, 28, 89–90, 89
paralysis, 161–2
parasites, 162, 162
parvovirus, 163
pedigree dogs, buying, 25
pedigrees, 113–14
Pekingese, 12, 22, 27, 28, 90–1, 90, 150, 182
Pembroke Corgi, 106, 106
penis, 18
peritonitis, 163
pet shops, 29
Pharaoh Hound, 91, 91
pheromones, 14
phobias, 140
Phoenicians, 12
pills, giving, 155, 155
play, 19, 114, 118, 118
pneumonia, 163
Pointer, 27, 93, 93, 185, 187, 187
poisons, 163
Pomeranian, 28, 93–5, 93
Poodle, 27, 94, 95, 149–50, 150, 164, 171, 181
pounds, choosing dogs from, 24–5
powdered medication, 155
pregnancy, 171
prolapse, 163
Pug, 12, 26, 28, 95, 95, 136
Puli, 95, 95
pulling on the lead, 131–2, 139–40, 139
punishment: bad behavior, 137
    housetraining puppies, 123
puppies, 111–25
    buying, 29
    car travel, 124–5
    chewing, 140
    and children, 27, 114
    choosing, 24–8, 30–1
    collars and leads, 118–19
    collecting, 113–14
    diet, 114, 115–16
    docking tails, 172
    equipment, 113
    feeding, 172, 174
    grooming, 119–23, 120–2
    handrearing, 175, 175
    health, 116
    housetraining, 123, 123
    introduction to other pets, 115
    learning its name, 116–17

obedience training, 129–37
    and older dogs, 165
    play, 118, 118
    safety in the home, 112–13
    shows, 181
    sleep, 114
    teething, 116
    training, 112, 117–18, 119
    vaccinations, 124
    weaning, 174–5
    whelping, 171–2
    worms, 116, 163
Pyrenean Mountain Dog, 96, 97

quarantine, 164, 165

rabies, 163–4, 165
    vaccination, 116, 125
Rameses VI, tomb of, 11
rectal prolapse, 163
rectal thermometers, 154, 155
release word, training, 130
reproduction, 18, 18
resentment of handling, 143
respiration, 16
Retriever trials, 186–7
retrieving, training, 135, 135
rheumatism, 164
Rhodesian Ridgeback, 96, 97, 118
ribcage, 15
rickets, 164
road accidents, 156, 156
roaming dogs, 140
Romans, 12
Rottweiler, 27–8, 96, 97
round worms, 162, 163
running lines, 140

safety, 112–13, 157
St Bernard, 14, 22, 97–8, 97
Saluki, 12, 98, 98
Samoyed, 98–9, 98
sarcoptic mange, 162
scent: anal glands, 151
    marking, 14
scent hounds, 25
Schipperke, 27, 28, 99, 99
Schnauzer, 28, 99–100, 99
Scottish Deerhound, 16, 61, 61
Scottish Terrier, 27, 28, 100, 100
scurf, 149
Sealyham Terrier, 28, 100, 100, 136
season, 18, 22, 169–71
semimoist foods, 148
senses, 13
sex play, 164
shaking hands, 136–7
shampoo, bathing dogs, 152
sheep, chasing, 125, 143
sheep ticks, 162, 162
shelters, choosing dogs from, 24–5
Shetland Sheepdog, 28, 100, 101
Shih Tzu, 27, 28, 101, 101, 149

shock, 164
shorthaired breeds, 26–7
    grooming, 122
shoulders, 15–16
showing, 12, 179–85, *181–4*
    choosing puppies for, 31
    handling, 183–4
    preparation for, 182–3
Siberian Husky, 101, *101*
sickness, 152, 158–64
sight hounds, 25
Silky Terrier, 39, *39*
'sit!', training, 131, 132, *132*, 133
'sit and stay', training, 133
skeleton, 14–16, *15*
skin: eczema, 160
    healthy dogs, 154
    puppies, 30–1
skulls, 14–15
Skye Terrier, 102, *102*
sleep, 114, 153
slip collars *see* choke chains
Sloughi, 102–3, *102*
smell, sense of, 13–14, *13*
snapping, 143
Soft-coated Wheaten Terrier, 103, *103*
Spaniel trials, 187
Spaniels, 12, *113*, 164
spaying, 22
sperm, 18
spine, 15
Spitz breeds, 26
Staffordshire Bull Terrier, 26, 103–4, *103*
'stay!', training, 133–5
stealing food, 142, *142*
stomach, 17
stud dogs, 22, 169–71, *169*
Sussex Spaniel, 104, *104*
Swedish Vallhund, 104, *104*, 180

tails, docking, 172

tapeworms, *162*, 163
tartar, 149
teeth, 16–17, *17*, 149
teething, puppies, 116
temperament: breeding dogs, 169
    and obedience training, 128
temperature: healthy dogs, 154–5, *154*
    panting to control, 16, *16*
terriers, 15–16, 26, 148, 183, *184*
territories, 22, 145
Tervueren, 43, *43*
testicles, 18
thermometers, 154, 155
threat signals, 13
Tibetan Spaniel, 104–5, *105*
Tibetan Terrier, 105, *105*
ticks, 162, *162*
tidbits, 149
tie, 171
Tomarctus, 10
toy dogs, 12, 26, 119, 148
Toy Manchester Terrier, 64–5, *64*
toys, 113, *113*, 140
training: curing bad habits, 137–45
    housetraining, 123, *123*
    lead training, 119
    obedience, 127–37
    preparation for shows, 183
    puppies, 117–18, 119
    tricks, 135–7, *136*
tranquilizers, 140
travel, 165
    car, 124–5, 145
    travel sickness, 125, 158–9
tricks, training, 135–7, *136*
tumors, 164

umbilical hernia, 31, 161
undershot jaws, 15
United States of America, 125, 164, 180, 181,
    182, 183–4, 187

urine, 18, 123
    urinating indoors, 145
uterus, 18, *18*

vaccinations, 114, 116, 124, 169
vagina, 18
    prolapse, 163
vertebrae, 15
veterinarians, 157–8, *158*
vision, 13
vitamins, 148, 149
vomiting, 160, 164
vulva, 18

'wait!', training, 133–4, *134*
walking at heel, 131–3, *132*
wandering dogs, 140
warts, 164
watchdogs, 27–8
water, drinking, 148, 149
weaning, 174–5
Weimaraner, 26, 28, 105–6, *105*
Welsh Corgi, 28
    Cardigan, 106, *106*
    Pembroke, 106, *106*
Welsh Springer Spaniel, 106–7, *107*
Welsh Terrier, 107, *107*
West Highland White Terrier, 27, 107–8, *108*
whelping, 171–2
whining, 14
Whippet, 26, 108, *108*
whipworms, *162*, 163
wire brushes, 120–2
wolves, 10, 11–12
worming, 114, 116
worms, 30, 160, *162*, 163
wounds, 'fly strike', 163

Yorkshire Terrier, 28, 108, *108*, *109*, 149, *182*